£2

EICOSANOIDS, ASPIRIN, AND ASTHMA

LUNG BIOLOGY IN HEALTH AND DISEASE

Executive Editor

Claude Lenfant
Director, National Heart, Lung and Blood Institute
National Institutes of Health
Bethesda, Maryland

1. Immunologic and Infectious Reactions in the Lung, *edited by Charles H. Kirkpatrick and Herbert Y. Reynolds*
2. The Biochemical Basis of Pulmonary Function, *edited by Ronald G. Crystal*
3. Bioengineering Aspects of the Lung, *edited by John B. West*
4. Metabolic Functions of the Lung, *edited by Y. S. Bakhle and John R. Vane*
5. Respiratory Defense Mechanisms (in two parts), *edited by Joseph D. Brain, Donald F. Proctor, and Lynne M. Reid*
6. Development of the Lung, *edited by W. Alan Hodson*
7. Lung Water and Solute Exchange, *edited by Norman C. Staub*
8. Extrapulmonary Manifestations of Respiratory Disease, *edited by Eugene Debs Robin*
9. Chronic Obstructive Pulmonary Disease, *edited by Thomas L. Petty*
10. Pathogenesis and Therapy of Lung Cancer, *edited by Curtis C. Harris*
11. Genetic Determinants of Pulmonary Disease, *edited by Stephen D. Litwin*
12. The Lung in the Transition Between Health and Disease, *edited by Peter T. Macklem and Solbert Permutt*
13. Evolution of Respiratory Processes: A Comparative Approach, *edited by Stephen C. Wood and Claude Lenfant*
14. Pulmonary Vascular Diseases, *edited by Kenneth M. Moser*
15. Physiology and Pharmacology of the Airways, *edited by Jay A. Nadel*
16. Diagnostic Techniques in Pulmonary Disease (in two parts), *edited by Marvin A. Sackner*
17. Regulation of Breathing (in two parts), *edited by Thomas F. Hornbein*
18. Occupational Lung Diseases: Research Approaches and Methods, *edited by Hans Weill and Margaret Turner-Warwick*
19. Immunopharmacology of the Lung, *edited by Harold H. Newball*
20. Sarcoidosis and Other Granulomatous Diseases of the Lung, *edited by Barry L. Fanburg*

21. Sleep and Breathing, *edited by Nicholas A. Saunders and Colin E. Sullivan*

22. *Pneumocystis carinii* Pneumonia: Pathogenesis, Diagnosis, and Treatment, *edited by Lowell S. Young*

23. Pulmonary Nuclear Medicine: Techniques in Diagnosis of Lung Disease, *edited by Harold L. Atkins*

24. Acute Respiratory Failure, *edited by Warren M. Zapol and Konrad J. Falke*

25. Gas Mixing and Distribution in the Lung, *edited by Ludwig A. Engel and Manuel Paiva*

26. High-Frequency Ventilation in Intensive Care and During Surgery, *edited by Graziano Carlon and William S. Howland*

27. Pulmonary Development: Transition from Intrauterine to Extrauterine Life, *edited by George H. Nelson*

28. Chronic Obstructive Pulmonary Disease: Second Edition, Revised and Expanded, *edited by Thomas L. Petty*

29. The Thorax (in two parts), *edited by Charis Roussos and Peter T. Macklem*

30. The Pleura in Health and Disease, *edited by Jacques Chrétien, Jean Bignon, and Albert Hirsch*

31. Drug Therapy for Asthma: Research and Clinical Practice, *edited by John W. Jenne and Shirley Murphy*

32. Pulmonary Endothelium in Health and Disease, *edited by Una S. Ryan*

33. The Airways: Neural Control in Health and Disease, *edited by Michael A. Kaliner and Peter J. Barnes*

34. Pathophysiology and Treatment of Inhalation Injuries, *edited by Jacob Loke*

35. Respiratory Function of the Upper Airway, *edited by Oommen P. Mathew and Giuseppe Sant'Ambrogio*

36. Chronic Obstructive Pulmonary Disease: A Behavioral Perspective, *edited by A. John McSweeny and Igor Grant*

37. Biology of Lung Cancer: Diagnosis and Treatment, *edited by Steven T. Rosen, James L. Mulshine, Frank Cuttitta, and Paul G. Abrams*

38. Pulmonary Vascular Physiology and Pathophysiology, *edited by E. Kenneth Weir and John T. Reeves*

39. Comparative Pulmonary Physiology: Current Concepts, *edited by Stephen C. Wood*

40. Respiratory Physiology: An Analytical Approach, *edited by H. K. Chang and Manuel Paiva*

41. Lung Cell Biology, *edited by Donald Massaro*

42. Heart–Lung Interactions in Health and Disease, *edited by Steven M. Scharf and Sharon S. Cassidy*

43. Clinical Epidemiology of Chronic Obstructive Pulmonary Disease, *edited by Michael J. Hensley and Nicholas A. Saunders*

44. Surgical Pathology of Lung Neoplasms, *edited by Alberto M. Marchevsky*

45. The Lung in Rheumatic Diseases, *edited by Grant W. Cannon and Guy A. Zimmerman*

46. Diagnostic Imaging of the Lung, *edited by Charles E. Putman*
47. Models of Lung Disease: Microscopy and Structural Methods, *edited by Joan Gil*
48. Electron Microscopy of the Lung, *edited by Dean E. Schraufnagel*
49. Asthma: Its Pathology and Treatment, *edited by Michael A. Kaliner, Peter J. Barnes, and Carl G. A. Persson*
50. Acute Respiratory Failure: Second Edition, *edited by Warren M. Zapol and Francois Lemaire*
51. Lung Disease in the Tropics, *edited by Om P. Sharma*
52. Exercise: Pulmonary Physiology and Pathophysiology, *edited by Brian J. Whipp and Karlman Wasserman*
53. Developmental Neurobiology of Breathing, *edited by Gabriel G. Haddad and Jay P. Farber*
54. Mediators of Pulmonary Inflammation, *edited by Michael A. Bray and Wayne H. Anderson*
55. The Airway Epithelium, *edited by Stephen G. Farmer and Douglas Hay*
56. Physiological Adaptations in Vertebrates: Respiration, Circulation, and Metabolism, *edited by Stephen C. Wood, Roy E. Weber, Alan R. Hargens, and Ronald W. Millard*
57. The Bronchial Circulation, *edited by John Butler*
58. Lung Cancer Differentiation: Implications for Diagnosis and Treatment, *edited by Samuel D. Bernal and Paul J. Hesketh*
59. Pulmonary Complications of Systemic Disease, *edited by John F. Murray*
60. Lung Vascular Injury: Molecular and Cellular Response, *edited by Arnold Johnson and Thomas J. Ferro*
61. Cytokines of the Lung, *edited by Jason Kelley*
62. The Mast Cell in Health and Disease, *edited by Michael A. Kaliner and Dean D. Metcalfe*
63. Pulmonary Disease in the Elderly Patient, *edited by Donald A. Mahler*
64. Cystic Fibrosis, *edited by Pamela B. Davis*
65. Signal Transduction in Lung Cells, *edited by Jerome S. Brody, David M. Center, and Vsevolod A. Tkachuk*
66. Tuberculosis: A Comprehensive International Approach, *edited by Lee B. Reichman and Earl S. Hershfield*
67. Pharmacology of the Respiratory Tract: Experimental and Clinical Research, *edited by K. Fan Chung and Peter J. Barnes*
68. Prevention of Respiratory Diseases, *edited by Albert Hirsch, Marcel Goldberg, Jean-Pierre Martin, and Roland Masse*
69. *Pneumocystis carinii* Pneumonia: Second Edition, Revised and Expanded, *edited by Peter D. Walzer*
70. Fluid and Solute Transport in the Airspaces of the Lungs, *edited by Richard M. Effros and H. K. Chang*
71. Sleep and Breathing: Second Edition, Revised and Expanded, *edited by Nicholas A. Saunders and Colin E. Sullivan*
72. Airway Secretion: Physiological Bases for the Control of Mucous Hypersecretion, *edited by Tamotsu Takishima and Sanae Shimura*

73. Sarcoidosis and Other Granulomatous Disorders, *edited by D. Geraint James*
74. Epidemiology of Lung Cancer, *edited by Jonathan M. Samet*
75. Pulmonary Embolism, *edited by Mario Morpurgo*
76. Sports and Exercise Medicine, *edited by Stephen C. Wood and Robert C. Roach*
77. Endotoxin and the Lungs, *edited by Kenneth L. Brigham*
78. The Mesothelial Cell and Mesothelioma, *edited by Marie-Claude Jaurand and Jean Bignon*
79. Regulation of Breathing: Second Edition, Revised and Expanded, *edited by Jerome A. Dempsey and Allan I. Pack*
80. Pulmonary Fibrosis, *edited by Sem Hin Phan and Roger S. Thrall*
81. Long-Term Oxygen Therapy: Scientific Basis and Clinical Application, *edited by Walter J. O'Donohue, Jr.*
82. Ventral Brainstem Mechanisms and Control of Respiration and Blood Pressure, *edited by C. Ovid Trouth, Richard M. Millis, Heidrun F. Kiwull-Schöne, and Marianne L. Schläfke*
83. A History of Breathing Physiology, *edited by Donald F. Proctor*
84. Surfactant Therapy for Lung Disease, *edited by Bengt Robertson and H. William Taeusch*
85. The Thorax: Second Edition, Revised and Expanded (in three parts), *edited by Charis Roussos*
86. Severe Asthma: Pathogenesis and Clinical Management, *edited by Stanley J. Szefler and Donald Y. M. Leung*
87. *Mycobacterium avium*–Complex Infection: Progress in Research and Treatment, *edited by Joyce A. Korvick and Constance A. Benson*
88. Alpha 1–Antitrypsin Deficiency: Biology • Pathogenesis • Clinical Manifestations • Therapy, *edited by Ronald G. Crystal*
89. Adhesion Molecules and the Lung, *edited by Peter A. Ward and Joseph C. Fantone*
90. Respiratory Sensation, *edited by Lewis Adams and Abraham Guz*
91. Pulmonary Rehabilitation, *edited by Alfred P. Fishman*
92. Acute Respiratory Failure in Chronic Obstructive Pulmonary Disease, *edited by Jean-Philippe Derenne, William A. Whitelaw, and Thomas Similowski*
93. Environmental Impact on the Airways: From Injury to Repair, *edited by Jacques Chrétien and Daniel Dusser*
94. Inhalation Aerosols: Physical and Biological Basis for Therapy, *edited by Anthony J. Hickey*
95. Tissue Oxygen Deprivation: From Molecular to Integrated Function, *edited by Gabriel G. Haddad and George Lister*
96. The Genetics of Asthma, *edited by Stephen B. Liggett and Deborah A. Meyers*
97. Inhaled Glucocorticoids in Asthma: Mechanisms and Clinical Actions, *edited by Robert P. Schleimer, William W. Busse, and Paul M. O'Byrne*
98. Nitric Oxide and the Lung, *edited by Warren M. Zapol and Kenneth D. Bloch*

99. Primary Pulmonary Hypertension, *edited by Lewis J. Rubin and Stuart Rich*
100. Lung Growth and Development, *edited by John A. McDonald*
101. Parasitic Lung Diseases, *edited by Adel A. F. Mahmoud*
102. Lung Macrophages and Dendritic Cells in Health and Disease, *edited by Mary F. Lipscomb and Stephen W. Russell*
103. Pulmonary and Cardiac Imaging, *edited by Caroline Chiles and Charles E. Putman*
104. Gene Therapy for Diseases of the Lung, *edited by Kenneth L. Brigham*
105. Oxygen, Gene Expression, and Cellular Function, *edited by Linda Biadasz Clerch and Donald J. Massaro*
106. Beta$_2$-Agonists in Asthma Treatment, *edited by Romain Pauwels and Paul M. O'Byrne*
107. Inhalation Delivery of Therapeutic Peptides and Proteins, *edited by Akwete Lex Adjei and Pramod K. Gupta*
108. Asthma in the Elderly, *edited by Robert A. Barbee and John W. Bloom*
109. Treatment of the Hospitalized Cystic Fibrosis Patient, *edited by David M. Orenstein and Robert C. Stern*
110. Asthma and Immunological Diseases in Pregnancy and Early Infancy, *edited by Michael Schatz, Robert S. Zeiger, and Henry N. Claman*
111. Dyspnea, *edited by Donald A. Mahler*
112. Proinflammatory and Antiinflammatory Peptides, *edited by Sami I. Said*
113. Self-Management of Asthma, *edited by Harry Kotses and Andrew Harver*
114. Eicosanoids, Aspirin, and Asthma, *edited by Andrew Szczeklik, Ryszard J. Gryglewski, and John R. Vane*
115. Fatal Asthma, *edited by Albert F. Sheffer*

ADDITIONAL VOLUMES IN PREPARATION

Inflammatory Mechanisms in Asthma, *edited by Stephen T. Holgate and William W. Busse*

Biology of Lung Cancer, *edited by Madeleine A. Kane and Paul A. Bunn, Jr.*

Pulmonary Edema, *edited by Michael A. Matthay and David H. Ingbar*

The Lung at Depth, *edited by Claes Lundgren and John N. Miller*

Lung Tumors, *edited by Christian Brambilla and Elizabeth Brambilla*

Five-Lypoxygenase Products in Asthma, *edited by Jeffrey M. Drazen, Sven-Erik Dahlén, and Tak H. Lee*

Diagnostic Pulmonary Pathology, *edited by Philip Cagle*

Immunotherapy of Asthma, *edited by Jean Bousquet and Hans Yssel*

Rhinitis, *edited by Robert M. Maclerio, Stephen R. Durham, and Niels Mygind*

Interleukin-5: From Molecule to Drug Target for Asthma, *edited by Colin Sanderson*

Viral Infections of the Lung, *edited by Raphael Dolin and Peter F. Wright*

Pediatric Asthma, *edited by Shirley J. Murphy, H. William Kelly, and Bernie C. McWilliams*

LAM and Other Diseases Characterized by Smooth Muscle Proliferation, *edited by Joel Moss*

Control of Breathing in Health and Disease, *edited by Murray D. Altos and Yoshikazu Kawakani*

Physiological Basis of Ventilatory Support, *edited by John J. Marini and Arthur S. Slutsky*

Complexity in Structure and Function of the Lung, *edited by Michael P. Hlastala and H. Thomas Robertson*

Human Immunodeficiency Virus and the Lung, *edited by Mark J. Rosen and James M. Beck*

The opinions expressed in these volumes do not necessarily represent the views of the National Institutes of Health.

EICOSANOIDS, ASPIRIN, AND ASTHMA

Edited by

Andrzej Szczeklik
Ryszard J. Gryglewski

Jagiellonian University School of Medicine
Krakow, Poland

John R. Vane

William Harvey Research Institute
St. Bartholomew's Hospital and The Royal London
School of Medicine and Dentistry
Queen Mary Westfield College
University of London
London, England

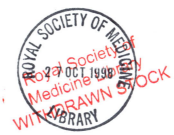

MARCEL DEKKER, INC.   NEW YORK · BASEL · HONG KONG

1998

ISBN: 0-8247-0146-1

The publisher offers discounts on this book when ordered in bulk quantities. For more information, write to Special Sales/Professional Marketing at the address below.

This book is printed on acid-free paper.

Marcel Dekker, Inc.
270 Madison Avenue, New York, New York   10016
http://www.dekker.com

Current printing (last digit):
10   9   8   7   6   5   4   3   2   1

Printed in the United States of America

INTRODUCTION

In the preface of the book *Aspirin and the Salicylate* (1), Michael Whitehouse points out that "the sheer tonnage of aspirin consumed each day and the number of its formulations in the marketplace are indeed remarkable statistics." Added to this daily consumption is the fact that aspirin and the salicylates appear to have been used for more than 2400 years for a variety of indications, all of which have a definitive inflammation component.

In the early days, the salicylates were extracted from various plant components such as willow and poplar bark. During the nineteenth century, salicylic acid was isolated and purified, which led to a more "rational," albeit more extensive, use of this compound. It was not long before its side effects—stomach irritation, ulceration, and even bleeding—were recognized.

A new era started in 1897, when a chemist at the Bayer Company in Germany chemically synthesized acetylsalicylic acid in an attempt to find a less irritating pain reliever to help his father, who was suffering from rheumatism. He accomplished this by adding one acetyl molecule to salicylic acid. This attracted the attention of the Bayer Company, which eventually registered acetylsalicylic acid under the name aspirin. By the early part of this century, aspirin had become the most widely used medication in the world. In the

United States alone, as many as 30 billion tablets are used each year. Whether this is enough, too much, or not enough may be debated, but it is estimated that as many as 10,000 of the deaths from heart attack and stroke that occur each year could be avoided if victims took aspirin on a regular basis.

Of course, there is a tradeoff. Aspirin, like most drugs, has side effects, some very serious. One is hypersensitivity reactions in many organs, including the airways. In fact, in view of the consumption of aspirin, one might expect that the prevalence of asthma would be higher by several orders of magnitude.

Fortunately, however, aspirin intolerance manifested by airway reactivity has a low prevalence. Although the mechanisms of airway reactivity leading to asthma attacks are complex, remarkable advances in understanding these mechanisms came in the early 1970s from the discovery, in Krakow, of the role of cyclooxygenase and the Nobel prize-winning discovery by John Vane of the mechanisms of the anti-inflammatory properties of acetylsalicylic acid. It was these discoveries that paved the way to development of therapeutic approaches for aspirin-induced asthma.

Thus, it was a remarkable opportunity when Drs. Szczeklik, Gryglewski, and Vane, the pioneers in the field, accepted by invitation to edit this volume for the Lung Biology in Health and Disease series. The authors they, in turn, invited come from many countries but together they constitute a unique roster of experts. As the executive editor of this series, I want to express my deepest appreciation for their contribution. The importance and significance of this volume will be recognized by all.

Claude Lenfant, M.D.
Bethesda, Maryland

Reference

1. Rainsford KD. Aspirin and the Salicylate. Butterworth, London, 1984.

PREFACE

This volume results from discussions among the members of the European Network on Aspirin-Induced Asthma (AIANE) and of the Jagiellonian Medical Research Center (JMRC). The discovery of an essential link between inhibition of cyclooxygenase (COX) in aspirin-sensitive patients and the precipitation of asthma attacks was made in Krakow a quarter of a century ago. Today Krakow serves as the coordinating center of AIANE. It is clear that aspirin-induced asthma (AIA), which affects about 10% of adult asthmatics, is not a simple, immune-type hypersensitivity to salicylates. Even now, when the COX-dependent mechanism that triggers the adverse reaction to nonsteroidal anti-inflammatory drugs (NSAIDs) in AIA has been firmly established, its molecular basis still remains a mystery.

In this book, Sir John Vane presents new data on the mechanism of action of NSAIDs on COX-1 and COX-2. Over the last few years, new pathways of arachidonic acid metabolism have been discovered. Some of them may be relevant to the mechanisms of AIA. To the well-known pathways of cyclooxygenation and lipoxygenation, the cytochrome P450–dependent pathway was added. John McGiff, who greatly contributed to the understanding of this third pathway, analyzes it with Michael Balazy. Isoprostanes constitute another class of eicosanoids generated by the nonenzymatic oxidation of phospholipids. Paola Patrignani and associates discuss the interesting possibility of the participation of COX-2 in the biosynthesis of isoprostanes by human monocytes. Intracellular localization of eicosanoid-forming enzymes in the endoplasmic reticulum or in the perinuclear envelope, comprehensively reviewed by Thomas Brock and Marc Peters-Golden, permits a better understanding of the intracellular metabolism of eicosanoids between eosinophils, mast cells, and epithelial cells in asthma.

Inhibition of cyclooxygenase in the airways of AIA patients sets off the chain of reactions that result in asthma. It is not known, however, which isoform of COX is a target for NSAID in this clinical syndrome. Kenneth Wu describes the expression of cyclooxygenase genes, while Peter Barnes and associates concentrate on their expression in airway cells. Daniel Picot reports on recent achievements of crystallography in the understanding of the three-dimensional structure of both cyclooxygenases. Daniel Simmons presents the phenomenon of NSAID-induced apoptosis, which is important for the antitumor action of aspirin but might also be of significance for NSAID-induced asthmatic attacks.

The basic mechanisms operating in asthma, which are of special relevance for AIA, include: genetic influences, as discussed by William Cookson; viruses, presented by Gert Folkerts and Frans Nijkamp; "intrinsic" factors, explored by Leonardo Fabbri and associates; eicosanoids, summarized by Paul O'Byrne; ion airway transport, reviewed by Sebastiano Bianco and associates; and autoimmunity, promulgated by Michel Joseph and associates. As far as the protective mediators are concerned, John Oates and associates discuss the role of PGE_2, and Ryszard Gryglewski and associates present evidence for the pneumoprotective action of endogenous nitric oxide.

An overview of the mechanisms operating in AIA is given by Andrezej Szczeklik, while Shuaib Nasser and Tak Lee concentrate on the participation of cysteinyl–leukotrienes, which over the last few years have emerged as the principal mediators of asthma. They seem to be of special importance in AIA, as evidenced by the efficacy of antileukotriene drugs, and the pathogenic role of 5-lipoxygenase products in animal models, as discussed by Colin Funk and associates.

The cellular source of leukotrienes is vividly disputed. Eosinophils and mast cells are considered the best candidates, as judged by Barbro Dahlén. To solve this problem innovative techniques are required. Bronchoalveolar lavage (BAL), which follows bronchial instillation of aspirin-like drugs, offers such a possibility, as presented by Esther Langmack and Sally Wenzel, while Anthony Sampson proposes bronchial biopsies coupled with sensitive immunochemical methods as another option. Klaus Rabe and Gordon Dent describe pharmacological intervention in generation of leukotrienes by eosinophils.

Practicing physicians will find a rich panorama of clinical symptoms of AIA, based on the largest data base developed by AIANE, presented in this volume by Ewa Nizankowska and associates. Special attention is given to the nasal passages, where the syndrome seems to originate, and to nasal polyposis, a classical manifestation of AIA. This topic is summarized by Niels Mygind and César Picado, and their associates. AIA patients cannot be cured, but pharmacological treatment improves their quality of life. Corticosteroids, discussed by Ryszard Dworski and Philippe Godard and associates, are required to control the disease in at least half of the patients, while desensitization with aspirin offers additional benefit to some, according to Donald Stevenson.

We found it exciting and enjoyable to coordinate the work of so many distinguished colleagues who contributed to this book. We hope the reader will share with us some of this excitement and pleasure.

Andrzej Szczeklik
Ryszard J. Gryglewski
John R. Vane

CONTRIBUTORS

Claus Bachert, M.D.   Professor, Department of Otolaryngology, University Hospital, Ghent, Belgium

Michael Balazy, Ph.D.   Associate Professor, Department of Pharmacology, New York Medical College, Valhalla, New York

Peter J. Barnes, M.D., D.Sc., F.R.C.P.   Professor and Head, Department of Thoracic Medicine, National Heart and Lung Institute, Imperial College School of Medicine, London, England

Joanna B. Bartus, M.D.   Department of Pharmacology, Jagiellonian University School of Medicine, Krakow, Poland

Bianca Beghé, M.D.   Section of Respiratory Diseases, Department of Clinical and Experimental Medicine, University of Ferrara, Ferrara, Italy

Maria G. Belvisi, Ph.D.   Lecturer, Department of Thoracic Medicine, National Heart and Lung Institute, Imperial College of Medicine, London, England

Sebastiano Bianco, M.D.   Professor, Institute of Cardiovascular and Respiratory Diseases, University of Milan, Milan, Italy

Grażyna Bochenek, M.D., Ph.D.   Department of Medicine, Jagiellonian University School of Medicine, Krakow, Poland

Regina M. Botting, B.Pharm., Ph.D.   The William Harvey Research Institute, St. Bartholomew's Hospital and The Royal London School of Medicine and Dentistry, Queen Mary Westfield College, University of London, London, England

Jean Bousquet, M.D.   Professor, Department of Respiratory Diseases, Hôpital Arnaud de Villeneuve, INSERM U454, Montpellier, France

Thomas G. Brock, Ph.D.   Research Investigator, Division of Pulmonary and Critical Care Medicine, Department of Internal Medicine, University of Michigan, Ann Arbor, Michigan

Gaetano Caramori, M.D.   Section of Respiratory Diseases, Department of Clinical and Experimental Medicine, University of Ferrara, Ferrara, Italy

Pascal Chanez, M.D., Ph.D.   Department of Respiratory Diseases, Hôpital Arnaud de Villeneuve, INSERM U454, Montpellier, France

Claude Chavis, Ph.D.   Department of Respiratory Diseases, Hôpital Arnaud de Villeneuve, INSERM U454, Montpellier, France

Xin-Sheng Chen, Pharm.D.   Research Associate, Center for Experimental Therapeutics, University of Pennsylvania, Philadelphia, Pennsylvania

William O. C. M. Cookson, M.D., Ph.D.   Wellcome Senior Clinical Research Fellow, Nuffield Department of Medicine, John Radcliffe Hospital, Oxford, England

Ronald Dahl, M.D.   Professor, Department of Respiratory Diseases, Aarhus University Hospital, Aarhus, Denmark

Barbro Dahlén, M.D., Ph.D.   Division of Respiratory Medicine, Department of Internal Medicine, Karolinska Institute, Stockholm, Sweden

Gordon Dent, Ph.D.   Research Associate, Krankenhaus Grosshansdorf, Grosshansdorf, Germany

Mariusz Duplaga, M.D.   Department of Medicine, Jagiellonian University School of Medicine, Krakow, Poland

Ryszard Dworski, M.D.   Assistant Professor, Division of Allergy, Pulmonary, and Critical Care Medicine, Department of Medicine, Vanderbilt University School of Medicine, Vanderbilt Medical Center, Nashville, Tennessee

Leonardo M. Fabbri, M.D.   Associate Professor of Respiratory Medicine, Section of Respiratory Diseases, Department of Clinical and Experimental Medicine, University of Ferrara, Ferrara, Italy

Gert Folkerts, Ph.D.   Departments of Pharmacology and Pathophysiology, Utrecht University, Utrecht, The Netherlands

Colin D. Funk, Ph.D.   Associate Professor, Department of Pharmacology and Center for Experimental Therapeutics, University of Pennsylvania, Philadelphia, Pennsylvania

Philippe Godard, M.D.   Professor, Department of Respiratory Diseases, Hôpital Arnaud de Villeneuve, INSERM U454, Montpellier, France

Ryszard J. Gryglewski, M.D.   Professor and Head, Department of Pharmacology, Jagiellonian University School of Medicine, Krakow, Poland

David D. Hagaman, M.D.   Department of Pulmonary and Allergy, St. Thomas Hospital, Nashville, Tennessee

Charles G. Irvin, Ph.D.   Professor, Department of Medicine, National Jewish Center for Immunology and Respiratory Medicine, Denver, Colorado

Ewa Janowska, M.D.   Department of Pathophysiology, Jagiellonian University School of Medicine, Krakow, Poland

Michel Joseph, Ph.D.   Director of Research, CNRS, Institut Pasteur, INSERM U416, Lille, France

Howard R. Knapp, M.D., Ph.D.   University of Iowa School of Medicine, Iowa City, Iowa

Esther L. Langmack, M.D.   Research Fellow, Department of Medicine, National Jewish Medical and Research Center, Denver, Colorado

Per L. Larsen, M.D. Associate Professor, Department of Otolaryngology, Hillerød Hospital, Hillerød, Denmark

Philippe Lassalle, M.D. Institut Pasteur, INSERM U416, Lille, France

Tak H. Lee, M.D., Sc.D., F.R.C.Path., F.R.C.P. Professor, Department of Allergy and Respiratory Medicine, Guy's Hospital, London, England

Torben Lildholdt, M.D. Associate Professor, Department of Otolaryngology, Vejle Hospital, Vejle, Denmark

Cristina Mapp, M.D. Assistant Professor, Department of Occupational Diseases, University of Padua, Padua, Italy

John C. McGiff, M.D. Professor and Chairman, Department of Pharmacology, New York Medical College, Valhalla, New York

Jane A. Mitchell, Ph.D. Lecturer, Department of Thoracic Medicine, National Heart and Lung Institute, Imperial College of Medicine, London, England

Joaquim Mullol, M.D., Ph.D. Senior Investigator, Institut de Recevie di Sunyer, Hospital Clinic, Barcelona, Spain

John J. Murray, M.D., Ph.D. Associate Professor, Division of Allergy, Pulmonary, and Critical Care Medicine, Departments of Medicine and Pharmacology, Vanderbilt University School of Medicine, Vanderbilt Medical Center, Nashville, Tennessee

Niels Mygind, M.D. Associate Professor, Department of Respiratory Diseases, Aarhus University Hospital, Aarhus, Denmark

S. M. Shuaib Nasser, M.B., B.S., M.R.C.P. Senior Registar and Lecturer, Department of Allergy and Clinical Immunology, Addenbrooke's Hospital, Cambridge, England

Robert Newton, Ph.D. Lecturer, Department of Thoracic Medicine, National Heart and Lung Institute, Imperial College School of Medicine, London, England

Frans P. Nijkamp, Ph.D. Professor and Head, Departments of Pharmacology and Pathophysiology, Utrecht University, Utrecht, The Netherlands

Ewa Niżankowska, M.D., Ph.D. Professor, Department of Medicine, Jagiellonian University School of Medicine, Krakow, Poland

John A. Oates, M.D. The Thomas F. Frist, Sr. Professor of Medicine and Professor, Division of Clinical Pharmacology, Department of Pharmacology, Vanderbilt University School of Medicine, Vanderbilt Medical Center, Nashville, Tennessee

Paul M. O'Byrne, M.B., F.R.C.P.I., F.R.C.P.(C) Professor, Department of Medicine, McMaster University, Hamilton, Ontario, Canada

Roberto Padovano, D.Sc. Researcher, Department of Pharmacology, University of Chieti "G. D'Annunzio," Chieti, Italy

Maria Rosaria Panaro, D.Sc. Researcher, Department of Pharmacology, University of Chieti "G. D'Annunzio," Chieti, Italy

Paola Patrignani, Ph.D. Assistant Professor, Department of Pharmacology, University of Chieti "G. D'Annunzio," Chieti, Italy

Carlo Patrono, M.D. Researcher, Department of Pharmacology, University of Chieti "G. D'Annunzio," Chieti, Italy

Marc Peters-Golden, M.D. Professor, Division of Pulmonary and Critical Care Medicine, Department of Internal Medicine, University of Michigan, Ann Arbor, Michigan

César Picado, M.D., Ph.D. Professor of Medicine, Head of Pneumology Section, Hospital Clinic, Barcelona, Spain

Daniel Picot, Ph.D. Institut de Biologie Physico-Chimique, Centre National de la Recherche Scientifique, Paris, France

Klaus F. Rabe, M.D., Ph.D. Krankenhaus Grosshansdorf, Grosshansdorf, Germany

Giulia Renda, M.D. Researcher, Department of Pharmacology, University of Chieti "G. D'Annunzio," Chieti, Italy

L. Jackson Roberts II, M.D. Division of Clinical Pharmacology, Department of Pharmacology, Vanderbilt University School of Medicine, Vanderbilt Medical Center, Nashville, Tennessee

Maria Robuschi, M.D. Associate Professor, Institute of Pulmonary Diseases, University of Milan, Milan, Italy

Maria Teresa Rotondo, D.Sc. Researcher, Department of Pharmacology, University of Chieti "G. D'Annunzio," Chieti, Italy

Anthony P. Sampson, Ph.D. Lecturer in Immunopharmacology, Southampton General Hospital, Southampton, England

Giovanna Santini, D.Sc. Researcher, Department of Pharmacology, University of Chieti "G. D'Annunzio," Chieti, Italy

Maria Gina Sciulli Researcher, Department of Pharmacology, University of Chieti "G. D'Annunzio," Chieti, Italy

Piersante Sestini, M.D. Institute of Pulmonary Diseases, University of Siena, Siena, Italy

James R. Sheller, M.D. Associate Professor of Medicine, Division of Allergy, Pulmonary, and Critical Care Medicine, Department of Medicine, Vanderbilt University School of Medicine, Vanderbilt Medical Center, Nashville, Tennessee

Daniel L. Simmons, Ph.D. Associate Professor of Biochemistry, Department of Chemistry and Biochemistry, Brigham Young University, Provo, Utah

Donald D. Stevenson, M.D. Senior Consultant, Division of Allergy, Asthma and Immunology, Scripps Clinic, La Jolla, California

Andrzej Szczeklik, M.D. Professor and Chairman, Department of Medicine, Jagiellonian University School of Medicine, Krakow, Poland

Andre-Bernard Tonnel, M.D. Professor, Institut Pasteur, INSERM U416, Lille, France

Yuan-Po Tu, M.D., D.V.M. Staff Physician, Everett Clinic, Everett, Washington

Wojciech Uracz, M.D., Ph.D. Associate Professor, Department of Pharmacology, Jagiellonian University School of Medicine, Krakow, Poland

Isabelle Vachier, Ph.D. Department of Respiratory Diseases, Hôpital Arnaud de Villeneuve, INSERM U454, Montpellier, France

Andriano Vaghi, M.D. Pneumology Division, Santa Corona Hospital, Garbagnate, Italy

John R. Vane, F.R.S., B.Sc., D.Phil., D.Sc. Honorary President, The William Harvey Research Institute, St. Bartholomew's Hospital and The Royal London School of Medicine and Dentistry, Queen Mary Westfield College, University of London, London, England

Sally E. Wenzel, M.D. Associate Professor, Department of Medicine, National Jewish Medical and Research Center, Denver, Colorado

Pawel P. Wolkow, M.D. Department of Pharmacology, Jagiellonian University School of Medicine, Krakow, Poland

Kenneth Kun-yu Wu, M.D., Ph.D. Roy and Phyllis Huffington Chair, and Professor and Director, Division of Hematology and Vascular Biology Research Center, University of Texas Medical School at Houston, Houston, Texas

CONTENTS

Introduction   Claude Lenfant   *iii*
Preface   *v*
Contributors   *ix*

1.   Mechanism of Action of Antiinflammatory Drugs   **1**
     John R. Vane and Regina M. Botting

    I.   Synthesis of Prostaglandins   1
   II.   Inhibition of Prostaglandin Synthesis   1
  III.   Two Isoenzymes   3
  IV.   Physiological and Pathological Functions of COX-1
          and COX-2   3
   V.   COX-2/COX-1 Inhibitory Ratios of NSAIDs   8
  VI.   Assessment of Selectivity   8
 VII.   Selective COX-2 Inhibitors   11
VIII.   Conclusions   16
         References   16

2. **Pathways of Arachidonate Metabolism**   **25**
   John C. McGiff and Michael Balazy

   I.   Introduction   25
   II.   Cyclooxygenases   25
   III. Lipoxygenases   26
   IV.   Eicosanoid Synthesis, Release, and Metabolism   28
   V.   Hormones and Phospholipases   33
   VI.   Prostanoids Affect Gene Transcription   35
   VII. Prostaglandin Receptors   36
   VIII. Endothelial-Derived Hyperpolarizing Factor: An
         Eicosanoid?   38
         References   38

3. **Cytochromes P450 and Arachidonic Acid Metabolism**   **45**
   Michael Balazy and John C. McGiff

   I.   Introduction   45
   II.   Characterization of CYP450   46
   III. Metabolism of Eicosanoids by CYP450   51
   IV.   Metabolism of Arachidonic Acid by CYP450   56
   V.   Phospholipid-Bound CYP450 Eicosanoids and
         Potential Role in Signal Transduction   65
   VI.   Conclusions   68
         References   68

4. **Mechanisms of Isoprostane Biosynthesis in Humans**   **77**
   Paola Patrignani, Roberto Padovano, Maria Gina Sciulli,
   Giovanna Santini, Maria Rosaria Panara, Maria Teresa
   Rotondo, Giulia Renda, and Carlo Patrono

   I.   Introduction   77
   II.   Cyclooxygenase-Dependent Formation of
         8-epi-PGF$_{2\alpha}$ by Human Blood Cells   79
   III. Conclusions   86
         References   87

5. **Intracellular Localization of Eicosanoid-Forming Enzymes**   **91**
   Thomas G. Brock and Marc Peters-Golden

   I.   Introduction   91
   II.   Researching Enzyme Localization   92

III.	Enzyme Locales: Our Current Understanding	93
IV.	The Nuclear Envelope as an Integrated Site of Action	99
V.	Consequences of Nuclear Localization	101
VI.	Unanswered Questions	103
	References	104

6. Cyclooxygenase-2 Expression in Airway Cells   **111**
*Peter J. Barnes, Maria G. Belvisi, Robert Newton,
and Jane A. Mitchell*

I.	Introduction	111
II.	Prostanoids in Airways	112
III.	Induction of COX-2 in Airway Cells	114
IV.	Regulation of COX-2	117
V.	Relevance in Asthma	121
	References	123

7. Cyclooxygenase Gene Expression and Regulation   **129**
Kenneth Kun-yu Wu

I.	Introduction	129
II.	COX-1 Gene Expression	131
III.	Up-regulation of COX-1 Expression	132
IV.	Induction of COX-2 Gene Expression	133
V.	Pathophysiological Implications of COX Induction	137
VI.	COX-1 and COX-2 Gene Deletion in Mice	138
VII.	COX Overexpression by Gene Transfer	139
	References	140

**8. NSAID-Induced Apoptosis: A New Therapeutic Activity
of Competitive Cyclooxygenase Inhibitors?**   **145**
Daniel L. Simmons

I.	Introduction	145
II.	The Role(s) of COXs in Apoptosis	148
	References	155

9. The Three-Dimensional Structure of Cyclooxygenases   **161**
Daniel Picot

I.	Introduction	161
II.	Structure Determination	162

III.   The Structure of PGHS-I and PGHS-II   164
IV.   Catalytic Mechanism   170
V.   Structural Basis of the Mechanism of Inhibition
        of the Cyclooxygenases   173
VI.   Flurbiprofen   174
VII.   Iodosuprofen   176
VIII.   Indomethacin   178
IX.   RS-104897   178
X.   Aspirin   178
XI.   SC-558   180
XII.   RS-57067   180
XIII.   PGHS-II Without Inhibitor   181
XIV.   Conclusions   182
        References   183

**10.   The Role of 5-Lipoxygenase Products in a Mouse Model of
        Allergic Airway Inflammation   187**
*Colin D. Funk, Xin-Sheng Chen, Charles G, Irvin,
Yuan-Po Tu, and James R. Sheller*

I.   Introduction   187
II.   Asthma, Airways Hyperresponsiveness, and
        Leukotrienes   187
III.   5LO Products, B Lymphocytes, and the Immune
        Response   191
IV.   A Murine System of Antigen-Driven
        Hyperresponsiveness: Model Characterization   192
V.   Diminished Airway Responsiveness and Eosinophilia
        in 5LO-Deficient Mice Using a Mouse Model of
        Allergic Airway Inflammation   193
VI.   Conclusions   195
        References   198

11.   Genetic Influences on Asthma   201
William O. C. M. Cookson

I.   Introduction   201
II.   Finding Genes   202
III.   Genes Influencing Asthma   203
IV.   HLA   206
V.   The T-Cell Receptor   208
VI.   Whole Genome Screens for Atopy and Asthma   210

VII.   Conclusions   210
       References   211

12. **Intrinsic Asthma**   **215**
     Leonardo M. Fabbri, Gaetano Caramori, Bianca Beghè,
     and Cristina Mapp

       I.   Introduction   215
       II.   Classification of Asthma   216
       III. Epidemiology of Intrinsic Asthma   217
       IV.   Pathogenesis and Pathology of Intrinsic Asthma   218
       V.   Conclusions   224
             References   224

13. **Viral Infection and Asthma: The Modulatory Role of**
     Nitric Oxide on Prostaglandin H Synthase   **231**
     Gert Folkerts and Frans P. Nijkamp

       I.   Introduction   231
       II.   Overview of the Release and Interaction of NO on
             Prostaglandin H Synthase   232
       III. Prostaglandin E_2 as an Epithelium-Derived Relaxing
             Factor   235
       IV. PGE_2 in Animal Models of Airway
             Hyperresponsiveness   236
       V.   NO as an Epithelium-Derived Relaxing Factor   236
       VI.   NO and Virus-Induced Airway Hyperresponsiveness   238
       VII. Functional Effects of NO Acting on Prostaglandin H
             Synthase   240
       VIII. Hypothesis on the Interaction of NO on PGHS in
             the Respiratory Airways   242
             References   245

14. **The Pharmacology of Prostaglandin E_2: Actions in Human**
     Diseases Involving the Mast Cell   **253**
     John A. Oates, John J. Murray, David D. Hagaman,
     James R. Sheller, Ryszard Dworski, L. Jackson Roberts II,
     and Howard R. Knapp

       I.   Introduction   253
       II.   Pilot Study   254
       III. Misoprostol Trial in Idiopathic Anaphylactoid Attacks 255

IV. Misoprostol Effect on Late-Phase Allergic
     Bronchoconstriction   255
 V. Conclusion   256
     References   257

**15. Eicosanoids in the Pathogenesis of Exercise- and
     Allergen-Induced Asthma**   **259**
Paul M. O'Byrne

   I. Introduction   259
  II. Exercise-Induced Bronchoconstriction   260
 III. Exercise Refractoriness   260
  IV. Allergen-Induced Airway Responses   261
   V. Investigating the Role of a Mediator in Asthma   262
  VI. Cysteinyl Leukotrienes and Exercise Bronchoconstriction 262
 VII. Inhibitory Prostaglandins and Exercise
       Refractoriness   264
VIII. Cysteinyl Leukotrienes and Allergen Responses   265
  IX. Conclusions   268
       References   268

**16. Endotoxin-Induced Acute Respiratory Distress Syndrome
     in Nitric Oxide-Deficient Rats**   **273**
*Pawel P. Wolkow, Ewa Janowska, Joanna B. Bartus,
Wojciech Uracz, and Ryszard J. Gryglewski*

   I. Introduction   273
  II. Methods   274
 III. Results   276
  IV. Discussion   279
       References   280

17. Eicosanoid Regulation by Glucocorticoids in Asthma **283**
Ryszard Dworski

   I. Introduction   283
  II. Effects of GC on Eicosanoid Metabolism in Cells
       Relevant to Asthma In Vitro   284
 III. Eicosanoid Involvement in the Inflammatory
       Responses in Asthma   286
  IV. Regulation of AA Metabolism by GC in Asthmatics
       In Vivo   287

| | V. | Conclusion | 292 |
| | | References | 292 |

18. Mechanisms of Aspirin-Induced Asthma   299
Andrzej Szczeklik

	I.	Introduction	299
	II.	Clinical Presentation	299
	III.	Allergic Mechanism	301
	IV.	Platelet Mechanism	301
	V.	The Cyclooxygenase Theory	301
	VI.	Involvement of Leukotrienes	302
	VII.	Release of Mediators at Site of the Reaction	304
	VIII.	PGE$_2$ and the Switch in Eicosanoid Metabolism	305
	IX.	Aspirin Desensitization	307
	X.	Chronic Inflammation of Airways	308
	XI.	Concluding Remarks	309
		References	309

19. Leukotrienes in Aspirin-Sensitive Asthma   317
S. M. Shuaib Nasser and Tak H. Lee

	I.	History of Aspirin-Induced Reactions	317
	II.	Clinical Presentation	318
	III.	Epidemiology	319
	IV.	Relevance of Anticyclooxygenase Activity	320
	V.	Cysteinyl Leukotriene Release in ASA	321
	VI.	Antileukotriene Drugs	323
	VII.	Aspirin Desensitization	326
	VIII.	Cellular Source of Cysteinyl Leukotrienes	328
	IX.	The Future	331
		References	332

**20. Mast Cell and Eosinophil Responses After Indomethacin
in Asthmatics Tolerant and Intolerant to Aspirin   337**
Esther L. Langmack and Sally E. Wenzel

	I.	Introduction	337
	II.	The Eosinophil Response in AIA	338
	III.	The Mast Cell Response in AIA	343
	IV.	The Role of Prostaglandins in AIA	344
	V.	Conclusions	347
		References	348

21. Aspects of Mechanisms in Aspirin-Intolerant Asthma   **351**
Barbro Dahlén

    I.   Introduction   351
    II. Bronchial Provocations for Diagnosis and Mechanistic
        Studies   351
    III. Plasma Levels of ASA and SA During Intolerance
        Reactions   353
    IV. Leukotrienes as Mediators of Aspirin-Induced
        Bronchoconstriction   355
    V.   Evidence for Mast Cell Activation During
        Aspirin-Induced Bronchoconstriction   357
    VI. Leukotrienes as Mediators of Persistent Airway
        Obstruction in Aspirin-Intolerant Asthmatics   360
    VII. Concluding Remarks   363
        References   364

**22. Aspirin-Intolerant Asthma: New Insights from Bronchial
Mucosal Biopsies**   **371**
Anthony P. Sampson

    I.   Introduction   371
    II. Profile of Leukocytes in AIA Bronchial Biopsies   372
    III. Expression of Cysteinyl-LT Synthetic Pathway
        Enzymes in AIA Bronchial Biopsies   374
    IV. The Cellular Source of Cysteinyl-LT Overproduction
        in AIA   377
    V. LTC_4 Synthase Expression Correlates Uniquely with
        Bronchial Responsiveness to Inhaled Lysine-Aspirin   379
    VI. Suppression of Cysteinyl-LT Synthesis by Endogenous
        PGE_2 380
    VII. Cytokine Regulation of Cysteinyl-LT Production   382
    VIII. A New Model of Aspirin-Sensitive Asthma   383
        References   384

**23. Pharmacological Intervention in Generation of Leukotrienes
by Eosinophils**   **391**
Klaus F. Rabe and Gordon Dent

    I.   Introduction   391
    II. Eosinophils as a Source of Leukotrienes   391
    III. Physiological Significance of Leukotriene Production
        by Eosinophils   395

	IV.	Modulation of Eosinophil Leukotriene Production	400
	V.	Concluding Remarks	409
		References	409

24. Airway Ion Transport Mechanisms and Aspirin in Asthma   **419**
Sebastiano Bianco, Maria Robuschi, Andriano Vaghi,
and Piersante Sestini

	I.	Introduction	419
	II.	The Inhalation Challenge Test for Aspirin-Induced Asthma	419
	III.	Bronchial Obstructive Responses to Pyrazolone Derivatives	421
	IV.	Bronchial Hypersensitivity to Hydrocortisone	423
	V.	Prevention of Aspirin-Induced Bronchoconstriction by Drugs Affecting Ion Transport Mechanisms	424
	VI.	Furosemide	427
	VII.	Chromones	429
	VIII.	Protective Activity of Furosemide and Aspirin-like Drugs	430
	IX.	Conclusion	432
		References	432

25. Role of Autoantibodies Against Endothelial Cells in Severe Asthma   **439**
Philippe Lassalle, Michel Joseph, and Andre-Bernard Tonnel

	I.	Introduction	439
	II.	Autoimmune Features in Severe Asthma and More Particularly AIA	441
	III.	Involvement of Antiendothelial Antibodies	442
	IV.	Conclusion	449
		References	449

26. Clinical Course of Aspirin-Induced Asthma: Results of AIANE   **451**
Ewa Niżankowska, Mariusz Duplaga, Grażyna Bochenek,
and Andrzej Sczczeklik

| | I. | The AIANE Project | 451 |
| | II. | Software Tool Development | 452 |

III.	The AIANE Database Structure	452
	References	470

27. Nasal Polyposis   **473**
Niels Mygind, Ronald Dahl, Per L. Larsen, Torben Lildholdt, and Claus Bachert

I.	Introduction	473
II.	Occurrence and Prevalence	474
III.	Etiology	474
IV.	Anatomy and Histology	476
V.	Pathogenesis: Immune Inflammation	479
VI.	Clinical Presentation	484
VII.	Diagnosis	485
VIII.	Treatment	485
IX.	Conclusions	487
	References	488

28. The Nose in Aspirin-Sensitive Asthma   **493**
César Picado and Joaquim Mullol

I.	Introduction	493
II.	Nasal Polyps, Chronic Rinosinusitis, and Aspirin-Sensitive Asthma	493
III.	Arachidonic Acid Metabolites in Nasal and Bronchial Secretions in Aspirin-Sensitive Patients	496
IV.	Effects of Aspirin on the Release of Mast Cells and Eosinophil Products in the Nose and Airways	498
V.	Clinical Manifestations	499
VI.	Diagnosis of Aspirin Sensitivity	499
VII.	Treatment of Rhinosinusitis and Nasal Polyposis in Aspirin-Sensitive Patients	500
VIII.	Summary	502
	References	503

29. The Role of Glucocorticoids in the Modulation of Eicosanoid Metabolism in Asthma   **507**
Isabelle Vachier, Pascal Chanez, Claude Chavis, Jean Bousquet, and Philippe Godard

I.	Introduction	507
II.	Mechanisms of Glucocorticoid Action	508

III. Effects of Glucocorticoids on Arachidonic Acid
Metabolism In Vitro   512
IV. Inhibition of Eicosanoid Biosynthesis In Vivo   514
V. Conclusions   516
References   516

30. Desensitization in Aspirin-Induced Asthma   **523**
Donald D. Stevenson

I. Introduction   523
II. ASA Desensitization Procedures   524
III. ASA Cross-Sensitivity and Desensitization   526
IV. Treatment with ASA Desensitization   529
V. Pathogenesis of ASA Desensitization   532
References   535

Author Index   539
Subject Index   597

EICOSANOIDS, ASPIRIN, AND ASTHMA

1

Mechanism of Action of Antiinflammatory Drugs

JOHN R. VANE and REGINA M. BOTTING

The William Harvey Research Institute
St. Bartholomew's Hospital and The Royal
   London School of Medicine and Dentistry
Queen Mary Westfield College
University of London
London, England

I. Synthesis of Prostaglandins

Almost any type of chemical or mechanical stimulus releases prostaglandins. The key enzyme in their synthesis is prostaglandin endoperoxide synthase (PGHS) or cyclooxygenase (COX), which possesses two catalytic sites. The first, a cyclooxygenase active site, converts arachidonic acid to the endoperoxide PGG_2. The second, a peroxidase active site, then converts the PGG_2 to another endoperoxide PGH_2. Prostaglandin H_2 is further processed by specific isomerases to form prostaglandins, prostacyclin, and thromboxane A_2. Cyclooxygenase activity has long been studied in preparations from sheep seminal vesicles and a purified, enzymatically active COX was isolated in 1976 (1). We now know that cyclooxygenase exists in at least two isoforms, COX-1 and COX-2.

II. Inhibition of Prostaglandin Synthesis

Twenty-five years ago, Vane proposed that the mechanism of action of the aspirin-like drugs (nonsteroidal anti-inflammatory drugs; NSAIDs) was through the inhibition of prostaglandin biosynthesis (2), and there is now a general

1

acceptance of the theory. The inhibition by aspirin is due to the irreversible acetylation of the cyclooxygenase site of PGHS, leaving the peroxidase activity of the enzyme unaffected. In contrast to this unique irreversible action of aspirin, other NSAIDs such as ibuprofen or indomethacin produce reversible or irreversible COX inhibition by competing with the substrate, arachidonic acid, for the active site of the enzyme.

The inhibition of prostaglandin synthesis by NSAIDs has been demonstrated in a wide variety of systems, ranging from microsomal enzyme preparations, cells, and tissues to whole animals and humans. For instance, the concentration of PGE_2 is about 20 ng/ml in the synovial fluid of patients with rheumatoid arthritis (3). This decreases to zero in patients taking aspirin, which is a good clinical demonstration of the effect of this drug on prostaglandin synthesis. Over the last two decades, several new drugs have reached the market based on COX-1 enzyme screens.

Garavito and his colleagues (4) have determined the three-dimensional structure of COX-1, providing a new understanding for the actions of COX inhibitors. Each dimer of COX-1 comprises three independent folding units: an epidermal growth factor–like domain, a membrane-binding motif, and an enzymatic domain. The sites for peroxidase and cyclooxygenase activity are adjacent but spatially distinct. The conformation of the membrane-binding motif strongly suggests that the enzyme integrates into only a single leaflet of the lipid bilayer and is thus a monotopic membrane protein. Three of the helices of the structure form the entrance to the cyclooxygenase channel and their insertion into the membrane could allow arachidonic acid to gain access to the active site from the interior of the bilayer. The cyclooxygenase-active site is a long, hydrophobic channel, and Picot et al. (4) provide evidence to suggest that some of the aspirin-like drugs, such as flurbiprofen, inhibit COX-1 by excluding arachidonate from the upper portion of the channel. Tyrosine 385 and serine 530 are at the apex of the long active site. Aspirin irreversibly inhibits COX-1 by acetylation of the serine 530, thereby excluding access of arachidonic acid (4). The S(–) stereoisomer of flurbiprofen interacts via its carboxylate with arginine 120, thereby placing the second phenyl ring within van der Waals' contact of tyrosine 385. There may be a number of other subsites for drug binding in this narrow channel.

The three-dimensional structure of COX-2 has also now been published (5). It closely resembles the structure of COX-1, except that the COX-2 active site is slightly larger and can accommodate bigger structures than those that are able to reach the active site of COX-1. A secondary internal pocket of COX-2 contributes significantly to the larger volume of the active site in this enzyme, although the central channel is also bigger by 17%. Selectivity for COX-2 inhibitors is dependent on the presence of Val at position 523 instead of the Ile found in COX-1 (6).

III. Two Isoenzymes

The constitutive isoform, COX-1, has clear physiological functions. Its activation leads, for instance, to the production of prostacyclin, which is antithrombogenic when released by the endothelium (7) and cytoprotective when released by the gastric mucosa (8). It is also COX-1 in platelets that leads to thromboxane A_2 production, causing aggregation of the platelets to prevent inappropriate bleeding (9). The existence of the inducible isoform, COX-2, was first suspected when Needleman and his group showed that cytokines induced the expression of COX protein (10) and that bacterial lipopolysaccharide increased the synthesis of prostaglandins in human monocytes in vitro (11) and in mouse peritoneal macrophages in vivo (12). This increase was inhibited by dexamethasone and associated with de novo synthesis of new COX protein. A year or so later, COX-2 was identified as a distinct isoform encoded by a different gene from COX-1 (13–17). The human COX-2 gene at 8.3 kb is similar to the COX-2 gene of mouse and chicken, but smaller than the 22-kb human COX-1 gene. The amino acid sequence of its cDNA shows a 60% homology with the sequence of the noninducible enzyme, with the mRNA for the inducible enzyme being approximately 4.5 kb and that of the constitutive enzyme being 2.8 kb. However, both enzymes have a molecular weight of 71 kDa and similar active sites for the natural substrate and for blockade by NSAIDs. The inhibition by the glucocorticoids of the expression of COX-2 is an additional aspect of the anti-inflammatory action of the corticosteroids. The levels of COX-2, normally very low in cells, are tightly controlled by a number of factors including cytokines, intracellular messengers, and availability of substrate.

COX-2 is induced by inflammatory stimuli and by cytokines in migratory and other cells, suggesting that the anti-inflammatory actions of NSAIDs are due to the inhibition of COX-2, whereas the unwanted side effects such as irritation of the stomach lining and toxic effects on the kidney are due to inhibition of the constitutive enzyme, COX-1 (18).

IV. Physiological and Pathological Functions of COX-1 and COX-2

COX-1 performs a "housekeeping" function to synthesize prostaglandins that regulate normal cell activity. The concentration of the enzyme largely remains stable, but small (two- to fourfold) increases in expression can occur in response to stimulation with hormones or growth factors (19,20). Normally, little or no COX-2 is found in resting cells but its expression can be increased dramatically after exposure of cells to bacterial lipopolysaccharides, phorbol esters, cytokines, or growth factors. However, "constitutive" levels of COX-2 have been detected in some organs such as the brain and in uterine tissues during gestation.

A. In the Gastrointestinal Tract

The so-called "cytoprotective" action of prostaglandins in preventing gastric erosions and ulceration is mainly brought about by endogenously produced prostacyclin and PGE_2, which reduce gastric acid secretion and exert a direct vasodilator action on the vessels of the gastric mucosa. In addition to these major actions, prostanoids stimulate the secretion of viscous mucus as a protective barrier and gastric fluid as well as duodenal bicarbonate (21).

In most species, including humans, the bulk of the protective prostaglandins are synthesized by COX-1 although small quantities of COX-2 are also expressed in the stomach of the rat (22). It is, therefore, hard to explain why mice rendered deficient in the gene for COX-1 do not develop spontaneous gastric bleeding or erosions (23). Perhaps compensatory protective mechanisms, such as the synthesis of nitric oxide, take over the protective role of the prostaglandins.

It is interesting that COX-2 is highly expressed in human and animal colon cancer cells as well as in human colorectal adenocarcinomas (24,25). The consequent increase in synthesis of prostaglandins (mainly PGE_2), can be prevented with NSAIDs, including some that are selective inhibitors of COX-2. Epidemiological studies have established a strong link between ingestion of aspirin and a reduced risk of developing colon cancer (26,27). It has also been reported that sulindac causes reduction of prostaglandin synthesis and regression of adenomatous polyps which would otherwise develop into rectal carcinomas unless surgically removed (28).

Support for the close connection between COX-2 and colon cancer has come from studies in mice with a mutation of the APC gene. These animals develop a condition similar to familial adenomatous polyposis characterized by the presence of large numbers of intestinal polyps. However, mice carrying the APC mutation made deficient in the COX-2 gene have very few intestinal polyps indicating that COX-2 is involved in polyp formation and in neoplasia of the colon (29).

B. In the Kidney

The cortex of normal kidneys produces both PGE_2 and PGI_2 whereas the renal medulla synthesizes mostly PGE_2. Both of these prostanoids are potent vasodilators, while PGE_2 in addition inhibits reabsorption of sodium and chloride from the ascending limb of the loop of Henle (30). Prostaglandins also attenuate the reabsorption of sodium by vasopressin in the collecting ducts, thus further increasing urine flow (31).

Maintenance of normal kidney function is dependent on prostaglandins both in animal models of disease states and in patients with congestive heart failure, liver cirrhosis, or renal insufficiency. Patients are therefore at risk of renal ischemia when prostaglandin synthesis is reduced by NSAIDs.

Those kidney cells that synthesize prostaglandins contain mostly COX-1, but low levels of COX-2 mRNA have also been measured (32). Cultured rat mesangial cells increase production of PGI_2 and PGE_2 after induction of COX-2 with cytokines or growth factors (33). It is possible that the PGI_2 formed by mesangial cells directly stimulates renin secretion as a feedback control for inhibition of salt reabsorption. Up-regulation of COX-2 expression has been observed in kidneys, in the macula densa, following salt deprivation (32). Thus, prostaglandin production in the normal kidney is probably driven by the activity of COX-1, whereas kidneys subject to either inflammatory or other challenges induce COX-2.

Mice that lack the gene for production of COX-1 appear healthy and do not show significant signs of kidney pathology. This is in accord with the finding that inhibition of COX-1 by NSAIDs does not alter renal function under normal physiological conditions. However, in COX-2 (−/−) null mice the kidneys failed to manifest the normal further kidney development after birth with the result that the animals died within 8 weeks of birth (34).

C. In the Lungs

Prostaglandins have important actions on the tone of the bronchial tree and on the diameter of the pulmonary blood vessels. The airways of most species, including humans, are constricted by $PGF_{2\alpha}$, TXA_2, PGD_2, and PGI_2 whereas PGE_2 is a weak bronchodilator. Asthmatics are 8000 times more sensitive to the bronchoconstrictor action of inhaled $PGF_{2\alpha}$ than healthy subjects. Pulmonary blood vessels are constricted by $PGF_{2\alpha}$ and TXA_2, but in some species they are dilated by PGE_2. The vasoconstrictor responses to $PGF_{2\alpha}$ are potentiated by hypoxia. Prostacyclin is a potent vasodilator of the pulmonary circulation in humans and other species. Blood levels of prostacyclin increase 15- to 20-fold in anaesthetized patients with artificial ventilation. This endothelium-derived prostacyclin is well placed to function as a local vasodilator and to prevent the formation of microthrombi (35).

Mediators of inflammation such as bradykinin, histamine, and 5-hydroxytryptamine all release prostaglandins from lung tissue. Histamine releases $PGF_{2\alpha}$ from human lung fragments by stimulating H_1 receptors. Lungs of asthmatics produce more histamine than normal lungs, which correlates with the greater number of mast cells found in asthmatic lungs (36).

Airway hyperreactivity, a feature of allergic asthma, is associated with inflammation of the airways. Increased expression of COX-2 mRNA and of enzyme protein, with no change in COX-1 levels, has been detected in pulmonary epithelial cells, airway smooth muscle cells, pulmonary endothelial cells, and alveolar macrophages treated with LPS or proinflammatory cytokines. In the carrageenin-induced pleurisy model of inflammation, levels of COX-2 protein increased maximally at 2 hr in the cell pellets of pleural exudate (37). This could be accounted for by induction of COX-2 found in all mast cells, in about 65% of resident mononuclear leukocytes, and in approximately 8% of extravasated neutrophils present in the exudate (38). However, lung tissue can also express COX-2 constitutively. COX-2 mRNA was weakly expressed in unstimulated rat isolated perfused lungs and this could be up-regulated by nitric oxide (NO) donors (39). Human lungs obtained from accident victims (40) and human, cultured, pulmonary epithelial cells expressed more constitutive COX-2 than constitutive COX-1 (41,42). Interestingly, hypoxia induces COX-2 gene expression in isolated, perfused lungs of the rat without affecting the mRNA for COX-1 (39). This induction of the COX-2 gene by hypoxia was inhibited by NO donors, which may represent one of the mechanisms of the beneficial effect of inhaled NO in pulmonary hypertension.

Inflammatory stimuli cause differential release of prostaglandins from various regions of the lungs. Human, cultured, pulmonary epithelial cells stimulated with LPS, IL-1β, TNFα, or a mixture of cytokines synthesize mainly PGE_2 together with smaller amounts of $PGF_{2\alpha}$, PGI_2, and TXA_2. This prostaglandin production can be suppressed by dexamethasone (43). Exposure to environmental pollutants from car exhausts can also induce the COX-2 gene and increase COX-2 protein levels in human, cultured airway epithelial cells, and results in an increased formation of PGE_2 and $PGF_{2\alpha}$ (44). Administration of LPS to rat isolated perfused lungs caused delayed bronchoconstriction accompanied by the release of TXA_2 and PGI_2, which could be blocked with dexamethasone, a selective COX-2 inhibitor, or a thromboxane receptor antagonist. Human lungs contain the highest levels of thromboxane synthase of any major organ and severe trauma can increase pulmonary TXA_2 production in humans (45). PGE_2 and TXB_2, in addition to COX-2 protein, could be detected in the inflammatory exudate produced by injection of carrageenin into the rat pleural cavity (46).

Thus, it seems likely that COX-2 is up-regulated in the inflamed lungs of asthmatic patients resulting in increased production of bronchoconstrictor prostaglandins which exert an exaggerated effect on the bronchiolar smooth muscle that has become hyperreactive to constrictor agents.

D. In the Brain and Spinal Cord

The brain contains high concentrations of PGD_2 which, when injected into the preoptic area, induces sleep. PGE_2 is also distributed widely throughout the brain, although intracerebral injections of PGE_2, as opposed to PGD_2, reduce the amount of sleep (47). PGD and PGE synthases have also been identified in brain tissue as have receptors for both PGD_2 and PGE_2.

Brains of neonates have higher levels of cerebral prostanoids than those of adult animals (48). These prostaglandins are made mostly by "constitutive" COX-2 and are likely to be important in the regulation of cerebral blood flow in the newborn (49,50).

COX-1 is distributed in neurones throughout the brain but it is most abundant in forebrain, where prostaglandins may be involved in complex integrative functions, such as control of the autonomic nervous system, and in sensory processing (51,52). COX-2 mRNA is induced in brain tissue and in cultured glial cells by pyrogenic substances such as LPS and IL-1 (53,54). However, low levels of COX-2 immunoreactivity and COX 2 mRNA have been detected in neurons of the forebrain without previous stimulation by proinflammatory substances (51,52,55). These "basal" levels of COX-2 are particularly high in neonates and are probably induced by physiological nervous activity. Intense nerve stimulation, leading to seizures, induces COX-2 mRNA in discrete neurons of the hippocampus (56), whereas acute stress raises levels in the cerebral cortex (51). COX-2 mRNA is also constitutively expressed in the spinal cord of normal rats and is likely to be involved with processing of nociceptive stimuli (57).

Fever is produced by an injection of PGE_2 into the preoptic area (58). Endogenous, fever-producing PGE_2 is thought to originate from COX-2 induced by LPS or IL-1 in endothelial cells lining the cerebral blood vessels (54). Selective inhibitors of COX-2 such as NS-398 are potent antipyretic agents (59).

E. In Gestation and Parturition

Prostaglandins are important for inducing uterine contractions during labor. NSAIDs such as indomethacin will thus delay premature labor by inhibiting this production of prostaglandins (60). Furthermore, prostaglandins synthesized by COX-1 are apparently essential for the survival of fetuses during parturition, since the majority of offspring born to homozygous COX-1 knockout mice do not survive (61). This high mortality of the pups may be due to premature closure of the ductus arteriosus. Expression of COX-1 is much greater than that of COX-2 in fetal hearts, kidneys, lungs, and brains as well as in the decidual lining of the uterus (60,62). Constitutive COX-1 in the amnion could also contribute prostaglandins for the maintenance of a healthy pregnancy (63). In human amnion cells, COX-1 mRNA is increased by human chorionic gonadotrophin (64).

Female COX-2 knockout mice are mostly infertile, producing very few offspring due to a reduction in ovulation (65). Both COX-1 and COX-2 are expressed in the uterine epithelium at different times in early pregnancy and may be important for implantation of the ovum and in the angiogenesis important for establishment of the placenta (66). Prostaglandins originating from COX-2 may play a role in the birth process since COX-2 mRNA in the amnion and placenta increases markedly immediately before and after the start of labor (62). Glucocorticoids, EGF, IL-1β, and IL-4 all stimulate COX-2 production in human amnion cells (67,68), and glucocorticoids can cause premature labor in pregnant sheep possibly by inducing progesterone-metabolizing enzymes, which reduce progesterone levels below those needed to maintain pregnancy (69). It is possible that preterm labor could be caused by an intrauterine infection resulting in release of endogenous factors that increase prostaglandin production by up-regulating COX-2 (68). Selective inhibitors of COX-2 reduce prostaglandin synthesis in fetal membranes and should be useful in delaying premature labor without the side effects of indomethacin (60).

V. COX-2/COX-1 Inhibitory Ratios of NSAIDs

Individual NSAIDs show different potencies against COX-1 compared with COX-2 and this nicely explains the variations in the side effects of NSAIDs at their anti-inflammatory doses. Drugs with high potency against COX-2, and therefore a lower COX-2/COX-1 activity ratio, will have anti-inflammatory activity with fewer side effects in the stomach and kidney. Garcia Rodriguez and Jick (70), Langman et al. (71), and Henry et al. (72) have published a comparison of epidemiological data of the side effects of NSAIDs. Piroxicam and indomethacin were among those with the highest gastrointestinal toxicity. These drugs have a much higher potency against COX-1 than against COX-2 (73). Thus, when epidemiological results are compared with COX-2/COX-1 ratios, there is a parallel relationship between gastrointestinal side effects and COX-2/COX-1 ratios (Fig. 1). COX-2/COX-1 ratios provide a useful comparison of relative values for a series of NSAIDs tested in the same system. However, the COX-2/COX-1 ratio for a particular NSAID will vary according to whether it is measured on intact cells, cell homogenates, purified enzymes, or recombinant proteins expressed in bacterial, insect, or animal cells. It will also vary when measured in different types of cells derived from various species.

VI. Assessment of Selectivity

A number of methods have thus been described for determining the ED_{50} values for NSAIDs against COX-2 and COX-1, leading to the aforesaid variable

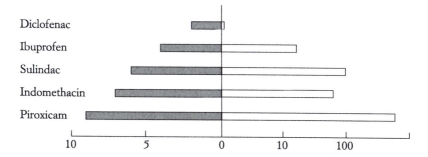

Figure 1 Comparison of gastric damage and cyclooxygenase selectivity of nonsteroidal anti-inflammatory drugs. The left side represents the ranking of gastrointestinal toxicity for anti-inflammatory doses of the NSAIDs taken from the epidemiological study of Henry et al. (72). The right side represents log COX-2/COX-1 activity ratios determined in intact cells by measuring IC_{50} values of the NSAIDs as $\mu M/l$. (Data taken from Ref. 75.)

values for the COX-2/COX-1 ratio. Table 1 shows values for indomethacin that vary between 0.07 (74) and 60 (75). Clearly, cultures of cells from animals (first group) give relatively high values whereas microsomal human enzyme preparations (middle group) give a different set. Some of the reasons for variation have been identified. For example, Laneuville et al. (76) added drug and substrate to the human microsomal enzyme at the same time but noted that several NSAIDs, including indomethacin, take 10–20 min to produce a full enzyme inhibition. When the drug was incubated for 20 min with the enzyme before adding substrate (77), indomethacin was far more potent (especially on COX-2) and the ratio was reduced to 3.5. Other conditions that will lead to variation in results are the presence of protein in the medium and the several hours taken to induce COX-2 in cells.

Some examples of the experimental systems in which COX-2/COX-1 ratios of NSAIDs have been estimated are listed in Table 2. Inhibition of COX-1 is measured in unstimulated cells, whereas animal or human cells stimulated with bacterial lipopolysaccharide or interleukin-1 provide a source of COX-2.

Whole blood from humans shows promise as an assay, using platelets for COX-1 activity and inducing COX-2 in monocytes (78,79). Even so, the ratios show variation. Out of line with all other assays is that of Grossman et al. (74), using human washed platelets and leukocytes. Not only were the ratios they obtained substantially different from previous measurements, but the individual drugs were several orders of magnitude higher in potency than those obtained by others. This is most likely linked to the lack of protein in the medium.

Table 1 Inhibition of COX-1 and COX-2 by Indomethacin, Determined Using Different Models

COX-2 IC$_{50}$ (μM)	COX-1 IC$_{50}$ (μM)	COX-2/COX-1 Ratio	Ref.	
145	6.6	22	Meade et al., 1993 (96)	
1.7	0.028	60	Mitchell et al., 1993 (75)	ae
0.006	0.0002	30	Engelhardt et al., 1996 (81)	
0.009	0.0015	6	Klein et al., 1994 (97)	
0.97	7.4	1.3	Futaki et al., 1994 (98)	
>1000	13	>75	Laneuville et al., 1994 (76)	
1.4	0.6	2.3	O'Neill et al., 1994 (99)	he
0.9	0.1	9	Gierse et al., 1995 (100)	
0.1	0.35	3.5	Churchill et al., 1996 (77)	
0.36	0.7	0.51	Patrignani et al., 1994 (78)	
0.0012	0.017	~0.07	Grossman et al., 1995 (74)	hc
1.7	0.13	12.5	Young et al., 1996 (79)	

ac = animal cell cultures; he = human enzyme preparations; hc = human cells.

Churchill et al. (77) tested a series of drugs including meloxicam and nimesulide against microsomes prepared from insect cells transfected with human recombinant COX-1 and COX-2 (Table 3).

Despite these methodological variations the ratios still fall into three broad groups; high ratios for indomethacin, naproxen, and piroxicam, approxi-

Table 2 Examples of Experimental Models Used to Determine Inhibition of COX-1 and COX-2 by NSAIDs

Source of COX-1	Source of COX-2 (LPS or IL-1-stim)	Ref.
B.A.E.C.	Mouse macrophages	Mitchell et al., 1993 (75)
G.P. macrophages	G.P. macrophages	Engelhardt et al., 1996 (81)
Human platelets	Rat mesangial cells	Klein et al., 1994 (97)
Human gastric mucosa	Human leukocytes	Tavares and Bennett, 1993 (101)
Human platelets	Human whole blood	Patrignani et al., 1994 (78)
Human whole blood	Human whole blood	Young et al., 1996 (79)
Human platelets	Human leukocytes	Grossman et al., 1995 (74)
Human enzyme	Human enzyme	Churchill et al., 1996 (77)

B.A.E.C. = bovine aortic endothelial cells; G.P. = guinea pig; LPS = lipopolysaccharide; IL-1 = interleukin-1.

Table 3 Comparison of the Selectivity of Meloxicam with Other NSAIDs Using Human Recombinant COX-2 and COX-1 in a Microsomal Assay System

NSAID	COX-1 IC_{50} (μm)	COX-2 IC_{50} (μM)	COX-2/COX-1 ratio
Naproxen	2.7	~50	18.5
Ibuprofen	13.9	~80	5.8
Indomethacin	0.10	0.35	3.5
6-MNA	>100	NA	—
Diclofenac	0.059	0.031	0.5
Nimesulide	~50	9.4	0.2
Meloxicam	36.6	0.49	0.01

NA = less than 20% inhibition at 300 μM. 6-MNA = 6-methoxy-2-naphthyl acetic acid, active metabolite of nabumetone.
Source: Data taken from Ref. 77.

mately equiactivity on the two enzymes for diclofenac and ibuprofen, and selectivity for COX-2 for nimesulide, meloxicam, MK-966, and celecoxib. Thus, most of the results published so far support the hypothesis that the unwanted side effects of NSAIDs are due to their ability to inhibit COX-1 whereas their anti-inflammatory (therapeutic effects) are due to inhibition of COX-2.

VII. Selective COX-2 Inhibitors

A. Meloxicam

Meloxicam, which has a selectivity toward COX-2 of up to 100-fold over COX-1 (depending on the test system), is being marketed this year around the world for use in rheumatoid arthritis and osteoarthritis (80; Fig. 2). It has a COX-2/COX-1 ratio of about 0.01 on human recombinant enzymes (77) and about 0.33 in guinea pig peritoneal macrophages (81). Meloxicam is a potent inhibitor of adjuvant arthritis in rats at doses that only weakly affect the synthesis of prostaglandins in the gastric mucosa and kidneys (82). In double-blind trials in more than 5000 patients with osteoarthritis and rheumatoid arthritis, meloxicam in doses of 7.5 mg and 15 mg was comparable in efficacy to standard NSAIDs such as naproxen 750–1000 mg, piroxicam 20 mg, and diclofenac 100 mg slow release. Both doses of meloxicam produced significantly fewer gastrointestinal adverse effects than the standard NSAIDs ($p < 0.05$). Discontinuation of treatment due to gastrointestinal side effects was also significantly less frequent with meloxicam. Perforations, ulcerations, and bleedings occurred in fewer meloxicam-treated patients than in patients treated with piroxicam, diclofenac, or naproxen. The frequency of adverse events with meloxicam was significantly less at $p < 0.05$ when compared to piroxicam and naproxen (80).

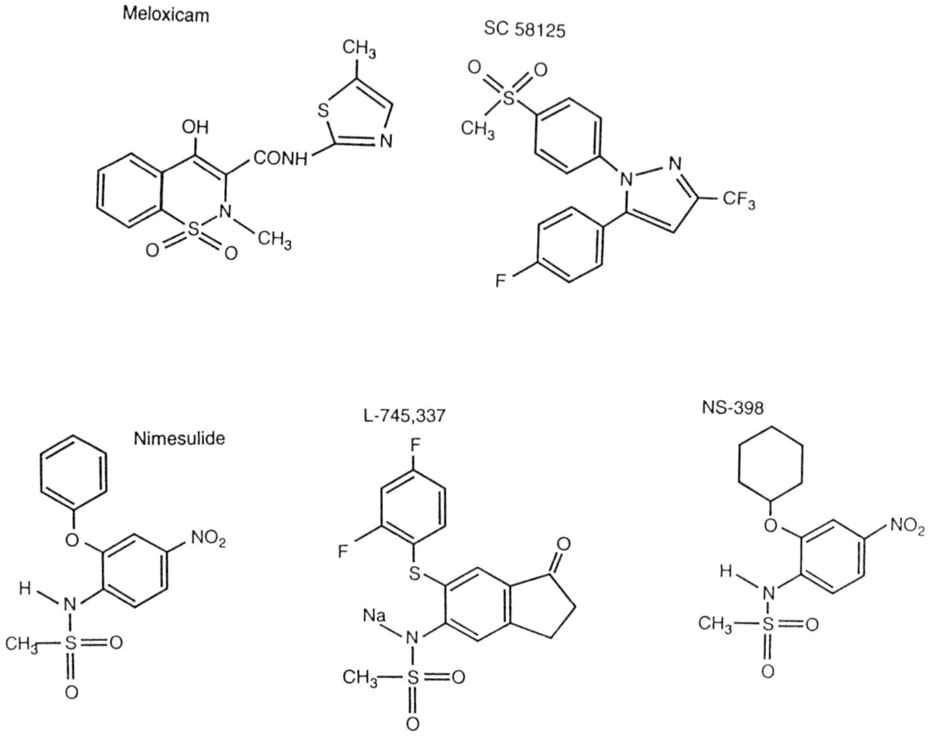

Figure 2 Selective COX-2 inhibitors. Meloxicam and nimesulide are marketed in several countries.

B. Nimesulide

Nimesulide was patented in 1974 in Belgium and in the United States and is currently sold in several European countries for the relief of pain associated with inflammatory conditions (Fig. 2). It has an unusual pharmacological profile compared to other NSAIDs in that it inhibits weakly the bovine seminal vesicle microsomal cyclooxygenase with 1/1000 of the activity of indomethacin (83), while reducing the inflammation of rat adjuvant arthritis and carrageenin paw edema at similar doses to indomethacin, diclofenac, or piroxicam. In limited clinical trials for its use in acute and chronic inflammation in patients, it was more effective than placebo or had comparable anti-inflammatory activity to established NSAIDs (84–86). Epidemiological data suggested that, in long-term therapeutic use at anti-inflammatory doses (100 mg twice daily), it caused no more serious gastrointestinal symptoms than placebo (87). This unusual

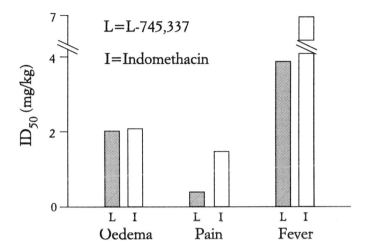

Figure 3 Comparison of in vivo ID_{50} values (mg/kg) for L-745,337 (L) and indomethacin (I) to inhibit inflammation in rats. The parameters measured were edema, pain, and fever. Indomethacin produced stomach lesions with an ED_{50} of 14.5 mg/kg whereas L-745,337 did not cause lesions up to 30 mg/kg. (Data taken from Ref. 91.)

profile became understandable when nimesulide was shown to be a selective inhibitor of COX-2 with 10- to 20-fold greater potency against this enzyme than against COX-1 (88). Moreover, nimesulide seems safe to use in aspirin-sensitive asthmatics. Nine recent studies in over 1000 NSAID-intolerant patients demonstrated the absence of allergic reactions in 90–100% of patients receiving therapeutic doses of nimesulide (89).

C. Celecoxib

Other nonsteroidal anti-inflammatory compounds that have greater selectivity for COX-2 over COX-1 are in clinical development (90,91). Monsanto/Searle have made inhibitors, such as SC 58125 (Fig. 2), that are some 400-fold more potent in vitro against COX-2 than against COX-1. One of these, celecoxib (SC 58635), is an effective analgesic in humans for moderate to severe pain following tooth extraction (92). In phase II placebo-controlled, double-blind trials in 25 centers in the United States, patients with osteoarthritis of the knee were treated for 2 weeks with twice-daily doses of 40 mg, 100 mg, or 200 mg celecoxib. Assessments made by physicians and patients indicated significantly greater improvement on all doses of celecoxib than on placebo and withdrawal for lack of efficacy was greater on placebo than on celecoxib. The incidence of adverse reactions and withdrawal from the study due to adverse reactions was similar in placebo and celecoxib-treated groups. In a phase II placebo-controlled, double-blind study, patients with rheumatoid arthritis were treated for 4 weeks with twice-daily doses of 40 mg, 200 mg, or 400 mg of celecoxib. Duration of morning stiffness was significantly better on all doses of celecoxib than on placebo and the number of painful joints was significantly less at the two highest doses than on placebo. No serious adverse events or changes in renal parameters were reported on celecoxib. Celecoxib is currently in phase III trials in arthritic patients (93).

D. L-475,337, L-758,115, and MK-966

In whole-cell assays, the selective COX-2 inhibitor from Merck-Frosst L475,337 (Fig. 2), inhibited COX-2 with an IC_{50} of 20 nM, but was inactive on COX-1 even at doses of 10 μM (COX-2/COX-1 ratio of 1/500). It reduced carrageenin-induced rat paw edema with an ED_{50} of 2 mg/kg (91). Oral doses of L-475,337 reduced carrageenin hyperalgesia in the rat paw with ED_{50} values similar to piroxicam and indomethacin (0.37, 0.51, and 1.47 mg/kg, respectively). It did not cause stomach lesions at doses of up to 30 mg/kg whereas the ED_{50} for the ulcerogenic actions of piroxicam and indomethacin was 14 mg/kg (94; Fig. 3). No gastrointestinal bleeding was detected in a ^{51}Cr excretion assay in monkeys at doses of 10 mg/kg given twice daily for 5 days. Indomethacin and flurbiprofen had a significant effect in this test at 5 mg/kg given for 1 day (91). Furthermore, no obvious stomach lesions were found in rats at doses that reduced PGE_2 levels in the inflammatory exudate from the pleural cavity.

Another lead compound reported by Merck-Frosst was the methyl sulfone, L-758115 (Fig. 4), which in whole cells had an IC_{50} for COX-2 of 3.38 μM and for COX-1 of >100 μM demonstrating a COX-2/COX-1 ratio of less than 0.03. In the rat carrageenin paw edema model of inflammation, L-758115 had an oral ID_{50} of 0.16 mg/kg without any adverse gastrointestinal effects (93). A similar selective COX-2 inhibitor from Merck-Frosst, MK-966, is currently undergoing phase IIb/III clinical trials.

E. New Selective COX-2 and Dual COX-2/5LO Inhibitors

Several pharmaceutical companies have new selective COX-2 inhibitors under investigation (93; Fig. 4). Parke-Davis is conducting clinical studies on CI-1004, a combined COX-2 and 5-lipoxygenase inhibitor, which has no gastric toxicity in rats or monkeys and is well tolerated in humans in single doses of up to 100 mg. This drug inhibits recombinant human COX-2 with an IC_{50} of 0.48 μM and has no apparent activity against COX-1. PD 098120-003 is another COX-2 inhibitor from Parke-Davis that has no effect on COX-1 and does not cause any gastrointestinal toxicity.

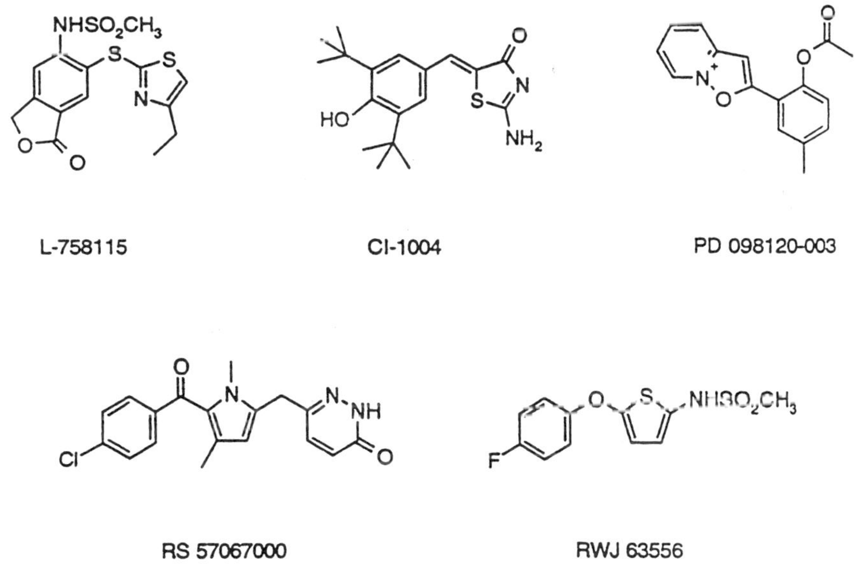

L-758115 CI-1004 PD 098120-003

RS 57067000 RWJ 63556

Figure 4 Selective COX-2 inhibitors in preclinical studies. (Reproduced from Ref. 93 with permission.)

RS-57067000, a compound from Roche Bioscience, has a very weak effect on COX-1 and does not cause gastric erosions in the rat in doses up to 200 mg/kg. The COX-2/COX-1 ratio for this compound on human recombinant enzymes is less than 0.0006.

Other companies are developing dual COX-2/5-lipoxygenase inhibitors as anti-inflammatory drugs. Johnson and Johnson are currently evaluating RWJ 63556, which inhibits LTB$_4$ production in human leukocytes with an IC$_{50}$ of 1.02 μM and has a COX-2/COX-1 ratio of less than 0.18 determined on human peripheral leukocytes. Procter and Gamble have presented data on PGV 20229, which has no gastrointestinal toxicity in dogs and inhibits leukotriene biosynthesis in RBL-2 cells. The COX-2/COX-1 ratio of PGV 20229 has been quoted as 0.03 measured on human platelets for COX-1 and on human monocytes for COX-2.

As well as benefiting arthritic patients, these selective inhibitors may demonstrate new therapeutic potential, slowing down tumor growth, preventing premature labor, and ameliorating some of the symptoms of asthma.

VIII. Conclusions

As mentioned previously, COX-2 levels can be increased in the lung by hypoxia and a variety of inflammatory stimuli. Up-regulation of COX-2 with simultaneous down-regulation of COX-1 by LPS has also been reported (95). The cyclooxygenase products formed by the lung consist mostly of the weak bronchodilator PGE_2, together with the potent bronchoconstrictor prostanoids $PGF_{2\alpha}$ and TXA_2. Surprisingly, clinical studies in more than 1000 patients show that the selective COX-2 inhibitor nimesulide is well tolerated in aspirin-sensitive asthmatics (89). This means, presumably that a COX-1 inhibitor brings about asthma in these patients through the release of a bronchoconstrictor, perhaps by making more arachidonic acid available for leukotriene biosynthesis. Thus, selective inhibition of COX-2 may well avoid the aspirin intolerance in these patients.

Acknowledgments

The William Harvey Research Institute is supported by grants from the ONO Pharmaceutical Company, Schwarz Pharma Ltd., and the Servier International Research Institute.

References

1. Hemler M, Lands WEM, Smith WL. Purification of the cyclooxygenase that forms prostaglandins: demonstration of two forms of iron in the holoenzyme. J Biol Chem 1976; 251:5575–5579.
2. Vane JR. Inhibition of prostaglandin synthesis as a mechanism of action for the aspirin-like drugs. Nature 1971; 231:232–235.
3. Higgs GA, Vane JR, Hart FD, Wojtulewski JA. Effects of anti-inflammatory drugs on prostaglandins in rheumatoid arthritis. In: Robinson HJ, Vane JR, eds. Prostaglandin Synthase Inhibitors. New York: Raven Press, 1974:165–173.
4. Picot D, Loll PJ, Garavito RM. The X-ray crystal structure of the membrane protein prostaglandin H_2 synthase-1. Nature 1994; 367:243–249.
5. Luong C, Miller A, Barnett J, Chow J, Ramesha C, Browner MF. Flexibility of the NSAID binding site in the structure of human cyclooxygenase-2. Nature Struct Biol 1996; 3:927–933.
6. Gierse JK, McDonald JJ, Hauser SD, Rangwala SH, Koboldt CM, Seibert K. A single amino acid difference between cyclooxygenase-1 (COX-1) and -2 (COX-2) reverses the selectivity of COX-2 specific inhibitors. J Biol Chem 1996; 271:15810–15814.
7. Moncada S, Gryglewski R, Bunting S, Vane JR. An enzyme isolated from arteries transforms prostaglandin endoperoxides to an unstable substance that inhibits platelet aggregation. Nature 1976; 263:663–665.

8. Whittle BJR, Higgs GA, Eakins KE, Moncada S, Vane JR. Selective inhibition of prostaglandin production in inflammatory exudates and gastric mucosa. Nature 1980; 284:271–273.

9. Funk CD, Funk LB, Kennedy ME, Pong AS, Fitzgerald GA. Human platelet/erythroleukemia cell prostaglandin G/H synthase: cDNA cloning, expression, and gene chromosomal assignment. FASEB J 1991; 5:2304–2312.

10. Raz A, Wyche A, Needleman P. Temporal and pharmacological division of fibroblast cyclooxygenase expression into transcriptional and translational phases. Proc Natl Acad Sci USA 1989; 86:1657–1661.

11. Fu JY, Masferrer JL, Seibert K, Raz A, Needleman P. The induction and suppression of prostaglandin H$_2$ synthase (cyclooxygenase) in human monocytes. J Biol Chem 1990; 265:16737–16740.

12. Masferrer JL, Zweifel BS, Seibert K, Needleman P. Selective regulation of cellular cyclooxygenase by dexamethasone and endotoxin in mice. J Clin Invest 1990; 86: 1375–1379.

13. Xie W, Chipman JG, Robertson DL, Erikson RL, Simmons DL. Expression of a mitogen-responsive gene encoding prostaglandin synthase is regulated by mRNA splicing. Proc Natl Acad Sci USA 1991; 88:2692–2696.

14. Xie W, Robertson DL, Simmons DL. Mitogen-inducible prostaglandin G/H synthase: a new target for nonsteroidal antiinflammatory drugs. Drug Devel Res 1992; 25:249–265.

15. O'Banion MK, Sadowski HB, Winn V, Young DA. A serum- and glucocorticoid-regulated 4-kilobase mRNA encodes a cyclooxygenase-related protein. J Biol Chem 1991; 266:23261–23267.

16. Kujubu DA, Fletcher BS, Varnum BC, Lim RW, Herschman HR. TIS10, a phorbol ester tumor promoter-inducible mRNA from Swiss 3T3 cells, encodes a novel prostaglandin synthase/cyclooxygenase homologue. J Biol Chem 1991; 26:12866–12872.

17. Sirois J, Richards JS. Purification and characterisation of a novel, distinct, isoform of prostaglandin endoperoxide synthase induced by human chorionic gonadotropin in granulosa cells of rat preovulatory follicles. J Biol Chem 1992; 267:6382–6388.

18. Vane J. Towards a better aspirin. Nature 1994; 367:215–216.

19. DeWitt DL. Prostaglandin endoperoxide synthase: regulation of enzyme expression. Biochim Biophys Acta 1991; 1083:121–134.

20. Wu KK, Sanduja R, Tsai A-L, Ferhanoglu B, Loose-Mitchell DS. Aspirin inhibits interleukin 1-induced prostaglandin H synthase expression in cultured endothelial cells. Proc Natl Acad Sci USA 1991; 88:2384–2387.

21. Whittle BJR, Vane JR. Prostanoids as regulators of gastrointestinal function. In: Johnston LR, ed. Physiology of the Gastrointestinal Tract. Vol I, 2nd ed. New York: Raven Press, 1987:143–180.

22. Kargman S, Charleson S, Cartwright M, Frank J, Riendeau D, Mancini J, Evans J, O'Neill GP. Characterization of prostaglandin G/H synthase 1 and 2 in rat, dog, monkey and human gastrointestinal tracts. Gastroenterology 1996; 111:445–454.

23. Langenbach R, Morham SG, Tiano HF, Loftin CD, Ghanayem BI, Chulada PC, Mahler JF, Lee CA, Goulding EH, Kluckman KD, Kim HS, Smithies O. Pro-

staglandin synthase 1 gene disruption in mice reduces arachidonic acid-induced inflammation and indomethacin-induced gastric ulceration. Cell 1995; 83:483–492.

24. Kutchera W, Jones DA, Matsunami N, Groden J, McIntyre TM, Zimmerman GA, White RL, Prescott SM. Prostaglandin H synthase 2 is expressed abnormally in human colon cancer: evidence for a transcriptional effect. Proc Natl Acad Sci USA 1996; 93:4816–4820.

25. Gustafson-Svärd C, Lilja I, Hallböök O, Sjödahl R. Cyclooxygenase-1 and cyclo-oxygenase-2 gene expression in human colorectal adenocarcinomas and in azoxy-methane induced colonic tumours in rats. Gut 1996; 38:79–84.

26. Thun MJ, Hamboodiri MM, Heath CWJ. Aspirin use and reduced risk of fatal colon cancer. N Engl J Med 1991; 325:1593–1596.

27. Luk GD. Prevention of gastrointestinal cancer—the potential role of NSAIDs in colorectal cancer. Schweiz Med Wochenschr 1996; 126:801–812.

28. Nugent KP, Spigelman AD, Phillips RKS. Tissue prostaglandin levels in familial adenomatous polyposis patients treated with sulindac. Dis Colon Rectum 1996; 39:659–662.

29. Oshima M, Dinchuk JE, Kargman SL, Oshima H, Hancock B, Kwong E, Trzaskos JM, Evans JF, Taketo MM. Suppression of intestinal polyposis in $Apc^{\Delta716}$ knockout mice by inhibition of cyclooxygenase 2 (COX-2). Cell 1996; 87:803–809.

30. Stokes JB. Effect of prostaglandin E_2 on chloride transport across the rabbit thick ascending limb of Henle. Selective inhibition of the medullary portion. J Clin Invest 1979; 64:495–502.

31. Orloff J, Zusman R. Role of prostaglandin E (PGE) in the modulation of action of vasopressin on water flow in the urinary bladder of the toad and mammalian kidney. J Membr Biol 1978; 40:297–304.

32. Harris RC, McKanna JA, Akai Y, Jacobson HR, Dubois RN, Breyer MD. Cyclooxygenase-2 is associated with the macula densa of rat kidney and increases with salt restriction. J Clin Invest 1994; 94:2504–2510.

33. Nüsing RM, Klein T, Pfeilschifter J, Ullrich V. Effect of cyclic AMP and prostaglandin E_2 on the induction of nitric oxide- and prostanoid-forming pathways in cultured rat mesangial cells. Biochem J 1996; 313:617–623.

34. Morham SG, Langenbach R, Loftin CD, Tiano HF, Vouloumanos N, Jennette JC, Mahler JF, Kluckman KD, Ledford A, Lee CA, Smithies O. Prostaglandin synthase 2 gene disruption causes severe renal pathology in the mouse. Cell 1995; 83:473–482.

35. Bakhle YS, Ferreira SH. Lung metabolism of eicosanoids. In: Fishman A, Fisher AB, eds. Handbook of Physiology. Bethesda, MD: American Physiological Society, 1985:365–386.

36. Holgate ST. The pathophysiology of bronchial asthma and targets for its drug treatment. Agents Actions 1986; 18:281–287.

37. Tomlinson A, Appleton I, Moore AR, Gilroy DW, Willis D, Mitchell JA, Willoughby DA. Cyclo-oxygenase and nitric oxide synthase isoforms in rat carrageenin-induced pleurisy. Br J Pharmacol 1994; 113:693–694.

38. Hatanaka K, Harada Y, Kawamura M, Ogino M, Saito M, Katori M. Cell types expressing COX-2 in rat carrageenin-induced pleurisy. Jpn J Pharmacol 1996; 71 (Suppl I):304P.

39. Chida M, Voelkel NF. Effects of acute and chronic hypoxia on rat lung cyclooxygenase. Am J Physiol 1996; 270:L872–L878.
40. O'Neill GP, Ford-Hutchinson AW. Expression of mRNA for cyclooxygenase-1 and cyclooxygenase-2 in human tissues. FEBS Lett 1993; 330:156–160.
41. Asano K, Lilly CM, Drazen JM. Prostaglandin G/H synthase-2 is the constitutive and dominant isoform in cultured human lung epithelial cells. Am J Physiol 1996; 271:L126–L131.
42. Walenga RW, Kester M, Coroneos E, Butcher S, Dwivedi R, Statt C. Constitutive expression of prostaglandin endoperoxide G/H synthase (PGHS)-2 but not PGHS-1 in human tracheal epithelial cells in vitro. Prostaglandins 1996; 52:341–359
43. Mitchell JA, Belvisi MG, Akarasereenont P, Robbins RA, Kwon O-J, Croxtall J, Barnes PJ, Vane JR. Induction of cyclo-oxygenase-2 by cytokines in human pulmonary epithelial cells: regulation by dexamethasone. Br J Pharmacol 1994; 113: 1008–1014.
44. Samet JM, Reed W, Ghio AJ, Devlin RB, Carter JD, Dailey LA, Bromberg PA, Madden MC. Induction of prostaglandin H synthase 2 in human airway epithelial cells exposed to residual oil fly ash. Toxicol Appl Pharmacol 1996; 141:159–168.
45. Uhlig S, Nüssing R, von Bethmann A, Featherstone RL, Klein T, Brasch F, Müller K-M, Ullrich V, Wendel A. Cyclooxygenase-2-dependent bronchoconstriction in perfused rat lungs exposed to endotoxin. Mol Med 1996; 2:373–383.
46. Harada Y, Hatanaka K. Kawamura M, Saito M, Ogino M, Majima M, Ohno T, Ogino K, Yamamoto K, Taketani Y, Yamamoto S, Katori M. Role of prostaglandin H synthase-2 in prostaglandin E_2 formation in rat carrageenin-induced pleurisy. Prostaglandins 1996; 51:19–33.
47. Hayaishi O. Molecular mechanisms of sleep-wake regulation: roles of prostaglandins D_2 and E_2. FASEB J 1991; 5:2575–2581.
48. Jones SA, Adamson SL, Bishai I, Lees J, Engelberts D, Coceani F. Eicosanoids in third venticular cerebrospinal fluid of fetal and newborn sheep. Am J Physiol 1993; 264:R135–R142.
49. Peri KG, Hardy P, Li DY, Varma DR, Chemtob S. Prostaglandin G/H synthase-2 is a major contributor of brain prostaglandins in the newborn. J Biol Chem 1995; 270:24615–24620.
50. Chemtob S, Beharry K, Rex J, Varma DR, Aranda JV. Prostanoids determine the range of cerebral blood flow autoregulation of newborn piglets. Stroke 1990; 21: 777–784.
51. Yamagata K, Andreasson KI, Kaufman WE, Barnes CA, Worley PF. Expression of a mitogen-inducible cyclooxygenase in brain neurons; regulation by synaptic activity and glucocorticoids. Neuron 1993; 11:371–386.
52. Breder CD, Dewitt D, Kraig RP. Characterization of inducible cyclooxygenase in rat brain. J Comp Neurol 1995; 355:296–315.
53. Breder CD, Saper CB. Expression of inducible cyclooxygenase mRNA in the mouse brain after systemic administration of bacterial lipopolysaccharide. Brain Res 1996; 713:64–69.
54. Cao C, Matsumura K, Yamagata K, Watanabe Y. Endothelial cells of the brain vasculature express cyclooxygenase-2 mRNA in response to systemic interleukin-

1β: a possible site of prostaglandin synthesis responsible for fever. Brain Res 1996; 733:263–272.

55. Cao C, Matsumura K, Yamagata K, Watanabe Y. Induction by lipopolysaccharide of cyclooxygenase-2 mRNA in rat brain; its possible role in the febrile response. Brain Res 1995; 697:187–196.

56. Marcheselli VL, Bazan NG. Sustained induction of prostaglandin endoperoxide synthase-2 by seizures in hippocampus. J Biol Chem 1996; 271:24794–24799.

57. Beiche F, Scheuerer S, Brune K, Geisslinger G, Goppelt-Struebe M. Up-regulation of cyclooxygenase-2 mRNA in the rat spinal cord following peripheral inflammation. FEBS Lett 1996; 390:165–169.

58. Milton AS. Antipyretic actions of aspirin. In: Vane JR, Botting RM, eds. Aspirin and Other Salicylates. London: Chapman and Hall, 1992:213–244.

59. Futaki N, Yoshikawa K, Hamasaka Y, Arai I, Higuchi S, Iizuka H, Otomo S. NS-398, a novel non-steroidal anti-inflammatory drug with potent analgesic and antipyretic effects which causes minimal stomach lesions. Gen Pharmacol 1993; 24: 105–110.

60. Bennett P, Slater D. COX-2 expression in labour. In: Vane J, Botting J, Botting R, eds. Improved Nonsteroid Anti-inflammatory Drugs. COX-2 Enzyme Inhibitors. Lancaster, UK: Kluwer Academic Publishers, and London: William Harvey Press, 1996:167–188.

61. Langenbach R, Morham SG, Tiano HF, Loftin CD, Ghanayem BI, Chulada PC, Mahler JF, Lee CA, Goulding EH, Kluckman KD, Kim HS, Smithies O. Prostaglandin synthase 1 gene disruption in mice reduces arachidonic acid-induced inflammation and indomethacin-induced gastric ulceration. Cell 1995; 83:483–492.

62. Gibb W, Sun M. Localization of prostaglandin H synthase type 2 protein and mRNA in term human fetal membranes and decidua. J Endocrinol 1996; 150:497–503.

63. Trautman MS, Edwin SS, Collmer D, Dudley DJ, Simmons D, Mitchell MD. Prostaglandin H synthase-2 in human gestational tissues: regulation in amnion. Placenta 1996; 17:239–245.

64. Toth P, Li X, Lei ZM, Rao CV. Expression of human chorionic gonadotropin (hCG)/luteinizing hormone receptors and regulation of the cyclooxygenase-1 gene by exogenous hCG in human fetal membranes. J Clin Endocrinol Metab 1996; 81:1283–1288.

65. Dinchuk JE, Car BD, Focht RJ, Johnston JJ, Jaffee BD, Covington MB, Contel NR, Eng VM, Collins RJ, Czerniak PM, Gorry SA, Trzaskos JM. Renal abnormalities and an altered inflammatory response in mice lacking cyclooxygenase II. Nature 1995; 378:406–409.

66. Chakraborty I, Das SK, Wang J, Dey SK. Developmental expression of the cyclo-oxygenase-1 and cyclo-oxygenase-2 genes in the peri-implantation mouse uterus and their differential regulation by the blastocyst and ovarian steroids. J Mol Endocrinol 1996; 16:107–122.

67. Zakar T, Hirst JJ, Milovic JE, Olson DM. Glucocorticoids stimulate the expression of prostaglandin endoperoxide H synthase-2 in amnion cells. Endocrinology 1995; 136:1610–1619.

68. Spaziani EP, Lantz ME, Benoit RR, O'Brien WF. The induction of cyclooxygenase-2 (COX-2) in intact human amnion tissue by interleukin-4. Prostaglandins 1996; 51:215–223.

69. McLaren WJ, Young IR, Wong MH, Rice GE. Expression of prostaglandin G/H synthase-1 and -2 in ovine amnion and placenta following glucocorticoid-induced labour onset. J Endocrinol 1996; 151:125–135.

70. Garcia Rodriguez LA, Jick H. Risk of upper gastrointestinal bleeding and perforation associated with individual non-steroidal anti-inflammatory drugs. Lancet 1994; 343:769–772.

71. Langman MJS, Weil J, Wainwright P, Lawson DH, Rawlins MD, Logan RFA, Murphy M, Vessey MP, Colin Jones DG. Risks of bleeding peptic ulcer associated with individual non-steroidal anti-inflammatory drugs. Lancet 1994; 343: 1075–1078.

72. Henry D, Lim LL-Y, Rodriguez LAG, Gutthann SP, Carson JL, Griffin M, Savage R, Logan R, Moride Y, Hawkey C, Hill S, Fries JT. Variability in risk of gastrointestinal complications with individual non-steroidal anti-inflammatory drugs: results of a collaborative meta-analysis. Br Med J 1996; 312:1563–1566.

73. Vane JR, Botting RM. New insights into the mode of action of anti-inflammatory drugs. Inflamm Res 1995; 44:1–10.

74. Grossman CJ, Wiseman J, Lucas FS, Trevethick MA, Birch PJ. Inhibition of constitutive and inducible cyclooxygenase activity in human platelets and mononuclear cells by NSAIDs and Cox 2 inhibitors. Inflamm Res 1995; 44:253–257.

75. Mitchell JA, Akarasereenont P, Thiemermann C, Flower RJ, Vane JR. Selectivity of nonsteroidal antiinflammatory drugs as inhibitors of constitutive and inducible cyclooxygenase. Proc Natl Acad Sci USA 1993; 90:11693–11697.

76. Laneuville O, Breuer DK, DeWitt DL, Hla T, Funk CD, Smith WL. Differential inhibition of human prostaglandin endoperoxide H synthases-1 and -2 by nonsteroidal anti-inflammatory drugs. J Pharmacol Exp Ther 1994; 271:927–934.

77. Churchill L, Graham AG, Shih C-K, Pauletti D, Farina PR, Grob PM. Selective inhibition of human cyclo-oxygenase-2 by meloxicam. Inflammopharmacology 1996; 4:125–135.

78. Patrignani P, Panara MR, Greco A, Fusco O, Natoli C, Iacobelli S, Cipollone F, Ganci A, Créminon C, Maclouf J, Patrono C. Biochemical and pharmacological characterization of the cyclooxygenase activity of human blood prostaglandin endoperoxide synthases. J Pharmacol Exp Ther 1994; 271:1705–1712.

79. Young JM, Panah S, Satchawatcharaphong C, Cheung PS. Human whole blood assays for inhibition of prostaglandin G/H synthases-1 and -2 using A23187 and lipopolysaccharide stimulation of thromboxane B_2 production. Inflamm Res 1996; 45:246–253.

80. Barner A. Review of clinical trials and benefit/risk ratio of meloxicam. Scand J Rheumatol 1996; 25 (Suppl 102):29–37.

81. Engelhardt G, Bögel R, Schnitzer Chr, Utzmann R. Meloxicam: influence on arachidonic acid metabolism. Part I. In vitro findings. Biochem Pharmacol 1996; 51:21–28.

82. Engelhardt G, Homma D, Schlegel K, Utzmann R, Schnitzler C. Anti-inflammatory, analgesic, antipyretic and related properties of meloxicam, a new non-steroi-

dal anti-inflammatory agent with favourable gastrointestinal tolerance. Inflamm Res 1995; 44:423–433.

83. Böttcher I, Schweizer A, Glatt M, Werner H. A sulphonamidoindanone CGP 28237 (ZK 34228), a novel non-steroidal anti-inflammatory agent without gastrointestinal ulcerogenicity in rats. Drugs Exp Clin Res 1987; 13:237–245.

84. Weissenbach R. Clinical trials with nimesulide, a new non-steroid anti-inflammatory agent, in rheumatic pathology. J Int Med Res 1981; 13:237–245.

85. Pais JM, Rosteiro FM. Nimesulide in the short-term treatment of the inflammatory process of dental tissues: a double-blind controlled trial against oxyphenbutazone. J Int Med Res 1983; 11:149–154.

86. Emami Nouri E. Nimesulide for treatment of acute inflammation of the upper respiratory tract. Clin Ther 1984; 6:142–150.

87. Fusetti G, Magni E, Armandola MC. Tolerability of nimesulide. Epidemiological data. Drugs 1993; 46 (Suppl 1):277–280.

88. Rabasseda X. Nimesulide: a selective cyclooxygenase 2 inhibitor antiinflammatory drug. Drugs Today 1996; 32 (Suppl D):1–23.

89. Senna GE, Passalacqua G, Andri G, Dama AR, Albano M, Fregonese L, Andri L. Nimesulide in the trreatment of patients intolerant of aspirin and other NSAIDs. Drug Safety 1996; 14:94–103.

90. Seibert K, Zhang Y, Leahy K, Hauser S, Masferrer J, Perkins W, Lee L, Isakson P. Pharmacological and biochemical demonstration of the role of cyclooxygenase 2 in inflammation and pain. Proc Natl Acad Sci USA 1994; 91:12013–12017.

91. Chan C-C, Boyce S, Brideau C, Ford-Hutchinson AW, Gordon R, Guay D, Hill RG, Li C-S, Mancini J, Penneton M, Prasit P, Rasori R, Riendeau D, Roy P, Tagari P, Vickers P, Wong E, Rodger IW. Pharmacology of a selective cyclooxygenase-2 inhibitor, L745,337: a novel nonsteroidal anti-inflammatory agent with an ulcerogenic sparing effect in rat and nonhuman primate stomach. J Pharmacol Exp Ther 1995; 274:1531–1537.

92. Hubbard RC, Mehlisch DR, Jasper DR, Nugent MJ, Yu S, Isakson PC. SC-58635, a highly selective inhibitor of COX-2, is an effective analgesic in an acute post-surgical pain model. J Invest Med 1996; 44:293A.

93. Parnham MJ. COX-2 inhibitors at the 8th International Conference of the Inflammation Research Association. Exp Opin Invest Drugs 1997; 6:79–82.

94. Boyce S, Chan C-C, Gordon R, Li C-S, Rodger IW, Webb JK, Rupniak NMJ, Hill RG. L-745,337: a selective inhibitor of cyclooxygenase-2 elicits antinociception but not gastric ulceration in rats. Neuropharmacology 1994; 33:1609–1611.

95. Liu SF, Newton R, Evans TW, Barnes PJ. Differential regulation of cyclo-oxygenase-1 and cyclo-oxygenase-2 gene expression by lipopolysaccharide treatment in vivo in the rat. Clin Sci 1996; 90:301–306.

96. Meade EA, Smith WL, DeWitt DL. Differential inhibition of prostaglandin endoperoxide synthase (cyclooxygenase) isozymes by aspirin and other non-steroidal anti-inflammatory drugs. J Biol Chem 1993; 268:6610–6614.

97. Klein T, Nüsing RM, Pfeilschifter J, Ullrich V. Selective inhibition of cyclooxygenase 2. Biochem Pharmacol 1994; 48:1605–1610.

98. Futaki N, Takahashi S, Yokoyama M, Arai S, Higuchi S, Otomo S. NS-398, a new anti-inflammatory agent, selectively inhibits prostaglandin G/H synthase/cyclo-oxygenase (COX-2) activity in vitro. Prostaglandins 1994; 47:55–59.

99. O'Neill GP, Mancini JA, Kargman S, Yergey J, Kwan MY, Falgueyret JP, Abramovitz M, Kennedy BP, Ouellet M, Cromlish W, Culp S, Evans JF, Ford-Hutchinson AW, Vickers PJ. Overexpression of human prostaglandin G/H synthase-1 and -2 by recombinant vaccinia virus: inhibition by nonsteroidal anti-inflammatory drugs and biosynthesis of 15-hydroxyeicosatetraenoic acid. Mol Pharmacol 1994; 45:245–254.

100. Gierse JK, Hauser SD, Creely DP, Koboldt C, Rangwala SH, Isakson PC, Seibert K. Expression and selective inhibition of the constitutive and inducible forms of human cyclo-oxygenase. Biochem J 1995; 305:479–484.

101. Tavares IA, Bennett A. Activity of nimesulide on constitutive and inducible prostaglandin cyclo-oxygenase. Int J Tissue React 1993, 15:49 (abstract).

2

Pathways of Arachidonate Metabolism

JOHN C. MCGIFF and MICHAEL BALAZY

New York Medical College
Valhalla, New York

I. Introduction

Three enzyme systems—cyclooxygenases (COX), lipoxygenases (LOX), and cytochrome P450-dependent monooxygenases (CYP450)—generate lipid mediators (eicosanoids*) from arachidonic acid (AA) via oxygenase reactions that are regiospecific and stereospecific (1). As the oxygenase that transforms AA to PGH_2 possesses two enzymatic sites and activities, COX ($AA \rightarrow PGG_2$) and peroxidase ($PGG_2 \rightarrow PGH_2$) (2), the combined activity is sometimes called PGH synthase (PGHS), although COX is used more frequently.

II. Cyclooxygenases

Two isoforms of COX, COX-1 and COX-2, having 60% amino acid identity, have been identified; each is encoded by a different gene (3). COX-1 gene expression is regulated developmentally and, once expressed, is sustained (4), whereas COX-2 is usually expressed transiently after induction by either

---

*Eicosanoids refers to any of the myriad of C-20 products arising from AA metabolism.

mitogens, proinflammatory cytokines, or lipopolysaccharide (LPS) (2). Under physiological conditions, COX-2 protein is said to be undetectable. However, COX-2 mRNA has been detected in several tissues at low levels, using the highly sensitive reverse transcription-polymerase chain reaction (RT-PCR) (5). Moreover, COX-2 is scattered throughout the cells of the renal medullary thick ascending limb (mTAL), being present in *ca.* 15% of cells under normal conditions (Carlos Vio, personal communication). COX-2 mRNA and protein are greatly increased in inflammation—for example, in joint synovia of patients with rheumatoid arthritis and in activated monocytes (2,6). COX-1 activity, on the other hand, remains relatively unaffected by inflammation (2). Developmental regulation of COX-1 results in manyfold elevation in COX-1 levels during the neonatal period and beyond.

Posttranscriptional stabilization of COX-2 mRNA contributes importantly to prolonged COX-2 expression as activation of COX-2 gene transcription is transient. COX-2 mRNA is less stable than that of COX-1, peaking within 4–6 h in response to induction, and declining over 24 h (2). Thus, enhanced stability of the COX-2 transcript is a major factor in prolonged activity of COX-2. As glucocorticoids suppress COX-2 activity, a potential mechanism for their effect may relate to posttranscriptional factors. Ristimäki et al. (7), having examined this possibility, have demonstrated that glucocorticoids destabilize the COX-2 transcript, contributing to their inhibitory effect on COX-2.

The constitutive enzyme, COX-1, is found in most, but not all, tissues and is expressed to the highest degree in seminal vesicles, platelets, endothelium, renal collecting tubules, monocytes, and gastric mucosa at which sites COX-1 performs a housekeeping function by responding rapidly to changes in local conditions affecting water excretion, gastric acidity, and vascular integrity, to name a few (2). The kinetic properties of COX-1 and -2 as indicated by V_{max} and K_m are virtually indistinguishable; each is subject to suicide inactivation (2,8). Nonetheless, differences are evident in the active sites of COX-1 and COX-2 in terms of their utilization of fatty acids and susceptibility to inhibition by aspirin-like drugs. The latter difference between COX-1 and -2 lends itself to therapeutic exploitation in terms of differential inhibition of the COX isoforms (9). Drugs are now available to suppress COX-2 and, thereby, dampen the inflammatory response while not affecting COX-1. Sparing COX-1 reduces the toxicity of aspirin-like drugs, lessening gastric bleeding, delayed parturition, and salt and water retention, to name several untoward effects, among many, of these drugs.

III. Lipoxygenases

Mammalian LOXs are designated by positional specificity relative to oxygenation of AA; three principle forms are recognized: 5-, 12-, and 15-LOXs. For

12-LOX, three isoforms exist, a leukocyte, a platelet, and an epithelial enzyme. LOXs may have two or more positional specificities. The leukocyte-type 12-LOX resembles 15-LOX as it also can oxygenate AA at C-15 depending on reaction conditions and demonstrates 80–90% sequence homology with 15-LOX as opposed to 60–70% with the platelet-type 12-LOX (10,11).

With respect to the importance of eicosanoid stereospecificity, the (S) and (R) enantiomers of 12-HETE are illustrative as they demonstrate crucial differences in their origin and in their biological properties, differences that reside in the planar orientation of the hydroxyl group attached to C-12. 12(R)-Hydroxyeicosatetraenoic acid (HETE) is a CYP450 product (12) whereas 12(S)-HETE is formed by the several isoforms of 12-LOX via a peroxy intermediate, 12-hydroperoxy-eicosatrienoic acid (HPETE) (11). 12(R)-HETE is generated by the cornea and, possibly, the vasculature and bronchial epithelium and has been shown to affect transport and vasomotion (1,12). 12(S)-HETE, first described in platelets (13), acts as a second messenger in the cellular events initiated by angiotensin II (AII) in the vasculature, adrenal zona glomerulosa, and juxtaglomerular apparatus, thereby, participating, respectively, in AII-induced vasoconstriction, steroidogenesis, and inhibition of renin secretion (14–16).

The synthesis of leukotrienes (LTs) is initiated by 5-LOX, which converts AA to 5-HPETE followed by dehydration of 5-HPETE to form LTA_4 (17). There are two principal pathways of LTA_4 metabolism either via LTA_4 hydrolase to form LTB_4 (18) or via LTC_4 synthase to form LTC_4 (19). LTA_4 hydrolase is found in many tissues in which 5-LOX is absent (20). For example, the small intestine has the highest activity of LTA_4 hydrolase but lacks 5-LOX. However, LTA_4 hydrolase is a dual-function enzyme, possessing aminopeptidase activity; the activity in some tissues may be directed toward metabolism of peptides, cleaving the N-terminal amino acid of the peptide (21). Activated leukocytes, capable of producing an abundance of LTA_4, can serve as sources of LTA_4 to cells that lack 5-LOX, resulting in generation of LTC_4 by these cells (20). This type of cell-cell interaction is apparently essential to the progression of some forms of inflammatory disease. LTA_4 hydrolase is inactivated by its product, LTB_4, which influences enzyme activity by covalent modification of the hydrolase. LTB_4 is catabolized via an ω-oxidation pathway in human leukocytes to 20-OH-LTB_4 and then 20-COOH-LTB_4. LTB_4 is also catabolized to 12-oxo-LTB_4 by other cells as well as via peroxisomal β oxidation (20).

LTB_4 turnover is critical to the magnitude and duration of inflammation as it induces a series of events resulting in recruiting cells of the immune system to the site of its synthesis, an essential event in the inflammatory response (22). A priori, containment or extinction of inflammation by inducing the enzymes that catabolize LTB_4 should be possible. The peroxisome-proliferator-activated receptors (PPARs) regulate expression of genes governing lipid catabolic enzymes including those that degrade LTB$_4$, viz., ω- and β-oxidation pathways (22). The PPARα subtype is found in tissues such as the liver and immune system that display high rates of lipid degradation. As LTB$_4$ stimulates PPARα, it serves in a negative feedback mechanism that controls the inflammatory response by modulating its own levels. Targeting this mechanism could result in the development of drugs that modify the PPARα to control the progression of inflammation.

The cysteinyl LTs—LTC$_4$, LTD$_4$, and LTE$_4$—contract smooth muscle and are produced in excess in bronchial asthma, constricting the airways in this disease (23). The cysteinyl LTs have been shown to be formed in the human lung in response to IgE challenge (24). The highest expression of 5-LOX, and the greatest capacity to synthesize LTs, reside in cells of myeloid origin: leukocytes, eosinophils, monocytes, and macrophages (25). Activation of 5-LOX requires the presence of an 18-kDa nuclear membrane-associated protein, 5-LOX activating protein (FLAP), which binds released AA for presentation to 5-LOX (26). Translocation of 5-LOX to the nuclear membrane, effected by a calcium-dependent mechanism, results in "transfer" of AA from FLAP to 5-LOX with generation of 5-HPETE and subsequent formation of LTA$_4$. LTA$_4$ is conjugated to reduced glutathione by microsomal LTC$_4$ synthase found in eosinophils, mast cells, and monocytes (23). Platelets, endothelium, and vascular smooth muscle also can synthesize LTC$_4$ from LTA$_4$ via cell-cell transfer as 5-LOX is absent in these cells (27). Lam et al. have reported that LTC$_4$ formed by eosinophils is released into the extracellular space via a probenecid-sensitive export carrier (28). LTC$_4$ can be acted upon by γ glutamyl transpeptidase to form LTD$_4$, which, in turn, can be converted to LTE$_4$ by a dipeptidase (23).

CYP450-dependent monooxygenase metabolism of AA is addressed at length in Chapter 3.

IV. Eicosanoid Synthesis, Release, and Metabolism

Generation of eicosanoids can be reduced to three successive steps: (1) release of AA followed by (2) conversion of AA via an oxygenase to a metabolite that is (3) transformed in a tissue-specific manner to a product that characterizes the tissue/cell.

1. *The first step involves release of esterified AA from storage in phospholipids in response to activation of a phospholipase.* Cholesterol esters and triglycerides can also serve as sources of AA; they have been mainly overlooked although they may be the principal "precursor lipid" in some cells such as those of ovarian follicles (29) and renal interstitium (30). As prostaglandins are synthesized on demand, the release of AA must be rapid and controlled. Thus,

the response to a stimulus such as AII occurs within seconds, is proportional to the strength of the stimulus, and declines rapidly on withdrawal of the stimulus (31). In a classic study, Anggärd et al. demonstrated vanishingly low levels of tissue prostanoids in the kidney under resting conditions (32).

Phospholipases

The rate-limiting step in the synthesis of eicosanoids is the release of AA from tissue stores, mainly membrane glycerophospholipids, by acylhydrolases of which the most prominent is phospholipase A_2 (PLA_2) (33). Activation of acylhydrolases, then, is key to the regulation of the AA cascade; these are subject to control, either directly or indirectly, by local and systemic factors of which glucocorticoids have received the greatest attention. Untransformed but free AA has been suggested to act as a second messenger in some tissues, for example, in regulating ion channels in the nephron (34). Free AA may activate sphingomyelin hydrolysis in response to tumor necrosis factor α (TNF), resulting in generation of ceramide, a signal for the cytokines TNF and interleukin-1 (IL-1) (35).

The rapid response of tissues to hormonal stimulation is strikingly evident in the capacity of the kidney to release prostanoids. A several-hundred-fold elevation of PGE_2 above basal levels occurs within 2 min in response to norepinephrine challenge (31). As the cellular concentration of free AA, under basal conditions, is submicromolar, which is maintained by an AA-specific reacylation mechanism (36), arachidonyl selective lipases must be rapidly activated when stimulated. In view of the fact that oleic acid is the most abundant unsaturated fatty acid (by a factor of three or more) in mammalian cell phospholipids and is released in negligible amounts in response to activation of PLA_2 (37), the requirement for selectivity of the acylhydrolase regarding release of AA is evident.

The phospholipase that has commanded the greatest interest in the AA cascade is a Ca^{2+}-dependent, 85-kDa cytosolic (c) PLA_2 (37). This acylhydrolase selectively cleaves phospholipids having AA in the *sn*-2 position, responds to hormonal stimuli by releasing AA that is converted to eicosanoids, and is activated at physiological concentrations of calcium (38). $cPLA_2$ also demonstrates lysophosphatidyl transacylase activity (37). Diverse stimuli can activate $cPLA_2$: cytokines, thrombin, mitogens, LPS, and hormones through association with G-protein-coupled receptors (GPCR). $cPLA_2$, thus far, is the only PLA_2 that demonstrates selectivity with respect to arachidonyl phospholipids (37).

Activation of $cPLA_2$ by a stimulus is dependent on a severalfold elevation of cytosolic Ca^{2+} from resting levels of less than 100 nM to levels of 300 nM or more associated with ten-fold or greater activity of $cPLA_2$ (39). Based on immunofluorescent findings, $cPLA_2$ is translocated from the cytosol to the endoplasmic reticulum and nuclear membrane in response to elevation of intracellular Ca^{2+} (40). Translocation of $cPLA_2$ dovetails with the primary localization of COX-1 (endoplasmic reticulum) and COX-2 (the nuclear membrane) as well as FLAP in the nuclear membrane, suggesting that these sites are the major cellular loci for metabolism of AA after release by PLA_2 (2). Phosphorylation of serine and, possibly, tyrosine residues of PLA_2 is associated with activation of PLA_2 that can be blocked by staurosporin and other inhibitors of protein kinase C (PKC) (37). PKC has been suggested to stimulate mitogen-activated protein (MAP) kinase, which is responsible for phosphorylation of a serine residue (Ser-505) of PLA_2 (37). Based on mutational studies, Ser-505 appears critical to the PKC response (41).

In contrast to phospholipase C-β species, regulation of PLA_2 activity by a G-protein through a direct effect is uncertain, although ongoing studies may resolve this question. However, an indirect effect of G-protein on PLA_2 via MAP kinase-dependent phosphorylation of $cPLA_2$ probably occurs. The cytokines IL-1 and TNF activate $cPLA_2$ posttranslationally as well as by transcriptional means, possibly, via a mechanism involving NF-κB (42).

HETEs and EETs Are Stored

In contrast to prostanoids, a fraction of HETEs derived from either LOX or CYP450 can be stored in phospholipids and neutral lipids. Of the eicosanoids, only epoxides (epoxyeicosatrienoic acids = EETs) and HETEs can be incorporated into cellular lipids (43). Alkaline hydrolysis of neutral lipids and phospholipids yielded 333 ng/g wet weight of EETs in the human renal cortex (44), values similar to those found in rabbit (45) and rat kidneys (46) and 10-fold higher than those reported for HETEs in the rabbit renal cortex (30). Human platelet lipids on hydrolysis also yielded greater quantities of EETs than HETEs (100:1) (47). EETs and HETEs are probably not formed after esterification of AA as, based on the study of Karara et al., oxidation of AA by CYP450 preceded acylation (48). Cellular membrane characteristics regarding permeability and properties of membrane-bound enzymes can be affected by EETs and HETEs esterified to glycerolipids (49). Incorporation of 12- and 15-HETEs into phospholipids was shown by Gordon and Spector to reduce prostaglandin biosynthetic capacity and to result in release of altered second messengers, respectively (50). EETs and HETEs, after release from phospholipids, can participate in transmembrane signaling as either intracellular or intercellular messengers.

The HETEs incorporated into renal lipids represent a preformed or storage pool of CYP450-derived eicosanoids that can be released by specific agonists via receptor-mediated stimulation of one or more phospholipases.

20-HETE, a potent eicosanoid having diverse biological properties, is released into renal plasma and tubular fluid from storage in phospholipids and triglycerides in response to AII (30). Inhibition of CYP450-AA metabolism with a mechanism-based inhibitor, 17-octadecynoic acid, which abolished basal renal efflux of 20-HETE and the subterminal HETEs (16-, 17-, 18-, and 19-HETEs), did not prevent AII-induced release of HETEs from the rabbit kidney (30). In the rabbit renal medulla, the largest quantities of esterified HETEs were found in neutral lipids, although in the cortex, HETEs were found to be incorporated mainly in phospholipids. In the rat kidney, 85–90% of endogenous 20-HETE was esterified to phosphatidylcholine and phosphatidylethanolamine (51). Thus, P450 HETEs are stored and are subject to release by peptide activation of acylhydrolases.

2. *The second step relates to conversion of AA by tissue oxygenases to AA metabolites, such as PGH_2 and LTA_4 for COX and 5-LOX, respectively.*

3. *The third step involves tissue specific transformation of the initial AA products of oxygenases; e.g., PGH_2 to TxA_2 and PGI_2, which characterize platelets and vascular endothelium, respectively, and LTA_4 by neutrophils to LTB_4 or by eosinophils to LTC_4* (20). Each tissue has a characteristic profile of eicosanoids that can be altered by departure from the resting state, such as that imposed by either deprivation or excessive intake of sodium as well as, more strikingly, by disease.

Several CYP450-AA metabolites can be metabolized by COX to products such as prostaglandin analogs of 20-HETE and 5,6-EET resulting in the acquisition of new properties (52,53). A compelling hypothesis resulted from the recognition that 20-HETE, generated by the renal mTAL, modulates the cotransporter (Na^+-K^+-$2Cl^-$) located in the luminal surface of that nephron segment (54) and upon extrusion contraluminally into the medullary interstitium can be transformed by COX to prostaglandin analogs of 20-HETE that are vasoactive (55). This metabolic sequence has been hypothesized to serve as the basis of a mechanism linking changes in transport in the mTAL and proximal tubules, the principal renal sites of 20-HETE synthesis, to changes in local (medullary) blood flow (43).

Despite lead sentences in reviews (usually by clinicians) that COX-1 is ubiquitous, it is not, although it is found in many tissues/cells. There are cells/tissues that are devoid of COX-1 but may be stimulated by eicosanoids produced by other cell types, assuming that the nonproducing cell possesses the requisite receptor, be it PGE_2 (EP), PGI_2 (IP), thromboxane A_2 (TxP), $PGF_{2\alpha}$ (FP), or PGD_2 (DP). Eicosanoids may stimulate either the cell of origin, in which case they act in an autocrine fashion, or adjacent cells to act in a paracrine mode. To do this, prostaglandins must be extruded from the cell of origin to stimulate membrane receptors of that cell or contiguous cells.

Although PGH$_2$ is usually rapidly converted by a mix of synthases, isomerases, and reductases to PGI$_2$, PGE$_2$, PGD$_2$, PGF$_{2\alpha}$, and TxA$_2$ that characterize a particular cell type, there are pathological conditions that result in the uncoupling of PGH$_2$ from enzymes such as PGI$_2$ synthase. The uncoupling has been shown, in a rat model of aortic coarctation hypertension, to depend on induction of either a 12- or 15-LOX, and production of corresponding HPETEs, 12- and 15-HPETEs that have the capacity to inhibit PGI$_2$ synthase and, thereby, promote increased tissue levels of the contractile eicosanoid, PGH$_2$, resulting in increased vascular tone (56). There are additional factors integral to this vascular mechanism involving diminished nitric oxide (NO) production and increased activity of PKC. These factors have been linked to elevation of vascular tone and heightened response to pressor agents in the aortic coarctation model of hypertension (57).

Prostanoids: Release and Uptake

Whether prostaglandins act as circulating hormones seems unlikely under physiological conditions because of rapid metabolism locally as well as a pulmonary prostaglandin uptake-catabolizing mechanism that prevents prostaglandins in the venous blood, on passage across the lungs, from entering the systemic circulation (58). PGI$_2$ is not subject to uptake by the lungs and could enter the systemic circulation to act as a circulating hormone (59). Further, lung disease, particularly diseases producing venous-arterial shunting of blood, will bypass the uptake mechanism allowing entry of the prostaglandin into the systemic circulation. As prostanoids have limited ability to diffuse across plasma membranes and as the rate of release of prostanoids from stimulated tissues is exceedingly rapid, a transporter has been postulated to facilitate eicosanoid entry (extrusion) into the extracellular space. Kanai et al. (60) have isolated and cloned a prostaglandin transporter from several tissues. (The relationship of the transporter to the uptake mechanism is unclear.) The latter functions to clear prostaglandins from biological fluids and has been well defined in the lungs as the critical step in metabolizing/degrading prostanoids (60). This mechanism prevents prostaglandins' acting as circulating hormones upon release from organs that have considerable prostaglandin synthetic capacity such as the kidney or gastrointestinal tract. Indeed, as noted above, PGI$_2$ could function as a circulating hormone as it is not a substrate for the pulmonary uptake mechanism although it is susceptible to catabolism by the principal degradative enzyme, 15-hydroxy prostaglandin dehydrogenase (15-OH PGDH), located in the cytosol (59). Furosemide and aspirin-like drugs such as indomethacin also block prostaglandin uptake/secretion. This uptake mechanism (transporter) is also found in the proximal tubules, choroid plexus, and ciliary body (61,62). In the proximal tubules, it may serve as a delivery system for prostaglandins from plasma into the tubular fluid (63).

V. Hormones and Phospholipases

In most target tissues, phospholipase C (PLC) is the signal transduction pathway linked to AII receptors (64). In rat renal mesangial cells, AII induced phosphoinositide hydrolysis and associated prostaglandin synthesis; products of the latter, particularly PGE_2, oppose the contractile action of AII on the glomerular epithelial and mesangial cells (65). On the other hand, stimulation of an apical receptor in proximal tubules by AII in the nM–μM range which produces natriuresis involves PLA_2 and the production of a CYP450 arachidonate epoxide, 5,6-EET (66). Higher concentrations of AII have been reported in tubular fluid than in plasma (nM vs. pM) (67). To evaluate PLA_2 activity in response to challenge with AII, lysophosphatidylcholine was measured as its precursor, phosphatidylcholine, is the most abundant phospholipid, in excess of 30% of total phospholipids (68). Thus, renal lipase stimulation by AII results in (1) production of vasodilator prostanoids via sequential activation of PLC and diacylglycerol lipase in glomerular mesangial cells (65) and (2) formation of an epoxide via activation of PLA_2 which is coupled to the CYP450 pathway in the proximal tubules (66). A PLC is also present in the proximal tubules but is not involved in AII signaling. It is activated by bradykinin, however, resulting in IP_3 generation and an increase in cytosolic Ca^{2+} derived from intracellular stores (68). These events are associated with a natriuresis in response to bradykinin. The increase in proximal tubular cytosolic Ca^{2+} produced by nM–μM AII is postulated to be mediated by 5,6-EET via stimulation of voltage-sensitive Ca^{2+} channels, which, in turn, inhibits transcellular sodium movement (66).

Model Systems and Lipid Mediators

In pM concentrations, AII, acting at the blood site of the proximal tubules, stimulates a different signal transduction pathway operating through adenylate cyclase (64). In the basolateral compartment of the proximal tubules, AII (pM to nM) inhibits adenylate cyclase activity and the resulting decline in cAMP affects Na^+/H^+ exchange on the luminal surface of the proximal tubules. Changes in cAMP regulate Na^+/H^+ exchange in this nephron segment, accounting for absorption of ca. 70% of the filtered load of sodium (69). What is lacking in this schema, involving AII, cAMP, and sodium transport, is the lipid mediator/modulator that a general concept of regulatory systems appears to require as an integral component. Indeed, an interaction of cAMP with the CYP450 system has been described in the mTAL (70); namely, cAMP stimulates production of CYP450 AA metabolism resulting in increased formation of 20-HETE, the principal eicosanoid produced in the mTAL and in the proximal tubules. 20-HETE affects transepithelial sodium movement by modulating the Na^+-H^+-$2Cl^-$ cotransporter of the mTAL (71) and, perhapsy, the Na^+ pump (Na^+-H^+-ATPase) in the proximal tubules (72).

The weight of evidence indicates that construction of models of cellular regulatory systems involves a lipid mediator as a key component of these systems together with protein kinases, G proteins, phospholipases, and other essential links that function coordinately in transporting epithelia, endothelium, and secretory cells. The species of eicosanoid involved in the regulatory mechanism is not fixed as has been shown in the mTAL after challenge with either LPS, cytokines, or AII, each of which stimulates production of TNF by the mTAL (73). Increased production of TNF by the mTAL is associated with expression of COX-2 (74) and suppression of CYP450 AA metabolism. The pivotal role of NO, after induction by TNF in this "switching mechanism," is addressed at length in Chapter 3. It involves induction of nitric oxide synthase (NOS) by TNF, the latter generated in situ, resulting in production of NO that either directly or after conversion to peroxynitrite via interaction of NO with superoxide anion stimulates production of prostaglandins (75) and, possibly, dampens formation of 20-HETE (76). The molecular bases of these divergent effects of NO or an NO derivative on COX and CYP450 remain to be defined.

Of the hormones involved in the regulation of extracellular fluid volume through affecting salt and water balance, AII and its congeners, such as AI, III, and A(1-7), occupy a central position as they can influence renal tubular function at several nephron sites, both proximally and distally, and also regulate vasomotion and act on the heart. These multiple sites of action of angiotensins are coupled through G proteins and lipases to the generation of eicosanoids from all three classes of oxygenases: (1) PGE_2 in the glomerulus, where the vasoconstrictor action of AII is modulated by PGE_2 (65); (2) 12- and, perhaps, 15-LOX in the vasculature and adrenal zona glomerulosa as well as in the renal afferent arteriole, the latter a major site of renal renin production that is inhibited by stimulation of 12-HETE by AII (14–16); and (3) 20-HETE in the preglomerular circulation (77) and key segments of the nephron, the proximal tubules (78), and mTAL (79). Production of 5,6-EET by the proximal tubules, as noted, is also stimulated by AII (66).

Within a cell type it is possible to distinguish more than one signaling pathway that responds to AII. In rat ventricular myocytes two distinct and parallel signaling pathways were identified, each linked to different angiotensin receptors, AT_1 and AT_2, and different phospholipases, PLA_2 and PLC, respectively (80). The first signaling pathway operated through AT_1 receptors and was linked to activation of PLA_2 and AA release. AA did not undergo transformation by the cells used in this study, rat cultured neonatal ventricular myocytes. The second signaling system proceeded through AII stimulation of AT_2 receptors, which activates phosphoinositide-specific PLC with production of inositol phosphates and mobilization of intracellular Ca^{2+}. The latter, in turn, may activate Ca^{2+}-dependent lipases such as cPLA2, an example of "crosstalk" between two signaling pathways present in the same cell that are activated by a single agonist acting on different receptors of the cell. The release of AA in the absence of discernible oxygenase activity suggests that AA itself acts as a signaling agent. In some tissues such as the heart, untransformed AA may modulate critical steps involved in excitation-contraction coupling. In addition to short-term immediate effects of AA, long-term effects on tissue function may be effected through AA activation of a PKC isoform (80) that alters gene expression.

In cells expressing COX-1, induction of COX-2 can occur in response to TNF and other inflammatory and/or mitogenic stimuli. The two forms of COX "represent two independently operating prostanoid biosynthetic systems," which use different pools of AA that respond to different agonists and oriented to different loci of activity: nucleus (COX-2) and cell membrane (COX-1). The latter differences reflect primary sites of activity: COX-1 within the endoplasmic reticulum and COX-2 on the nuclear envelope (2,81).

VI. Prostanoids Affect Gene Transcription

The capacity of prostanoids to affect gene transcription has been well defined in terms of the regulation of TNF and lymphotoxin production by T cells that can be activated to produce these cytokines by exposure to concavalin A (82). T cells do not generate prostanoids, unlike macrophages, which are responsible for most of the prostanoids produced by cells of the immune system. An inhibitory effect of PGE_2 on T-cell gene transcription when activated by mitogens/antigens was demonstrated by nuclear run-on experiments, indicating suppression of cytokine mRNA and associated inhibition of the biological activity of TNF and lymphotoxin. The possibility of inhibition by PGE_2 of a posttranscriptional as well as transcriptional mechanism was suggested as the degree of suppression of biological activity of the cytokines exceeded the reduction in transcription. There are two important features of these studies relative to eicosanoid-dependent mechanisms. The first relates to specificity of the prostanoid component. Only PGE_2, not other prostanoids nor leukotrienes, inhibited TNF and lymphotoxin production by T cells. The second feature relates to observations regarding PGE_2 and the immune system. A general conclusion cannot be drawn from these findings, namely, that PGE_2 is always immunosuppressive (82). PGE_2 can also act as an immunostimulant with respect to other cytokines and other cell types. This consideration also applies to general concepts regarding proliferative and proinflammatory actions of prostanoids as there are experimental conditions from which opposite conclusions can be drawn. Some of the apparent contradictions in the broad spectrum of actions of a prostanoid have been resolved by identification of receptor subtypes, particularly PGE_2 receptors, which are multiple and coupled to different signaling systems.

VII. Prostaglandin Receptors

The conventional prostaglandin receptor is a cell surface receptor that is specific for each of the several classes of prostanoids. These have been designated FP, IP, TP, EP, and DP for $PGF_{2\alpha}$, PGI_2, TxA_2, PGE_2, and PGD_2, respectively (83). They had been characterized pharmacologically according to specificity as well as the rank order of their response to agonists and inhibition by antagonists. This approach has distinguished several subtypes of EP receptors, which differ in their coupling to G-proteins and linkage to signaling systems. It is possible to separate prostanoid receptors into two major branches according to their effects on adenylate cyclase and phosphatidylinositol hydrolysis (83). The first receptor branch (IP, DP, EP_2, and EP_4), activates adenylate cyclase (producing relaxation of smooth muscle) and the second branch either stimulates PI hydrolysis (FP, EP_{3D}, TP) or inhibits adenylate cyclase (EP_{3A}) (producing contriction of smooth muscle). The TxA_2 receptor was the first to be purified and its cDNA cloned (84). Based on homology screening of mouse cDNA libraries, structural identification of seven types and subtypes of prostanoid receptors has been accomplished. Homology among prostanoid receptors is only 20–30%. They are all members of the G-protein-coupled receptor rhodopsin-type superfamily and fit the general model for G-protein-coupled receptors: seven transmembrane domains, an extracellular amino terminus, and an intracellular carboxyl terminus (85). In the seventh transmembrane domain, an arginine is conserved in all prostanoid receptors and was suggested to be the binding site of the prostanoid carboxyl. Indeed, point mutation of the arginine in the TP receptor produced loss of ligand-binding capability.

Activation of nuclear receptors by AA metabolites has been studied in terms of PPARγ, the peroxisome proliferator-activated receptor, one of the nuclear receptor superfamily including those for retinoid, steroid, and thyroid hormones (86). PGD_2 and its metabolite, PGJ_2, alone among the many eicosanoids tested, were shown to activate the PPARγ receptor. These findings have been extended to PGA_2 and metabolites of PGJ_2, which have been proposed to act on a nuclear prostanoid receptor (PPARγ). The binding of cyclopentenone prostanoids to this nuclear receptor produces specific gene expression related to cell growth and differentiation. Forman et al. (87) have proposed that the PPARγ receptor in adipocytes is related to adipocyte development and glucose homeostasis and, therefore, might be targeted for development of drugs directed toward amelioration of diabetes and other diseases of metabolism. Indeed, a correlation exists between binding affinity of the thiazolidinedione class of antidiabetic drugs to PPARγ and their antidiabetic potency.

PGE (EP) Receptors

PGE (EP) receptors, unlike those of the other prostanoids, have a widespread distribution and multiple subtypes and possess varied and even opposing actions because of coupling via G-proteins to a number of signal transduction pathways that effect Ca^{2+} mobilization and either stimulation or inhibition of adenylate cyclase (88). The recognition of the several EP receptor subtypes within a tissue or even a cell explains seemingly paradoxical actions of PGE_2. The EP_2 and EP_3 receptors are responsible for PGE_2 stimulation and inhibition of cAMP formation, respectively, and, thereby, promotion of sodium excretion and inhibition of the action of AVP in the mTAL and collecting tubules. EP_1 receptors, via a Gs-protein linkage, stimulate PLC and result in Ca^{2+} mobilization and PKC activation, the latter acting as a negative regulator of EP_1 receptor activity by decreasing PGE_2 binding affinity to the EP receptor and dissociation of the G-protein from the receptor (88). EP_2 receptors are found in the glomerulus, and evoke cAMP accumulation associated with inhibition of contractile responses to pressor hormones. There are three isoforms of EP_3 receptors, which result from alternative splicing of a single gene transcript resulting in protein isoforms having different primary structures and different functions. The wide-ranging functional effects of EP_3 receptors anticipate the functional requirements of the several isoforms as the EP_3 receptor is involved in lipolysis, uterine contraction, salt and water excretion, inhibition of gastric secretion, and modulation of neurotransmitter release (83). Localization of the structural expression of renal EP receptors has been achieved through in situ hybridization and indicates the diverse effects of the renal actions of PGE_2 via stimulation of EP receptors (89). Thus, the localization of EP_1 to the papillary collecting tubule, EP_3 to the glomerular mesangium, and EP_3 to the mTAL and CCTs corresponds to the activities of PGE_2 on water reabsorption, glomerular filtration, and ion transport.

There is precedent for distinct TxA_2/PGH_2 receptor subtypes based on the use of receptor antagonists. The controversy associated with possible TxA_2 subtypes, viz., vascular versus platelet, may be partially resolved by the application of molecular biological techniques. Thus, a placental (84) and an endothelial isoform of the human TxA_2/PGH_2 receptor have been cloned (90); both isoforms are found in platelets (91) and, probably, the kidney (92,93).

VIII. Endothelial-Derived Hyperpolarizing Factor: An Eicosanoid?

Of the vasodilator effectors produced by the endothelium, NO occupies a unique position (94). However, a hyperpolarizing factor that has many of the properties of an eicosanoid may be of greater importance than NO in several regional vasculatures. Several recent studies have pointed to a CYP450 AA metabolite as the leading candidate to account for the activity of the endothelial-derived hyperpolarizing (EDHF) (95). To appreciate the magnitude of the contribution of EDHF to vascular dilator mechanisms, two recent studies based on examination of the several components of the rat renal (96) and coronary vasodilator (97) responses to bradykinin have disclosed either a major (renal) or dominant (coronary) contribution of a CYP450 AA metabolite to the vasodilator actions of bradykinin. This AA metabolite stimulated Ca^{2+}-activated K^+ channels and demonstrated many of the properties of an epoxide, particularly those of 5,6-EET (95).

The application of selective phospholipase inhibitors to an analysis of AA-releasing mechanisms and their contribution to formation of EDHF has disclosed important contributions of both PLC and the $cPLA_2$ to the generation of EDHF. Thus inhibition of either PLC or $cPLA_2$ abolished the coronary vasodilator response to bradykinin as did inhibition of CYP450 AA metabolism (98). Further, diacylglycerol was not a source of AA as inhibition of diacylglycerol lipase did not affect the coronary vasodilator action of bradykinin. However, release of AA from diacylglycerol is important to prostaglandin formation, as bradykinin-stimulated synthesis of prostacyclin was attenuated by RHC 80267, inhibitor of diacylglycerol lipase (98). The release of AA for conversion to EDHF in the rat heart, then, involves sequential stimulation of PLC and PLA_2.

Acknowledgments

The research in this review was supported by National Institutes of Health Grant HL34300. We wish to thank Melody Steinberg for editorial assistance.

References

1. Proctor KG, Capdevila JH, Falck JR, Fitzpatrick FA, Mullane KM, McGiff JC. Cardiovascular and renal actions of cytochrome P-450 metabolites of arachidonic acid. Blood Vessels 1989; 26:53–64.
2. Otto JC, Smith WL. Prostaglandin endoperoxide synthases-1 and -2. J Lipid Mediators Cell Signal 1995; 12:139–156.

3. Xie W, Chipman JG, Robertson DL, Erikson RL, Simmons DL. Expression of a mitogen-responsive gene encoding prostaglandin synthase is regulated by mRNA splicing. Proc Natl Acad Sci USA 1991; 88:2692–2696.

4. Brannon TS, North AJ, Wells LB, Shaul PW. Prostacyclin synthesis in ovine pulmonary artery is developmentally regulated by changes in cyclooxygenase-1 gene expression. J Clin Invest 1994; 93:2230–2235.

5. O'Neill GP, Ford-Hutchinson AW. Expression of mRNA for cyclooxygenase-1 and cyclooxygenase-2 in human tissues. FEBS Lett 1993; 330:156–160.

6. Sano H, Hla T, Maier JAM, Crofford LJ, Case JP, Maciag T, Wilder RL. In vivo cyclooxygenase expression in synovial tissue of patients with rheumatoid arthritis and osteoarthritis and rats with adjuvant and streptococcal cell wall arthritis. J Clin Invest 1992; 89:97–108.

7. Ristimäki A, Narko K, Hla T. Down-regulation of cytokine-induced cyclo-oxygenase-2 transcript isoforms by dexamethasone: evidence for post-transcriptional regulation. Biochem J 1996; 318:325–331.

8. Smith WL. Prostanoid biosynthesis and mechanisms of action. Am J Physiol 1992; 263:F181–F191.

9. Laneuville, O, Breuer DK, DeWitt DL, Hla T, Funk CD, Smith WL. Differential inhibition of human prostaglandin endoperoxide H synthases-1 and -2 by non-steroidal anti-inflammatory drugs. J Pharmacol Exp Ther 1994; 271:927–934.

10. Kuhn H, Thiele B-J. Arachidonate 15-lipoxygenase. J Lipid Mediators Cell Signal 1995; 12:157–170.

11. Yoshimoto T, Yamamoto S. Arachidonate 12-lipoxygenase. J Lipid Mediators Cell Signal 1995; 12:195–212.

12. Schwartzman ML, Balazy M, Masferrer J, Abraham NG, McGiff JC, Murphy RC. 12(R)-Hydroxyicosatetraenoic acid: A cytochrome P450-dependent arachidonate metabolite that inhibits Na^+, K^+-ATPase in the cornea. Proc Natl Acad Sci USA 1987; 84:8125–8129.

13. Hamberg M, Samuelsson B. Prostaglandin endoperoxides. Novel transformations of arachidonic acid in human platelets. Proc Natl Acad Sci USA 1974; 71:3400–3404.

14. Stern N, Golub M, Nozawa K, Berger M, Knoll E, Yanagawa N, Natarajan R, Nadler JL, Tuck ML. Selective inhibition of angiotensin II-mediated vasoconstriction by lipoxygenase blockade. Am J Physiol 1989; 257:H434–H443.

15. Nadler JL, Natarajan R, Stern N. Specific action of the lipoxygenase pathway in mediating angiotensin II-induced aldosterone synthesis in isolated adrenal glomerulosa cells. J Clin Invest 1987; 80:1763–1769.

16. Antonipillai I, Nadler JL, Robin EC, Horton R. The inhibitory role of 12- and 15-lipoxygenase products on renin release. Hypertension 1987; 10:61–66.

17. Borgeat P, Hamberg M, Samuelsson B. Transformation of arachidonic acid and homo-gamma-linolenic acid by rabbit polymorphonuclear leukocytes. Monohydroxy acids from novel lipoxygenases. J Biol Chem 1976; 251:7816–7820.

18. Radmark O, Shimizu T, Jornvall H, Samuelsson B. Leukotriene A_4 hydrolase in human leukocytes. Purification and properties. J Biol Chem 1984; 259:12339–12345.

19. Murphy RC, Hammarstrom S, Samuelsson B. Leukotriene C: a slow-reacting substance from murine mastocytoma cells. Proc Natl Acad Sci USA 1979; 76:4275–4279.

20. Yokomizo T, Uozumi N, Takahashi T, Kume K, Izumi T, Shimizu T. Leukotriene A_4 hydrolase and leukotriene B_4 metabolism. J Lipid Mediator Cell Signal 1995; 12:321–332.

21. Haeggstrom JZ, Wetterholm A, Vallee BL, Samuelsson B. Leukotriene A_4 hydrolase: an epoxide hydrolase with peptidase activity. Biochem Biophys Res Commun 1990; 173:431–437.

22. Devchand PR, Keller H, Peters JM, Vazquez M, Gonzalez FJ, Wahli W. The $PPAR\alpha$-leukotriene B_4 pathway to inflammation control. Nature 1996; 384:39–43.

23. Lam BK, Penrose JF, Xu K, Austen KF. Leukotriene C_4 synthase. J Lipid Mediators Cell Signal 1995; 12:333–341.

24. Lewis RA, Austen KF, Drazen JM, Clark DA, Marfat A, Corey EJ. Slow reacting substances of anaphylaxis: identification of leukotriene C-1 and D from human and rat sources. Proc Natl Acad Sci USA 1980; 77:3710–3714.

25. Vickers PJ. 5-Lipoxygenase-activating protein (FLAP). J Lipid Mediators Cell Signal 1995; 12:185–194.

26. Miller DK, Gillard JW, Vickers PJ, Sadowski S, Leveille C, Mancini JA, Charleson P, Dixon RAF, Ford-Hutchinson AW, Fortin R, Gauthier JY, Rodkey J, Rosen R, Rouzer C, Sigal IS, Strader CD, Evans JF. Identification and isolation of a membrane protein necessary for leukotriene synthesis. Nature 1990; 343:278–281.

27. Feinmark SJ, Cannon PJ. Endothelial cell leukotriene C_4 synthesis result from transfer of leukotriene A_4 synthesized by polymorphonuclear leukocytes. J Biol Chem 1986; 261:16466–16472.

28. Lam BK, Xu K, Atkins MB, Austen KF. Leukotriene C_4 uses a probenecid-sensitive export carrier that does not recognize leukotriene B_4. Proc Natl Acad Sci USA 1992; 89:11598–11602.

29. Kuehl FA, Jr. Prostaglandins, cyclic nucleotides and cell function. Prostaglandins 1974; 5:325–340.

30. Carroll MA, Balazy M, Huang D-D, Rybalova S, Falck JR, McGiff JC. Cytochrome P450–derived renal HETEs: Storage and release. Kidney Int 1977; 51:1696–1702.

31. Quilley J, McGiff JC. Eicosanoids. In: Swales JD, ed. Textbook of Hypertension. London: Blackwell Scientific Publications, 1994:314–327.

32. Anggärd E, Bohman SO, Griffin JE III, Larsson C, Maunsbach AB. Subcellular localization of the prostaglandin system in the rabbit renal papilla. Acta Physiol Scand 1972; 84:231–246.

33. Gronich JH, Bonventre JV, Nemenoff RA. Purification of a high-molecular-mass form of phospholipase A_2 from rat kidney activated at physiological calcium concentrations. Biochem J 1990; 271:37–43.

34. Nishizuka Y. Intracellular signaling by hydrolysis of phospholipids and activation of protein kinase C. Science 1992; 258:607–614.

35. Jayadev S, Linardic M, Hannun YA. Identification of arachidonic acid as a mediator of sphingomyelin hydrolysis in response to tumor necrosis factor α. J Biol Chem 1994; 269:5757–5763.

36. Irvine RF. How is the level of free arachidonic acid controlled in mammalian cells? Biochem J 1982; 204:3–16.

37. Clark JD, Shievella AR, Nalefski EA, Lin L-L. Cytosolic phospholipase A_2. J Lipid Mediators Cell Signal 1995; 12:83–117.

38. Gronich JH, Bonventre JV, Nemenoff RA. Identification and characterization of a hormonally regulated form of phospholipase A_2 in rat renal mesangial cells. J Biol Chem 1988; 263:16645–16551.
39. Clark JD, Lin L-L, Kriz RW, Ramesha CS, Sultzman LA, Lin AY, Milona N, Knopf JL. A novel arachidonic acid-selective cytosolic PLA_2 contains a Ca^{2+}-dependent translocation domain with homology to PKC and GAP. Cell 1991; 64:1043–1051.
40. Regier MK, DeWitt DL, Schindler MS, Smith WL. Subcellular localization of prostaglandin endoperoxide synthase-2 in murine 3T3 cells. Arch Biochem Biophys 1993; 301:439–444.
41. Lin L-L, Wartmann M, Lin AY, Knopf JL, Seth A, Davis RJ. $cPLA_2$ is phosphorylated and activated by MAP kinase. Cell 1993; 72:269–278.
42. Tay A, Maxwell P, Li Z, Goldberg H, Skorecki K. Isolation of promoter for cytosolic phospholipase A_2 ($cPLA_2$). Biochim Biophys Acta 1994; 1217:345–347.
43. McGiff JC. Cytochrome P-450 metabolism of arachidonic acid. Annu Rev Pharmacol Toxicol 1991; 31:339–369.
44. Karara A, Dishman E, Jacobson H, Falck JR, Capdevila JH. Arachidonic acid epoxygenase. Stereochemical analysis of the endogenous epoxyeicosatriencoic acids of human kidney cortex. FEBS Lett 1990; 268:227–230.
45. Falck JR, Schueler VJ, Jacobson HR, Siddhanta AK, Pramanik B, Capdevila J. Arachidonate epoxygenase: identification of epoxyeicosatrienoic acids in rabbit kidney. J Lipid Res 1987; 28:840–846.
46. Takahashi K, Capdevila J, Karara A, Falck JR, Jacobson HR, Badr KF. Cytochrome P-450 arachidonate metabolites in rat kidney: characterization and hemodynamic responses. Am J Physiol 1990; 258:F781–F789.
47. Zhu Y, Schieber EB, McGiff JC, Balazy M. Identification of arachidonate P-450 metabolites in human platelet phospholipids. Hypertension 1995; 25:854–859.
48. Karara A, Dishman E, Blair I, Falck JR, Capdevila JH. Endogenous epoxyeicosatrienoic acids. Cytochrome P-450 controlled stereoselectivity of the hepatic arachidonic acid epoxygenase. J Biol Chem 1989; 264:19822–19827.
49. Capdevila JH, Kishore V, Dishman E, Blair IA. A novel pool of rat liver inositol and ethanolamine phospholipids contains epoxyeicosatrienoic acids (EETs). Biochem Biophys Res Commun 1987; 146:638–644.
50. Gordon JA, Spector AA. Effects of 12-HETE on renal tubular epithelial cells. Am J Physiol 1987; 253:C277–C285.
51. Zhu Y, McGiff JC, Balazy M. Identification of 20-Hydroxyeicosatetraenoic acid in rat kidney phospholipids. Presented at 43rd ASMS Conference on Mass Spectrometry and Allied Topics, Atlanta, GA, May 1995.
52. Carroll MA, Balazy M, Margiotta P, Falck JR, McGiff JC. Renal vasodilator activity of 5,6-epoxyeicosatrienoic acid depends upon conversion by cyclooxygenase and release of prostaglandins. J Biol Chem 1993; 268:12260–12266.
53. Schwartzman ML, Falck JR, Yadagiri P, Escalante B. Metabolism of 20-hydroxyeicosatetraenoic acid by cyclooxygenase: formation and identification of novel endothelium-dependent vasoconstrictor metabolites. J Biol Chem 1989; 264:11658–11662.
54. Escalante B, Erlij D, Falck JR, McGiff JC. Effect of cytochrome P450 arachidonate metabolites on ion transport in rabbit kidney loop of Henle. Science 1991; 251:799–802.

55. Carroll MA, Pilar Garcia M, Falck JR, McGiff JC. Cyclooxygenase dependency of the renovascular actions of cytochrome P450-derived arachidonate metabolites. J Pharmacol Exp Ther 1992; 260:104–109.
56. Lin L, Balazy M, Pagano PJ, Nasjletti A. Expression of prostaglandin H_2-mediated mechanism of vascular contraction in hypertensive rats. Circ Res 1994; 74:197–205.
57. Pucci ML, Tong X, Miller KB, Guan H, Nasjletti A. Calcium- and protein kinase C–dependent basal tone in the aorta of hypertensive rats. Hypertension 1995; 25: 752–757.
58. McGiff JC, Terragno NA, Strand JC, Lee JB, Lonigro AJ, Ng KKF. Selective passage of prostaglandins across the lung. Nature 1969; 223:742–745.
59. Wong PY-K, McGiff JC, Sun FF, Malik KU. Pulmonary metabolism of prostacyclin (PGI_2) in the rabbit. Biochem Biophys Res Commun 1978; 83:731–738.
60. Kanai N, Lu R, Striano JA, Bao Y, Wolkoff AW, Schuster VL. Identification and characterization of a prostaglandin transporter. Science 1995; 268:866–869.
61. Bito LZ, Salvador EV. Effects of anti-inflammatory agents and some other drugs on prostaglandin biotransport. J Pharmacol Exp Ther 1976; 198:481–488.
62. Bito LZ, Davson H, Salvador EV. Inhibition of in vitro concentrative prostaglandin accumulation by prostaglandins, prostaglandin analogues and by some inhibitors of organic anion transport. J Physiol (Lon) 1976; 256:257–271.
63. Irish JM. Secretion of prostaglandin E2 by rabbit proximal tubules. Am J Physiol 1979; 237:F268–F273.
64. Douglas JG, Romero M, Hopfer U. Signaling mechanisms coupled to the angiotensin receptor of proximal tubular epithelium. Kidney Int 1990; 38:S-43–S-47.
65. Dunn MJ, Scharschmidt LA. Prostaglandins modulate the glomerular actions of angiotensin II. Kidney Int 1987; 31:S-95–S-101.
66. Madhun ZT, Goldthwait DA, McKay D, Hopfer U, Douglas JG. An epoxygenase metabolite of arachidonic acid mediates angiotensin II-induced rises in cytosolic calcium in rabbit proximal tubule epithelial cells. J Clin Invest 1991; 88:456–461.
67. Braam B, Mitchell KD, Fox J, Navar LG. Proximal tubular secretion of angiotensin II in rats. Am J Physiol 1993; 264:F891–F898.
68. Andreatta-van Leyen S, Romero MF, Khosla MC, Douglas JG. Modulation of phospholipase A_2 activity and sodium transport by angiotensin-(1-7). Kidney Int 1993; 44:932–936.
69. Liu FY, Cogan MG. Angiotensin II stimulates early proximal bicarbonate absorption in the rat by decreasing cyclic adenosine monophosphate. J Clin Invest 1989; 84:83–92.
70. Schwartzman M, Ferreri NR, Carroll MA, Songu-Mize-E, McGiff JC. Renal cytochrome P450-related arachidonate metabolite inhibits (Na^+-K^+)ATPase. Nature 1985; 314:620–622.
71. Escalante B, Erlij D, Falck JR, McGiff JC. Cytochrome P-450 arachidonate metabolites affect ion fluxes in rabbit medullary thick ascending limb. Am J Physiol 1994; 266:C1775–C1782.
72. Pedrosa Ribeiro CM, Dubay GR, Falck JR, Mandel LJ. Parathyroid hormone inhibits Na^+-K^+-ATPase through a cytochrome P-450 pathway. Am J Physiol 1994; 266:F497–F505.

73. Escalante BA, Ferreri NR, Dunn CE, McGiff JC. Cytokines affect ion transport in primary cultured thick ascending limb of Henle's loop cells. Am J Physiol 1994; 266:C1568–C1576.
74. Ferreri NR, Escalante BA, Zhao Y, An S-J, McGiff JC. Angiotensin II induces TNF production by the thick ascending limb: functional implications. Am J Physiol 1997. In press.
75. Salvemini D, Misko TP, Masferrer JL, Seibert K, Currie MG, Needleman P. Nitric oxide activates cyclooxygenase enzymes. Proc Natl Acad Sci USA 1993; 90:7240–7244.
76. Khatsenko OG, Gross SS, Rifkind AB, Vane JR. Nitric oxide is a mediator of the decrease in cytochrome P450-dependent metabolism caused by immunostimulants. Proc Natl Acad Sci USA 1993; 90:11147–11151.
77. Zou A-P, Imig JD, Kaldunski M, Ortiz de Montellano PR, Sui Z, Roman RJ. Inhibition of renal vascular 20-HETE production impairs autoregulation of renal blood flow. Am J Physiol 1994; 266:F275–F282.
78. Omata K, Abraham NG, Laniado Schwartzman M. Renal cytochrome P-450-arachidonic acid metabolism: localization and hormonal regulation in SHR. Am J Physiol 1992; 262:F591–F599.
79. Carroll MA, Sala A, Dunn CE, McGiff JC, Murphy RC. Structural identification of cytochrome P450-dependent arachidonate metabolites formed by rabbit medullary thick ascending limb cells. J Biol Chem 1991; 266:12306–12312.
80. Lokuta AJ, Cooper C, Gaa ST, Wang HE, Rogers TB. Angiotensin II stimulates the release of phospholipid-derived second messengers through multiple receptor subtypes in heart cells. J Biol Chem 1994; 269:4832–4838.
81. Morita I, Schindler M, Regier MK, Otto JC, Hori T, DeWitt DL, Smith WL. Different intracellular locations for prostaglandin endoperoxide H synthase-1 and -2. J Biol Chem 1995; 270:10902–10908.
82. Ferreri NR, Starr T, Askenase PW, Ruddle NH. Molecular regulation of tumor necrosis factor-α and lymphotoxin production in T cells. J Biol Chem 1992; 267:9443–9449.
83. Coleman RA, Smith WL, Narumiya S. International union of pharmacology classification of prostanoid receptors: properties, distribution, and structure of the receptors and their subtypes. Pharmacol Rev 1994; 46:205–229.
84. Hirata M, Hayashi Y, Ushikubi F, Yokota Y, Kageyama R, Nakanishi S, Narumiya S. Cloning and expression of cDNA for a human thromboxane A_2 receptor. Nature (Lond) 1991; 389:617–620.
85. Narumiya S. Structures, properties and distributions of prostanoid receptors. Adv Prosta Thromb Leuko Res 1995; 23:17–22.
86. Funk DC, Furci L, Moran N, FitzGerald GA. A point mutation in the seventh hydrophobic domain of the human thromboxane A_2 receptor allows discrimination between agonist and antagonist binding sites. Mol Pharmacol 1993; 44:934–939.
87. Forman BM, Tontonoz P, Chen J, Brun RP, Spiegelman BM, Evans RM. 15-deoxy-$\Delta^{12,14-}$ prostaglandin J_2 is a ligand for the adipocyte determination factor PPARγ. Cell 1995; 83:803–812.
88. Negishi M, Sugimoto Y, Ichikawa A. Prostaglandin E receptors. J Lipid Mediators Cell Signal 1995; 12:379–391.

89. Ushikubi F, Hirata M, Narumiya S. Molecular biology of prostanoid receptors; an overview. J Lipid Mediators Cell Signal 1995; 12:343–359.
90. Raychowdhury MK, Yukawa M, Collins LJ, McGrail SH, Kent KC, Ware JA. Alternative splicing produces a divergent cytoplasmic tail in the human endothelial thromboxane A_2 receptor. J Biol Chem 1994; 268:19256–19261.
91. Hirata T, Ushikubi F, Kakizuka A, Okuma M, Narumiya S. Two thromboxane A_2 receptor isoforms in human platelets. J Clin Invest 1996; 97:949–956.
92. Bresnahan BA, Le Breton GC, Lianos EA. Localization of authentic thromboxane A_2/prostaglandin H_2 receptor in the rat kidney. Kidney Int 1996; 49:1207–1213.
93. Abe T, Takeuchi K, Takahashi N, Tsutsumi E, Taniyama Y, Abe K. Rat kidney thromboxane receptor: molecular cloning, signal transduction and intrarenal expression localization. J Clin Invest 1995; 96:657–664.
94. Furchgott RF, Zawadzki JV. The obligatory role of endothelial cells in the relaxation of arterial smooth muscle by acetylcholine. Nature 1980; 288:373–376.
95. Quilley J, Fulton D, McGiff JC. Hyperpolarizing factors. Biochem Pharmacol 1997 (in press).
96. Fulton D, McGiff JC, Quilley J. Contribution of NO and cytochrome P450 to the vasodilator effect of bradykinin in the rat kidney. Br J Pharmacol 1992; 107:722–725.
97. Fulton D, Mahboubi K, McGiff JC, Quilley J. Cytochrome P450-dependent effects of bradykinin in the rat heart. Br J Pharmacol 1995; 114:99–102.
98. Fulton D, McGiff JC, Quilley J. Role of phospholipase C and phospholipase A_2 in the nitric oxide–independent vasodilator effect of bradykinin in the rat perfused heart. J Pharmacol Exp Ther 1996; 278:518–526.

3

Cytochromes P450 and Arachidonic Acid Metabolism

MICHAEL BALAZY and JOHN C. MCGIFF

New York Medical College
Valhalla, New York

I. Introduction

Hemoproteins play a fundamental role in oxidative transformations of arachidonic acid. Cyclooxygenases 1 and 2 (COX-1 and COX-2), which metabolize arachidonic acid to prostaglandin H_2 (PGH$_2$), and peroxidases, which convert various hydroperoxyeicosatetraenoic acids (HPETEs) to hydroxyeicosatetraenoic acids (HETEs), contain an iron protoporphyrin IX ring and a histidine nitrogen as a proximal iron ligand (1,2). This feature is shared by a large family of molecules functioning in oxygen transport such as hemoglobins, myoglobins, or cytochromes involved in the mitochondrial respiratory chain. The other, relatively small number of the hemoprotein family has been characterized as having *cysteine* sulfur as a proximal iron ligand. Unlike heme-histidine proteins, the heme-cysteinate proteins can bind carbon monoxide irreversibly when heme iron is in the reduced state. The hemoprotein-carbon monoxide complex produces a characteristic peak at 450 nm (called a red-shifted Soret band), which results from the absorbance of light by the electron-rich cysteinate ligand in *trans* position to carbon monoxide. The protein of this characteristic peak, first described by Omura and Sato in 1964 (3), is named

P450 because its carbon monoxide complexes absorb light at 450 nm. This distinctive spectral feature of heme-thiolate proteins has been found only in three classes of enzymes: the cytochromes P450 (CYP450), nitric oxide synthases, and chloroperoxidase (4).

A variety of unique CYP450 enzymes has been identified to play a crucial role at critical points of the arachidonic acid cascade. These heme-thiolate proteins, having multiple functions, are found in abundance in the endoplasmatic reticulum of the liver, kidney, and to a lesser extent, the lung, intestine, and vascular system. The CYP450 enzyme system has been found in almost all mammalian tissues. CYP450 can act purely as a monooxygenase by binding and activating molecular oxygen and inserting single oxygen into an eicosanoid substrate. The CYP450 monooxygenases play an important role in metabolism of prostaglandins and leukotrienes generating, typically, ω- and ω-1-hydroxylated analogs. Arachidonic acid is also a substrate for various monooxygenases of liver and kidney that biosynthesize a variety of monohydroxylated compounds like 20- and 19-HETE as well as 16-, 17-, and 18-HETEs (Fig. 1). CYP450 monooxygenases are also known to insert oxygen into arachidonate double bonds generating four epoxyeicosatrienoic acids (EETs) (Fig. 2). A single purified CYP450 isozyme can perform both arachidonate hydroxylation and epoxidation of double bonds. The common feature of all CYP450 monooxygenases is the absolute requirement for CYP450 reductase and NAD(P)H.

In contrast to monooxygenases, another unique group of heme-thiolate proteins functions as peroxide isomerases and does not require reductase and NADPH. The specialized hemoproteins, prostacyclin synthase and thromboxane synthase, are members of this group and react with PGH_2 to rearrange is peroxy bridge via a complex mechanism forming prostacyclin (PGI_2) and thromboxane A_2 (TxA_2).

CYP450 enzymes have been the subject of numerous reviews and excellent volumes have been published recently that provide a comprehensive picture of their structure and mechanism (2,5). Various aspects of pharmacology, biochemistry, chemistry, and molecular biology of CYP450-mediated metabolism of arachidonic acid and eicosanoids have been extensively reviewed (6–11).

II. Characterization of CYP450

A. Nomenclature

Early work on CYP450-mediated oxidation of eicosanoids was complicated by the inconsistent description of various CYP450 isoforms (isozymes). The CYP450-metabolizing prostaglandin was typically labeled after the tissue

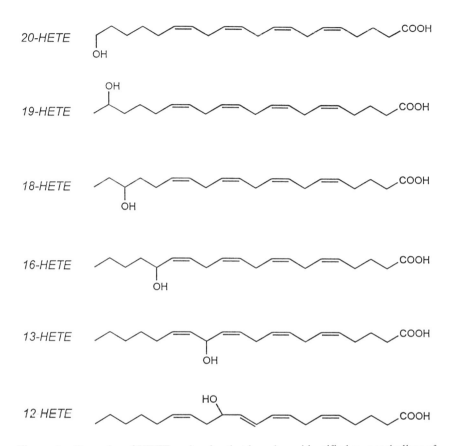

Figure 1 Examples of HETE molecules that have been identified as metabolites of arachidonic acid by cytochrome P450 hydroxylases in mammalian tissues.

origin of the enzyme and the nature of the substrate. For example, $CYP450_{ka}$ was described as a kidney enzyme with specificity for ω-hydrolysis of PGA_1 (12), whereas an enzyme purified from the lung of pregnant rabbits, $CYP450_{PG\omega}$, was described as an ω-hydroxylase capable of oxidizing several prostaglandins (13). Often, the cytochromes were labeled or named after the specific inducing agents such as $CYP450_{PB-1}$, which has been described as a hepatic enzyme induced by phenobarbitol. It was difficult to understand, when using this nomenclature, whether these enzymes were similar or differed substantially. Recently, a consistent nomenclature for CYP450 enzymes has been adopted that is based on the gene from which they are transcribed (14). For example, the fatty acid oxygenase enzyme is termed CYP4A1, which defines the enzyme

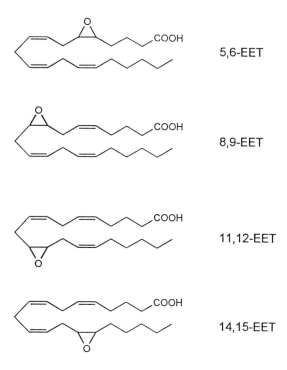

5,6-EET

8,9-EET

11,12-EET

14,15-EET

Figure 2 Metabolism of arachidonic acid by cytochrome P450 epoxygenases leads to four epoxides (EETs).

as a CYP from family 4, subfamily A, member 1. Nebert et al. have published a new nomenclature and compared it with the older (14).

B. The Catalytic Cycle

The CYP450 has unusual catalytic properties. Its complex catalytic activity consists of several distinct steps, collectively known as the CYP450 catalytic cycle (15). The initial step requires binding of the eicosanoid substrate to the enzyme. In the microsomal system, most of the reactions begin with the transfer of electrons from NAD(P)H to NADPH-CYP450 reductase and then to CYP450, resulting in the reduction of the CYP450 from the ferric to the ferrous (Fe^{2+}) state. To initiate the oxidative reaction, oxygen is bound to the ferrous CYP450 and forms an $[Fe^{2+}(O_2)]$ intermediate with the substrate still present. Transfer of the second electron then occurs with the probable involvement of cytochrome b_5 as an additional electron donor in mammalian microsomal systems. The next step involves splitting of the oxygen-oxygen bond with the uptake of two protons and the generation of an activated oxygen, perhaps an iron-oxene species, and release of water. In 1957, using oxygen 18 and water labeled with oxygen 18, Mason established that the monooxygenases transfer one atom of molecular oxygen into the substrate and reduce the other to a molecule of water (16). Oxygen insertion into the substrate is believed to involve hydrogen abstraction from the substrate and recombination of the resulting transient hydroxyl and carbon radicals to give the product. Dissociation of the oxidized product then restores the CYP450 to the starting ferric state. The fatty acid ω-hydroxylase system of mammalian liver is composed of three major components—the hemoprotein P450, NADPH-dependent CYP450 reductase, and a heat-stable factor identified as phosphatidylcholine. This phospholipid is believed to facilitate the flow of electrons from NAD(P)H to the CYP450 reductase and then to CYP450.

C. Inducibility

A characteristic feature of the CYP450 enzymes is their facile inducibility. Continuous exposure, but often a single dose of drugs (phenobarbital, clofibrate, ethanol), and a large number of chemicals (pollutants, carcinogens, dietary additives, cosmetics), have been shown to readily induce a specific CYP450 isozyme or a whole family of CYP450 isozymes in mammals (17). Pregnancy, neonatal hyperoxia, and diabetes are known to induce CYP450 in the liver, kidney, and lung (5). For example, in lung microsomes from pregnant rabbits a major CYP450 can be isolated that is negligible in males or nonpregnant females (18). This P450 ($P450_{PG\omega}$), which oxidizes prostaglandins at the ω carbon, is induced 50- to 100-fold during pregnancy and represents 15–30% of the total lung microsomal CYP450 in pregnant rabbits (18). The lungs and nasal tissues contain appreciable amounts of CYP450; these sites may be important in oxidation that occurs when compounds enter the pulmonary system. Two CYP isozymes were recently identified through cDNA cloning of human pulmonary CYP450s. Little is known about their catalytic activities except that one of them, CYP 2F1, is involved in activation of the pneumotoxin 3-methylindole (19). The effect of asthma on lung CYP450 isozymes remains to be investigated. CYP450s metabolically activate a variety of compounds such as polycyclic aromatic hydrocarbons to highly toxic, mutagenic, and carcinogenic products such as various epoxides and quinones. These toxic metabolites can be formed in the blood vessel wall and can initiate atherosclerosis by injuring the endothelial and smooth muscle cells (20).

D. Inhibitors

The catalytic cycle of CYP450 contains three steps that are particularly vulnerable to inhibition: (1) binding of the substrate, (2) binding of molecular oxygen subsequent to the first electron transfer, and (3) the catalytic step in which the substrate is actually oxidized. Inhibitors of CYP450 reductase also have been described (21). Many chemicals, drugs, and natural compounds have been tested as CYP450 inhibitors and have been reviewed in detail by Ortiz de Montellano and Correia (22). The more recent development of mechanism-based irreversible inhibitors (suicide substrates) for CYP450 enzymes has greatly enhanced the potential specificity and utility of CYP450 inhibitors. The ω-hydroxylation of arachidonic acid mediated by CYP4A isozymes can be inhibited by 17-octadecynoic acid (17-ODYA) (23). The ω-hydroxylations of leukotriene B_4 (LTB$_4$), prostaglandins and fatty acids are effectively inhibited by various acetylenic analogs of long- and short-chain unsaturated fatty acids (22). These compounds have frequently been used as pharmacological tools to unravel the contribution of CYP450 enzymes to vascular function (24,25). Novel compounds are being designed and synthesized with the aim of achieving selective inhibition of either one of the two most common reactions mediated by CYP450: ω-hydroxylation and olefinic epoxidation (J. R. Falck, personal communication). One promising compound, dibromododecenoic acid (DBDD), inhibits arachidonate hydroxylase with high specificity (26).

E. Interactions with Nitric Oxide

The chemical and spectral properties of nitric oxide–heme complexes of CYP450 enzymes have been known since the early 1960s but only recently have these interactions been studied in living systems. Nitric oxide (NO), a molecule of great physiological and pathophysiological significance, inhibits CYP450 monooxygenases by initial reversible binding of the nitrogen to the iron with subsequent time-dependent irreversible inactivation of the enzymes by an undefined mechanism (27). Bacterial lipopolysaccharide (LPS) and a diverse array of other immunostimulants and cytokines suppress the metabolism of endogenous and exogenous substances by reducing activity of the hepatic CYP450 mixed-function oxidase system (28). Although this effect of immunostimulants was first described almost 40 years ago, the mechanism is obscure. Immunostimulants are also known to cause NO overproduction by cells via induction of NO synthase. In vitro treatment of hepatic microsomes with NO, produced either by chemical decomposition of 3-morpholinosydnonimine or by NO synthase, substantially suppressed CYP450-dependent oxygenation reactions (29). This effect of NO was seen with hepatic microsomes prepared from two species (rat and chicken) and after exposure to chemicals that induce distinct molecular isoforms of CYP450 (β-naphthoflavone, 3-methylcholanthrene, and phenobarbital). Spectral studies indicated that NO reacts in vitro with both Fe^{2+}- and Fe^{3+}-hemes in microsomal CYP450. In vivo, LPS diminished the phenobarbital-induced dealkylation of 7-pentoxyresorufin by rat liver microsomes and reduced the apparent CYP450 content as measured by carbon monoxide binding. These LPS effects were associated with induction of NO synthesis; LPS-induced NO synthesis showed a strong positive correlation with the severity of CYP450 inhibition. The decrease in both hepatic microsomal CYP450 activity and carbon monoxide binding caused by LPS was largely prevented by the selective NO synthase inhibitor N-ω-nitro-L-arginine methyl ester. These findings implicate NO overproduction as a major factor mediating the suppression of hepatic metabolism by immunostimulants such as LPS (29). CYP2E1, which efficiently metabolizes arachidonic acid into 18-HETE and 19-HETE (30), rapidly loses catalytic activity by interacting with NO, which is attributed to formation of a relatively stable NO-heme complex (31). These observations indicate that the CYP450-mediated hepatic and renal metabolism of eicosanoids and arachidonic acid may be particularly sensitive to LPS-induced NO synthesis. Very little is known about these interactions in vivo, and the study of the effect of NO on CYP450-mediated prostaglandin and arachidonic acid metabolism is further complicated by the observation that NO activates cyclooxygenase, possibly via formation of peroxynitrite (32).

III. Metabolism of Eicosanoids by CYP450

Microsomal fractions from various tissues are a significant source of CYP450 and show specificity of the redox status of the heme iron and a requirement for NADPH for complex transformation of eicosanoids. The reactions depend critically on the substrate eicosanoid structure and mediate NADPH-dependent (monooxygenases) or NADPH-independent mechanisms (isomerases).

A. Metabolism of PGH$_2$ by CYP450 Isomerases—Prostacyclin and Thromboxane Synthases

The two enzymes described in this section belong to the CYP450 family because they share a significant degree of homology of the amino acid sequence with those of classical CYP450s. However, they do not catalyze monooxygenation reactions and do not even catalyze oxidation reactions. Rather, the CYP450 enzymatic machinery is used for highly complex and specialized isomerization of the peroxide bridge of PGH$_2$ into PGI$_2$ or TxA$_2$. Ullrich and Graf observed in the early 1980s that PGI and TxA synthases are hemoproteins with CYP450 characteristics (33). PGI synthase was originally purified from microsomes of porcine aorta as a homogenous 49.2-kDa ferric protein showing visible and electron-paramagnetic resonance spectra similar to those reported for CYP450 from the liver (34). It was noted that chemical reduction of PGI synthase protein with dithionite ($Na_2S_2O_4$) in the presence of carbon monoxide very slowly shifted the Soret band to 450 nm, a hallmark of the heme-thiolate protein. In contrast to microsomal CYP450 monooxygenases, full activity of PGI synthase does not require an external source of electrons (NADPH and CYP450 reductase) for a cage radical mechanism proposed for both PGI and TxA synthases (35). PGH_2 initially binds to the PGI synthase heme iron with its C-9 oxygen followed by free radical rearrangement to the prostacyclin structure. More recently, the cDNAs for bovine and human endothelial PGI synthases have been cloned (36,37). The amino acid sequence of PGI synthase showed the presence of the heme and conserved cysteine, typical of all CYP450s, and a 33.8% identity to human cholesterol 7α-hydroxylase, a member of the CYP450 7-gene family, and only 15.4% to human TxA synthase (37). PGI synthase is widely expressed in human tissues and is particularly abundant in lung, heart, ovary, skeletal muscle, and prostate (38). PGI synthase has a half-life ≤ 5 min and "suicide" inactivation accompanies catalysis by isolated PGI synthase and endothelial cells (39). PGI synthase is inhibited by lipid peroxides (15-HPETE) (40) but is not sensitive to carbon monoxide, hydrogen peroxide, superoxide, hydroxyl radical, NO, and nitrogen dioxide (41). Interestingly, PGI_2 synthesis is rapidly and irreversibly blocked by peroxynitrite (IC_{50} of $50\,\mu M$), a product of the spontaneous reaction of NO with superoxide (41). Hypochlorite, a cytotoxic substance released by activated neutrophils, also inhibits PGI synthase with IC_{50} of $7\,\mu M$ (41). The interplay among lipid peroxides, peroxynitrite, hypochlorite, and PGI_2 synthesis is complex and not fully understood despite intensive investigation.

Spectral studies of human platelet microsomes showed a CYP450-type hemoprotein identified as TxA synthase (42). PGH_2 binds to the active site of TxA synthase with its C-11 oxygen at the heme iron; oxygen or oxene transfer may then occur (35). TxA synthase generates equal amounts of TxA_2, 8-*trans*-12-hydroxyheptadecatrienoic acid (8-*trans*-HHT), and malondialdehyde with a molecular activity of about 50 turnovers per second. The cDNA coding for the human platelet and lung TxA synthases was cloned, sequenced, and shown to code for cysteine-heme coordinated hemoproteins with $\leq 35\%$ overall amino acid identity to members of the CYP450 3-gene family (43). Several compounds containing an imidazole or pyridine group strongly bind to TxA synthase iron Fe^{3+} (44). A protein structure with 533 amino acids (60.4 kDa) was deduced from the sequence of the platelet cDNA. It is interesting to note that 8-*iso*-PGH_2—an autoxidation product of arachidonic acid and a major precursor of isoprostaglandins—is quantitatively transformed by TxA synthase into 8-*cis*-HHT and malondialdehyde without TxA_2 formation. PGI synthase also converts 8-*iso*-PGH_2 into 8-*cis*-HHT and malondialdehyde; only trace amounts (1.5%) of the corresponding prostacyclin derivative are formed (35).

B. Metabolism of HPETEs by CYP450

HPETEs are unstable lipoxygenase metabolites that are further converted into corresponding HETEs by abundant hydroperoxidases. Another route of metabolism was proposed to be mediated by a CYP450 isozyme. Liver microsomes from phenobarbital-treated rats convert 15S-HPETE into epoxyalcohols and their trihydroxy hydrolysis products (45,46). The involvement of CYP450 has been suggested, likely because purified CYP 2B1 gives products similar to those generated by phenobarbital-induced microsomes. The transformation of 15HPETE by CYP 2B1 is stereoselective leading to different sets of metabolites from 15S and 15R HPETE molecules (46). These products are most likely to be generated in tissues that express both lipoxygenase and CYP450 such as kidney, lung, skin, cornea, or endothelium. There is no evidence as yet for the natural occurrence of CYP450-dependent stereoselective transformations of HPETEs in mammalian tissues.

C. Metabolism of Prostaglandins and Lipoxygenase Products by CYP450 via NADPH-Dependent Mechanism

Specific CYP450s of the endoplasmic reticulum are important in mediating the ω-oxidation of prostaglandins. Recent studies have suggested that specific isozymes from the CYP 4A family, namely CYP 4A1 and 4A3, play an important role in this process (47,48). The metabolism of prostaglandins is complex. A major route for prostaglandins is via 15-hydroxy-prostaglandin dehydrogenase and Δ^{13}-reductase followed by β-oxidation from the carboxyl terminus. Various CYP450 often further metabolize the 13,14-dehydro-15-keto form of prostaglandins into ω-hydroxy products (11). This hydroxylation occurs in the liver, the lungs, and the renal cortex of several species (11). In pregnancy, CYP450 enzymes are induced leading to elevation of ω-hydroxy prostaglandins in the lung (18). Further oxidation of the ω-hydroxyl leads to an ω-carboxy metabolite of prostaglandin that can be measured in urine (Fig. 3). Seminal vesicles of several species metabolize PGE_2 via uncharacterized CYP450 isozymes into 18-, 19-, and 20-hydroxy-PGE_2 (49,50). 19- and 20-hydroxy PGE_2 are biologically active yet their physiological function remains unknown. In the isolated perfused rabbit kidney, PGI_2 is metabolized into several products including 5-hydroxy-6-keto-$PGF_{1\alpha}$ which suggested epoxidation of PGI_2 via the renal epoxygenase pathway (51).

Leukotrienes originate from enzymatic oxidation of arachidonic acid by 5-lipoxygenase and contain 5-hydroxyl with conjugated triene as a common structural feature. The metabolism of the cysteinyl leukotriene C_4 (LTC_4), initially involves peptidases that sequentially remove amino acids from the glutathionyl portion of the LTC_4 to form the cysteine adduct, LTE_4 (Fig. 4). The liver is a major organ for extraction of leukotrienes from the blood. Subsequent

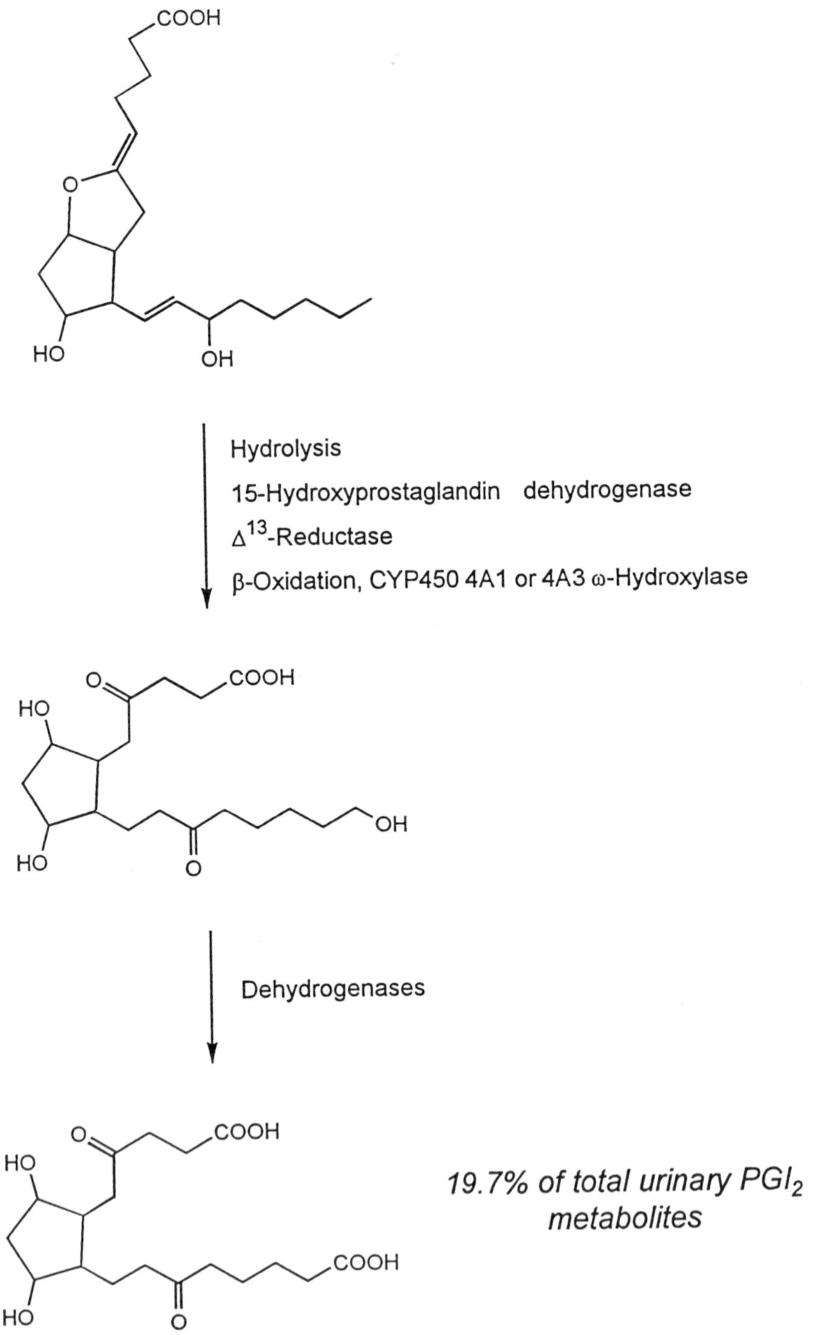

Figure 3 Cytochrome P450 4A1 or 4A3 metabolizes 6,15-diketo-13,14-dihydro-PGF$_{1\alpha}$ at the ω carbon in metabolism of prostacyclin forming a major urinary metabolite, 2,3-dinor-6,15-diketo-13,14-dihydro-20-carboxy-PGF$_{1\alpha}$ (114).

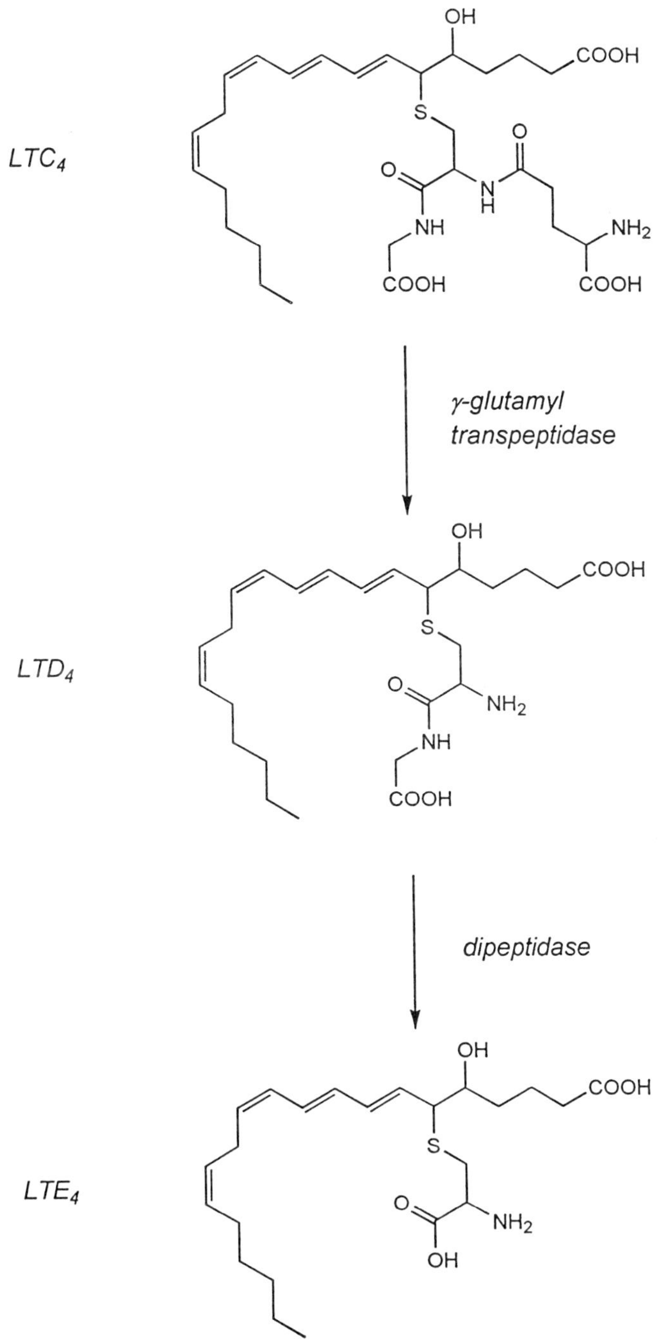

Figure 4 Metabolism of LTC$_4$ by peptidases forms LTD$_4$ and LTE$_4$.

ω-oxidation of LTE_4 is carried by a specific, as yet unidentified, CYP 450 isozyme in the endoplasmic reticulum of the liver (52). This step is characteristic and critical to metabolism of the 20-carbon arachidonyl moiety of leukotrienes in human subjects. Following ω-hydroxylation, the 20-carboxy-LTE_4 undergoes β-oxidation from the methyl terminus, which leads to the major urinary metabolites: 14-carboxy-LTE_3 and 16-carboxy-Δ^{13}-LTE_4 (52) (Fig. 5). Leukotrienes are important mediators in asthma and aspirin-induced asthma (53,54). Measurement of urinary LTE_4 has been widely used to assess whole-body cysteinyl leukotriene production in vivo in human subjects (55). However, measurement of the major urinary metabolites of LTE_4 may be more appropriate if synthesis of LTC_4 is periodic rather than continuous (56). Unfortunately, very little is known about the kinetics of LTC_4 formation in humans and methods have yet to be developed to measure the major urinary LTE_4 metabolites.

The metabolism of LTB_4 occurs within neutrophils by the unique CYP450 isoforms that have been designated $CYP450_{LTB\omega}$ (57,58). These enzymes metabolize LTB_4 to 20-hydroxy-LTB_4 via an NADPH-dependent mechanism. The metabolism of 20-hydroxy-LTB_4 to 20-carboxy-LTB_4 also occurs within neutrophils. The intermediate aldehyde, 20-oxo-LTB_4, is formed by the same $CYP450_{LTB\omega}$ in the presence of NADPH. The oxidation of 20-oxo-LTB_4 to 20-carboxy-LTB_4 involves an NAD^+-dependent aldehyde dehydrogenase found in neutrophil microsomes (59,60).

The metabolism of LTB_4 in the liver involves initial ω-hydroxylation by a specific CYP450, having high homology to $CYP450_{LTB\omega}$, followed by alcohol and aldehyde dehydrogenases to 20-carboxy LTB_4 (61). Metabolism of LTB_4 in hepatocytes is inhibited by ethanol, which also diverts metabolism into 3-hydroxy-LTB_4 as a partial β-oxidation product (62) and which retains biological activity similar to that of 20-hydroxy-LTB_4. Several unique β-oxidation products of 20-hydroxy-LTB_4 were characterized in the liver, including 18-carboxy-LTB_4, 16-carboxy-LTB_3, and 18-tauro-LTB_4 (63).

12S-HETE originating from platelets is ω-hydroxylated by neutrophils via transcellular metabolism into 12,20-DiHETE, possibly by a $CYP450_{LTB\omega}$ in the human neutrophil (64,65). Human neutrophil microsomes also metabolize lipoxins at the ω-carbon (66).

IV. Metabolism of Arachidonic Acid by CYP450

Fatty acids have long been known to be substrates for CYP450. In 1932, Verkade et al. described enzymatic ω-hydroxylation of palmitic acid long before microsomes were identified as a source of CYP450 (67). The metabolism of polyunsaturated fatty acids is somewhat more complex largely due to the

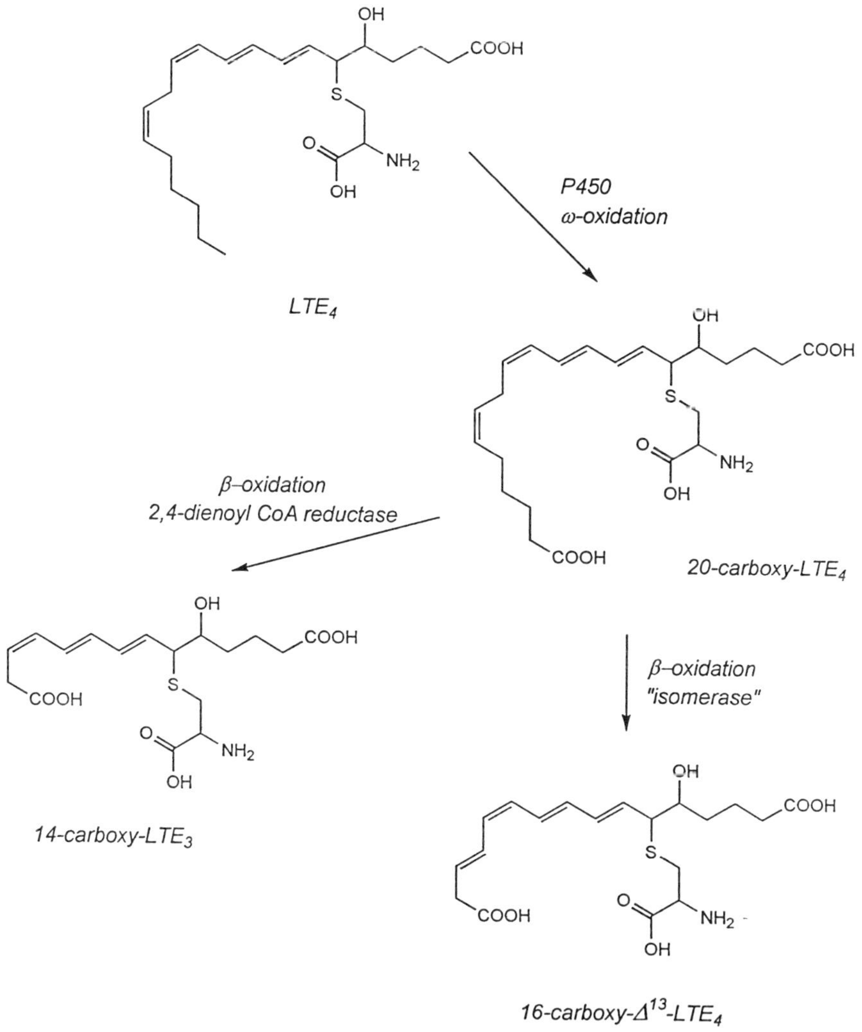

Figure 5 Metabolism of LTE$_4$ in humans leads to formation of 14-carboxy-LTE$_3$ and 16-carboxy-Δ^{13}-LTE$_4$ via an initial ω-oxidation by CYP450 forming 20-carboxy-LTE$_4$, which is further metabolized by β-oxidative processes (52).

additional oxidations involving double bonds. The studies on arachidonic acid monooxygenation over the past 15 years yielded substantial information about three distinct reactions mediated by CYP450: (1) epoxidation of double bonds; (2) allylic (lipoxygenase-like HETE generation) and bisallylic hydroxylations; (3) terminal and subterminal hydroxylations.

A. Epoxygenase Metabolites

Occurrence

Epoxidation of each of the four double bonds of arachidonic acid by CYP450 epoxygenase leads to generation of an epoxyeicosatrienoic acid (EET or EpETrE) (Fig. 2); the four EETs were named according to the carbons bearing the epoxide: 14,15-, 11,12-, 8,9-, and 5,6-EET. These epoxides are all of *cis* configuration and can be separated into optical isomers (9). Typically, all four EETs, as a mixture of regioisomers, have been detected in microsomal preparations of the kidney, liver, lung, and endothelial cells when incubated with arachidonic acid. The relative proportion of individual isomers and the stereochemistry of EETs have been established chromatographically; these properties largely depend on the species and tissue origin of the microsomal preparation. For example, rat liver microsomes generate four EETs, which account for about 85% of total products, whereas rat kidney microsomes generate 35% of EETs and 65% of ω/ω-1 hydroxy metabolites (HETEs) (9). The EETs often show a high degree of optical purity particularly when derived from liver microsomes of rats treated with phenobarbital (9). The 5,6-EET, a potent vasorelaxant (6), is formed in lesser amounts than the EETs that have the epoxy group closer to the terminal end. As expected from the model studies, the 5,6 double bond of arachidonic acid has limited access to the prosthetic heme ferryl oxygen, which explains lower epoxidation rate of this double bond. Unlike other EETs, the 5,6-EET can exist in the equilibrium of three forms, the epoxide, the diol, and the lactone, their relative proportion depending critically on the pH of the solution, which somehow complicates the detection of 5,6-EET. The EETs can be formed by several purified or cloned CYP450 isozymes from CYP subfamilies A, B, C, and E (9,68). However, no mammalian isozyme has revealed a high degree of regiospecificity for epoxidation of a single double bond of arachidonic acid nor any other polyunsaturated fatty acid. CYP450 epoxygenase commonly has some degree of hydroxylase activity. For example, isolated purified CYP2E1 from rabbit liver generates all epoxides except 5,6-EET in addition to ω-1 and ω-2 metabolites (19- and 18-HETE) (30). Thus, arachidonic acid epoxidation, although it can be highly enantioselective, generally shows limited regioselectivity (9). Rat renal CYP4A2 has been recently cloned and expressed in insect cells; it generates only one EET, 11,12-EET, upon incubation with arachidonic acid (69). Yet, this isozyme simultaneously produced high amounts of ω/ω-1 hydroxy metabolites. High stereo- and regiospecificity of arachidonic acid epoxidation can be achieved by mutated (F87V) bacterial CYP450$_{BM-3}$, which generates a single metabolite, 14R,15S-EET (70). The EETs may also be formed nonenzymatically by oxidation of arachidonic acid with peroxynitrite or its decomposition product, nitrogen dioxide (71).

Metabolism

Very little is known about the metabolic fate of the EETs in vivo. Available studies suggest that the EETs may be subject to numerous transformations but their significance in vivo is not known. The EETs can be hydrolyzed nonenzymatically or by abundant epoxide hydrolases into corresponding vicinal dihydroxy analogs (DiHETrE). The EETs are poor substrates for the microsomal form of epoxide hydrolase whereas cytosolic mouse liver epoxide hydrolase shows particular activity toward 14,15-EET (1260 nmol/min/mg protein) but low activity for 5,6-EET (69 nmol/min/mg protein) (72). Several recent observations describe the occurrence of DiHETrE in the human and rat urine. 5,6-EET along with its diol form were detected in rat urine and its levels were significantly higher in rats fed a high-salt diet than the levels of other EET regioisomers (73). EETs are increased in the urine of women with pregnancy-induced hypertension (74) and in patients with unstable coronary artery disease; they are further increased in the latter during coronary angioplasty (75). Measurement of EETs and DiHETrEs in urine by gas chromatography/mass spectrometry (GC/MS) is a noninvasive, specific, and sensitive method for analysis of CYP450 epoxygenase metabolites in humans. DiHETrEs measured in urine most likely derive from the kidney since after systemic administration of radiolabeled 14,15-EET negligible radioactivity was found in urine (74).

Another metabolic route for epoxides is by conjugation with glutathione. Two isoforms of rat hepatic glutathione transferase are particularly efficient in conjugation of EETs into hydroxyglutathione compounds with K_m values of 10 μM and V_{max}, resulting in conjugation of 25–60 nmol of EET/min/mg purified enzyme (76). The enzyme was most active toward 14,15-EET whereas the other EETs were less efficiently conjugated with glutathione. It is not known whether the EET-glutathione conjugates have biological activity, analogous to sulfidopeptide leukotrienes, or whether this process inactivates EETs.

Several EETs are substrates for enzymes that metabolize arachidonic acid. 5,6-EET, which is a poor substrate for cytosolic and microsomal epoxide hydrolase, has a unique metabolic fate. Cyclooxygenase metabolizes 5,6-EET into 5,6-epoxy-PGH$_2$, which can be further converted into 5,6-epoxy prostaglandins E, D, and F (77). The latter is converted via intramolecular hydrolysis of the epoxide into a PGI analog, 5-hydroxy-PGI$_1$. The 5,6-epoxy-PGE$_1$ has vasorelaxing activity comparable to that of PGE$_2$ (78). It is interesting that the 5,6-EET, when injected arterially into perfused rabbit kidney, stimulates the release of prostacyclin and PGE$_2$, possibly via releasing arachidonic acid from phospholipid stores and its subsequent transformation by cyclooxygenase (78). Human platelets metabolize 5,6-EET into a variety of products including an epoxy-thromboxane and 12-lipoxygenase metabolite, 5,6-epoxy-12S-HETrE (Fig. 6) (79). The metabolites derived from cyclooxygenase-mediated metabolism of 5,6-EET do not show PGH/TxA agonist activity in platelets. An unidentified rat platelet metabolite of 5,6-EET displays constrictor activity in the perfused kidney (80). Cyclooxygenase metabolizes 8,9-EET into 11R-hydroxy-8,9-EET without cyclization into a prostaglandin structure (81). Other EETs are not metabolized by cyclooxygenase because of unfavorable olefin configuration. Further metabolism of EETs is possible by lipoxygenases, ω- or β hydroxylation, and epoxidation.

B. Hydroxylase Metabolites—Allylic and Bisallylic Oxidations

HETE molecules can be formed by lipoxygenases, cyclooxygenases, and CYP450 monooxygenases and contain a characteristic *cis,trans* conjugated double bond and a vicinal hydroxyl. Incubation of arachidonic acid with rat liver microsomes generates a complex mixture of HETE molecules (Fig. 1) (82–84). The six conjugated diene HETEs generated by microsomes, 5-, 8-, 9-, 11-, 12-, and 15-HETE, are structurally similar to the HETEs generated by lipoxygenase, but their biosynthesis does not involve formation of a hydroperoxide as HPETE intermediates have not been detected. The precise mechanism by which HETE molecules are generated via P450 monooxygenation is not known. Lipoxygenase-dependent metabolism of arachidonic acid generates HETEs with high stereospecificity. Stereochemical analysis of the hydroxyl group revealed that the microsomal CYP450-derived HETEs are all nearly racemic with the exception of 12-HETE, which is generated with high abundance of the 12R-HETE isomer (9). This isomer is formed in the psoriatic skin and cornea and is a powerful stereospecific inhibitor of Na$^+$-K$^+$-ATPase in the cornea (85). Recently, a unique group of HETEs was isolated and characterized from liver microsomes of phenobarbital-treated rats. This new hydroxylation mechanism occurs at either one of the three methylene carbons that separate double bonds in the arachidonic acid chain (84). This leads to generation of a mixture containing 7-, 10-, and 13-HETE, which were named bisallylic HETEs because of this unique structural feature. These HETEs are unstable and in mildly acidic conditions spontaneously convert into conjugated diene-containing HETEs. For example, 13-HETE is rearranged into 11-HETE and 15-HETE with retention of configuration and retention of the original hydroxyl oxygen

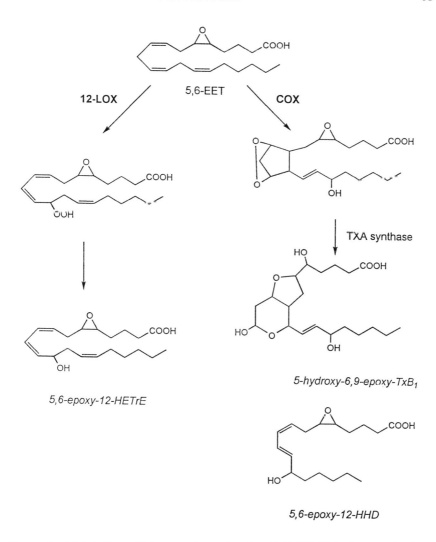

Figure 6 Metabolism of 5,6-epoxyeicosatrienoic acid (5,6-EET) by human platelets. Lipoxygenase (LOX) activity results in 5,6-epoxy-12-hydroxy-eicosatrienoic acid (5,6-epoxy-12-HETrE); cyclooxygenase (COX) and TxA synthase metabolites are 5,6-epoxy-PGH$_1$, 5-hydroxy-6,9-epoxy-thromboxane A$_1$ and 5,6-epoxy-12-hydroxy-heptadecadienoic acid (5,6-epoxy-12-HHD).

(84). This represents a novel mechanism involving HETEs but it remains to be defined whether or not this is a central mechanism in formation of conjugated diene HETEs by CYP450.

C. Terminal Carbon and Subterminal Hydroxylations

Occurrence

20-HETE is a major eicosanoid produced by incubating arachidonic acid with hepatic as well as renal cortical and inner medullary (82) and intestinal (86) microsomal preparations. 19-HETE, an ω-1 hydroxylase metabolite, is often detected with 20-HETE. Recently, the cDNA of CYP 4A2, a major isoform in the rat kidney, was cloned and sequenced and expressed using baculovirus and Sf9 insect cells (69). The expressed CYP4A2 efficiently metabolizes arachidonic acid into 20-HETE and 19-HETE and their formation is maximal at the CYP450 hemeprotein to CYP reductase ratio of 1:14. Understanding the physiological roles of 20-HETE and subterminal HETEs has been greatly enhanced with the recent development of a sensitive, specific, and selective method for quantitative measurement based on isotopic dilution GC/MS (26,87,88). The emerging observations indicate that hormonal stimulation of renal epithelial cells or the intact kidney releases 20-HETE and often other HETEs. For example, the isolated perfused rat kidney stimulated with endothelin 1 (ET-1) releases three- to fourfold higher amounts of 20-HETE relative to control and the release paralleled the constrictor response evoked by ET-1 suggesting that release of 20-HETE is associated with stimulation of the ET-1 receptor in the kidney (26). The perfused rabbit kidney responded to stimulation with angiotensin II (Ang II) by releasing 16-, 17-, 18-, 19-, and 20-HETEs whereas vasopressin and bradykinin were without effect on HETE efflux (88). Isolated rat medullary thick ascending limb (mTAL) cells selectively form 20-HETE (2.4 pg/μg protein, 260% of the control value) as the only HETE molecule following brief stimulation with Ang II (50 pM) again suggesting that the release of 20-HETE may be induced by stimulation of the Ang II receptor in the mTAL (89). Stimulation of the kidney in vivo by Ang II resulted in increased levels of 20-HETE in the urine (90). 20-HETE and 16-HETE can be formed on incubation of arachidonic acid with the unstimulated human neutrophil (91,92). Human neutrophils stimulated with fMLP, PAF, or calcium ionophore, A23187, generate 20-HETE (1.2–5.7 pg/10^6 cells) but the amount of 20-HETE is far less than products of the 5-lipoxygenase pathway of arachidonic acid metabolism formed by the neutrophil (93). 16-HETE inhibits neutrophil adhesion and aggression, possibly via release from phospholipid stores (92). In a recent study, Sacerdoti et al. have reported detection of 16-HETE in urine from cirrhotic patients (94). 16-HETE, 17-HETE, and 18-HETE have also been detected as products of arachidonic acid in rat liver microsomes, particularly after treatment of animals with β-naphthoflavone (83). Microsomal fractions isolated from monkey seminal vesicles catalyze formation of 18R-HETE (50) as well as purified reconstituted CYP2E1, which, in addition to 18R-HETE (100% optical purity), generates 19S- and 19R-HETE in proportion 3:1 (30).

Metabolism

20-HETE is metabolized by ram seminal vesicles into ω-hydroxy-PGH$_2$ with subsequent conversion into ω-hydroxy-prostaglandins. The vasoconstrictor properties of 20-HETE were found to be dependent upon activation by endothelial cyclooxygenase (95). Human platelets metabolize 20-HETE into a complex mixture of new metabolites formed by 12-lipoxygenase (12,20-Di-HETE) as well as cyclooxygenase. The identification of 11-hydroxy metabolite of 20-HETE as the most abundant platelet cyclooxygenase metabolite suggests that 20-HETE is less efficiently cyclized to an endoperoxide intermediate by cyclooxygenase than is arachidonate (96). The urinary excretion of 20-HETE in humans is in the low pg/ml range. However, treatment of urine with β-glucuronidase resulted in a 13- to 28-fold increase in its concentration. This suggests 20-HETE is excreted primarily as a glucuronide conjugate (97). The biochemical steps leading to its generation and tissue of origin of the glucuronic acid transferase required for this transformation have not been identified. One of the metabolites of arachidonic acid generated by renal microsomes was characterized as 20-carboxy-arachidonic acid (20-carboxy-AA) (82), which was later shown to inhibit the Na$^+$-K$^+$-2Cl$^-$ transporter in the mTAL but, unlike 20-HETE, was devoid of vasoactivity (98). The 20-carboxy-AA most likely resulted from a two-step oxidation of 20-HETE, which initially required generation of 20-oxo-AA, possibly via NADP-dependent alcohol dehydrogenase, and subsequently, oxidation of the aldehyde to 20-carboxy-AA, catalyzed by NAD$^+$-dependent aldehyde dehydrogenase. The biochemical steps leading to formation of 20-carboxy-AA are poorly characterized.

D. Biological Activity of CYP450 Arachidonate Metabolites

Arachidonic acid metabolites derived from P450 monooxygenation have prominent biological activities (6,10,99) (Table 1). These include vascular activity, renal tubular activity (100), stimulation of peptide hormone release from endocrine cells, inhibition of renal Na$^+$-K$^+$-ATPase, inhibition of arachidonate-induced platelet aggregation in vivo and inhibition of Ca^{2+} influx into platelets, mobilization of Ca^{2+} from aortic smooth muscle cells and anterior pituitary cells, mitogenic activity in the proximal tubules, dilatation of the intestinal microcirculation, and inhibition of renin release from cortical slices.

Table 1 Biological Actions of CYP450-Derived Arachidonate Metabolites

Eicosanoid	Biological activity
20-HETE	Constrictor of isolated rat aorta; modulates Na^+-K^+-$2Cl^-$ cotransporter in mTALH cells, induces $^{45}Ca^{2+}$ mobilization in renal arterial smooth muscle cells in vitro; inhibits platelet aggregation in vitro and thromboxane biosynthesis; stimulates erythropoietin-dependent stem cell growth in the human bone marrow; is mitogenic in proximal tubules in the nanomolar range; blocks rat renal apical 70 pS K^+ channel in mTALH in vitro
19S-HETE	Weak constrictor of rat aorta; stimulates Na^+-K^+-ATPase
18-HETE, 17-HETE	Weak vasodilators in the isolated rabbit kidney; inhibitors of ATPase
18R-HETE	Contracts guinea pig lung strip, relaxes guinea pig arteries
16R-HETE	Inhibits neutrophil aggregation and adhesion
12R-HETE	Inhibits Na^+-K^+-ATPase, proinflammatory mediator
5,6-EET	Inhibits platelet aggregation in vitro; inhibits TxA formation in vivo; increases somatostatin release in vitro from hypothalamic median eminence; increases insulin release in vitro from pancreatic islets; increases $^{45}Ca^{2+}$ efflux from anterior pituitary and canine aortic smooth muscle; activates K^+ channels in isolated vascular smooth muscle cells; inhibits vasopressin stimulated water flow in toad bladder in vitro
8,9-EET	Increases glucagon release from pancreatic islets, increases intestinal blood flow; inhibits vasopressin stimulated water flow in toad bladder
11,12-EET	Inhibits Na^+-K^+-ATPase; inhibits vasopressin stimulated water flow in toad bladder
14,15-EET	Inhibits cyclooxygenase; inhibits platelet aggregation; inhibits renin release; inhibits ^{86}Rb uptake in renal epithelial cells; activates Na^+/H^+ exchange; promotes tumor cell adhesion to endothelium; promotes mitogenesis; increases glucagon release from pancreatic islets

Several mechanisms have been proposed to explain the biological actions of EETs and HETEs: (1) activation by cyclooxygenase; (2) release of arachidonic acid from lipid stores with subsequent formation of vasorelaxing prostanoids; (3) mobilization of calcium; (4) modulation of cotransporters and inhibition of K^+ channels; (5) interaction with specific receptors or PGH/TxA receptor; (6) inhibition of Na^+-K^+-ATPase; (7) activation of adenylate cyclase;

(8) an emerging area suggests incorporation/release from cellular phospholipids. There is no evidence of cell activation via G-proteins. Specific receptors for EETs or HETEs have yet to be characterized (101).

V. Phospholipid-Bound CYP450 Eicosanoids and Potential Role in Signal Transduction

Capdevila et al. (102,103) described EETs esterified to rat hepatic phospholipids (>92% of total liver EETs). More recently, they reported that rat plasma LDL fraction contains EETs that are predominantly incorporated in phosphatidylcholine (PC) and phosphatidylethanolamine (PE) (104). These findings set a clear precedent for the enzymatic incorporation of EETs into phospholipids in mammalian systems. In the rat kidney, EETs are constituent components of rat renal phospholipid pool with the highest concentration in phosphatidylinositol (105). EETs readily incorporate into phospholipids of mastocytoma cells and the distribution of 14,15-EET was highest in PE and PC. EET-labeled phospholipids in these cells have a long half-life (34.9 ± 7 hr) and incorporation into cellular phospholipids protects the EETs from hydrolysis. Interestingly, the rate for calcium ionophore-stimulated release of 14,15-EET from cellular phospholipids exceeded that for arachidonic acid (106). These findings, however, have attracted little attention in terms of potential participation of EET-containing phospholipids in signal transduction mechanisms.

The four EETs are also found in phospholipids of human and rat platelets (87). The origin of these EETs is of particular interest as the identification of P450 monooxygenase in platelets has not been well established and EETs may originate from other biochemical sources. We observed that stimulation of human platelets by thrombin or platelet-activating factor results in release of these EETs in the amount of 1.8–2.3 pg/10^6 cells (87). This suggests that stimulation of either the thrombin or PAF receptor of platelets is linked to generation of EETs. As we have reported, the EETs are esterified in phospholipid pools of platelets; therefore, the EETs may originate from phospholipid stores rather than from agonist-stimulated biosynthesis (87).

20-HETE is a product of arachidonic acid and a CYP450 ω-hydroxylate of the 4A gene family and is an abundant microsomal CYP450-derived eicosanoid in the rat kidney. Very little is known about the metabolic fate of 20-HETE in the kidney in vivo. We observed that stimulation of the rat renal slices with calcium ionophore results in accumulation of 20-HETE, which is readily detectable by GC/MS. This release could not be inhibited with ETYA, an inhibitor of oxidative arachidonate metabolism, suggesting involvement of phospholipase A_2 in the release of 20-HETE (107,108). The isolated perfused kidney challenged with Ang II or ET-1 rapidly releases 20-HETE into the perfusion fluid (26,109). We investigated several mechanisms by which 20-HETE might be formed and released from the kidney. Since the hormone-mediated release of endogenous 20-HETE could not be inhibited by pretreatment of the kidney with the CYP450 inhibitors DBDD or 17-ODYA, it is unlikely that the release of arachidonic acid is coupled to CYP450-mediated metabolism. It is also unlikely that 20-HETE is generated in situ from arachidonate phospholipids since these phospholipids are not substrates for the recombinant CYP 450 4A2.

We have investigated the possibility that 20-HETE might be formed from arachidonic acid by CYP450 in the absence of stimulus and transformed to an active form, a coenzyme A thioester, which subsequently, via coupling with *lyso*-phospholipids, formed a phospholipid pool from which 20-HETE can be released upon hormonal stimulation (Fig. 7). We found that the concentration of free 20-HETE in the rat kidney was low [0.26 ± 0.08 ng/μmol phosphorus (P)] and increased almost 10-fold (2.42 ± 0.4 ng/μmol P) upon mild alkaline hydrolysis of renal total lipids ($n = 9$) indicating that 85–90% of *endogenous* 20-HETE was in the esterified form. Analysis of complex renal lipids by normal-phase high-performance liquid chromatography, followed by saponification of fractionated lipids and GC/MS analyses, revealed that the major forms containing endogenous 20-HETE were PC and PE with a molar ratio of 2.5.

The endogenous phospholipids containing 20-HETE coeluted with biosynthetically prepared 20-HETE-PE and 20-HETE-PC. Radiolabeled 20-HETE rapidly incorporated into renal slices in a time- and concentration-dependent manner. The total amount of radioactivity incorporated into the phospholipids was 60–70% during 0.5–1 hr incubation. The predominant form containing 20-HETE was PC whereas at incubations longer than 2 hr the predominant form was 20-HETE-PE. The amount of 20-HETE in PI + PS was 1.7% after 30 min and did not increase with incubation time. 20-HETE incorporated into two tritium-labeled PC species. Treatment of these 20-HETE-PCs with phospholipase C generated diglycerides containing 20-HETE (20-HETE-DAGs), which were analyzed by mass spectrometry. The spectra indicated that the two major PC forms containing 20-HETE were: 1-*O*-hexadecyl-2-(20-HETE)-3-glycero-PC and 1-stearoyl-2-(20-HETE)-3-glycero-PC. Various lipoxygenase-derived HETE molecules have been shown to be incorporated into cellular phospholipids of the kidney (110); however, the incorporation of a HETE molecule into an ether form of a PC has not been previously reported. These unique phospholipids may be involved in a number of metabolic transformations like generation of 20-HETE, 20-HETE-DAG, and 20-HETE-glycerophosphatidic acid (20-HETE-PA), depending on the phospholipase involved (Fig. 7). Ang II stimulation of a kidney tissue labeled with 20-HETE released

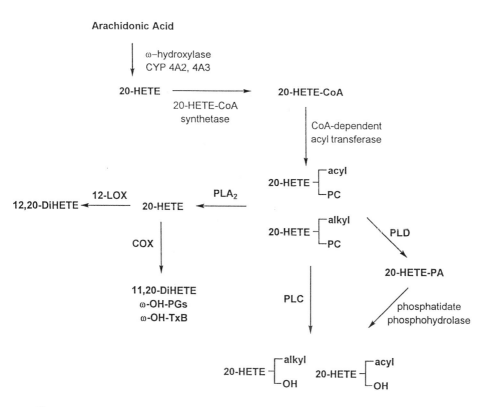

Figure 7 Hypothetical sequence of events leading to the incorporation of 20-HETE into the major phospholipids of the rat kidney. Acyl and alkyl indicate an ester and ether linkage at the *sn*-1 position of the glycerolipid backbone, respectively. PC, phosphatidylcholine; PA, phosphatidic acid.

10–20% of incorporated radioactivity. HPLC analysis of released radioactive compounds showed an accumulation of 20-HETE and 20-HETE DAG. These results suggest that 20-HETE may participate in the PC-mediated signaling pathway induced by Ang II in the kidney. That Ang II activation of the kidney releases 20-HETE and messengers containing 20-HETE raises the possibility that the ω-hydroxyl modification in these signaling molecules could thereby alter their function. The biological activity and function of such hydroxylated PAs and DAGs are unknown. 20-HETE-PA may be the main precursor of 20-HETE-DAG in the kidney. The production of DAG from PC may result from the phospholipase D and phosphatidic acid phosphohydrolase pathway rather than from the phospholipase C pathway.

VI. Conclusions

Metabolism of eicosanoids and arachidonic acid by multiple CYP450 isozymes displays complex chemistry, dependence on biosynthesis of cofactors, regulation by sex hormones, chemical environment, such as the presence of inducers and inhibitors (pollutants, nitric oxide, dietary components), disease, and age (4,5,15,111,112). These multiple factors and their interactions make studies of CYP-mediated metabolism exceptionally difficult. Much remains to be learned about the factors controlling regio- and stereospecificity in CYP450-catalyzed reactions, as well as the chemical identity of the potent oxidant molecule that is necessary for oxygen insertion into arachidonic acid molecules (15). The unusual catalytic properties of CYP450 contribute to the regulation of its own activities, as with competitive inhibition by alternative substrates, mechanism-based inactivation, and effects of other lipophobic substances (4). CYP450 may undergo suicide inactivation during catalytic turnover through an interaction of the active oxygen species with the hemoprotein active center (113). The biological activity of CYP450 metabolites has not been examined in terms of specific receptors that mediate their responses. Of great interest will be establishing the role of newly detected phospholipid-bound cytochrome CYP450-derived arachidonic acid metabolites in signal transduction mechanisms evoked by hormones and profiling the biological activity of novel mediators released from these phospholipids.

Acknowledgments

The preparation of this review was assisted by grants from the National Institutes of Health HL 34300 and the American Heart Association, New York State affiliate, 950325. We wish to thank Melody Steinberg for editorial assistance.

References

1. Picot D, Loll PJ, Garavito RM. The X-ray crystal structure of the membrane protein prostaglandin H_2 synthase-1. Nature 1994; 367:243–249.
2. Ortiz de Montellano PR, ed. Cytochrome P450. Structure, Mechanism and Biochemistry, 2nd ed. New York: Plenum Press, 1995.
3. Omura T, Sato R. The carbon monoxide-binding pigment of liver microsomes. J Biol Chem 1964; 239:2370–2385.
4. Mansuy D, Renaud JP. Heme-thiolate proteins different form cytochromes P450 catalyzing monooxygenations. In: Ortiz de Montellano PR, ed. Cytochrome P450: Structure, Mechanism, and Biochemistry, 2nd ed. New York: Plenum Press, 1995: 537–574.

5. Schenkman JB, Greim H, eds. Cytochrome P450, Handbook of Experimental Pharmacology, vol 105. Berlin: Springer Verlag, 1993:3–728.
6. McGiff JC. Cytochrome P-450 metabolism of arachidonic acid. Annu Rev Pharmacol Toxicol 1991; 31:339–369.
7. Fitzpatrick FA, Murphy RC. Cytochrome P450 metabolism of arachidonic acid: formation and biological actions of "epoxygenase"-derived eicosanoids. Pharmacol Rev 1989; 40:229–241.
8. Oliw EH. Oxygenation of polyunsaturated fatty acids by cytochrome P450 monooxygenases. Prog Lipid Res 1994; 33:329–354.
9. Capdevila JH, Zeldin D, Makita K, Karara A, Falck JR. In: Cytochrome P450 and the metabolism of arachidonic acid and oxygenated eicosanoids. Ortiz de Montellano PR, ed. Cytochrome P450: Structure, Mechanism and Biochemistry, 2nd ed. New York: Plenum Press, 1995:443–471.
10. Schwartzman ML, McGiff JC. Renal cytochrome P450. J Lipid Mediators Cell Signal 1995; 12:229–242.
11. Hanss JG, Taylor GW. Metabolism and toxicology of the prostaglandins. In: Vane JR, O'Grady J, eds. Therapeutic Applications of Prostaglandins. London: Edward Arnold, 1993:37–48.
12. Tanaka S, Imaoka S, Kusunose E, Kusunose M, Maekawa M, Funare Y. ω- and (ω-1)-hydroxylation of arachidonic acid, lauric acid and prostaglandin A_1 by multiple forms of cytochrome P450 purified from rat heparic microsomes. Biochim Biophys Acta 1990; 1043:177–181.
13. Williams DE, Hale SE, Okita RT, Masters BSS. A prostaglandin ω-hydroxylase cytochrome P-450 (P-450$_{PG-\omega}$) purified from lungs of pregnant rabbits. J Biol Chem 1984; 259:14600–14608.
14. Nebert DW, Nelson DR, Coon MJ, Estabrook RW, Feyereisen R, Fujii-Kuriyama Y, Gonzelez FJ, Guengerich FP, Gunsalus IC, Johnson EF, Loper JC, Sato R, Waterman MR, Waxman DJ. The P450 superfamily: update on new sequences, gene mapping, and recommended nomenclature. DNA Cell Biol 1991; 10:1–14.
15. Porter TD, Coon MJ. Cytochrome P-450. J Biol Chem 1991; 266:13469–13472.
16. Mason HS. Mechanisms of oxygen metabolism. Adv Enzymol 1957; 19:79–233.
17. Whitlock JP, Jr., Denison MS. Induction of cytochrome P450 enzymes that metabolize xenobiotics. In: Ortiz de Montellano, ed. Cytochrome P450, 2nd ed. New York: Plenum Press, 1995:367–390.
18. Muerhoff SA, Williams DE, Reich NO, CaJacob CA, Ortiz de Montellano PR, Masters BSS. Prostaglandin and fatty acid ω- and (ω-1) in oxidation in rabbit lung. J Biol Chem 1989; 264:749–756.
19. Thornton-Manning Jr., Ruangyuttikarn W, Gonzalez FJ, Yost GS. Metabolic activation of the pneumotoxin, 3-methylindole, by vaccinia-expressed cytochrome P450s. Biochem Biophys Res Commun 1991; 181:100–107.
20. Thurman MJ, Albrecht JH, Krueger MA, Erickson RR, Cherwitz DL, Park SS, Grelbein MV, Holtzman JL. Induction of cytochrome CYPIA1 and formation of toxic metabolites of benzocalpyrene by rat aorta: a possible role in atherogenesis. Proc Natl Acad Sci USA 1994; 91:5397–5401.

21. Shiiki S, Fuchimoto S, Orita K. A comparison of the antitumor effects of natural human tumor necrosis factor α and β: the roles of arachidonic acid metabolism and intracellular cAMP. Jpn J Clin Oncol 1990; 20:252–258.
22. Ortiz de Montellano PR, Correia MA. Inhibition of cytochrome P450 enzymes. In: Ortiz de Montellano PR, ed. Cytochrome P450: Structure, Mechanism, and Biochemistry, 2nd ed. New York: Plenum Press, 1995:305–364.
23. Zou AP, Ma YM, Sui ZM, Ortiz de Montellano PR, Clark JE, Masters BS, Roman RJ. Effects of 17-octadecynoic acid, a suicide substrate inhibitor of cytochrome P450 fatty acid ω-hydroxylase, on renal function in rats. J Pharmacol Exp Ther 1994; 268:474–481.
24. Fulton D, Mahboubi K, McGiff JC, Quilley J. Cytochrome P450-dependent effects of bradykinin in the rat heart. Br J Pharmacol 1995; 114:99–102.
25. Corriu C, Feletou M, Canet E, Vanhoutte PM. Inhibitors of the cytochrome P450-monooxygenase and endothelium-dependent hyperpolarizations in the guinea-pig isolated carotid artery. Br J Pharmacol 1996; 117:607–610.
26. Oyekan A, Balazy M, McGiff JC. Renal oxygenase: Differential contributions to vasoconstriction induced by endothelin-I and angiotensin II. Am J Physiol 1997; 273:R293–R300.
27. Wink DA, Osawa Y, Darbyshe JF, Jones CR, Eshenaur SC, Ninis RW. Inhibition of cytochromes P450 by nitric oxide and a nitric oxide releasing agent. Arch Biochem Biophys 1993; 300:115–123.
28. Shedlofsky SI, Israel BC, McClain CJ, Hill DB, Blouin RA. Endotoxin administration to humans inhibits hepatic cytochrome P450-mediated drug metabolism. J Clin Invest 1994; 94:2209–2214.
29. Khatsenko OG, Gross SS, Rifkind AB, Vane JR. Nitric oxide is a mediator of the decrease in cytochrome P450-dependent metabolism caused by immunostimulants. Proc Natl Acad Sci USA 1993; 90:11147–11151.
30. Laethem RM, Balazy M, Falck JR, Laethem CL, Koop DR. Formation of 19(S)-, 19(R)-, and 18(R)-hydroxyeicosatetraenoic acids by alcohol-inducible cytochrome P450 2E1. J Biol Chem 1993; 268:12912–12918.
31. Gergel D, Misik V, Reisz P, Cederbaum AI. Inhibition of rat and human cytochrome P4502E1 catalytic activity and reactive oxygen radical formation by nitric oxide. Arch Biochem Biophys 1997; 337:239–250.
32. Landino LM, Crews BC, Timmons MD, Morrow JD, Marnett LJ. Peroxynitrite, the coupling product of nitric oxide and superoxide, activates prostaglandin biosynthesis. Proc Natl Acad Sci USA 1996; 93:15069–15074.
33. Ullrich V, Graf M. Prostacyclin and thromboxane synthase as P-450 enzymes. Trends Pharmacol Sci 1984; 5:352–5.
34. Ullrich V, Castle L, Weber P. Spectral evidence for the cytochrome P450 nature of prostacyclin synthase. Biochem Pharmacol 1981; 30:2033–2040.
35. Hecker M, Ullrich V. On the mechanism of prostacyclin and thromboxane A₂ biosynthesis. J Biol Chem 1989; 264:141–150.
36. Hara S, Yokoyama C, Brugger R, Lottspeich F, Ullrich V, Tanabe T. Molecular cloning and expression of prostacyclin synthase from endothelial cells. Adv Prostaglandin Thromboxane Leukot Res 1995; 23:121–123.

37. Miyata A, Hara S, Yokoyama C, Inoue H, Ullrich V, Tanabe T. Molecular cloning and expression of human prostacyclin synthase. Biochem Biophys Res Commun 1994; 200:1728–1734.
38. Gryglewski RJ. Role of prostacyclin in cardiovascular homeostasis. In: Carrtin M, Paoletti R, Braquet P, Christen Y, eds. Endogenous Factors of Cardiovascular Regulation and Protection. Amsterdam: Excerpta Medica, 1990:21–59.
39. Wade ML, Voelkel NF, Fitzpatrick FA. "Suicide" inactivation of prostaglandin I_2 synthase: characterization of mechanism based inactivation with isolated enzyme and endothelial cells. Arch Biochem Biophys 1995; 321:453–458l.
40. Gryglewski RJ, Bunting S, Moncada S, Vane JR. Arterial walls are protected against deposition of platelet thrombi by a substance (prostaglandin X) which they make from prostaglandin endoperoxides. Prostaglandins 1976; 12:685–713.
41. Zou MH, Ullrich V. Peroxynitrite formed by simultaneous generation of nitric oxide and superoxide selectively inhibits bovine aortic prostacyclin synthase. FEBS Lett 1996; 382.101–104.
42. Haurand M, Ullrich V. Isolation and characterization of thromboxane synthase from human platelets as a cytochrome P450 enzyme. J Biol Chem 1985; 260:15059–15067.
43. Yokoyama C, Miyata A, Ihara H, Ullrich V, Tanabe T. Molecular cloning of human platelet thromboxane. A synthase. Biochem Biophys Res Commun 1991; 178: 1479–1484.
44. Hecker M, Maurand M, Ullrich V, Terao S. Spectral studies on structure activity relationships of thromboxane synthase inhibitors. Eur J Biochem 1986; 157:217–223.
45. Weiss RM, Arnold JL, Estabrook RW. Transformation of an arachidonic acid hydroperoxide into epoxyhydroxy and trihydroxy fatty acids by liver microsomal cytochrome P-450. Arch Biochem Biophys 1987; 252:334–338.
46. Chang MS, Boeglin WE, Guengerich FP, Brash AR. Cytochrome P450-dependent transformations of 15R- and 15S-hydroperoxyeicosatetraenoic acids: stereoselective formation of epoxy alcohol products. Biochemistry 1996; 35:464–471.
47. Kupfer D, Jansson I, Faureau I, Theoharides AD, Schenkman JB. Regioselective hydroxylation of prostaglandins by constitutive forms of cytochrome P450 from rat liver: formation of a novel metabolite by a female-specific P450. Arch Biochem Biophys 1988; 261:186–195.
48. Aoyama T, Hardwick JP, Imaoka S, Funae Y, Gelboir HV, Gonzales FJ. Clofibrate-inducible rat hepatic P450s IVA1 and IVA3 catalyze the ω- and (ω-1)-hydroxylation of fatty acids and the ω-hydrolation of prostaglandins E, and $F_{2\alpha}$. J Lipid Res 1990; 31:1477–1482.
49. Oliw EH, Fahlstadius P, Hamberg M. Biosynthesis of 19-hydroxy and 20-hydroxy E prostaglandins in seminal fluids. Adv Prostaglandin Thromboxane Leukot Res 1987; 17:39–43.
50. Oliw EH. Biosynthesis of 18(R_D)-hydroxyeicosatetraenoic acid from arachidonic acid by microsomes of monkey seminal vesicles. J Biol Chem 1989; 264:17845–17853.
51. Wong PY, Malik KU, Taylor BM, Schneider WP, McGiff JC, Sun FF. Epoxidation of prostacyclin in the rabbit kidney. J Biol Chem 1985; 260:9150–9153.

52. Sala A, Voelkel NF, Maclouf J, Murphy RC. Leukotriene E_4 elimination and metabolism in normal human subjects. J Biol Chem 1990; 265:21771–21778.
53. Arm JP, Lee TH. Evidence for a specific role of leukotriene E_4 in asthma and airway hyperresponsiveness. Adv Prostaglandin Thromboxane Leukot Res 1994; 22:227–240.
54. Szczeklik A. Aspirin-induced asthma: an update and novel findings. Adv Prostaglandin Thromboxane Leukot Res 1994; 22:185–198.
55. Manning PJ, Rokach J, Malo JL, Ethier D, Cartier A, Girard Y, Charleson S, O'Byrne PM. Urinary leukotriene E_4 levels during early and late asthmatic responses. J Allergy Clin Immunol 1990; 86:211–220.
56. Murphy RC, FitzGerald GA. Current approaches to estimation of eicosanoid formation in vivo. Adv Prostaglandin Thromboxane Leukot Res 1994; 22:341–348.
57. Hansson G, Lindgren JA, Dahlen SE, Hedqvist P, Samuelsson B. Identification and biological activity of novel ω-oxidized metabolites of leukotriene B_4 from human leukocytes. FEBS Lett 1981; 130:107–112.
58. Kikuta Y, Kusunose E, Endo K, Yamamoto S, Sogawa K, Fujii-Kuriyama Y, Kusunose M. A novel form of cytochrome P-450 family 4 in human polymorphonuclear leukocytes. J Biol Chem 1993; 268:9376–9380.
59. Soberman RJ, Okita RT, Fitzsimmons B, Rokach J, Spur B, Austen KF. Stereochemical requirements for substrate specificity of LTB_4 20-hydroxylase. J Biol Chem 1987; 262:12421–12427.
60. Sumimoto H, Minakama S. Oxidation of 20-hydroxyleukotriene B_4 to 20-carboxyleukotriene B_4 by human neutrophil microsomes. Role of aldehyde dehydrogenase and leukotriene B_4 ω-hydroxylase (cytochrome P-450$_{LTB\omega}$) in leukotriene B_4 ω-oxidation. J Biol Chem 1990; 265:4348–4353.
61. Kikuta Y, Kusunose E, Kondo T, Yamamoto S, Kinoshita, Kusunose M. Cloning and expression of a novel form of leukotriene by ω-hydroxylase from human liver. FEBS Lett 1994; 348:70–74.
62. Wheelan P, Sala A, Folco G, Nicosia S, Falck JR, Bhatt RK, Murphy RC. Stereochemical analysis and biological activity of 3-hydroxy-leukotriene B_4: a metabolite from ethanol treated rat hepatocytes. J Pharmacol Exp Ther 1994; 271:1514–1519.
63. Shirley MA, Murphy RC. Metabolism of leukotriene B_4 in isolated hepatocytes: Involvement of 2,4-dienoyl CoA reductase in leukotriene B_4 metabolism. J Biol Chem 1990; 265:16288–16295.
64. Wong PY-K, Westlund P, Hamberg M, Gramstrom E, Chao PWH, Samuelsson B. ω-Hydroxylation of 12-L-hydroxy-5,8,10,14-eicosatetraenoic acid in human polymorphonuclear leukocytes. J Biol Chem 1984; 259:2683–2686.
65. Marcus AJ, Safier LB, Ullman HL, Broekman MJ, Islam N, Oglesby TD, Gorman RR. 12S,20-dihydroxyeicosatetraenoic acid: a new eicosanoid produced by thrombin- or collagen-stimulated platelets. Proc Natl Acad Sci USA 1984; 81:903–907.
66. Sumimoto H, Isobe R, Mizukami Y, Minakami S. Formation of novel 20-hydroxylated metabolite of lipoxin A_4 by human neutrophil microsomes. FEBS Lett 1993; 315:205–210.
67. Verkade PE, Elzas M, Lee J, Wolff MH. Untersuchungen über den Fettstoffwechsel. Proc Roy Acad Sci Amsterdam 1932; 35:251–266.

68. Laethem RM, Balazy M, Koop DR. Epoxidation of unsaturated fatty acids by cytochromes P450 2C2 and P450 2CAA. Drug Metab Dispos 1996; 24:664–668.

69. Wang MH, Stec DE, Balazy M, Mastyugin V, Yang CS, Roman RJ, Schwartzman ML. Cloning, sequencing, and cDNA-directed expression of the rat renal CYP4A2: Arachidonic acid ω-hydroxylation and 11,12-epoxidation by CYP4A2 protein. Arch Biochem Biophys 1996; 336:240–250.

70. Graham-Lorence S, Truan G, Peterson JA, Falck JR, Wei S, Helvig C, Capdevila JH. An active site substitution, F87V, converts cytochrome P450 BM-3 into a regio- and stereoselective (14S,15R)-arachidonic acid epoxygenase. J Biol Chem 1997; 272:1127–1135.

71. Balazy M. Peroxynitrite and arachidonic acid. Identification of arachidonate epoxides. Pol J Pharmacol 1994; 46:593–600.

72. Chacos N, Capdevila J, Falck JR, Manna S. The reaction of arachidonic acid epoxides with cytosolic epoxide hydrolase. Arch Biochem Biophys 1983; 223:639 648.

73. Capdevila JH, Wei S, Yan J, Karara A, Jacobson HR, Falck JR, Guengerich FP, DuBois RN. Cytochrome P-450 arachidonic acid epoxygenase. J Biol Chem 1992; 267:21720–21726.

74. Catella F, Lawson JA, Fitzgerald DJ, FitzGerald GA. Endogenous biosynthesis of arachidonic acid epoxides in human: Increased formation in pregnancy-induced hypertension. Proc Natl Acad Sci USA 1990; 87:5893–5897.

75. Catella F, Lawson JA, Fitzgerald DJ, Shipp E, FitzGerald GA. Biosynthesis of P450 products of arachidonic acid in human: Increased formation in cardiovascular disease. Adv Prostaglandin Thromboxane Leukot Res 1991; 21:193–196.

76. Spearman ME, Prough RA, Estabrook RW, Falck JR, Manna S, Murphy RC, Capdevila J. Novel glutathione conjugates formed from epoxyeicosatriencoic acids (EETs). Arch Biochem Biophys 1985; 242:225–230.

77. Oliw EH. Metabolism of 5(6) epoxyeicosatrienoic acid by ram seminal vesicles. Biochim Biophys Acta 1984; 793:408–415.

78. Carroll MA, Balazy M, Margiotta P, Falck JR, McGiff JC. Renal vasodilator activity of 5,6-epoxyeicosatrienoic acid depends upon conversion by cyclooxygenase and release of prostaglandins. J Biol Chem 1993; 268:12260–12266.

79. Balazy M. Metabolism of 5,6-epoxyeicosatetraenoic acid by the human platelet. J Biol Chem 1991; 266:23561–23567.

80. Fulton D, Balazy M, McGiff JC, Quilley J. Possible contribution of platelet cyclooxygenase to the renal vascular action of 5,6-epoxyeicosatrienoic acid. J Pharmacol Exp Ther 1996; 277:1195–1199.

81. Zhang JY, Prakash, Yamashita K, Blair IA. Regiospecific and enantioselective metabolism of 8,9-epoxyeicosatrienoic acid by cyclooxygenase. Biochem Biophys Res Commun 1992; 183:138–143.

82. Oliw EH, Lawson JA, Brash AR, Oates JA. Arachidonic acid metabolism in rabbit renal cortex. J Biol Chem 1981; 256:9924–9930.

83. Falck JR, Lumin S, Blair I, Dishman E, Martin MV, Waxman DJ, Guengerich FP, Capdevila JH. Cytochrome P-450-dependent oxidation of arachidonic acid to 16-, 17-, and 18-hydroxyeicosatetraenoic acids. J Biol Chem 1990; 265:10244–10249.

84. Brash AR, Boeglin WE, Capdevila JH, Yeola S, Blair IA. 7-HETE, 10-HETE and 13-HETE are major products of NADPH-dependent arachidonic acid metabolism

in rat liver microsomes: Analysis of their stereochemistry, and stereochemistry of their acid-catalyzed rearrangement. Arch Biochem Biophys 1995; 321: 485–492.

85. Schwartzman ML, Balazy M, Masferrer J, Abraham NG, McGiff JC, Murphy RC. 12(R)-hydroxyeicosatetraenoic acid: a cytochrome P450-dependent arachidonate metabolite that inhibits Na^+,K^+-ATPase in the cornea. Proc Natl Acad Sci USA 1987; 84:8125–8129.

86. Macica C, Balazy M, Falck JR, Mioskowski C, Carroll MA. Characterization of cytochrome P450-dependent arachidonic acid metabolism in rabbit intestine. Am J Physiol 1993; 265:G735–G741.

87. Zhu Y, Schieber EB, McGiff JC, Balazy M. Identification of arachidonate P-450 metabolites in human platelet phospholipids. Hypertension 1995; 25(part 2):854–859.

88. Carroll MA, Balazy M, Huang DD, Rybalova S, Falck JR, McGiff JC. Cytochrome P450-derived renal HETEs. Kidney Int 1997; 51:1696–1702.

89. Lu M, Zhu Y, Balazy M, Reddy KM, Falck JR, Wang WH. Effect of angiotensin II on the apical K^+ channel in the thick ascending limb of the rat kidney. J Gen Physiol 1996; 108:537–547.

90. Takizawa H, Balazy M, Zhu Y, Falck JR, Nasjletti A. 20-hydroxyeicosatetraenoic acid (20-HETE) mediates renal vasoconstriction in rats. (abstr). J Hypertension 1996; 14(Suppl):S39, P144.

91. Hatzelman A, Ullrich V. The ω-hydroxylation of arachidonic acid by human polymorphonuclear leukocytes. Eur J Biochem 1988; 173:445–452.

92. Bednar MM, Gross CE, Belosludtsev Y, Catella DT, Zhang CD, Falck JR, Balazy M. 16(R)Hydroxy-5,8,11,14-eicosatetraenoic acid. A new arachidonate metabolite in human polymorphonuclear leukocytes. Biochim Biophys Acta (in press).

93. Hill E, Murphy RC. Quantitation of 20-hydroxy-5,8,11,14-eicosatetraenoic acid (20-HETE) produced by human polymorphonuclear leukocytes using electron capture ionization gas chromatography/mass spectrometry. Biol Mass Spectrom 1992; 21:249–253.

94. Sacerdoti D, Balazy M, Angeli P, Gatta A, McGiff JC. Eicosanoid excretion in hepatic cirrhosis: predominance of 20-HETE. J Clin Invest 1997; 100:1264–1270.

95. Schwartzman ML, Falck JR, Yadagiri P, Escalante B. Metabolism of 20-hydroxyeicosatetraenoic acid by cyclooxygenase. J Biol Chem 1989; 264:11658–11662.

96. Hill E, Fitzpatrick F, Murphy RC. Biological activity and metabolism of 20-hydroxyeicosatetraenoic acid in the human platelet. Br J Pharmacol 1992; 106:267–274.

97. Prakash C, Zhang JY, Falck JR, Chauhan K, Blair IA. 20-hydroxyeicosatetraenoic acid is excreted as a glucuronide conjugate in human urine. Biochem Biophys Res Commun 1991; 180:445–449.

98. Escalante B, Erij D, Falck JR, McGiff J. Effect of cytochrome P450 metabolites on ion transport in rabbit kidney loop of Henle. Science 1991; 251:799–802.

99. Smith WL, Fitzpatrick FA. The eicosanoids: Cyclooxygenase, lipoxygenase, and epoxygenase pathways. In: Vance DE, Vance JE, eds. Biochemistry of Lipids, Lipoproteins and Membranes. Amsterdam: Elsevier, 1996:283–308.

100. Carroll MA, Balazy M, McGiff JC. Tubular and vascular actions of cytochrome P450-arachidonate metabolites. J Physiol Pharmacol 1993; 44(Suppl 2):37–49.

101. Wong PY, Lin KT, Yan YT, Ahern D, Iles J, Shen SY, Bhatt RK, Falck JR. 14(R), 15(S)-epoxyeicosatrienoic acid (14(R),15(S)-EET) receptor in guinea pig mononuclear cell membranes. J Lipid Mediat 1993; 6:199–208.

102. Capdevila JH, Kishore V, Dishman E, Blair IA. A novel pool of rat liver inositol and ethanolamine phospholipids contains epoxyeicosatrienoic acids (EETs). Biochem Biophys Res Commun 1987; 146:638–644.

103. Karara A, Dishman E, Falck JR, Capdevila JH. Endogenous epoxyeicosatrienoylphospholipids. J Biol Chem 1991; 266:7561–7569.

104. Karara A, Wei S, Spady D, Swift L, Capdevila JM, Falck JR. Arachidonic acid epoxygenase: structural characterization and quantification of epoxyeicosatrienoates in plasma. Biochem Biophys Res Commun 1992; 182:1320–1325.

105. Balazy M, McGiff JC. The distribution of arachidonate epoxides in rat kidney phospholipids. Am J Hypertension 1995; 8(part 2):114A (abstract).

106. Bernstrom K, Kayganich K, Murphy RC, Fitzpatrick FA. Incorporation and distribution of epoxyeicosatrienoic acids into cellular phospholipids. J Biol Chem 1992; 267:3686–3690.

107. Zhu Y, McGiff JC, Balazy M. Identification of 20-hydroxyeicosatetraenoic acid in rat kidney phospholipids. 43rd ASMS Conference on Mass Spectrometry and Allied Topics, Atlanta, GA, May 21–24, 1995.

108. Zhu Y, Falck JR, McGiff JC, Balazy M. New group of phospholipid mediators in the kidney. 10th International Conference on Prostaglandins and Related Compounds, Vienna, Austria, September 22–27, 1996.

109. Wang W, Lu M, Balazy M, Hebert SC. Phospholipase A_2 is involved in mediating the effect of extracellular Ca^{2+} on apical K^+ channels in rat TAL. Am J Physiol 1997; 273:F421–F429.

110. Spector AA, Gordon JA, Moore SA. Hydroxyeicosatetraenoic acids (HETEs). Prog Lipid Res 1988; 27:271–323.

111. Lund J, Zaphiropoulos PG, Mode A, Warner M, Gustafsson JA. Hormonal regulation of cytochrome P-450 gene expression. Adv Pharm 1991; 22:325–353.

112. Koley AP, Buters JTM, Robinson RC, Markowitz A, Friedman FK. Differential mechanisms of cytochrome P450 inhibition and activation by β napthoflavone. J Biol Chem 1997; 272:3149–3152.

113. Karuzina II, Archakov AI. The oxidative inactivation of cytochrome P450 in monooxygenase reactions. Free Radical Biol Med 1994; 16:73–97.

114. Rosenkranz B, Fischer C, Weimer KE, Frölich JC. Metabolism of prostacyclin and 6-keto-prostaglandin $F_{1\alpha}$ in man. J Biol Chem 1980; 255:10194–10198.

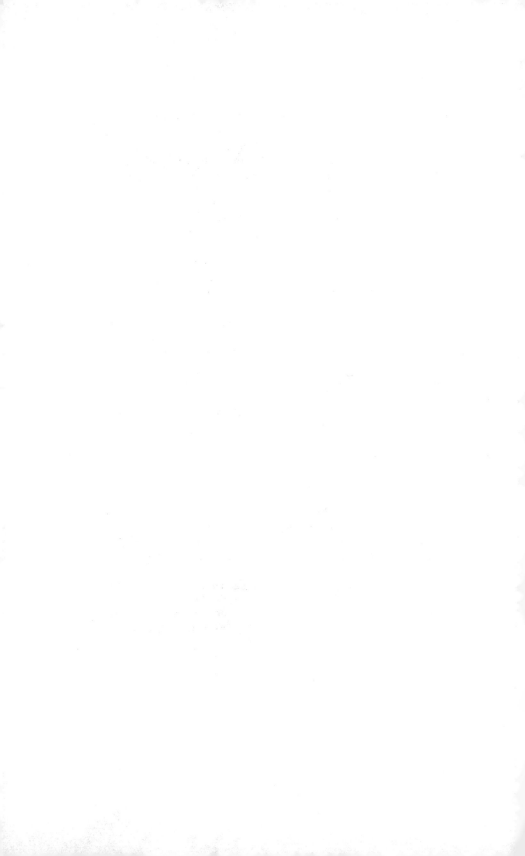

4

Mechanisms of Isoprostane Biosynthesis in Humans

PAOLA PATRIGNANI, ROBERTO PADOVANO, MARIA GINA SCIULLI, GIOVANNA SANTINI, MARIA ROSARIA PANARA, MARIA TERESA ROTONDO, GIULIA RENDA, and CARLO PATRONO

University of Chieti "G. D'Annunzio"
Chieti, Italy

I. Introduction

Isoprostanes represent a newly characterized family of vasoactive eicosanoids that are formed by a noncyclooxygenase, free-radical-catalyzed mechanism involving peroxidation of arachidonic acid (1). A mechanism to explain the formation of these compounds has been suggested by Morrow and Roberts (2) involving the formation of intermediates comprising arachidonoyl peroxyl radical isomers of arachidonic acid, which undergo endocyclization to form bicyclic endoperoxides. Four bicycloendoperoxide PG-like intermediates can be formed, which can be reduced to four PGF_2-like regioisomers. Each of these regioisomers can theoretically be comprised of eight racemic diasteroisomers. Thus, 64 different compounds can be potentially produced by this mechanism that are structurally isomeric with $PGF_{2\alpha}$ and are collectively referred to as F_2-isoprostanes. Factors involved in the reduction of the isoprostane endoperoxide intermediates in vivo, however, remain to be identified. The endoperoxide intermediates may, in part, escape reduction and rearrange to form PGE_2-like and PGD_2-like isoprostanes (3).

Unlike cyclooxygenase-derived prostanoids, F_2-isoprostanes are initially formed in situ on phospholipids, from which they are subsequently released preformed, presumably by phospholipases (4). They circulate in plasma and are excreted in urine. Differently, D_2/E_2-isoprostanes cannot be detected free in the circulation in physiological conditions but large quantities of D_2/E_2-isoprostanes can be detected esterified to tissue lipids that in some tissues exceed levels of F_2-isoprostanes. Studies performed in vitro have shown that D_2/E_2-isoprostanes, once released from tissue lipids, can be converted by cytosolic ketoreductases to F_2-isoprostanes (5). However, the occurrence of this phenomenon in vivo remains to be demonstrated.

Based on the mechanism of formation of isoprostanes, one compound 8-epi-$PGF_{2\alpha}$ (Fig. 1) would be expected to be formed. In fact, the formation of compounds with the side chains oriented *cis* in relation to the cyclopentane ring is highly favored. 8-epi-$PGF_{2\alpha}$ has been demonstrated to be one of the more abundant F_2-isoprostanes produced in vivo in humans (6). It is detectable in plasma in normal conditions both free and esterified (103 ± 19 and 345 ± 65 pmol/L, respectively) (7) and in urine (70 ± 34 pmol/mmol creatinine) (8).

8-epi-$PGF_{2\alpha}$ has attracted considerable attention because of its biological activities. It is a potent vasoconstrictor (1,9) that induces DNA synthesis in vascular smooth muscle cells through the interaction with receptors that are distinct from but closely related to thromboxane (TX)A_2/PGH_2 receptors (10). In fact, TXA_2/PGH_2 receptor antagonists are capable of reversing, at least in part, the constrictor and mitogenic effects of 8-epi-$PGF_{2\alpha}$ in vascular smooth muscle cells both in vitro and in vivo. However, in TXA_2/PGH_2 receptor-transfected COS-7 cells, 8-epi-$PGF_{2\alpha}$ displaced the binding of SQ 29548, a TXA_2/PGH_2 receptor antagonist, very weakly (10). In porcine and bovine coronary arteries, 8-epi-$PGF_{2\alpha}$ is a vasoconstrictor with a potency approximately twice that of $PGF_{2\alpha}$ but 5–20 times lower than U46619, a thromboxane mimetic (11).

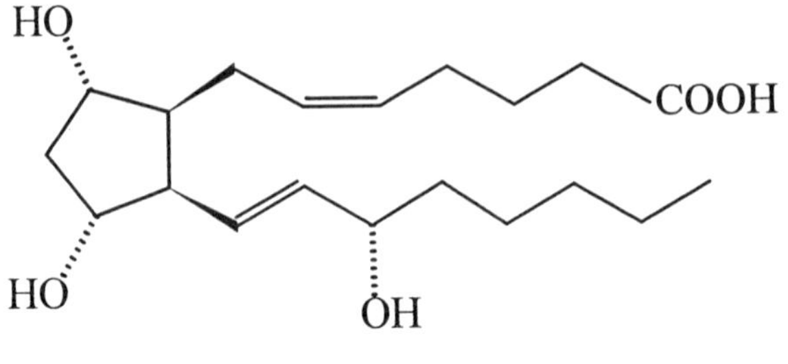

Figure 1   Chemical structure of 8-epi-$PGF_{2\alpha}$.

Several lines of evidence suggest that in human platelets, 8-epi-$PGF_{2\alpha}$ acts as a partial agonist of TXA_2/PGH_2 receptors (12–14): (1) it induces shape change, but not aggregation and the release reaction, that is blocked by SQ 29548; (2) it inhibits TXA_2-dependent aggregation induced by platelet agonists; (3) it potentiates the reversible primary aggregation induced by low doses of ADP.

Quantification of F_2-isoprostanes in urine and plasma may provide stable markers of oxidative reactions in human subjects, as they possess longer half-lives than hydroperoxides and/or reactive oxygen species.

In normal subjects, the urinary excretion of 8-epi-$PGF_{2\alpha}$ has been shown to significantly correlate with increasing age (8). 8-epi-$PGF_{2\alpha}$ excretion was not affected by the administration of two distinct nonsteroidal anti-inflammatory drugs (NSAIDs), aspirin (1 g as a single oral dose) and ibuprofen (400 mg tid, for 4 days) (8).

In addition to age, chronic cigarette smoking is associated with a reversible increase in the circulating plasma levels and urinary excretion of F_2-isoprostanes (7,15), consistent with the hypothesis that smoking can cause the oxidative modification of important biological molecules in vivo. Enhanced urinary excretion of 8-epi-$PGF_{2\alpha}$ in smokers can be suppressed by antioxidant vitamin therapy (15).

The biosynthesis of 8-epi-$PGF_{2\alpha}$ has been demonstrated elevated in several pathological conditions in humans in vivo: (1) type IIa hypercholesterolemia (16); (2) non-insulin-dependent diabetes mellitus (17); (3) hepatorenal syndrome (18).

Due to its biological activities, enhanced formation of 8-epi-$PGF_{2\alpha}$ may provide an aspirin-insensitive mechanism linking lipid peroxidation to amplification of platelet and vascular smooth muscle activation.

In this chapter, we will review the recent studies of 8-epi-$PGF_{2\alpha}$ biosynthesis in human platelets and monocytes in vitro that demonstrated cyclooxygenase-dependent mechanisms of formation. In addition, we will discuss the relevance of enzymatic versus nonenzymatic pathways in the biosynthesis of 8-epi-$PGF_{2\alpha}$ in the settings of platelet and monocyte activation in vivo in humans.

II. Cyclooxygenase-Dependent Formation of 8-epi-$PGF_{2\alpha}$ by Human Blood Cells

Prostaglandin endoperoxide synthase (PGHS) is the first enzyme in the pathway leading from arachidonic acid to prostanoids (PGs and TXs). PGHS is a bifunctional enzyme that exhibits both cyclooxygenase and peroxidase activities (19). It catalyzes the conversion of arachidonic acid to PGG_2 and PGG_2

to PGH$_2$. Two forms of PGHS have been identified. PGHS-1 is a constitutive enzyme present in most tissues including platelets, endothelial cells, and monocytes, whereas PGHS-2 has restricted tissue distribution and is expressed at a very low basal level but is highly inducible in response to mitogenic and inflammatory stimuli (19).

Prostanoid biosynthesis by platelets is dependent on the cyclooxygenase activity of PGHS-1. Recently, Praticò et al. (20), have demonstrated that activation of platelets by threshold concentrations of collagen, thrombin, and arachidonic acid resulted in formation of 8-epi-PGF$_{2\alpha}$ coincident with that of the PGHS-1 product TXB$_2$ and the 12-lipoxygenase product, 12-hydroxyeicosatetraenoic acid, as detected by selected ion monitoring assay using gas chromatography/mass spectrometry. The effect appeared selective for 8-epi-PGF$_{2\alpha}$ among the F$_2$-isoprostanes. The formation of 8-epi-PGF$_{2\alpha}$ was abolished by pretreatment of platelets with aspirin or indomethacin. 8-epi-PGF$_{2\alpha}$ represented only a minor product of the cyclooxygenase activity of platelets. In fact, activated platelets generated 8-epi-PGF$_{2\alpha}$ and TXB$_2$ in a molar ratio of approximately 1:1000.

However, the biosynthesis of 8-epi-PGF$_{2\alpha}$ in a PGHS-1-dependent fashion appears to contribute negligibly to the global formation of this prostanoid in vivo, as suggested by the failure of NSAIDs to depress urinary 8-epi-PGF$_{2\alpha}$ excretion in healthy subjects (8) as well as in patients with acute ischemic stroke (21), a condition associated with episodic platelet activation.

We have recently developed a radioimmunoassay for 8-epi-PGF$_{2\alpha}$ that was validated by direct and indirect comparison with other analytical procedures, i.e., enzyme immunoassay and gas chromatography/mass spectrometry (8). This assay has been applied to evaluate the biosynthesis of 8-epi-PGF$_{2\alpha}$ in human blood cells in vitro.

The endotoxin lipopolysaccharide (LPS) is a well-known stimulus for the cyclooxygenase activity of different cell types. LPS can induce a rapid release of arachidonic acid from membrane phospholipids (22) that could be utilized by the constitutive PGHS-1 to produce prostanoids. However, in monocytes, PGE$_2$ formation in response to LPS occurred after a lag time of several hours (23 and Fig. 2B) that correlated with the induction of a novel protein of approximately 72–74 kDa analyzed by Western blot (23 and Fig. 3) using specific rabbit polyclonal antibodies directed against the 19-amino-acid peptide derived from a unique region of PGHS-2 protein near the carboxyl-terminal (24) that is not present in PGHS-1. In contrast, unstimulated human monocytes contained only the PGHS-1 protein that was not significantly induced by LPS (10 μg/ml) up to 24 hr (Fig. 3). As shown in Figure 4, at 24 hr, LPS (0.01–10 μg/ml) stimulated PGE$_2$ formation by isolated human monocytes in a dose-dependent fashion that correlated with the mass of monocyte PGHS-2 analyzed by Western blot using specific anti-PGHS-2 antibodies. These results suggest

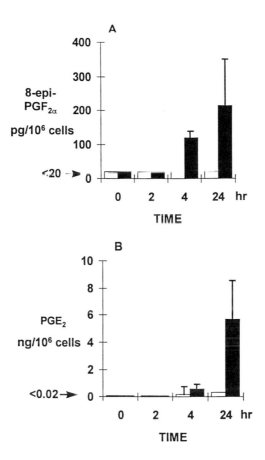

Figure 2 Time course of 8-epi-PGF$_{2\alpha}$ and PGE$_2$ production by LPS-stimulated human monocytes: 1 ml human monocyte suspension (3×10^6 cells) was incubated with saline (□) or LPS (10 μg/ml) (■) for 24 hr at 37°C. Supernatants were assayed for 8-epi-PGF$_{2\alpha}$ (A) and PGE$_2$ (B) by specific radioimmunoassay techniques.

that the formation of prostanoids by LPS-stimulated monocytes involves the cyclooxygenase activity of the inducible PGHS-2 but not of the constitutive PGHS-1. In accordance with our results, Reddy and Herschman (25) have recently demonstrated that PGHS-2 expression is necessary for endotoxin-induced prostanoid biosynthesis in macrophages. PGHS-1 present in these cells cannot utilize arachidonic acid released in response to endotoxin.

We have investigated whether 8-epi-PGF$_{2\alpha}$ formation is associated with the induction of PGHS-2 in human monocytes in response to LPS. We studied

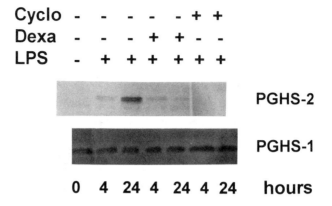

Figure 3 Effects of dexamethasone and cycloheximide on PGHS isozyme biosynthesis by LPS-stimulated human monocytes: 1 ml human monocyte suspension (3×10^6 cells) was incubated with saline or LPS ($10 \mu g/ml$) for 4 and 24 hr at 37°C both in the absence and in the presence of dexamethasone (Dexa, $2 \mu M$) or cycloheximide (Cyclo, $10 \mu g/ml$). Monocytes were lysed and proteins were analyzed by SDS-polyacrylamide gel electrophoresis and immunoblotting techniques using rabbit antibodies directed against PGHS-1 or the carboxyl-terminal of PGHS-2. Equal amounts of proteins ($10 \mu g$) were loaded in all lanes. Immune complexes were visualized by incubating the membranes with anti-rabbit IgG conjugated with horseradish peroxidase for 1 hr at room temperature. ECL substrates were used to reveal positive bands that were visualized after exposure to Hyperfilm ELC (Amersham).

the pharmacological modulation of monocyte 8-epi-PGF$_{2\alpha}$ formation by inhibitors of PGHS-2 biosynthesis (dexamethasone and cycloheximide) and a selective inhibitor of the cyclooxygenase activity of PGHS-2, 5-methanesulphonamido-6-(2,4-difluorothiophenyl)-1-indanone (L-745,337) (26,27).

Heparinized whole-blood samples were drawn from healthy volunteers, 48 hr following oral dosing with aspirin 300 mg to suppress platelet cyclooxygenase activity. One-milliliter aliquots were incubated with LPS (0.5–$50 \mu g/ml$) for 0–24 hr at 37°C. PGE$_2$ and 8-epi-PGF$_{2\alpha}$ were measured in separated plasma by previously validated radioimmunoassay techniques (7,8). Levels of both eicosanoids were undetectable (i.e., <60 pg/ml) at time 0. LPS ($10 \mu g/ml$) induced the formation of PGE$_2$ and 8-epi-PGF$_{2\alpha}$ in a time-dependent fashion. A lag time of several hours was required to detect both 8-epi-PGF$_{2\alpha}$ and PGE$_2$ in the medium of LPS-stimulated whole blood. At 24 hr of incubation, PGE$_2$ and 8-epi-PGF$_{2\alpha}$ production was significantly increased versus saline control. PGE$_2$ and 8-epi-PGF$_{2\alpha}$ averaged $10,480 \pm 4643$ and 295 ± 140 pg/ml (mean $\pm$ SD, $n = 6$), respectively. The production of PGE$_2$ and 8-epi-PGF$_{2\alpha}$ by LPS was dose-dependent. Enhanced prostanoid formation at 24 hr was associated

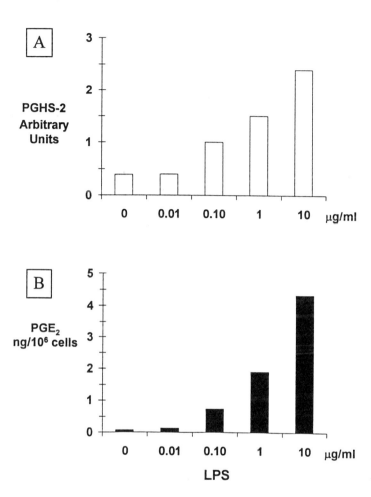

Figure 4 Dose-response curves for PGHS-2 expression and PGE_2 production in isolated human monocytes incubated with LPS: 1 ml human monocyte suspension (3×10^6 cells) was incubated with LPS (0.01–$10 \mu g/ml$) for 24 hr at 37°C. Supernatants were assayed for PGE_2 (B) by a specific radioimmunoassay technique. Monocytes were lysed and proteins were analyzed by SDS-polyacrylamide gel electrophoresis and immunoblotting techniques using rabbit antibodies directed against the carboxyl-terminal of PGHS-2 (A). Immune complexes were visualized by incubating the membranes with anti-rabbit IgG conjugated with horseradish peroxidase for 1 hr at room temperature. ECL substrates were used to reveal positive bands that were visualized after exposure to Hyperfilm ECL (Amersham). Protein bands were quantified on the film by densitometry using a Bio-Rad densitometer.

with the induction of a protein of approximately 72 kDa in lymphomonocytes analyzed by Western blot technique using anti-PGHS-1 antibodies (23).

To evaluate whether LPS-induced production of PGE_2 and 8-epi-$PGF_{2\alpha}$ in whole blood was dependent on newly synthesized PGHS-2 expressed by blood cells, we studied the effects of dexamethasone that has been reported to inhibit PGHS-2 biosynthesis. Dexamethasone ($2\,\mu M$) suppressed PGE_2 and 8-epi-$PGF_{2\alpha}$ production in LPS-stimulated whole blood by more than 80%.

Since dexamethasone might also affect prostanoid biosynthesis by inhibiting the release of arachidonic acid from membrane phospholipids and isoprostane release is dependent on phospholipase activity, we studied the effects of L-745,337, a selective inhibitor of the cyclooxygenase activity of human monocyte PGHS-2. L-745,337 inhibited PGE_2 and 8-epi-$PGF_{2\alpha}$ production in LPS-stimulated whole blood with similar dose-response curves (IC_{50} for PGE_2 and 8-epi-$PGF_{2\alpha}$ 1.6 and $1\,\mu M$, respectively), thus suggesting that 8-epi-$PGF_{2\alpha}$ formation is dependent on the cyclooxygenase activity of PGHS-2 in these circumstances.

Studies on isolated monocytes, lymphocytes, and neutrophils demonstrated that only monocytes respond to LPS by releasing PGE_2 and 8-epi-$PGF_{2\alpha}$ in a time-dependent fashion that was dependent on the expression of PGHS-2. In Figure 2A, the time-dependent formation of 8-epi-$PGF_{2\alpha}$ and PGE_2 by isolated human monocytes in response to LPS ($10\,\mu g/ml$) is shown.

To demonstrate that the production of PGE_2 and 8-epi-$PGF_{2\alpha}$ by isolated monocytes was dependent on the induction of PGHS-2 in response to LPS, we studied the effects of dexamethasone and cycloheximide. As shown in Figure 5, after 4 and 24 hr of incubation with LPS ($10\,\mu g/ml$), dexamethasone ($2\,\mu M$) and cycloheximide ($10\,\mu g/ml$) profoundly suppressed the production of both PGE_2 and 8-epi-$PGF_{2\alpha}$. The induction of the monocyte PGHS-2 protein was correspondingly suppressed by dexamethasone and cycloheximide (Fig. 3). Dexamethasone and cycloheximide had no detectable effect on the expression of monocyte PGHS-1 (Fig. 3).

Overall, these results suggest that the formation of 8-epi-$PGF_{2\alpha}$ by LPS-stimulated monocytes involves the cyclooxygenase activity of the inducible PGHS-2 but not of the constitutive PGHS-1.

To study whether the mechanism of formation of 8-epi-$PGF_{2\alpha}$ involved the generation of free radicals associated with the catalytic activity of PGHS-2 and consequently via the formation of peroxyl radical isomers, we evaluated the effects of the incubation of LPS-stimulated monocytes for 24 hr with three structurally distinct radical scavengers, vitamin E, mannitol, and deoxyribose, on the formation of PGE_2 and 8-epi-$PGF_{2\alpha}$. As shown in Table 1, the antioxidants failed to inhibit the formation of both PGE_2 and 8-epi-$PGF_{2\alpha}$.

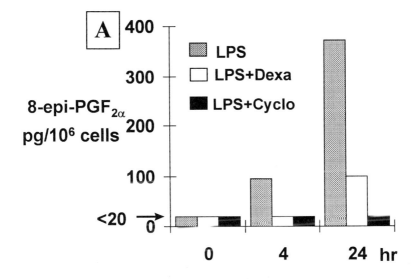

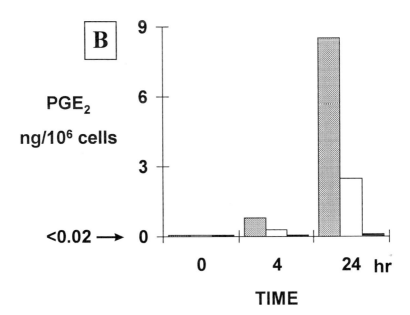

Figure 5 Effects of dexamethasone and cycloheximide on 8-epi-PGF$_{2\alpha}$ and PGE$_2$ production by LPS-stimulated human monocytes: 1 ml human monocyte suspension (3×10^6 cells) was incubated with LPS ($10 \mu g/ml$) for 4 and 24 hr at 37°C both in the absence and in the presence of dexamethasone (Dexa, $2 \mu M$) or cycloheximide (Cyclo, $10 \mu g/ml$). Supernatants were assayed for 8-epi-PGF$_{2\alpha}$ (A) and PGE$_2$ (B) by specific radioimmunoassay techniques.

Table 1 Effects of the Antioxidants Vitamin E, Mannitol, and Deoxyribose on PGE_2 and 8-epi-$PGF_{2\alpha}$ Formation in Isolated Human Monocytes Incubated for 24 hr with LPS (10 μg/ml)

Addition to monocytes	8-epi-$PGF_{2\alpha}$ (pg/10^6 cells)	PGE_2 (pg/10^6 cells)
LPS (10 μg/ml)	97 ± 41	3400 ± 1300
LPS + vitamin E (500 μM)	108 ± 44	3700 ± 2000
LPS + mannitol (5 mM)	102 ± 48	4100 ± 2200
LPS + deoxyribose (5 mM)	101 ± 50	3000 ± 1400

Values are mean ± SD, $n = 3$.

Recently, Praticò et al. (28), demonstrated the formation of PGE_2, TXB_2, and 8-epi-$PGF_{2\alpha}$ but not other F_2-isoprostanes by human monocytes in response to concanavalin A, the phorbol ester PMA, and LPS that was dependent on the cyclooxygenase activity of induced PGHS-2. Differently, monocytes stimulated with opsonized zymosan in the presence of low-density lipoprotein (LDL) produced 8-epi-$PGF_{2\alpha}$ and other F_2-isoprostanes but not PGE_2 or TXB_2 in a free-radical manner.

The formation of 8-epi-$PGF_{2\alpha}$ by a cyclooxygenase-dependent mechanism has been previously reported by others. Corey et al. (29) proposed a schema in which 8-epi-$PGF_{2\alpha}$ might be formed via the correspondent endoperoxide by a biomimetic cyclization, and Hecker et al. (30) demonstrated that 8-epi-$PGF_{2\alpha}$ is a product of the ram seminal vesicle PGHS.

Thus, three distinct mechanisms of F_2-isoprostane biosynthesis have been characterized in humans: (1) free-radical-catalyzed lipid peroxidation; (2) platelet PGHS-1, and (3) monocyte PGHS-2.

III. Conclusions

Several factors have been identified that can influence the rate of F_2-isoprostane biosynthesis in humans. These include chronic cigarette smoking, age, and complex metabolic disturbances. In addition, the potential for a cyclooxygenase-dependent component in F_2-isoprostane biosynthesis should be considered in the setting of platelet and monocyte activation. Although indirect pharmacological evidence suggests that free-radical-catalyzed lipid peroxidation is the prevailing mechanism of 8-epi-$PGF_{2\alpha}$ biosynthesis in healthy subjects, the relative contribution of the other mechanisms in various pathophysiological settings remains to be investigated. Thus, analytical measurements of 8-epi-$PGF_{2\alpha}$ excretion, as an index of in vivo lipid peroxidation, should take these novel findings into account and require rigorous testing of the underlying assumption.

References

1. Morrow JD, Hill KE, Burk RF, Nanmour TM, Badr KF, Roberts LJ II. A series of prostaglandin F_2-like compounds are produced in vivo in humans by a non-cyclooxygenase, free radical-catalyzed mechanism. Proc Natl Acad Sci USA 1990; 87:9383–9387.
2. Morrow JD, Roberts LJ II. The isoprostanes. Current knowledge and directions for future research. Biochem Pharmacol 1996; 51:1–9.
3. Morrow JD, Minton TA, Mukundan CR, Campbell MD, Zackert WE, Daniel VC, Badr KF, Blair IA, Roberts LJ II. Free radical-induced generation of isoprostanes in vivo. Evidence for the formation of D-ring and E-ring isoprostanes. J Biol Chem 1994; 269:4317–4326.
4. Morrow JD, Awad JA, Boss HJ, Blair IA, Roberts LJ II. Non-cyclooxygenase-derived prostanoids (F_2-isoprostanes) are formed in situ on phospholipids. Proc Natl Acad Sci USA 1992; 89:10721–10725.
5. Roberts LJ II, Morrow JD. The isoprostanes: novel markers of lipid peroxidation and potential mediators of oxidant injury. Adv Prostaglandin Thromboxane Leukot Res 1995; 23:219–224.
6. Morrow JD, Minton TA, Badr KF, Roberts LJ II. Evidence that the F_2-isoprostane, 8-epi-prostaglandin $F_{2\alpha}$, is formed in vivo. Biochim Biophys Acta 1994; 1210:244–248.
7. Morrow JD, Frei B, Longmire AW, Gaziano JM, Lynch SM, Shyr Y, Strauss WE, Oates JA, Roberts LJ II. Increase in circulating products of lipid peroxidation (F_2-isoprostanes) in smokers. Smoking as a cause of oxidative damage. N Engl J Med 1995; 332:1198–1203.
8. Wang Z, Ciabattoni G, Créminon C, Lawson J, FitzGerald GA, Patrono C, Maclouf J. Immunological characterization of urinary 8-epi-prostaglandin $F_{2\alpha}$ excretion in man. J Pharmacol Exp Ther 1995; 275:94–100.
9. Banerjee M, Kang KH, Morrow JD, Roberts LJ II, Newman JH. Effects of a novel prostaglandin, 8-epi-$PGF_{2\alpha}$, in rabbit lune in situ. Am J Physiol 1992; 263:H660–H663.
10. Fukunaga M, Makita N, Roberts LJ II, Morrow JD, Takahashi K, Badr KF. Evidence for the existence of F_2-isoprostane receptors on rat vascular smooth muscle cells. Am J Physiol 1993; 264:C1619–C1624.
11. Kromer BM, Tippins JR. Coronary artery constriction by the isoprostane 8-epi-prostaglandin $F_{2\alpha}$. Br J Pharmacol 1996; 119:1276–1280.
12. Morrow JD, Minton TA, Roberts LJ II. The F_2-isoprostane, 8-epi-$PGF_{2\alpha}$, a potent agonist of the vascular thromboxane/endoperoxide receptor, is a platelet thromboxane/endoperoxide receptor antagonist. Prostaglandins 1992; 44:155–163.
13. Yin K, Halushka PV, Yan YT, Wong PY. Antiaggregatory activity of 8-epi-prostaglandin $F_{2\alpha}$ and other F-series prostanoids and their binding to thromboxane A_2-/prostaglandin H_2 receptors in human platelets. J Pharmacol Exp Ther 1994; 270:1192–1196.

14. Praticò D, Smyth E, Violi F, FitzGerald GA. Local amplification of platelet function by 8-epi-$PGF_{2\alpha}$ is not modulated by thromboxane receptor isoforms. J Biol Chem 1996; 271:14916–14924.
15. Reilly M, Delanty N, Lawson JA, FitzGerald GA. Modulation of oxidant stress in vivo in chronic cigarette smoking. Circulation 1996; 94:19–25.
16. Alessandrini P, Bittolo Bon G, Bucciarelli A, Ciabattoni G, Costantini F, Davì G, De Cesare D, Mezzetti A, Minotti G, Patrono C. Vitamin E inhibits enhanced F_2-isoprostane biosynthesis in type IIa hypercholesterolemia. J Invest Med 1996; 44:224A (abstract).
17. Gopaul NK, Anggard EE, Mallet AI, Betteridge DJ, Wolff SP, Nourooz-Zadeh J. Plasma 8-epi-$PGF_{2\alpha}$ levels are elevated in individuals with non-insulin dependent diabetes mellitus. FEBS Lett 1995; 368:225–229.
18. Morrow JD, Moore KP, Awad JA, Ravenscraft MD, Marini G, Badr KF, Williams R, Roberts LJ II. Marked overproduction of non-cyclooxygenase derived prostanoids (F_2-isoprostanes) in the hepatorenal syndrome. J Lipid Mediat 1993; 6:417–420.
19. Smith WL, Garavito RM, DeWitt DL. Prostaglandin endoperoxide II synthases (cyclooxygenases)-1 and -2. J Biol Chem 1996; 271:33157–33160.
20. Praticò D, Lawson JA, FitzGerald GA. Cyclooxygenase-dependent formation of the isoprostane 8-epi-prostaglandin $F_{2\alpha}$. J Biol Chem 1995; 270:9800–9808.
21. Ciabattoni G, Patrono C, van Kooten F, Koudstaal PJ. Dissociation of platelet activation and lipid peroxidation in acute ischemic stroke. J Invest Med 1995; 43:292A (abstract).
22. Brown GP, Monik MM, Hunninghake GW. Human alveolar macrophage arachidonic acid metabolism. Am J Physiol 1988; 254:C809–C815.
23. Patrignani P, Panara MR, Greco A, Fusco O, Natoli C, Iacobelli S, Cipollone F, Ganci A, Créminon C, Maclouf J, Patrono C. Biochemical and pharmacological characterization of the cyclooxygenase activity of human blood prostaglandin endoperoxide synthases. J Pharmacol Exp Ther 1994; 271:1705–1712.
24. Habib A, Créminon C, Frobert Y, Grassi J, Pradelles P, Maclouf J. Demonstration of an inducible cyclooxygenase in human endothelial cells using antibodies raised against the carboxyl-terminal region of the cyclooxygenase-2. J Biol Chem 1993; 268:23448–23454.
25. Reddy ST, Herschman HR. Ligand-induced prostaglandin synthesis requires expression of the TIS10/PGS-2 prostaglandin synthase gene in murine fibroblasts and macrophages. J Biol Chem 1994; 269:15473–15480.
26. Panara MR, Greco A, Santini G, Sciulli MG, Rotondo MT, Padovano R, di Giamberardino M, Cipollone F, Cuccurullo F, Patrono C, Patrignani P. Effects of the novel anti-inflammatory compounds, N-[2-(cyclohexyloxy)-4-nitrophenyl]methanesulphonamide (NS-398) and 5-methanesulphonamido-6-(2,4-difluorothiophenyl)-1-indanone (L745,337), on the cyclo-oxygenase activity of human blood prostaglandin endoperoxide synthases. Br J Pharmacol 1995; 116:2429–2434.
27. Patrignani P, Santini G, Panara MR, Sciulli MG, Greco A, Rotondo MT, di Giamberardino M, Maclouf J, Ciabattoni G, Patrono C. Induction of prostaglandin endoperoxide synthase-2 in human monocytes associated with cyclo-oxygenase-dependent F_2-isoprostane formation. Br J Pharmacol 1996; 118:1285–1293.

28. Praticò D, FitzGerald GA. Generation of 8 epi-prostaglandin $F_{2\alpha}$ by human monocytes: Discriminant production by reactive oxygen species and prostaglandin endoperoxide synthase-2. J Biol Chem 1996; 271:8919–8924.
29. Corey EJ, Shih C, Shih N-Y, Shimoji K. Preferential formation of 8-epi-prostaglandin $F_{2\alpha}$ via the corresponding endoperoxide by a biomimetic cyclization. Tetrahedron Lett 1984; 25:5013–5016.
30. Hecker M, Ullrich V, Fisher C, Meese CO. Identification of novel arachidonic acid metabolites formed by prostaglandin H synthase. Eur J Biochem 1987; 169:113–123.

5

Intracellular Localization of Eicosanoid-Forming Enzymes

THOMAS G. BROCK and MARC PETERS-GOLDEN

University of Michigan
Ann Arbor, Michigan

I. Introduction

The eicosanoids are a structurally and functionally diverse group of metabolites of arachidonic acid (AA). The two best-studied groups of eicosanoids, those produced by the lipoxygenase and cyclooxygenase pathways, serve important regulatory roles both in normal cell functions and in the pathogenesis of a variety of inflammatory and immune processes. Furthermore, certain products of the 5-lipoxygenase pathway, the cysteinyl leukotrienes (1,2), as well as products of the cyclooxygenase pathway (3,4), are important in the pathogenesis of aspirin-induced asthma.

The basic pathways of eicosanoid formation have been recognized for many years. The substrate, AA, was known to be released from the sn-2 position of membrane phospholipids by phospholipase A_2 (PLA_2). Free AA could be converted to prostaglandin H_2 (PGH_2) by cyclooxygenase (COX) and further processed enzymatically to generate a variety of prostaglandins (PGs). Alternatively, free AA could be converted by 5-lipoxygenase (5-LO), in concert with the 5-LO activating protein (FLAP), to give leukotriene A_4 (LTA_4), which in turn could be enzymatically converted to assorted leukotrienes (LTs).

Because AA was known to be derived from cell membranes, and because its bioactive products were efficiently secreted from cells, it was generally assumed that the enzymes involved in both AA release and metabolism acted at or close to the plasma membrane. Furthermore, a change in the amount of eicosanoid produced by a given cell was generally assumed to result from either a change in the amount of a key enzyme (e.g., PLA_2, COX, 5-LO, or FLAP) or a change in enzyme activity (e.g., as a result of phosphorylation of PLA_2).

During the past few years, much has been learned about the intracellular localization of the enzymes involved in AA metabolism and eicosanoid production. A number of surprising findings have challenged the long-held assumptions noted above. In so doing, they have added greatly to our understanding of eicosanoid formation and have also raised a variety of novel questions that could not heretofore have been entertained. In this chapter, we will (1) discuss the methodological and conceptual complexities that must be considered if enzyme localization is to be understood; (2) review our current knowledge about the localization of the major enzymes involved in eicosanoid formation; and (3) discuss the potential consequences, both metabolic and nonmetabolic, of these new insights.

II. Researching Enzyme Localization

Our understanding of eicosanoid-forming enzymes, their actions, interactions, and localizations, is limited in part by methodological complexities. As one approach to determining localization, either enzyme activity or immunoreactive protein may be assayed in subcellular fractions prepared by any of a variety of methods that preserve the integrity of specific subcellular pools. Unfortunately, early studies examined these enzymes in whole-cell or tissue lysates, in crude subcellular fractions obtained by harsh techniques that disrupt intracellular membranes and structures, or only after subcellular fractions believed to be irrelevant (e.g., nuclei) were discarded. As a result, subtle aspects of intracellular distribution were missed. Improved fractionation schemes, combined with the use of marker proteins, have yielded better results; however, even under the best of circumstances data derived from cell fractionation can be compromised by population heterogeneity and intermixing of fractions. As an alternative to studying cell populations, individual cells may be evaluated directly by a variety of techniques. Immunoelectron microscopy has been used effectively for the localization of membrane-associated enzymes (5), and has also been applied to enzymes associated with cytosolic lipid bodies (6,7). However, this method has proven inadequate for detecting soluble proteins, presumably because of substantial losses resulting from sample fixation, sectioning, and washing (8). Immunocytochemistry and immunofluorescent microscopy have permitted the detection of soluble proteins, but these methods will also underestimate protein amounts because the permeabilization step that enhances the penetration of antibody into intracellular compartments will also allow a concomitant loss of protein. Because both approaches have their limitations, the complementary use of both cell fractionation and direct visualization techniques is desirable. Finally, the very process of removal of a cell from its environment, for study in vitro by any of the above methods, may alter enzyme distribution. As a result, it may be ideal to also attempt to evaluate the intracellular distribution of an enzyme in situ using immunohistochemical methods.

The issue of localization of the eicosanoid-forming enzymes is complicated further by a number of unanticipated features of these enzymes themselves. A given enzyme can exist in any of a number of different subcellular sites. Soluble pools can exist in the cytoplasm or the nucleoplasm, as well as within other membrane-delimited compartments. Bound pools could be associated with a variety of membrane surfaces, cytoskeletal or nuclear structures, DNA or lipid bodies. These pools may differ functionally, perhaps because of differences in enzyme conformation, degree of activation, or substrate availability. Different isoforms of a given enzyme may exist, and these could differ in spatial distribution. Further, pools can shift in response to external conditions, leading to significant changes in localization and function. For eicosanoid-forming enzymes, each of these possibilities has been recognized.

III. Enzyme Locales: Our Current Understanding

A. The Phospholipases A_2

The subcellular distribution of AA is certainly relevant to eicosanoid formation. AA can be found in all cell membranes. Intuitively, the plasma membrane would be expected to be the site of selective AA release for eicosanoid generation and secretion. However, early studies in mouse fibrosarcoma cells showed that the capacity for release and metabolism of recently incorporated AA correlated best with its presence in phospholipids of the nuclear envelope (9). These results suggested that membranes other than the plasma membrane could be important in eicosanoid formation.

The release of AA from phospholipids is achieved by the action of the PLA_2 enzymes, which, by definition, hydrolyze fatty acids preferentially from the *sn*-2 position. This release can occur both constitutively, as part of normal cellular "housekeeping," and inducibly, upon cell stimulation. An understanding of the regulation of AA release has been complicated by the existence of multiple forms of PLA_2, which can coexist within a given cell. These different gene products have been identified and characterized by biochemical, immunological, and molecular approaches. Although other forms are known, the best characterized are cytosolic PLA_2, the secretory PLA_2s, and the calcium-independent PLA_2s.

The so-called "cytosolic" PLA_2, or $cPLA_2$, appears to be a single protein, approximately 85 kDa in size, with biochemical characteristics that make it an ideal candidate to mediate agonist-stimulated intracellular AA release: it preferentially hydrolyzes AA, is activated by calcium at levels observed during cell stimulation (nM to low μM), and is resistant to reducing agents that are abundant intracellularly (10). In fact, $cPLA_2$ action has been implicated in eicosanoid formation in a number of experimental systems (e.g., 11–13).

As suggested by its name, $cPLA_2$ is localized primarily in the cytosol of resting cells (14); upon cell stimulation, it becomes membrane-bound (15). Initially, this membrane association was demonstrated by crude fractionation techniques that pooled different cell membranes; it was simply assumed that $cPLA_2$ acted at the plasma membrane. However, recent studies using appropriate disruption and fractionation techniques, as well as direct cell imaging, have revealed that $cPLA_2$ is localized primarily at the nuclear envelope and, to a lesser extent, the contiguous endoplasmic reticulum (ER) following cell stimulation (11,16–18). Membrane association is mediated by a calcium-dependent lipid-binding domain on $cPLA_2$ that is structurally similar to that on protein kinase C (19); however, it is unclear why $cPLA_2$ is preferentially targeted to the nuclear membrane. Phosphorylation of $cPLA_2$ can be triggered by a variety of agonists; phosphorylation is neither required for, nor the cause of, membrane association, although it does increase enzyme activity (e.g., 20,21). The consequence of the translocation of $cPLA_2$ to the nuclear envelope is the selective release of AA from that site (18). Prior or concomitant phosphorylation of $cPLA_2$ will enhance this result.

Remarkably, $cPLA_2$ has recently been demonstrated to be within the nucleus, rather than the cytosol, of endothelial cells growing in culture (22). In this experimental system, the enzyme is found in its expected site, the cytosol, only when growth stops due to contact inhibition. It seems likely that intranuclear $cPLA_2$ will act at the inner membrane of the nuclear envelope following cell stimulation, whereas cytosolic $cPLA_2$ will act at the outer membrane. These sites may differ both in AA content and in proximity to downstream enzymes. As a result, the movement of $cPLA_2$ from the cytosol into the nucleus has the potential to change both the amounts and types of AA metabolites generated upon cell stimulation.

The secretory PLA_2s ($sPLA_2$s) are a group of approximately 14-kDa enzymes found in inflammatory fluids and also in bee and snake venoms. In mammalian tissues, their expression is up-regulated by inflammatory stimuli. Because these PLA_2s require high (mM) levels of calcium for activity, and because they are inactivated by the reducing conditions commonly found within cells, it seems likely that these enzymes would be best suited to act extracellularly, at the cell surface. As their name implies, sPLA$_2$s are secreted from cells, and they may be found in the extracellular media or associated with the plasma membrane, presumably at the external face. In fact, an sPLA$_2$ is normally found in the lining fluid of the human respiratory tract (23). The sPLA$_2$s may interact directly with membranes to release fatty acids or they may interact with surface receptors to trigger specific responses (24,25). Because sPLA$_2$s hydrolyze fatty acids without selectivity, AA generation for eicosanoid synthesis is, at a minimum, inefficient. Nonetheless, sPLA$_2$s have been implicated in eicosanoid synthesis (26–28). An alternative role for this PLA$_2$ might be the generation of fatty acids that act as second messengers, triggering such diverse responses as mitogen-activated protein kinase activation (29) and heat shock gene transcription (30).

The calcium-independent PLA$_2$s (iPLA$_2$) are a group of soluble enzymes. The best-characterized isoforms [in macrophages (31) and myocardium (32,33)] differ in AA selectivity and in substrate preference. They are thought to mediate the deacylation process which is part of normal basal phospholipid turnover (34). In certain circumstances, their action may be stimulated by agonists (35), but it does not appear that they contribute significant amounts of substrate to eicosanoid formation (36). Both isoforms are described as "cytosolic." Like other PLA$_2$s, it is likely that they act at cellular membranes, but it is not known how membrane association might be regulated or if they act selectively at any particular membrane.

B. The Cyclooxygenases

The cyclooxygenase, or prostaglandin endoperoxide synthase, enzymes catalyze the insertion of molecular oxygen into AA, the rate-limiting step in its conversion to prostaglandins. It is now recognized that there are two isoforms, designated COX-1 and COX-2. The COX-1 form is constitutively present in most tissues and appears to be regulated only in exceptional cases. In contrast, the COX-2 form is not generally expressed constitutively but is inducible by a number of inflammatory, hormonal, or mitogenic stimuli; its induction is blocked by glucocorticoids.

The current paradigm holds that the differences in expression between COX-1 and COX-2 are linked to differences in the roles of their products. The constitutive expression of COX-1 is consistent with a role for COX-1-derived PGs in normal physiological functions, including the cytoprotection of the gastric lining, the preservation of renal blood flow, and the inhibition of intravascular platelet aggregation. In contrast, the PGs derived from COX-2 are thought to be responsible for inflammation, tumorigenesis, and parturition. Currently available nonsteroidal anti-inflammatory drugs (NSAIDs), including aspirin, inhibit the activity of both COX isoforms with similar potencies. It has therefore been proposed that the inhibition of COX-2 accounts for the therapeutic effects of NSAIDs, whereas inhibition of COX-1 leads to their undesirable renal and gastric toxicities.

Before distinct isoforms were recognized, COX was localized, not at the plasma membrane, but to the ER and nuclear membrane of 3T3 cells (5). Using isoform-specific antibodies, both COX-1 and COX-2 have recently been localized to the ER and the nuclear envelope. Early studies indicated that both enzymes were distributed similarly in 3T3 cells (37). However, in murine 3T3 cells and human and bovine endothelial cells, COX-1 is most abundant along the ER, while COX-2 is concentrated at the nuclear envelope, as revealed by immunofluorescent microscopy (38). Furthermore, their *activities* have been localized to these spatially distinct sites using a fluorescence-based assay to visualize cyclooxygenase/peroxidase activity in 3T3 cells (38). COX-1 has also been localized in lipid bodies (membrane-free, lipid-rich regions) within the cytoplasm of a variety of cell types (39), whereas soluble COX-2 has been reported within the nucleus (40). On the basis of these distinct sites of localization and enzymatic action, COX-1 and COX-2 have been suggested to represent distinct enzyme systems (41).

C. Enzymes Distal to the Cyclooxygenases

PGH_2, the product of both COX-1 and COX-2, can be metabolized to a broad array of potent lipid mediators by a variety of distal PG synthases. One of the prostanoids relevant to asthma is thromboxane (TxA_2), which increases airway and vascular smooth muscle tone as well as the aggregation of platelets. Its synthesis is dependent on the enzyme TxA_2 synthase. This enzyme is found in mononuclear phagocytes and platelets, as well as dendritic cells and some specialized epithelial cells (42). TxA_2 synthase activity has been demonstrated in isolated nuclei (43) and the enzyme has been localized immunologically to the ER as well (44).

PGD_2 is, like TxA_2, another bronchoconstrictor that may be relevant to asthma. PGD_2 is derived from PGH_2 by the action of PGD_2 synthase (also called PGD isomerase). This enzyme occurs in two forms, a glutathione-requiring form abundant in mast cells and a glutathione-independent form present in neural tissues. The glutathione-requiring form has been localized to the cytosol by a variety of techniques, including immunoelectron microscopy (45,46). The glutathione-independent form of PGD_2 synthase has been found at the rough ER and the outer nuclear membrane of glial cells (47) as well as the cytosol of brain and spinal cord tissue (45).

Unlike TxA_2 and PGD_2, which are bronchoconstrictive, the prostanoid PGE_2 is bronchoprotective (2,3,48), by virtue of its ability to relax smooth muscle and attenuate the function of inflammatory cells. PGE_2 is produced by epithelial cells, fibroblasts, and macrophages by the enzyme PGE_2 synthase (also called PGE isomerase). Apparently, the enzyme itself has never been carefully localized, although the ability of different cell compartments to generate PGE_2 from AA has been examined. Thus, the PGE_2 synthase "complex" is distributed primarily to the rough ER and partly to the nuclear membrane, but is absent from the plasma membrane, of goat vesicular gland (49). This activity requires COX, presumably COX-1, which also occurs at the ER and the nuclear envelope. Interestingly, two soluble forms of the enzyme have been purified from human brain; although they were both assumed to originate from the cytosol (50), this was not critically evaluated.

The enzyme PGI_2 synthase converts PGH_2 to prostacyclin (PGI_2), which is also bronchoprotective. This enzyme is abundant in tracheal epithelial cells, smooth muscle cells, endothelial cells, and fibroblasts. PGI_2 synthase has been localized to both the nuclear and plasma membranes of smooth muscle cells (51).

D. 5-Lipoxygenase (5-LO) and the 5-Lipoxygenase Activating Protein (FLAP)

The enzyme 5-LO carries out the first two catalytic steps in the synthesis of leukotrienes from AA, resulting in the generation of leukotriene A_4 (LTA_4). Although 5-LO can metabolize AA in the absence of FLAP, FLAP greatly enhances AA processing by 5-LO. Early studies found that, while 5-LO is soluble in resting cells, it quickly becomes membrane-associated following cell stimulation, apparently translocating from the cytosol to a membrane (52). Unlike $cPLA_2$, 5-LO was known to lack a protein kinase C–like, calcium-dependent lipid-binding domain, so its mechanism of membrane association was unknown. Subsequent studies showed that FLAP is an integral membrane protein (53) and that pharmacological agents that directly interact with FLAP block 5-LO translocation as well as LT synthesis (54). These findings suggested that FLAP functions as a docking protein, providing a site on the membrane that is necessary for both 5-LO membrane association and action. These early studies were not capable of resolving subcellular compartmentation; there was no a priori reason to do so at that time since it was generally assumed that AA processing occurred predominantly at the plasma membrane. However, when peritoneal macrophages were separated into nuclear as well as soluble and membrane fractions, FLAP was found predominantly in the nuclear fraction (16). Furthermore, 5-LO was found to translocate to the nuclear fraction in these cells. Consistent with this, 5-LO and FLAP were localized to the nuclear envelope of activated neutrophils by immunoelectron microscopy (8). Although initially surprising, these results indicating the nuclear envelope to be the site of AA metabolism by 5-LO and FLAP appear to reflect a universal phenomenon. Identical findings have now been reported for alveolar macrophages and blood monocytes (55), mast cells (56), and the rat basophilic leukemia (RBL) cell line (57). Finally, using immunoelectron microscopy, FLAP inhibition was found to have no effect on 5-LO translocation to the nuclear envelope despite inhibiting LT biosynthesis (55). These results indicate that FLAP does not serve as a docking protein for 5-LO; instead, in its known role as an AA-binding protein (58), it is thought to facilitate the presentation of substrate to 5-LO.

Attention was next directed at using appropriate techniques to localize 5-LO in unstimulated or resting cells of various types. Surprisingly, careful fractionation of unstimulated RBL cells, widely used to model mast cells, revealed abundant soluble 5-LO in the nuclear fraction, as well as in the cytosolic fraction (59). Direct visualization of RBL cells by immunofluorescent techniques as well as optical sectioning by confocal microscopy confirmed that 5-LO was distributed throughout the interior of nuclei. The nuclear pool of 5-LO, like the cytosolic pool, translocated to the nuclear envelope upon cell stimulation and was catalytically active as judged by cell-free assays (57). Nuclear 5-LO has subsequently also been noted in primary mouse mast cells (56). Abundant intranuclear 5-LO, predominantly in the euchromatin region, has also been demonstrated in resting alveolar macrophages from rats and humans by several techniques (55,59); importantly, this finding has been confirmed in situ by immunohistochemical staining of normal human lung tissue (60). Resting alveolar macrophages also have 5-LO within the cytosol but, curiously, only the nuclear 5-LO appears to translocate to the nuclear envelope upon cell stimulation (57). Unlike mast cells and alveolar macrophages, 5-LO is largely restricted to the cytoplasm of resting peritoneal macrophages (16), peripheral blood neutrophils (57), and monocytes (55). These observations have led to the conclusion that 5-LO distribution is cell type-dependent (61).

Several observations suggest that a static model cannot entirely account for the localization of 5-LO. Instead, a model in which enzyme localization is regulated and dynamic is favored. For example, blood monocytes, which have cytosolic 5-LO, are the precursors for all differentiated tissue macrophages. These include peritoneal macrophages, which similarly have only cytosolic 5-LO, and alveolar macrophages, which have both cytosolic and nuclear 5-LO. This means that nuclear accumulation of 5-LO is triggered by migration into the alveolar, but not the peritoneal, space. Second, when neutrophils move from the bloodstream into sites of inflammation (either the peritoneum or alveolus), their 5-LO rapidly moves from the cytosol into the nucleus (62). In contrast, when alveolar macrophages are incubated on fibronectin overnight, some of their nuclear 5-LO appears to move to the cytosol (Brock and Peters-Golden, unpublished results). These results indicate that, even within a given cell type, 5-LO distribution can be dictated by extracellular factors.

E. Enzymes Distal to 5-Lipoxygenase

5-LO both oxygenates AA to 5-HPETE and converts some of the 5-HPETE to LTA$_4$. The remainder of the first product, 5-HPETE, is rapidly converted to 5-HETE. 5-HETE has relatively weak chemoattractant and activating effects on leukocytes but can promote cell proliferation. In addition, 5-HETE can be further dehydrogenated to 5-oxo-ETE, a chemotactic factor with preferential activity for eisonophils that thus might play a role in recruiting eosinophils to the asthmatic airway. The second 5-LO product, LTA$_4$, is unstable and is nonenzymatically degraded unless acted on by downstream enzymes, such as those discussed below.

LTA$_4$ can be acted on by LTA$_4$ hydrolase to yield LTB$_4$, which is best known as a potent chemotactic agent and activator of leukocytes, but also has a number of other effects. The enzyme LTA$_4$ hydrolase is a soluble enzyme found in a variety of cell types. In alveolar macrophages, peritoneal macrophages, monocytes, and neutrophils, LTA$_4$ hydrolase is found only in the cytosol (Coffey and Peters-Golden, unpublished results). A unique feature of LTA$_4$ hydrolase is that it occurs in cells that have little or no 5-LO, including epithelial cells, fibroblasts, and endothelial cells. In this situation, it acts on LTA$_4$ released from neighboring cells in a transcellular fashion. In these cells, LTA$_4$ hydrolase also seems to be limited to the cytoplasm (63). Although this enzyme has only been localized to one intracellular site to date, the mouse LTA$_4$ hydrolase reportedly occurs in multiple forms (64), which raises the possibility of differences in regulation and localization of the different isoforms. Finally, LTA$_4$ hydrolase activity has also been detected extracellularly, apparently secreted from source cells (65). This activity was present in bronchoalveolar lavage fluid of normal individuals and activity was increased in smokers.

LTA$_4$ derived from the action of 5-LO can also be conjugated with glutathione, by LTC$_4$ synthase, to give rise to the cysteinyl LT, LTC$_4$. This substance, and its degradation products, LTD$_4$ and LTE$_4$, account for much of the bronchospasm, airway edema, and mucus hypersecretion characteristic of asthma. The enzyme LTC$_4$ synthase is abundant in mast cells (but not basophils), as well as in antigen-presenting cells. This enzyme has long been recognized as an integral membrane protein. Structurally, this enzyme shares homology with FLAP, raising the possibility that it, too, might be found predominantly at the nuclear envelope. Indeed, a perinuclear distribution has been observed in human alveolar macrophages, examined by immunohistochemistry in situ (66).

IV. The Nuclear Envelope as an Integrated Site of Action

An obvious theme to emerge from the studies reviewed above is that a number of key eicosanoid-forming enzymes act at the nuclear envelope of stimulated

Table 1 Summary of the Subcellular Localization of the Major Eicosanoid-Forming Enzymes

Eicosanoid-forming enzyme	Nucleoplasm	Nuclear envelope	ER	Lipid bodies	Cytoplasm	Plasma membrane	Extracellular
cPLA$_2$	(reported)	Most, upon activation	Some, upon activation	—	In resting cells	—	—
sPLA$_2$	—	—	—	—	—	Yes	Yes
iPLA$_2$	—	—	—	—	Yes	—	—
COX-1	—	Some	Most?	Yes	—	—	—
COX-2	(reported)	Most	Some	—	—	—	—
TxA$_2$ synthase	—	?	Yes	—	Yes	—	—
PGD$_2$ synthetase, glutathione-requiring	—	—	—	—	Yes	—	—
PGD$_2$ synthetase, glutathione-independent	—	Yes	Yes	—	Yes	—	—
PGE$_2$ synthase	—	Yes?	Yes	—	Yes?	—	—
PGI$_2$ synthase	—	Yes	—	—	—	Yes	—
5-LO	In some resting cells	Most, upon activation	Some, upon activation	—	In resting cells	—	—
FLAP	—	Most	Some	—	—	—	—
LTA$_4$ hydrolase	—	—	—	—	Yes	—	Yes
LTC$_4$ synthase	—	Most?	Some?	—	—	—	—

cells. This is true for cPLA$_2$, COX-1, COX-2, 5-LO, FLAP, and LTC$_4$ synthase (Table 1). The ER is an additional site of localization for some of these proteins, including COX-1, COX-2, TxA$_2$ synthase, PGD$_2$ synthase, PGE$_2$ synthase, FLAP, and perhaps LTC$_4$ synthase. In some cases, the ER may represent an extension of the outer membrane of the nuclear envelope; in others, it may represent a site of action that is distinct from the nuclear envelope. In any case, it is clear that crucial steps in AA release and metabolism occur deep within the cell, rather than peripherally at the plasma membrane.

V. Consequences of Nuclear Localization

A. Metabolic Consequences

It has long been recognized that different functional pools of AA exist within cells (67). For example, AA liberated in response to different stimuli often have different metabolic fates within a given cell type. In addition, the fact that pharmacological inhibition of one of the oxygenase pathways (e.g., COX) often fails to divert unmetabolized AA to the other oxygenase pathway (e.g., 5-LO) is also consistent with the notion that not all pools of AA are equally available to all metabolic routes. In view of this, it is attractive to speculate that one of the factors that distinguish different pools of substrate is the intracellular site at which it is liberated. For example, AA could be hydrolyzed from nuclear and plasma membrane phospholipids by the action of cPLA$_2$ and sPLA$_2$, respectively. It is also attractive to speculate that the degree of coupling of a given pool of AA to downstream metabolic enzymes might also be dictated, in part, by topographic proximity of the released fatty acid and the oxygenases. For example, AA derived by the action of cPLA$_2$ at the outer membrane of the nucleus may be efficiently passed by FLAP to 5-LO for the generation of LTA$_4$, which can in turn be efficiently processed by LTC$_4$ synthase, at the same site, to result in LTC$_4$ generation. On the other hand, AA liberated by sPLA$_2$ from the plasma membrane may be poorly coupled to metabolizing enzymes located at the nuclear envelope. As a result, this pool of AA may be better suited to function as a second messenger, triggering downstream responses, or to move to neighboring cells for transcellular metabolism. Does the available data support such a paradigm? While there are experimental systems in which eicosanoid formation depends on cPLA$_2$, but not sPLA$_2$, action, there certainly are other systems in which sPLA$_2$ action is, in fact, important for eicosanoid generation. Thus, experimental data neither clearly support nor refute this model. Nonetheless, it is teleologically plausible and might serve as a useful framework for future studies. If sPLA$_2$ action contributes plasma membrane-derived AA to eicosanoid-forming enzymes deep within the cell, then we must gain better understanding of the mechanisms controlling the intracellular movement of AA.

As noted above, inhibition of one oxygenase pathway typically does not result in processing of unmetabolized AA by the alternate oxygenase pathway. This, too, may be explained by the positioning of the rate-limiting enzymes in each of the pathways. An overly simplified topography might indicate that COX-1 is largely restricted to the ER, translocated 5-LO is predominantly at the outer membrane of the nuclear envelope, and COX-2 is primarily localized at the inner membrane of the nuclear envelope. Each of these enzymes, working at a different location, may be utilizing distinct AA pools. Only in the situation where 5-LO has moved into the nucleus and as a result would translocate to the inner membrane of the nuclear envelope upon activation would one find two AA-processing enzymes (i.e., 5-LO and COX-2) at the same site, where they could compete for a single AA pool. Inhibition of COX-2 by aspirin, in this scenario, could therefore shunt additional AA to the 5-LO pathway, resulting in an overproduction of LTs, as is seen in aspirin-induced asthma. Alternatively, the blockade of nuclear 5-LO by selective lipoxygenase inhibitors could lead to enhanced AA metabolism by COX-2 and elevated PG production.

The capacity of soluble $cPLA_2$ and 5-LO to be imported into the nucleus of resting cells adds several levels of complexity to the regulation of AA processing. Both of these enzymes are activated by calcium, and stimuli that increase cytosolic calcium may be ineffective in increasing intranuclear calcium (68). As a result, there may be a greater threshold for activation of these intranuclear enzyme pools; thus, nuclear $cPLA_2$ and 5-LO might be activated only by certain agonists or by higher doses of agonist. Consistent with this, alveolar macrophages, which have intranuclear 5-LO, require a higher dose of ionophore to trigger LT synthesis than do peritoneal macrophages, which have cytosolic 5-LO (69). Similarly, elicited peritoneal neutrophils, which have nuclear 5-LO, are less readily activated than are blood neutrophils, which have cytosolic 5-LO (62).

Finally, enzyme localization could theoretically affect the relationships among distal pathway proteins. The movement of 5-LO from the cytosol to the nucleus will distance this enzyme from the cytosol-localized LTA_4 hydrolase, potentially separating LTA_4 synthesis by 5-LO and LTA_4 metabolism by LTA_4 hydrolase. How does the colocalization of LTA_4 hydrolase with 5-LO affect 5-LO processing of AA? Transfected cells expressing 5-LO without LTA_4 hydrolase make very little LT, but instead release the 5-LO intermediate, 5-HETE; in cells expressing both 5-LO and LTA_4 hydrolase, LT generation increases dramatically (70). If the movement of 5-LO into the nucleus separates it from LTA_4 hydrolase to the extent that there is inefficient transfer of metabolites, then this movement may serve to change the profile of AA metabolites generated upon cell stimulation. In this way, then, the colocalization of enzymes may facilitate the processing of intermediates whereas their separation may hinder it.

B. Nonmetabolic Consequences

The realization that there are not only two isoforms of COX but that their predominant localizations (the ER for COX-1 and the nuclear membrane for COX-2) may differ suggests a more complicated model for AA processing than previously expected. The discovery that the positioning of 5-LO and cPLA$_2$ within the cell is regulated and that import into the nucleus is inducible suggests an additional level of complexity that far exceeds what is necessary simply to regulate eicosanoid production. One possible explanation might be that eicosanoids generated within the cell may have effects at their subcellular site of generation. That is, instead of being secreted from the cell and moving to a surface receptor on a target cell to trigger a response, eicosanoids may interact directly with soluble receptors close to the site of synthesis within the same cell. In support of this concept, soluble nuclear receptors for PG metabolites (71,72) as well as the lipoxygenase product LTB$_4$ (73) have recently been reported. In these studies, receptor-binding by eicosanoids triggered transcriptional activation and gene expression. The current paradigm would assume that these receptors would normally be responding to eicosanoids derived from extracellular sources. However, it is possible that eicosanoid receptors will exist in the nucleus of eicosanoid-generating cells themselves. Such receptors could act to regulate gene expression and could thereby control processes like cell motility, cell division, and apoptosis. Since both 5-LO (55) and COX-2 (40) proteins have been localized to the euchromatin region (the region of the nucleus containing actively transcribing genes), they could alternatively affect gene expression by themselves interacting with DNA, either directly or indirectly through a second transcription factor. Finally, these interactions of eicosanoids (or eicosanoid-forming enzymes) with biological targets within the compartment of synthesis may also occur in the cytoplasm. In this regard, it is notable that the 5-LO protein has a Src homology-3 binding domain and has been shown to interact with cytoskeletal elements (74). Interaction of eicosanoids or enzymes with such biological targets within the cytoplasm may alter cytosolic processes, like second-messenger pathways, cytoskeletal function, or endocytic/exocytic functions, as well as gene expression.

VI. Unanswered Questions

The importance of enzyme localization in eicosanoid generation, and the dynamic nature of 5-LO and cPLA$_2$ in particular, are only now becoming appreciated. Basic questions regarding how the localization of enzymes like 5-LO and cPLA$_2$ might be regulated, including their movement through the nuclear pore into the nucleus and the directional nature of translocation to a particular membrane, have yet to be answered. How AA and eicosanoids are trafficked into and out of the cell and between different enzymes and membranes is poorly understood. It seems likely that the positioning of downstream enzymes must affect the efficiency of different pathways, and that competition between different pathways might be influenced by enzyme localization. Still, these links between location and function remain to be demonstrated. Strong incentive to pursue such work will come from the possibility that a better understanding of enzyme localization may increase our knowledge about the pathogenesis of diseases such as aspirin-sensitive asthma.

References

1. Israel E, Fischer A, Rosenberg M, Lilly C, Callery J, Shapiro J, Cohn H, Rubin P, Drazen J. The pivotal role of 5-lipoxygenase products in the reaction of aspirin-sensitive asthmatics to aspirin. Am Rev Respir Dis 1993; 148:1447–1451.
2. Sestini P, Armetti L, Gambaro G, Pieroni M, Refini R, Sala A, Vaghi A, Folco G, Bianco S, Robuschi M. Inhaled PGE$_2$ prevents aspirin-induced bronchoconstriction and urinary LTE$_4$ excretion in aspirin-sensitive asthma. Am J Respir Crit Care Med 1996; 153:572–575.
3. Schafer D, Lindenthal U, Wagner M, Bolcskei P, Baenkler H. Effect of prostaglandin E$_2$ on eicosanoid release by human bronchial biopsy specimens from normal and inflamed mucosa. Thorax 1996; 51:919–923.
4. Szczeklik A, Sladek K, Dworski R, Nizankowska E, Soja J, Sheller J, Oates J. Bronchial aspirin challenge causes specific eicosanoid response in aspirin-sensitive asthmatics. Am J Respir Crit Care Med 1996; 154:1608–1614.
5. Rollins T, Smith W. Subcellular localization of prostaglandin-forming cyclooxygenase in Swiss mouse 3T3 fibroblasts by electron microscopic immunocytochemistry. J Biol Chem 1980; 255:4872–4875.
6. Dvorak A, Morgan E, Schleimer R, Ryeom S, Lichtenstein L, Weller P. Ultrastructural immunogold localization of prostaglandin endoperoxide synthase (cyclooxygenase) to non-membrane-bound cytoplasmic lipid bodies in human lung mast cells, alveolar macrophages, type II pneumocytes, and neutrophils. J Histochem Cytochem 1992; 40:759–769.
7. Dvorak A, Weller P, Harvey V, Morgan E, Dvorak H. Ultrastructural localization of prostaglandin endoperoxide synthase (cyclooxygenase) to isolated, purified fractions of guinea pig peritoneal macrophage and line 10 hepatocarcinoma cell lipid bodies. Int Arch Allergy Immunol 1993; 101:136–142.
8. Woods J, Evans J, Ethier D, Scott S, Vickers P, Hearn L, Charleson S, Heibein J, Singer I. 5-Lipoxygenase and 5-lipoxygenase activating protein are localized in the nuclear envelope of activated human leukocytes. J Exp Med 1993; 178:1935–1946.

9. Capriotti A, Furth E, Arrasmith M, Laposata M. Arachidonate released upon agonist stimulation preferentially originates from arachidonate most recently incorporated into nuclear membrane phospholipids. J Biol Chem 1988; 263:10029–10034.
10. Clark JD, Milona N, Knopf JL. Purification of a 110-kilodalton cytosolic phospholipase A_2 from the human monocytic cell line U937. Proc Natl Acad Sci USA 1990; 87:7707–7712.
11. Schievella A, Regier M, Smith W, Lin L. Calcium-mediated translocation of cytosolic phospholipase A_2 to the nuclear envelope and endoplasmic reticulum. J Biol Chem 1995; 270:30749–54.
12. Xu X, Rock C, Qiu Z, Leslie C, Jackowski S. Regulation of cytosolic phospholipase A_2 phosphorylation and eicosanoid production by colony-stimulating factor 1. J Biol Chem 1994; 269:31693–31700.
13. Brock TG, McNish RW, Coffey MJ, Ojo TC, Phare SM, Peters-Golden M. Effect of granulocyte-macrophage colony-stimulating factor on eicosanoid production by mononuclear phagocytes. J Immunol 1996; 156:2522–2527.
14. Alonso F, Henson P, Leslie C. A cytosolic phospholipase in human neutrophils that hydrolyzes arachidonoyl-containing phosphatidylcholine. Biochim Biophys Acta 1986; 878:273–280.
15. Channon J, Leslie C. A calcium-dependent mechanism for associating a soluble arachidonoyl-hydrolyzing phospholipase A_2 with membrane in the macrophage cell line RAW 264.7. J Biol Chem 1990; 265:5409–5413.
16. Peters-Golden M, McNish R. Redistribution of 5-lipoxygenase and cytosolic phospholipase A_2 to the nuclear fraction upon macrophage activation. Biochem Biophys Res Commun 1993; 196:147–153.
17. Glover S, Bayburt T, Jonas M, Chi E, Gelb M. Translocation of the 85-kDa phospholipase A_2 from cytosol to the nuclear envelope in rat basophilic leukemia cells stimulated with calcium ionophore or IgE/antigen. J Biol Chem 1995; 270:15359–15367.
18. Peters-Golden M, Song K, Marshall T, Brock T. Translocation of cytosolic phospholipase A_2 to the nuclear envelope elicits topographically localized phospholipid hydrolysis. Biochem J 1996; 318:797–803.
19. Clark J, Lin L, Kriz R, Ramesha C, Sultzman L, Lin A, Milona N, Knopf J. A novel arachidonic acid-selective cytosolic PLA_2 contains a Ca^{2+}-dependent translocation domain with homology to PKC and GAP. Cell 1991; 65:1043–1051.
20. Kramer R, Roberts E, Manetta J, Hyslop P, Jakubowski J. Thrombin-induced phosphorylation and activation of Ca^{2+}-sensitive cytosolic phospholipase A_2 in human platelets. J Biol Chem 1993; 268:26795–26804.
21. Rao G, Lassegue B, RW A, Griendling K. Angiotensin II stimulates phosphorylation of high-molecular-mass cytosolic phospholipase A_2 in vascular smooth-muscle cells. Biochem J 1994; 299:197–201.
22. Sierra-Honigmann M, Bradley J, Pober J. "Cytosolic" phospholipase A_2 is in the nucleus of subconfluent endothelial cells but confined to the cytoplasm of confluent endothelial cells and redistributes to the nuclear envelope and cell junctions upon histamine stimulation. Lab Invest 1996; 74:684–695.
23. Samet J, Madden M, Fonteh A. Characterization of a secretory phospholipase A_2 in human bronchoalveolar lavage fluid. Exp Lung Res 1996; 22:299–315.

24. Tohkin M, Kishino J, Ishizaki J, Arita H. Pancreatic-type phospholipase A_2 stimulates prostaglandin synthesis in mouse osteoblastic cells (MC3T3-E1) via a specific binding site. J Biol Chem 1993; 268:2865–2871.

25. Mukhopadhyay A, Stahl P. Bee venom phospholipase A_2 is recognized by the macrophage mannose receptor. Arch Biochem Biophys 1995; 324:78–84.

26. Murakami M, Kudo I, Inoue K. Molecular nature of phospholipases A_2 involved in prostaglandin I_2 synthesis in human umbilical vein endothelial cells: possible participation of cytosolic and extracellular type II phospholipases A_2. J Biol Chem 1993; 268:839–844.

27. Fonteh A, Bass D, Marshall L, Seeds M, Samet J, Chilton F. Evidence that secretory phospholipase A_2 plays a role in arachidonic acid release and eicosanoid biosynthesis by mast cells. J Immunol 1994; 152:5438–5446.

28. Reddy S, Herschman H. Transcellular prostaglandin production following mast cell activation is mediated by proximal secretory phospholipase A_2 and distal prostaglandin synthase 1. J Biol Chem 1996; 271:186–191.

29. Rao G, Baas A, Glasgow W, Eling T, Runge M, Alexander R. Activation of mitogen-activated protein kinases by arachidonic acid and its metabolites in vascular smooth muscle cells. J Biol Chem 1994; 269:32586–32591.

30. Jurivich D, Sistonen L, Sarge K, Morimoto R. Arachidonate is a potent modulator of human heat shock gene transcription. Proc Natl Acad Sci USA 1994; 91:2280–2284.

31. Ackermann E, Kempner E, Dennis E. Ca^{2+}-independent cytosolic phospholipase A_2 from macrophage-like P3381 cells: Isolation and characterization. J Biol Chem 1994; 269:9227–9233.

32. Hazen S, Stuppy R, Gross R. Purification and characterization of canine myocardial cytosolic phospholipase A_2: a calcium-independent phospholipase with absolute *sn*-2 regiospecificity for diradyl glycerophospholipids. J Biol Chem 1990; 265:10622–10630.

33. Hazen S, Hall C, Ford D, Gross R. Isolation of a human myocardial cytosolic phospholipase A_2 isoform. Fast atom bombardment mass spectroscopic and reverse-phase high pressure liquid chromatography identification of choline and ethanolamine glycerophospholipid substrates. J Clin Invest 1993; 91:2513–2522.

34. Balsinde J, Bianco I, Ackermann E, Conde-Frieboes K, Dennis E. Inhibition of calcium-independent phospholipase A_2 prevents arachidonic acid incorporation and phospholipid remodeling in P388D1 macrophages. Proc Natl Acad Sci USA 1995; 92:8527–8531.

35. Lehman J, Brown K, Ramanadham S, Turk J, Gross R. Arachidonic acid release from aortic smooth muscle cells induced by [Arg^8] vasopressin is largely mediated by calcium-independent phospholipiase A_2. J Biol Chem 1993; 268:20713–20716.

36. Balsinde J, Dennis E. Distinct roles in signal transduction for each of the phospholipase A_2 enzymes present in P338D1 macrophages. J Biol Chem 1996; 271:6758–6765.

37. Regier M, DeWitt D, Schindler M, Smith W. Subcellular localization of prostaglandin endoperoxide synthase-2 in murine 3T3 cells. Arch Biochem Biophys 1993; 301:439–444.

38. Morita I, Schindler M, Regier M, Otto J, Hori T, DeWitt D, Smith W. Different intracellular locations for prostaglandin endoperoxide H synthase-1 and -2. J Biol Chem 1995; 270:10902–10908.

39. Dvorak A, Morgan E, Tzizik D, Weller P. Prostaglandin endoperoxide synthase (cyclooxygenase): ultrastructural localization to nonmembrane-bound cytoplasmic lipid bodies in human eosinophils and 3T3 fibroblasts. Int Arch Allergy Immunol 1994; 105:245–250.

40. Coffey R, Hawkey C, Damstrup L. Graves-Deal R, Daniel V, Dempsey P, Chinery R, Kirkland S, DuBois R, Jetton T, Morrow J. Epidermal growth factor receptor activation induces nuclear targeting of cyclooxygenase-2, basolateral release of prostaglandins, and mitogenesis in polarizing colon cancer cells. Proc Natl Acad Sci USA 1997; 94:657–662.

41. Smith W, DeWitt D. Prostaglandin endoperoxide H synthases-1 and -2. Adv Immunol 1996; 62:167–215.

42. Nusing R, Sauter G, Fehr P, Durmuller U, Kasper M, Gudat F, Ullrich V. Localization of thromboxane synthase in human tissues by monoclonal antibody Tu 300. Virchows Arch A Pathol Anat Histopathol 1992; 421:249–254.

43. Matsumoto K, Morita I, Murota S. Arachidonic acid metabolism by nuclei of a retinoic acid– or vitamin D_3–differentiated human leukemia cell line HL-60. Prostaglandins Leukot Essent Fatty Acids 1994; 51:51–55.

44. Ruan K, Li P, Kulmacz R, Wu K. Characterization of the structure and membrane interaction of NH_2-terminal domain of thromboxane A_2 synthase. J Biol Chem 1994; 269:20938–20942.

45. Ujihara M, Urade Y, Eguchi N, Yayashi H, Ikai K, Hayaishi O. Prostaglandin D_2 formation and characterization of its synthetases in various tissues of adult rats. Arch Biochem Biophys 1988; 260:521–531.

46. Urade Y, Ujihara M, Horiguchi Y, Ikai K, Hayaishi O. The major source of endogenous prostaglandin D_2 production is likely antigen-presenting cells. Localization of glutathione-requiring prostaglandin D synthetase in histiocytes, dendritic, and Kupffer cells in various rat tissues. J Immunol 1989; 143:2982–2989.

47. Urade Y, Fujimoto N, Kaneko T, Konishi A, Mizuno N, Hayaishi O. Postnatal changes in the localization of prostaglandin D synthetase from neurons to oligodendrocytes in the rat brain. J Biol Chem 1987; 262:15132–15136.

48. Pavord I, Wong C, Williams J, Tattersfield A. Effect of inhaled PGE_2 on allergen-induced asthma. Am Rev Respir Dis 1993; 148:87–90.

49. Mukherjee E, Ghosh D. Subcellular localization of cyclo-oxygenase-prostaglandin E_2 synthetase complex in goat vesicular gland by catalytic activity analysis. Prostaglandins 1989; 38:557–563.

50. Ogorochi T, Ujihara M, Narumiya S. Purification and properties of prostaglandin H-E isomerase from the cytosol of human brain: identification as anionic forms of glutathione S-transferase. J Neurochem 1987; 48:900–909.

51. Smith W, DeWitt D, Allen M. Bimodal distribution of the prostaglandin I_2 synthase antigen in smooth muscle cells. J Biol Chem 1983; 258:5922–5926.

52. Rouzer CA, Kargman S. Translocation of 5-lipoxygenase to the membrane in human leukocytes challenged with ionophore A23187. J Biol Chem 1988; 263:10980–10988.

53. Dixon RAF, Diehl RE, Opas E, Rands E, Vickers P, Evans J, Gillard J, Miller D. Requirement of a 5-lipoxygenase-activating protein for leukotriene synthesis. Nature 1990; 343:282–284.

54. Rouzer CA, Ford-Hutchinson AW, Morton HE, Gillard JW. MK886, a potent and specific leukotriene biosynthesis inhibitor blocks and reverses the membrane association of 5-lipoxygenase in ionophore-challenged leukocytes. J Biol Chem 1990; 265:1436–1442.

55. Woods J, Coffey M, Brock T, Singer I, Peters-Golden M. 5-Lipoxygenase is located in the euchromatin of the nucleus in resting human alveolar macrophages and translocates to the nuclear envelope upon cell activation. J Clin Invest 1995; 95: 2035–2040.

56. Chen X-S, Naumann T, Kurre U, Jenkins N, Copeland N, Funk C. cDNA cloning, expression, mutagenesis, intracellular localization, and gene chromosomal assignment of mouse 5-lipoxygenase. J Biol Chem 1995; 270:17993–17999.

57. Brock TG, McNish RW, Peters-Golden M. Translocation and leukotriene synthetic capacity of nuclear 5-lipoxygenase in rat basophilic leukemia cells and alveolar macrophages. J Biol Chem 1995; 270:21652–21658.

58. Abramovitz M, Wong E, Cox M, Richardson C, Li C, Vickers P. 5-Lipoxygenase-activating protein stimulates the utilization of arachidonic acid by 5-lipoxygenase. Eur J Biochem 1993; 215:105–111.

59. Brock TG, Paine R, Peters-Golden M, Localization of 5-lipoxygenase to the nucleus of unstimulated rat basophilic leukemia cells. J Biol Chem 1994; 269:22059–22066.

60. Wilborn J, Bailie M, Coffey M, Burdick M, Strieter R, Peters-Golden M. Constitutive activation of 5-lipoxygenase in the lungs of patients with idiopathic pulmonary fibrosis. J Clin Invest 1996; 97:1827–1836.

61. Serhan C, Haeggston J, Leslie C. Lipid mediator networks in cell signaling: update and impact of cytokines. FASEB J 1996; 10:1147–1158.

62. Brock T, McNish R, Bailie M, Peters-Golden M. Rapid import of cytosolic 5-lipoxygenase into the nucleus of neutrophils following in vivo recruitment and in vitro adherence. J Biol Chem 1997; 272:8276–8280.

63. Ikai K, Okano H, Horiguchi Y, Sakamoto Y. Leukotriene A_4 hydrolase in human skin. J Invest Dermatol 1994; 102:253–257.

64. Medina J, Radmark O, Funk C, Haeggstrom J. Molecular cloning and expression of mouse leukotriene A_4 hydrolase cDNA. Biochem Biophys Res Commun 1991; 176:1516–1524.

65. Munafo D, Shindo K, Baker J, Bigby T. Leukotriene A_4 hydrolase in human bronchoalveolar lavage fluid. J Clin Invest 1994; 93:1042–1050.

66. Penrose J, Spector J, Lam B, Friend D, Xu K, Jack R, Austen K. Purification of human lung LTC_4 synthase and preparation of a polyclonal antibody. Am J Respir Crit Care Med 1995; 152:283–289.

67. Humes J, Sadowski S, Galavage M, Goldenberg M, Subers E, Bonney R, Kuehl F. Evidence for two sources of arachidonic acid for oxidative metabolism by mouse peritoneal macrophages. J Biol Chem 1982; 257:1591–1594.

68. Minamikawa T, Takahashi A, Fujita S. Differences in features of calcium transients between the nucleus and the cytosol in cultured heart muscle cells: analyzed by confocal microscopy. Cell Calcium 1995; 17:167–176.

69. Peters-Golden M, McNish RW, Hyzy R, Shelly C, Toews GB. Alterations in the pattern of arachidonate metabolism accompany rat macrophage differentiation in the lung. J Immunol 1990; 144:263–270.

70. Mancini J, Evans J. Coupling of recombinant 5-lipoxygenase and leukotriene A_4 hydrolase activities and transcellular metabolism of leukotriene A_4 in Sf9 insect cells. Eur J Biochem 1993; 218:477–484.

71. Forman B, Tontonoz P, Chen J, Brun R, Spiegelman B, Evans R. 15-Deoxy-delta 12, 14-prostaglandin J_2 is a ligand for the adipocyte determination factor PPAR gamma. Cell 1995; 83:803–812.

72. Kliewer S, Lenhard J, Willson T, Patel I, Morris D, Lehmann J. A prostaglandin J_2 metabolite binds peroxisome proliferator-activated receptor gamma and promotes adipocyte differentiation. Cell 1995; 83:813–819.

73. Devchand P, Keller H, Peters J, Vazquez M, Gonzalcz F, Wahli W. The PPAR α-leukotriene B_4 pathway to inflammation control. Nature 1996; 384:39–43.

74. Lepley RA, Fitzpatrick F. 5-lipoxygenase contains a functional Src homology 3-binding motif that interacts with the Src homology 3 domain of Grb2 and cytoskeletal proteins. J Biol Chem 1994; 269:24163–24168.

6

Cyclooxygenase-2 Expression in Airway Cells

PETER J. BARNES, MARIA G. BELVISI, ROBERT NEWTON,
and JANE A. MITCHELL

National Heart and Lung Institute
Imperial College School of Medicine
London, England

I. Introduction

Asthma is a chronic inflammatory disease and many inflammatory mediators are involved (1). These mediators include prostaglandins (PG), such as PGE_2, $PGF_{2\alpha}$, PGD_2, and thromboxane $(Tx)A_2$, which are products of cyclooxygenase. The role of eicosanoids in asthma is somewhat uncertain, as cyclooxygenase inhibitors have little effect on airway function in most patients with asthma, apart from the patients with aspirin-sensitive asthma, who are made worse by these drugs. Recently, a noncyclooxygenase pathway has been described that generates isoprostanes from arachidonic acid via a nonenzymatic peroxidation mechanism catalyzed by free radicals (2). Among the most prevalent isoprostanes are F2-isoprostanes, such as 8-epi-$PGF_{2\alpha}$, which is generated in humans (3). 8-Epi-$PGF_{2\alpha}$ is a potent constrictor of guinea pig and human airways in vitro, via activation of thromboxane (TP) receptors (4).

The discovery of an inducible form of cyclooxygenase (COX-2) is of particular interest in asthma as proinflammatory cytokines, such as IL-1β and TNFα, that induce this enzyme are present in the inflamed airway of asthmatic patients (5,6).

II. Prostanoids in Airways

There is considerable evidence that prostanoids production is increased in asthma and that these mediators exert many effects relevant to the pathophysiology of asthma (Fig. 1).

A. Prostanoid Production in Asthma

There is much evidence that prostaglandins and thromboxane are generated in asthmatic airways. Concentrations of PGD_2, $PGF_{2\alpha}$ in bronchoalveolar lavage fluid of asthmatic patients were over 10-fold higher than in nonasthmatic normal and atopic control subjects (7). Patients with elevated bronchoalveolar lavage fluid concentrations of PGD_2 are more likely to have nocturnal asthma (8). Allergen challenge is associated with increased excretion of a stable metabolite of TxA_2 within 2 hr after challenge, but not during the late response

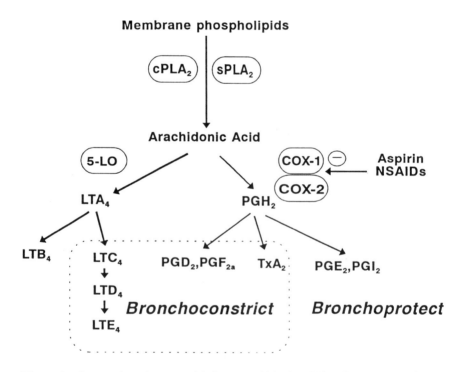

Figure 1   Generation of prostanoids from arachidonic acid involves the coordinated expression of phospholipase A_2 (PLA_2), and both secretory ($sPLA_2$) and cytosolic ($cPLA_2$) forms may be involved. Arachidonic acid is then transformed into prostanoids by cyclooxygenase-1 (COX-1) and COX-2.

(9,10). The cellular source of increased eicosanoid production in asthma is not certain, but many inflammatory cells that are activated in asthmatic airways, including mast cells, macrophages, and eosinophils, are capable of producing a range of prostanoids. In addition, structural cells such as airway epithelial cells and airway smooth muscle cells may also be a source of these mediators in the inflamed airway.

B. Prostanoid Effects on Airways

Prostanoids have potent effects on human airway function (Table 1). PGD_2 and $PGF_{2\alpha}$ are potent bronchoconstrictors in asthmatic subjects and increase the bronchoconstrictor response to other spasmogens (11,12). $PGF_{2\alpha}$ causes cough in asthmatic and normal subjects (13,14). The thromboxane mimetic U46619 is a potent bronchoconstrictor in asthmatic patients and this is mediated in part through the increased release of acetylcholine (15). Thromboxane is also a potent inducer of airway microvascular leakage in animal airways (16). PGE_2 has effects that are both beneficial and detrimental in asthma. Inhaled PGE_2 causes cough and sensitizes the cough reflex (13,17), and although it is a bronchodilator in human airways in vitro, it may induce bronchoconstriction due to activation of reflex bronchoconstriction (18). On the other hand, PGE_2 inhibits the release of acetylcholine from human airway nerves in vitro (19) and inhibits the contractile effect of histamine (20). PGE_2 also inhibits eosinophil release of mediators (21). Inhaled PGE_2 has an inhibitory effect on allergen- and exercise-induced bronchoconstriction in asthma (22,23). Endogenous PGE_2 may therefore be bronchoprotective in asthma and may even act as an endogenous anti-inflammatory mechanism (24). PGE_2 has been implicated in the refractoriness to exercise-induced asthma (23). Prostacyclin (PGI_2) appears to

Table 1 Effects of Prostanoids on Airway Function

Prostanoid	Airway effect
PGE_2	Bronchodilatation and bronchoprotection
	Inhibition of inflammatory cell activation
	Cough
	Vasodilatation
PGI_2	Vasodilatation
$PGF_{2\alpha}$	Bronchoconstriction
	Cough
	Mucus secretion
TxA_2	Bronchoconstriction
	Airway hyperresponsiveness
	Microvascular leakage

have relatively little direct effect on airway tone, although it may be more important in the regulation of bronchial blood flow (25).

C. Prostanoid Inhibitors in Asthma

The production of potent prostanoids in asthmatic patients and the airway effects demonstrated by these mediators suggest that they may play an important role in the pathophysiology of asthma. In animal studies, and particularly in guinea pigs, prostanoids appear to play a key role in airway inflammation in allergic asthma models. Thromboxane is a major bronchoconstrictor mediator in guinea pigs, suggesting that cyclooxygenase inhibitors or thromboxane antagonists may be useful in asthma therapy. However, cyclooxygenase inhibitors have not been shown to have any consistent beneficial effects in asthma. This might be because prostanoids have both beneficial and harmful effects on the airways, so that nonselective cyclooxygenase inhibitors, such as indomethacin and flurbiprofen, have no net effect. However, neither thromboxane synthase inhibitors nor potent thromboxane receptor antagonists have been found to inhibit induced asthma (26), although a thromboxane antagonist is reported to reduce airway hyperresponsiveness in asthmatic subjects (27).

III. Induction of COX-2 in Airway Cells

A.   Epithelial Cells

COX-2 protein and mRNA are induced in a human lung epithelial cell line (A549) and in primary human airway epithelial cells after exposure to the proinflammatory cytokines IFN-γ, IL-1β, TNFα, and a mixture of these cytokines (28–30) (Fig. 2). The expression of COX-2 protein is due to increased transcription, as it is blocked by the transcription blocker actinomycin D (29) and there appears to be coordinated regulation of cyctosolic (85 kDa) phospholipase A$_2$ (cPLA$_2$) (29,30). Induction of COX-2 is accompanied by the release of the COX metabolites PGE$_2$, PGF$_{2\alpha}$, 6-oxo-PGF$_{1\alpha}$ (reflecting PGI$_2$), and minimal amounts of TxB$_2$. The increased protein expression of COX-2 is preceded by an increase in COX-2 mRNA (measured by semiquantitative PCR) and an increased rate of transcription (measured by nuclear run-on assay) (31). PGE$_2$ is the predominant product of COX-2 in these cells.

There is little expression of COX-1 before or after cytokine stimulation and little expression of COX-2 before exposure to cytokines. Indeed, in vivo studies in rats indicate that induction of COX-2 by lipopolysaccharide results in suppression of COX-1 transcription (32).

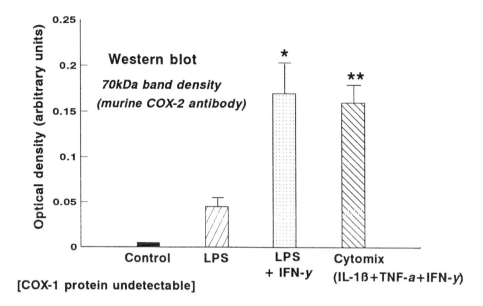

Figure 2 COX-2 expression in primary cultured human airway epithelial cells after exposure to lipopolysaccharide (LPS), LPS + interferon-γ (IFN-γ), and a mixture of cytokines (cytomix) containing interleukin-1β (IL-1β), tumor necrosis factor-α (TNFα), and IFN-γ. COX-2 was detected by Western blotting using a murine antibody to COX-2. *Significance of difference from control; *p < 0.05, **p < 0.01.

The induction of COX-2 and the release of prostaglandins are inhibited in A549 cells by the glucocorticoid dexamethasone (28,29). This is accompanied by a reduction in COX-2 mRNA (29).

The relevance of prostaglandin production in epithelial cells in asthma is not yet certain. Immunocytochemical studies have reported increased expression of COX-2 in epithelial cells of asthmatic patients (33). The in vitro studies suggest that the major prostanoid product of COX-2 in these cells is PGE_2, but whether it is beneficial or detrimental in asthma is not yet certain and studies with selective COX-2 inhibitors are needed. In vitro studies in animals suggest that epithelial production of PGE_2 may protect against bronchoconstriction induced by bradykinin, tachykinins and endothelin-1 (34–38).

B. Airway Smooth Muscle

Airway smooth muscle, including human airway smooth muscle, also produces prostanoids, including PGE_2, $PGF_{2\alpha}$, PGI_2, and TxB_2 (39,40). There is a very low basal expression of COX-1 and COX-2 in cultured rat and human airway smooth muscle in vitro, but COX-2 protein and mRNA increase after exposure to TNFα and IL-1β, whereas there is no increased expression of COX-1 (40,41) (Fig. 3). This is associated with increased production of PGE$_2$, 6-keto PGF$_{1\alpha}$, and TxB$_2$, and the pattern of prostanoids differs from epithelial cells in that 6-keto PGF$_{1\alpha}$ and PGE$_2$ are produced in equal amounts, whereas in epithelial cells PGE$_2$ predominates (40). The protein inhibitor cycloheximide inhibits COX-2 expression and PGE$_2$ release in these cells indicating that de novo protein synthesis is involved (Fig. 4). Indeed, there is a superinduction of COX-2 in the presence of cycloheximide, a phenomenon seen with other rapidly inducible genes such as inducible nitric oxide synthase (iNOS) that may relate to increased activation of the transcription factor nuclear factor-κB (NF-κB) (42).

The functional significance of COX-2 induction in airway smooth muscle cells is uncertain. PGE$_2$ and PGI$_2$ should exert a protective effect against bronchoconstrictors, such as leukotriene D$_4$ and histamine and acetylcholine. Furthermore, PGE$_2$ may have an inhibitory effect on the proliferation of airway smooth muscle (43). On the other hand, thromboxane increases proliferation of rabbit airway smooth muscle in vitro (44).

C. Inflammatory Cells

Many inflammatory cells may produce prostanoids at the inflammatory site. Macrophages may play a key role in asthmatic inflammation (45) and produce

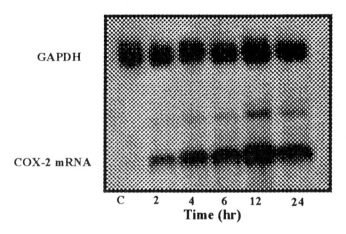

Figure 3 Northern blot showing expression of COX-2 mRNA in cultured human airway smooth muscle cells. There is a time-dependent induction of mRNA after exposure of smooth muscle cells to cytomix.

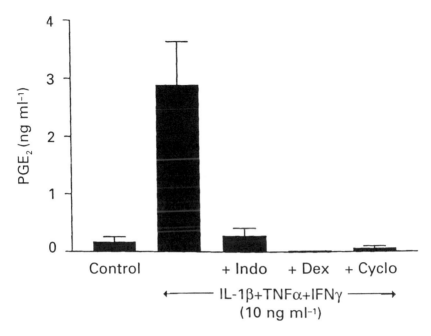

Figure 4 Induction of prostaglandin E_2 (PGE$_2$) release from cultured human airway smooth muscle cells after exposure to a mixture of interleukin-1β (IL-1β), tumor necrosis factor-α (TNFα), and interferon-γ (IFN-γ). Release of PGE$_2$ is blocked by indomethacin (Indo), dexamethasone (Dex), and cycloheximide (Cyclo).

multiple prostanoids. COX-2 is potently induced in animal and human alveolar macrophages in vitro by lipopolysaccharide (46,47). In contrast to epithelial cells and airway smooth muscle cells where PGE$_2$ is the main product of COX-2, the predominant product of COX-2 in alveolar macrophages is PGF$_{2\alpha}$ (48) (Fig. 5). COX-2 is also expressed in human blood monocytes after lipopolysaccharide exposure in vitro (47), and there is evidence for increased expression of COX-2 mRNA in monocytes from patients with asthma compared to normal controls (49). It is likely that COX-2 may also be induced in mast cells and eosinophils, which are also important sources of prostanoids in asthmatic airways.

IV. Regulation of COX-2

Induction of COX-2 appears to occur at a transcriptional level, indicating that transcription factors are involved. NF-κB is involved in the transcription of

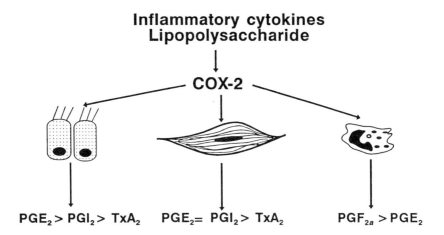

Inflammatory cytokines
Lipopolysaccharide

COX-2

$PGE_2 > PGI_2 > TxA_2$ $PGE_2= PGI_2 > TxA_2$ $PGF_{2a} > PGE_2$

Figure 5   Induction of COX-2 in different airway cells may result in the release of different patterns of prostanoid product. Epithelial cells (left), airway smooth muscle (center), and macrophage (right) release different profiles of prostanoids.

many immune and inflammatory genes (50) and appears to play a key role in chronic inflammatory diseases, such as asthma and rheumatoid arthritis (51, 52). NF-κB is activated in asthmatic airways, particularly in epithelial cells and macrophages (53). The human COX-2 gene has two putative NF-κB binding motifs in its upstream promoter region (54) (Fig. 6). The upstream κB site binds NF-κB (p65/p50 dimers) with a higher affinity than the downstream site. There is evidence that NF-κB is involved in the induction of COX-2 in murine macrophages in response to TNF-α, but IL-6 acting through another transcription factor (NF-IL6 or C/EBPβ) is also involved and may interact with NF-κB synergistically (55). Cyclic AMP may also affect transcription as there is a cyclic AMP response element adjacent to the NF-IL6 binding site. Exposure of epithelial cells to IL-1β is associated with massive induction of NF-κB that precedes the increased transcription of COX-2 (56), and NF-κB activates a reporter plasmid containing 917 bases of the upstream promoter of the COX-2 gene (31). Furthermore, the protein tyrosine phosphatase inhibitor phenylarsine oxide inhibits NF-κB activation and COX-2 expression, without affecting other transcription factors such as AP-1, Oct-1, and SP-1. NF-κB also regulates the expression of iNOS (57–59), and proinflammatory cytokines such as IL-1β and TNFα may therefore result in the coordinated expression of these two inducible genes. There may be a functional interaction between these genes. In a macrophage line, while indomethacin had no effect on nitrite formation, an NOS inhibitor, L-NMMA, increased the formation of

Human COX-2 gene

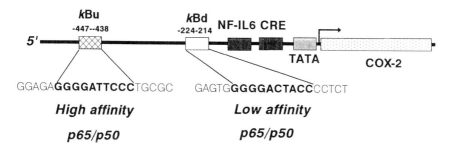

Figure 6 5'-Upstream promoter region of the human COX-2 gene showing two consensus sites for NF-κB binding. An upstream site has a high affinity for p65/p50 binding (κBu) and a downstream site has a lower affinity (κBd). There are also consensus sequences for binding of the transcription factors nuclear factor interleukin-6 (NF-IL6 or C/EBPβ) and cyclic AMP response element (CRE) binding protein.

prostanoids induced by lipopolysaccharide, suggesting that NO generated by iNOS has an inhibitory effect on COX-2 (60). This was confirmed by an increased amount of COX-2 protein in these cells after incubation with L-NMMA. However, others have reported that NO increases COX-2 expression in macrophages (61). These differences may relate to the amounts of endogenous NO generated.

The signal transduction pathways involved in the activation of COX-2 transcription are not yet certain. Mitogen-activated protein (MAP) kinases are involved in the activation of NF-κB and other transcription factors, such as C/EBPβ. There is evidence for the involvement of tyrosine kinases in the expression of COX-2 as tyrosine kinase inhibitors block COX-2 expression in response to IL-1β (62,63).

Effect of Glucocorticoids

The glucocorticoid dexamethasone potently inhibits COX-2 expression in epithelial cells and airway smooth muscle cells (28,40,64) and inhibits the expression of COX-2 in lung in vivo after induction by lipopolysaccharide (32) (Fig. 7). This effect of dexamethasone is partly mediated by inhibition of transcription of the COX-2 and cPLA$_2$ genes (29). Glucocorticoids potently inhibit NF-κB, by activating binding of the glucocorticoid receptor to the p65 subunit (65–67), and may also increase synthesis of the inhibitory protein IκB-α (68,69). This suggests that glucocorticoids inhibit COX-2 expression by

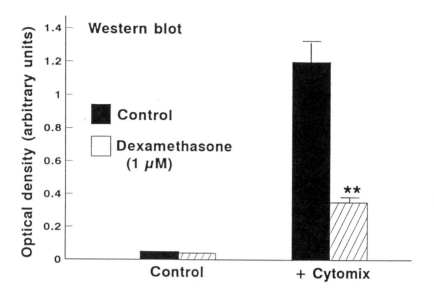

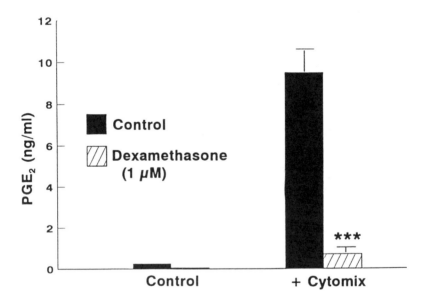

Figure 7 Effect of dexamethasone on expression of COX-2 protein (top) and of prostaglandin E_2 (PGE_2) (bottom) release from epithelial A549 cells after stimulation with cytomix. Significance of difference from control: **p < 0.01; ***p < 0.001.

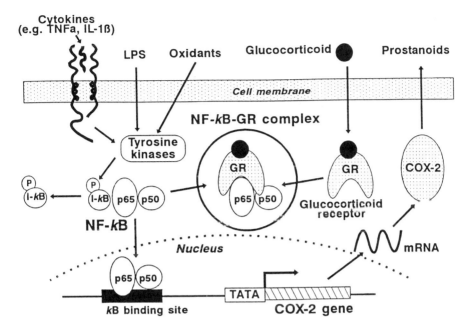

Figure 8 Inhibition of COX-2 by glucocorticoids probably involves the direct inhibition of nuclear factor-κB (NF-κB) by the activated glucocorticoid receptor (GR), which inhibits the induction of COX-2 by cytokines, such as interleukin-1 (IL-1β) and tumor necrosis factor-α (TNFα) and by lipopolysaccharide (LPS).

blocking the activation of NF-κB by proinflammatory cytokines (Fig. 8). However, there is also evidence that glucocorticoid may destablize COX-2 mRNA, providing evidence for a posttranscriptional control mechanism (70). Glucocorticoids are also effective in inhibiting the synthesis of proinflammatory cytokines, including IL-1β and TNFα, that may induce COX-2 in asthmatic airways (71).

V. Relevance in Asthma

Airway epithelial cells are increasingly recognized as an important source of inflammatory mediators in ashtma (72,73). These cells may be activated by oxidants in addition to inflammatory cytokines and this may be of relevance in asthmatic patients who may be exposed to inhaled oxidants such as ozone and nitrogen dioxide (57). These cells are also activated by rhinoviruses, which are the commonest mechanisms of acute exacerbations (74). All of these stimuli activate NF-κB, which, in turn, increases the transcription of inflammatory genes, such as iNOS, COX-2, and chemokines (51,52). The functional significance of the prostanoids released from airway epithelial cells in asthma is not yet clear, however. Thus, PGE_2, the major cyclooxygenase product of epithelial cells, may have beneficial effects in asthma (bronchodilator, protection against bronchoconstriction) (24), but also has potentially deleterious effects (sensitization and activation of airway sensory nerves, vasodilatation). In airway smooth muscle the expression of COX-2 may result in the formation of PGE_2, which should protect against bronchoconstriction and inhibit proliferation of airway smooth muscle, or of thromboxane, which causes bronchoconstriction, increases airway hyperresponsiveness, and increases airway smooth muscle proliferation.

Glucocorticoids are the most effective therapy available for asthma (75) and control inflammation, at least in part, by inhibiting the activation of NF-κB (71). This is likely to underlie the inhibitory effect of glucocorticoids on COX-2 expression in airway cells, resulting in a reduction in prostanoids. Since glucocorticoids are highly effective in controlling asthma it must be assumed that the result of COX-2 expression in asthma is detrimental, at least in the short term, and that deleterious effects of prostanoids outweigh any beneficial effects. However, the long-term effects of prostanoids may be different, and if steroids inhibit the potentially antimitogenic effect of PGE_2 on proliferation of airway smooth muscle, this may be a potential problem with long-term steroid therapy in asthma. Proliferation of airway smooth muscle is a feature of chronic asthma and may contribute to the irreversible airway narrowing that may occur in some patients (76). Several mitogenic agents, including platelet-derived growth factor (PDGF) and endothelin, are generated in asthmatic airways (77–79), and endogenous antiproliferative mechanisms, such as PGE_2, are presumably important in counteracting this structural change.

The recent development of selective COX-2 inhibitors, such as NS-398 and L-745,337, may have implications for asthma therapy (80–82). While nonselective inhibitors, such as aspirin and indomethacin, have little or no beneficial effect in asthma, it is possible that selective COX-2 inhibitors might be more effective by sparing the effects of prostanoids generated by COX-1, but inhibiting the production of prostanoids via COX-2. Whether this would favorably change the profile of prostanoids in asthma remains to be determined, however. Aspirin-sensitive asthma may be induced by all nonselective cyclooxygenase inhibitors, but whether this relates to inhibition of COX-1 or COX-2 is not yet certain. It is possible that selective COX-2 inhibitors may have less propensity to induce asthma and there are anecdotal reports that nonsteroidal anti-inflammatory drugs, such as nimesulide and meloxicam, that are more COX-2 selective are less likely to cause problems.

References

1. Barnes PJ, Chung KF, Page CP. Inflammatory mediators and asthma. Pharmacol Rev 1988; 40:49–84.
2. Morrow JD, Roberts LJ. The isoprostanes. Current knowledge and directions for future research. Biochem Pharmacol 1996; 51:1–9.
3. Awad JA, Morrow JD, Takahashi K, Roberts LJ, 2d. Identification of non-cyclooxygenase-derived prostanoid (F2-isoprostane) metabolites in human urine and plasma. J Biol Chem 1993; 268:4161–4169.
4. Kawikova I, Barnes PJ, Takahashi T, Tadjkarimi S, Yacoub MH, Balvisi MG. 8-epi-prostaglandin $F_{2\alpha}$, a novel non-cyclooxygenase derived prostaglandin, is a potent constrictor of guinea-pig and human airways. Am J Respir Crit Care Med 1996; 153:590–596.
5. Mitchell JA, Larkin S, Williams TJ. Cyclooxygenase-2: regulation and relevance in inflammation. Biochem Pharmacol 1995; 50.1535–1542.
6. Barnes PJ. Cytokines as mediators of chronic asthma. Am J Respir Crit Care Med 1994; 150:S42–S49.
7. Liu MC, Bleecker ER, Lichtenstein LM, Kagey Sobotka A, Niv Y, McLemore TL, Permutt S, Proud D, Hubbard WC. Evidence for elevated levels of histamine, prostaglandin D_2, and other bronchoconstricting prostaglandins in the airways of subjects with mild asthma. Am Rev Respir Dis 1990; 142:126–132.
8. Oosterhoff Y, Kauffman HF, Rutgers B, Zijlstra FJ, Koeter GH, Postma DS. Inflammatory cell number and mediators in bronchoalveolar lavage fluid and peripheral blood in subjects with asthma with increased nocturnal airways narrowing. J Allergy Clin Immunol 1995; 96:219–229.
9. Sladek K, Dworski R, Fitzgerald GA, Buitkus KL, Block FJ, Marney SR, Jr., Sheller JR. Allergen-stimulated release of thromboxane A_2 and leukotriene E_4 in humans. Effect of indomethacin. Am Rev Respir Dis 1990; 141:1441–1445.
10. Kumlin M, Dahlen B, Bjorck T, Zetterstrom O, Granstrom E, Dahlen SE. Urinary excretion of leukotriene E_4 and 11-dehydro-thromboxane B_2 in response to bronchial provocations with allergen, aspirin, leukotriene D_4, and histamine in asthmatics. Am Rev Respir Dis 1992; 146:96–103.
11. Hardy CC, Robinson C, Tattersfield AE, Holgate ST. The bronchoconstrictor effect of inhaled prostaglandin D_2 in normal and asthmatic men. N Engl J Med 1984; 311:210–213.
12. Fuller RW, Dixon CMS, Dollery CT, Barnes PJ. Prostaglandin D_2 potentiates airway responses to histamine and methacholine. Am Rev Respir Dis 1986; 133:252–254.
13. Nichol G, Nix A, Barnes PJ, Chung KF. Prostaglandin $F_{2\alpha}$ enhancement of capsaicin induced cough in man: modulation by beta$_2$-adrenergic and anticholinergic drugs. Thorax 1990; 45:694–698.
14. Stone RA, Barnes PJ, Fuller RW. Contrasting effects of $PGF_{2\alpha}$ and PGE_2 on the sensitivity of the human cough reflex. J Appl Physiol 1992; 73:92–99.
15. Saroea HG, Inman MD, O'Byrne PM. U46619-induced bronchoconstriction in asthmatic subjects is mediated by acetylcholine release. Am J Respir Crit Care Med 1995; 151:321–324.

16. Lotvall JO, Elwood W, Tokuyama K, Sakamoto T, Barnes PJ, Chung KF. Effect of thromboxane A_2 mimetic U 46619 on airway microvascular leakage in the guinea pig. J Appl Physiol 1991.

17. Chaudry NB, Fuller RW, Pride NB. Sensitivity of the human cough reflex: effect of inflammatory mediators prostaglandin E_2, bradykinin and histamine. Am Rev Respir Dis 1989; 40:137–141.

18. Walters EH, DAvies BH. Dual effect of prostaglandin E_2 on normal airways smooth muscle in vivo. Thorax 1982; 37:918–922.

19. Ellis JL, Conanan ND. Prejunctional inhibition of cholinergic responses by prostaglandin E_2 in human bronchi. Am J Respir Crit Care Med 1996; 154: 244–246.

20. Knight DA, Stewart GA, Thompson PJ. Prostaglandin E_2, but not prostacyclin inhibits histamine-induced contraction of human bronchial smooth muscle. Eur J Pharmacol 1995; 272:13–19.

21. Giembycz MA, Kroegel C, Barnes PJ. Platelet activating factor stimulates cyclo-oxygenase activity in guinea-pig eosinophils. J Immunol 1990; 144:3489–3497.

22. Pavord ID, Wong CS, Williams J, Tattersfield AE. Effect of inhaled prostaglandin E_2 on allergen-induced asthma. Am Rev Respir Dis 1993; 148:87–90.

23. Melillo E, Woolley KL, Manning PJ, Watson RM, O'Byrne PM. Effect of inhaled PGE_2 on exercise-induced bronchoconstriction in asthmatic subjects. Am J Respir Crit Care Med 1994; 149:1138–1141.

24. Pavord ID, Tattersfield AE. Bronchoprotective role for endogenous prostaglandin E_2. Lancet 1995; 344:436–438.

25. Hardy C, Robinson C, Lewis RA, Tattersfield AE, Holgate ST. Airway and cardiovascular responses to inhaled prostacyclin in normal and asthmatic subjects. Am Rev Respir Dis 1985; 131:18–21.

26. O'Byrne PM, Fuller RW. The role of thromboxane A_2 in the pathogenesis of airway hyperresponsiveness. Eur Respir J 1989; 2:782–786.

27. Aizawa H, Shigyo M, Nogami H, Hirose T, Hara N. BAY u3405, a thromboxane A_2 antagonist, reduces bronchial hyperresponsiveness in asthmatics. Chest 1996; 109:338–342.

28. Mitchell JA, Belvisi MG, Akarasereemom P, Robbins RA, Kowon OJ, Croxtell J, Barnes PJ, Vane JR. Induction of cyclo-oxygenase-2 by cytokines in human pulmonary epithelial cells: regulation by dexamethasone. Br J Pharmacol 1994; 113: 1008–1014.

29. Newton R, Kuitert LM, Slater DM, Adcock IM, Barnes PJ. Induction of $cPLA_2$ and COX-2 mRNA by proinflammatory cytokines is suppressed by dexamethasone in human airway epithelial cells. Life Sci 1997; 60:67–78.

30. Croxtall JD, Newman SP, Choudhury Q, Flower RJ. The concerted regulation of $cPLA_2$, COX2, and lipocortin 1 expression by IL-1β in A549 cells. Biochem Biophys Res Commun 1996; 220:491–495.

31. Newton R, Kuitert LME, Bergmann M, Adcock IM, Barnes PJ. Evidence for the involvement of NF-κB in the transcriptional control of cyclooxygenase-2 gene expression by interleukin-1β. Biochem Biophys Res Commun 1997; 237:28–32.

32. Liu SF, Newton R, Barnes PJ, Evans TW. Expression of inducible cyclooxygenase in lung. Clin Sci 1996; 90:301–306.

33. Springall DR, Meng Q-H, Redington AE, Howarth PH, Polak JM. Inflammatory genes in asthmatic airway epithelium: suppression by corticosteroids. Eur Respir J 1995; 8(Suppl 19):44S.
34. Frossard N, Stretton CD, Barnes PJ. Modulation of bradykinin responses in airway smooth muscle by epithelial enzymes. Agents Actions 1990; 31:204–209.
35. Frossard N, Rhoden KJ, Barnes PJ. Influence of epithelium on guinea pig airway responses to tachykinins: role of endopeptidase and cyclooxygenase. J Pharmacol Exp Ther 1989; 248:292–298.
36. Devillier P, Acker M, Advenier C, Regoli D, Frossard N. Respiratory epithelium releases relaxant prostaglandin E_2 through activation of substance P (NK_1) receptors. Am Rev Respir Dis 1991; 139:A351.
37. Battistini B, Filep J, Sirois P. Potent thromboxane-mediated in vitro bronchoconstrictor effect of endothelin in guinea pig. Eur J Pharmacol 1990; 178:141–142.
38. Goldie RG, Fernandes LB, Farmer SG, Hay DWP. Airway epithelium-derived inhibitory factor. Trends Pharmacol Sci 1990; 11:67–70.
39. Delamere F, Holland E, Patel S, Bennett J, Pavord I, Knox A. Production of PGE_2 by cultured bovine airways smooth muscle cells and its inhibition by cyclooxygenase inhibitors. Br J Pharmacol 1994; 111:983–988.
40. Belvisi MG, Saunders MA, Haddad E, Hirst SJ, Yacoub MH, Barnes PJ, Mitchell JA. Induction of cyclo-oxygenase-2 by cytokines in human cultured airway smooth muscle cells. Br J Pharmacol 1997; 120:910–916.
41. Vadas P, Stefanski E, Wloch M, Grouix B, van den Bosch H, Kennedy B. Secretory nonpancreatic phospholipase A_2 and cyclooxygenase-2 expression by tracheobronchial smooth muscle cells. Eur J Biochem 1996; 235:557–563.
42. Newton R, Adcock IM, Barnes PJ. Superinduction of NF-κB by actinomycin D and cycloheximide in epithelial cells. Biochem Biophys Res Commun 1996; 218: 518–523.
43. Johnson PR, Armour CL, Carey D, Black JL. Heparin and PGE2 inhibit DNA synthesis in human airway smooth muscle cells in culture. Am J Physiol 1995; 269: L514–9.
44. Noveral JP, Grunstein MM. Role and mechanism of thromboxane-induced proliferation of cultured airway smooth muscle cells. Am J Physiol 1992; 263: L555–61.
45. Lee TH, Lane SJ. The role of macrophages in the mechanisms of airway inflammation in asthma. Am Rev Respir Dis 1992; 145:S27–30.
46. O'Sullivan M, Huggins EM, Meade EA, DeWitt DL, McCall CE. Lipopolysaccharide induces prostaglandin H synthase-2 in alveolar macrophages. Biochem Biophys Res Commun 1992; 187:1123–1127.
47. Hempel S, Monick MM, Hunninghake GW. Lipopolysaccharide induces prostaglandin H synthase-2 protein and mRNA in human alveolar macrophages and blood monocytes. J Clin Invest 1994; 391–396.
48. Mitchell JA, Saunders MA, Bishop-Bailey D, Barnes PJ, Belvisi MG. Cyclo-oxygenase-2 (COX-2) in the lung. Am J Respir Crit Care Med 1996; 153:
49. Kuitert LM, Newton R, Barnes NC, Adcock IM, Barnes PJ. Eicosanoid mediator expression in mononuclear and polymorphonuclear cells in normal subjects and patients with atopic asthma and cystic fibrosis. Thorax 1996; 51:1223–1228.

50. Siebenlist U, Franzuso G, Brown R. Structure, regulation and function of NF-κB. Annu Rev Cell Biol 1994; 10:405–455.
51. Barnes PJ, Karin M. Nuclear factor-κB: a pivotal molecule in chronic inflammation. N Engl J Med 1997; 336:1066–1071.
52. Barnes PJ, Adcock IM. NF-κB: a pivotal role in asthma and a new target for therapy. Trends Pharmacol Sci 1997; 18:46–50.
53. Hart L, Krishnan VJ, Adcock IM, Barnes PJ, Chung KF. Activation of the transcription factor nuclear factor-κB in mild asthma. Am J Respir Crit Care Med 1997 (in press).
54. Appleby SB, Ristimaki A, Neilson K, Narko K, Hla T. Structure of the human cyclooxygenase-2 gene. Biochem J 1994; 302:723–727.
55. Yamamoto K, Arakawa T, Ueda N, Yamamoto S. Transcriptional roles of nuclear factor κB and nuclear factor-interleukin 6 in the tumor necrosis-α–dependent induction of cyclooxygenase-2 in MC3T3-E1 cells. J Biol Chem 1995; 270:31315–31320.
56. Newton R, Adcock IM, Barnes PJ. Stimulation of COX-2 message by cytokines or phorbol ester is preceded by a massive and rapid induction of NF-κB binding activity. Am J Respir Crit Care Med 1995; 151:A165.
57. Adcock IM, Brown CR, Kwon OJ, Barnes PJ. Oxidative stress induces NF-κB DNA binding and inducible NOS mRNA in human epithelial cells. Biochem Biophys Res Commun 1994; 199:1518–1524.
58. Xie Q, Kashiwarbara Y, Nathan C. Role of transcription factor NF-κB/Rel in induction of nitric oxide synthase. J Biol Chem 1994; 269:4705–4708.
59. Kleinert H, Euchenhofer C, Ihrig-Biedert I, Förstermann U. Glucocorticoids inhibit the induction of nitric oxide synthase II by down-regulating cytokine-induced activity of transcription factor nuclear factor-κB. Mol Pharmacol 1996; 49:15–21.
60. Swierkosz TA, Mitchell JA, Warner TD, Botting RM, Vane JR. Co-induction of nitric oxide synthase and cyclo-oxygenase: interactions between nitric oxide and prostanoids. Br J Pharmacol 1995; 114:1335–1342.
61. Salvemini D, Misko TP, Masferrer JL, Seibert K, Currie MG, Needleman P. Nitric oxide activates cyclooxygenase enzymes. Proc Natl Acad Sci USA 1993; 90:7240–7244.
62. Akarasereenont P, Bakhle YS, Thiemermann C, Vane JR. Cytokine-mediated induction of cyclo-oxygenase-2 by activation of tyrosine kinase in bovine endothelial cells stimulated by bacterial lipopolysaccharide. Br J Pharmacol 1995; 115:401–408.
63. Akarasereenont P, Thiemermann C. The induction of cyclo-oxygenase-2 in pulmonary epithelial cell culture (A549) activated by IL-1β is inhibited by tyrosine kinase inhibitors. Biochem Biophys Res Commun 1996; 220:181–185.
64. Newman SP, Flower RJ, Croxtall JD. Dexamethasone suppression of IL-1β-induced cyclooxygenase 2 expression is not mediated by lipocortin-1 in A549 cells. Biochem Biophys Res Commun 1994; 202:931–939.
65. Adcock IM, Brown CR, Gelder CM, Shirasaki H, Peters MJ, Barnes PJ. The effects of glucocorticoids on transcription factor activation in human peripheral blood mononuclear cells. Am J Physiol 1995; 37:C331–C338.
66. Ray A, Prefontaine KE. Physical association and functional antagonism between the p65 subunit of transcription factor NF-κB and the glucocorticoid receptor. Proc Natl Acad Sci USA 1994; 91:752–756.

67. Scheinman RI, Gualberto A, Jewell CM, Cidlowski JA, Baldwin AS. Characterization of the mechanisms involved in transrepression of NF-κB by activated glucocorticoid receptors. Mol Cell Biol 1996; 15:943–953.

68. Auphan N, DiDonato JA, Rosette C, Helmberg A, Karin M. Immunosuppression by glucocorticoids: inhibition of NF-κB activity through induction of IκB synthesis. Science 1995; 270:286–290.

69. Scheinman RI, Cogswell PC, Lofquist AK, Baldwin AS. Role of transcriptional regulation of IκBα in mediation of immunosuppression by glucocorticoids. Science 1995; 270:283–286.

70. Ristimaki A, Narko K, Hla T. Down-regulation of cytokine-induced cyclo-oxygenase-2 transcript isoforms by dexamethasone: evidence for post-transcriptional regulation. Biochem J 1996; 318:325–331.

71. Barnes PJ. Molecular mechanisms of steroid action in asthma. J Allergy Clin Immunol 1996; 97:159–168.

72. Devalia JL, Davies RJ. Airway epithelial cells and mediators of inflammation. Respir Med 1993; 6:405–408.

73. Levine SJ. Bronchial epithelial cell-cytokine interactions in airway epithelium. J Invest Med 1995; 43:241–249.

74. Zhu Z, Tang W, Ray A, Wu Y, Einarsson O, Landry ML, Gwaltney J, Elias JA. Rhinovirus stimulation of interleukin-6 in vivo and in vitro. Evidence for nuclear factor κB-dependent transcription activation. J Clin Invest 1996; 97:421–430.

75. Barnes PJ. Inhaled glucocorticoids for asthma. N Engl J Med 1995; 332:868–875.

76. Knox AJ. Airway re-modeling in asthma: role of airway smooth muscle. Clin Sci 1994; 86:647–652.

77. Hirst SJ, Barnes PJ, Twort CHL. Quantifying proliferation of cultured human and rabbit airway smooth muscle cells in response to serum and platelet-derived growth factor. Am J Respir Cell Mol Biol 1992; 7:574–581.

78. Hirst SJ, Barnes PJ, Twort CHC. PDGF isoform-induced proliferation and receptor expression in human cultured airway smooth muscle cells. Am J Physiol 1996; 14:L415–L428.

79. Glassberg MK, Engul A, Wanner A, Puett D. Endothelin binding and stimulation of mitogenesis in ovine airway smooth muscle cells. Am Rev Respir Dis 1992; 145:A124.

80. Gierse JK, Hauser SD, Creely DP, Koboldt C, Rangwala SH, Isakson PC, Seibert K. Expression and selective inhibition of the constitutive and inducible forms of human cyclooxygenase. Biochem J 1995; 305:479–484.

81. Futaki N, Takahashi S, Yokoyama M, Arai I, Higuchi S, Otomo S. NS-398 a new anti-inflammatory agent, selectively inhibits prostaglandin synthase cyclooxygenase (COX-2) activity in vitro. Prostaglandins 1994; 47:55–59.

82. Chan CC, Boyce S, Brideau C, Ford Hutchinson AW, Gordon R, Guay D, Hill Rg, Li CS, Mancini J, Penneton M, et al. Pharmacology of a selective cyclooxygenase-2 inhibitor, L-745,337: a novel nonsteroidal anti-inflammatory agent with an ulcerogenic sparing effect in rat and nonhuman primate stomach. J Pharmacol Exp Ther 1995; 274:1531–1537.

7

Cyclooxygenase Gene Expression and Regulation

KENNETH KUN-YU WU

University of Texas Medical School at Houston
Houston, Texas

I. Introduction

Cyclooxygenase (COX, also known as prostaglandin H synthase, PGHS) is a key enzyme in prostanoid biosynthesis (for a review see Ref. 1). It is a bifunctional enzyme comprising a COX activity that catalyzes the bisoxygenation of arachidonate to form prostaglandin G_2 (PGG_2) and a peroxidase activity that converts PGG_2 to PGH_2. PGH_2 is the common precursor for biologically active and physiological important prostanoids such as thromboxane A_2 (TXA_2), prostacyclin (PGI_2), PGE_2, $PGF_{2\alpha}$, and PGD_2. Two isoforms of COX have been identified and characterized. COX-1 isoform was originally purified from ram seminal vesicle (2,3). The purified enzyme in detergent was reported to be a dimer with a monomeric molecular weight of approximately 70 kDa. It is membrane associated and localized in the lumen of endoplasmic reticulum. The COX-1 cDNA was originally cloned from ram seminal vesicles (4–6). The ovine COX-1 cDNA codes for a 600-amino-acid (aa) polypeptide containing a 18-aa signal peptide at its amino terminus. Human and murine COX-1 cDNAs code for a 599-aa and 602-aa polypeptide, with a 17-aa and 20-aa signal peptide, respectively (7). Sequence comparison of COX-1 of these three species reveals an over 90% sequence identity. Site-directed mutagenesis of ovine COX-1 cDNA identified Tyr-385 as the active site and two histidine residues (His-388 and His-309) as the potential heme ligand (8,9). Ser-530 was identified as the acetylation site of aspirin, which earlier has been shown to irreversibly inhibit COX activity (10). It was postulated that acetylation of this serine residue introduces a bulky group into the substrate channel that interferes with the contact of arachidonate to the active site. This supposition was confirmed by X-ray crystallographic structure of COX-1 (11). The X-ray structure reveals a long substrate channel lined with hydrophobic residues. Tyr-385 is identified as the active site and His-388 as the heme ligand. Ser-530 is located in the vicinity of Tyr-385 and can exert spatial hinderance when it is acetylated or mutated to a more bulky amino acid residue.

COX-1 undergoes suicidal autoinactivation during catalysis (12). The mechanism by which the enzyme is inactivated is unclear. It was postulated that oxygen radicals generated during catalysis cause protein unfolding and proteolysis. The half-life of COX-1 activity during catalysis was estimated to be approximately 10 min (13,14). In response to the suicidal autoinactivation, the cells are endowed with mechanisms to replenish the enzyme by regulated de novo synthesis of COX-1.

COX-2 cDNA was cloned from src transformed chick embryo fibroblasts and phorbol-induced murine 3T3 fibroblasts (15,16). The murine COX-2 codes for a 604-aa polypeptide in which a 17-aa near the amino terminus is absent but an 18-aa insert near the carboxyl terminus that is absent in COX-1 sequence is present. Human COX-2 cDNA cloned from endothelial cells (17,18) also encodes a 604-aa polypeptide and, like murine COX-2, has a shorter signal peptide than COX-1 and an 18-aa insert near the carboxyl terminus. Sequence comparison between murine and human COX-2 cDNA shows about 60% identity. However, residues important in COX-1 catalytic activity are conserved in COX-2. The aspirin acetylation serine residue is also conserved. Interestingly, COX-2 is less sensitive to aspirin inhibition than COX-1. Studies on purified COX proteins and in cells have shown that the concentration of aspirin to inhibit 50% COX-2 activity (IC_{50}) is about 100-fold higher than that to inhibit 50% COX-1 activity (19,20). Moreover, 15(R)-hydroxyeicosatetraenoic acid (HETE) is generated by COX-2 treated with aspirin (19). These results suggest that despite a similar substrate binding pocket between these two isoforms of COX, the substrate channel of COX-1 is more rigid than that of COX-2 and more sensitive to the spatial hinderance of acetyl group on the serine residue. The substrate channel of COX-2 is thought to be more flexible, and when hindered by the acetyl group, arachidonate may enter the binding pocket at a different orientation, which leads to oxygenation at the C-15 position. COX-1 is also more sensitive than COX-2 to the inhibition by other commonly used nonsteroidal anti-inflammatory drugs (19,20). The mechanisms by which this differential inhibition occurs are less clear. However, several new compounds selectively inhibiting COX-2 activity have been developed (21,22). These compounds will be useful in probing differences in the substrate and heme-binding sites between COX-1 and COX-2. Moreover, they may offer better anti-inflammatory therapy with fewer undesirable side effects.

Expression and regulation of these two isoforms of COX differ considerably at the transcriptional level. These differences and their physiological and pathophysiological relevances are discussed in detail in the following sections.

II. COX-1 Gene Expression

COX-1 is constitutively expressed in almost all mammalian cells. The cellular level of COX-1 is low and varies somewhat from tissue to tissue. The human COX-1 gene spans 22 kb on the long arm of chromosome 9 and contains 11 exons (Fig. 1) that encode a 2.7-kb mRNA (23). The 5'-flanking region of human COX 1 gene does not contain a canonical TATA box or an initiator element (24). The 200-bp region upstream from the translation start codon ATG is G and C rich. Multiple transcription start sites have been identified by primer extension (24). These features are consistent with those of a house-

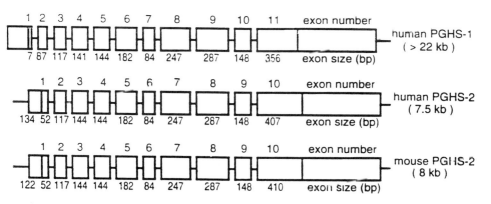

Figure 1 Comparison of human COX-1 and COX-2 genomic structures. Mouse COX-2 (PGHS-2) genomic structure is included as reference. Exons are shown as boxes and introns are shown as lines connecting boxes. Numbers shown above the boxes denote exon numbers and numbers shown below the boxes denote the length of nucleotides. The vertical lines within the exon 1 boxes denote the ATG start codon whereas the lines within the last exons correspond to the translational stop codon. (Reproduced from Ref. 40 with permission from Biochemical Biophysical Research Communications.)

keeping gene. We have analyzed the regulatory elements in the 2.1-kb 5'-flanking region. It bears putative binding sites for Sp1, GATA, AP2, PEA3, and shear stress response elements (SSRE). The promoter activity conferred by this 5'-flanking region was evaluated by constructing a ~2.0-kb fragment into a promoterless luciferase expression vector, pXP1, and transiently expressing the recombinant plasmid into cultured human umbilical vein endothelial cells (HUVEC) or NS-20 cells (24). pXP1 vector and pSV-luc (driven by SV40 early promoter) were included as the negative and positive control, respectively. To control the transfection variability, all the cells were cotransfected with pSV-LacZ in which β-galactosidase (β-gal) expression is driven by a SV40 early promoter. Both luciferase (luc) and β-gal activities were measured by highly sensitive chemiluminescent assays specifically for these two enzymes. The results were expressed as the ratio of luc activity to β-gal activity. This ~2.0-kb 5'-flanking DNA fragment conferred a promoter activity about 20% of that of pSV-luc. A series of 5-deletion mutants of this DNA fragment constructed into the promoterless luc expression vector (pXP1 and more recently pGL3-basic) were expressed in HUVEC to define the minimal promoter region. The promoter activity was retained in fragment (-744/-21). Further 5'- and 3'-deletion mutations identified two discrete regions important in basal promoter activity. DNase I foot printing analysis revealed that a Sp1 site in the proximal region was protected by Sp1 binding. Another Sp1 site at the distal region was considered to be important, too. These two Sp1 sites are separated by about 500 bp. Electrophoretic mobility shift assay coupled with competition with wild-type and Sp1 mutated Sp1 consensus sequences as well as super shift assay confirmed the binding of Sp1 and/or its immunoreactive proteins to these two regions. Mutation of these two Sp1 sites reduced the promoter activity by about 75% when compared to the wild-type promoter. These results indicate that two Sp1 sites are involved in basal COX-1 gene transcription. Additional transcriptional activators are likely to contribute to the full expression of this gene. This requires further investigation.

III. Up-regulation of COX-1 Expression

It is generally believed that COX-1 gene is constitutively expressed and is not inducible. However, several recent reports indicate that COX-1 expression is up-regulated by physiological agonists in a variety of cells including primary cultured cells such as HUVEC, bone marrow–derived mast cells (25,26), and transformed cells such as 3T3 EC osteoblasts and lung epithelial cells (27,28). Work from our laboratory showed that interleukin-1β (IL-1β) and phorbol 12-myristate 13-acetate (PMA) increased endothelial COX-1 mRNA levels in a time- and concentration-dependent manner (25). COX-1 mRNA was determined by Northern blot analysis and quantitative polymerase chain reaction

(PCR). In multiple experiments, densitometric analysis of COX-1 mRNA on Northern blots revealed a maximal twofold increase in COX-1 mRNA in HUVEC stimulated with IL-1β for 4 hr. The Northern blot results were corroborated by the competitive PCR quantitation of COX-1 mRNA levels. The basal COX-1 mRNA levels in passage 2 confluent HUVEC were 24.3 ± 10.6 amol/μg RNA. Treatment of these cells with PMA (50 nM) increased the COX-1 mRNA levels over the basal level by 1.7-fold (Fig. 2A). Stimulation of HUVEC with rIL-1β (50 U/ml) for 4 hr resulted in a maximal increase in COX-1 mRNA levels by 2.1-fold. COX-1 mRNA increments induced by PMA were suppressed by actinomycin D or cycloheximide. This contrasts to the superinduction of COX-2 gene expression by cycloheximide. Biologically active analogs of PMA such as 2-deoxyphorbol 13-phenyl acetate 20-acetate (dPPA) increased the HUVEC COX-1 mRNA levels to a similar extent as PMA whereas inactive phorbol analogs such as 4α-phorbol 12,13 didecanoate (PDD) had no stimulating effect. IL-1β and PMA increased the COX-1 protein levels in a time- and concentration-dependent manner in accordance with the increments of the COX-1 mRNA levels (25). IL-1β and PMA increased the 6-keto-PGF$_{1\alpha}$ content produced by HUVEC, and the maximal level of PGI$_2$ synthesis induced by these two agents was approximately twofold over the basal level. Biologically active PMA analogs such as dPPA increased PGI$_2$ synthesis whereas inactive analog, PDD, did not (Fig. 2B). These results indicate that endothelial COX-1 expression is induced by IL-1β and PMA. Our results further show that COX-1 expression induced by PMA is suppressed by protein kinase C inhibitors such as calphostin C and staurosporine (25).

Induction of COX-1 mRNA expression by PMA is correlated with the stimulation of COX-1 gene promoter activity by PMA in HUVEC transduced with 5'-flanking promoter/enhancer element of COX-1 gene in a luciferase expression vector as described in the previous section. PMA (50 nM, 4 hr incubation) increased the promoter activity conferred by the minimal promoter fragment by 1.8-fold over the basal activity. Mutations of either and both Sp1 binding sites did not abolish the increment in the promoter activity induced by PMA although the overall promoter activity was markedly reduced due to the loss of the basal promoter activity conferred by binding of Sp1 proteins to these two Sp1 binding sites in this promoter region. These studies provide strong evidence that PMA increases the transcription of COX-1 gene. PMA-induced transcriptional activation probably requires an interaction between Sp1 and other transcriptional activators.

IV. Induction of COX-2 Gene Expression

Except for cells in the central nervous system and gastric mucosa in which COX-2 expression is detected at the basal state (29,30), COX-2 gene is not

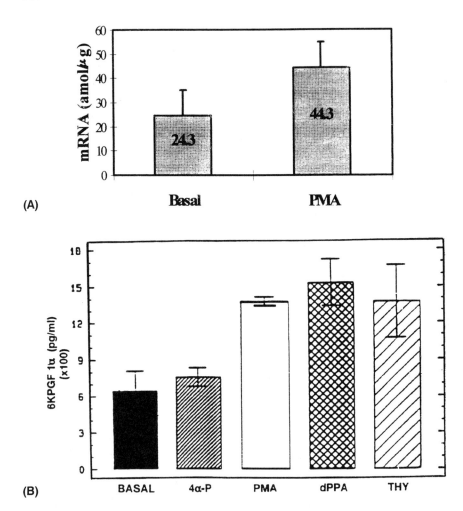

Figure 2 Stimulation of HUVEC COX-1 expression by PMA. (A) COX-1 mRNA levels in basal and PMA-stimulated HUVEC (passage 2) measured by competitive PCR. Each bar represents mean ± SD of four experiments. The numbers shown in the bars are the mean values in amol/μg RNA. (B) PGI$_2$ levels measured as 6-keto-PGF$_{1\alpha}$ by RIA in basal HUVEC and HUVEC treated with 100 nM 4α-P (4α phorbol 12,13-didecanoate), 100 nM PMA (phorbol 12-myristate 13-acetate), 100 nm dPPA (2-deoxyphorbol 13-phenylacetate 20-acetate), or 100 nm THY (thymeleatoxin) for 4 hr. Each bar represents mean value ± SD of four experiments. (B reproduced from Ref. 25, with permission.)

constitutively expressed but highly inducible. Induction of COX-2 expression by a variety of agonists has been reported in diverse types of cells and tissues in a variety of animal species (for a review see Ref. 31). A selective list of cell types and their inducing agents is shown in Table 1 (for a review see Ref. 31). COX-2 in a large repertoire of cells involved in inflammation are induced by inflammatory cytokines, raising the possibility that COX-2 induction plays a crucial role in generating inflammatory prostanoids (32,33). In vivo studies have provided strong evidence to support this. COX-2 induction has been shown to be involved in physiological functions such as ovulation. Rat granulosa cell COX-2 expression was reported to be inducible by sex hormones and COX-2 gene disruption mice failed to ovulate (34). COX-2 expressions in vascular endothelial cells, airway epithelial cells, and kidney tissues are induced by pathophysiological agents raising the possibility that COX-2 induction in these organs may play an important role in cytoprotection. COX-2 mRNA levels in human colon cancer tissues have been reported to be elevated. It has been implied that COX-2 may be involved in resistance to apoptosis (35). These studies indicate that COX-2 induction has diverse pathophysiological roles depending on the tissues and the circumstances under which its expression is induced.

The kinetics of COX-2 mRNA expressions induced by diverse agonists in a wide variety of cells and tissues is similar. COX-2 mRNA levels start to

Table 1 COX Gene Induction or Stimulation by Diverse Inducers in Different Cells and Different Animal Species[a]

Cells	Inducers
COX-1 Stimulation	
Human umbilical vein E.C.	PMA, IL-1β
Mouse bone marrow–derived mast cells	Stem cell factor and dexamethasone
Rat tracheal epithelial cells	PMA, EGF
Mouse osteoblastic MC3T3-E1 cells	Serum
COX-2 Induction	
Human umbilical vein E.C.	PMA, IL-1β
Human MØ	Endotoxin
Mouse 3T3 fibroblasts	PMA serum growth factors
Mouse MC3T3-E1 osteoblasts	Serum, growth factors, PGE_2
Rat mesangial cells	Endothelin-1
Rat vascular SMC	Serum
Rat ovary granulosa cells	Estrogen
Chick embryo fibroblasts	V-SRC oncogene

[a]For references, please see Ref. 31.

rise at about 30 min, reach a plateau at 2 hr, and decline rapidly 4 hr after addition of stimuli. The maximal COX-2 mRNA levels induced by these agonists are much higher than the COX-1 mRNA levels. By using quantitative competitive PCR procedures specific for COX-1 and COX-2 mRNAs, we have shown that maximal COX-1 mRNA levels in passage 1 cultured HUVEC induced by IL-1β or PMA are about 80 amol/μg RNA whereas maximal COX-2 mRNA levels induced by IL-1β or PMA are 580 and 2935 amol/μg RNA, respectively. Hence, it has been assumed that induction of COX-2 is accompanied by a "burst" of prostanoid biosynthesis. However, the arachidonate metabolic profile in COX-2-induced cells may vary with cell types. Several recent observations suggest that COX-2 utilizes a different pool of arachidonic acid. Furthermore, since COX-2 is localized in nucleus and at nuclear envelope and endoplasmic reticulum (ER) (36), it is possible that COX-2 at different locations may have different prostanoid synthetic profiles. This issue is of considerable importance in cells wherein prostanoids are synthesized by a final specific enzyme step. An example of this is prostacyclin synthesis in endothelial cells. PGH$_2$ generated via COX catalysis is further converted to PGI$_2$ by PGI synthase. PGI synthase is primarily bound to the ER membrane. It is unclear whether PGH$_2$ generated by the nuclear COX-2 will be as efficient as that generated by ER COX-2 or COX-1 for PGI$_2$ biosynthesis. It is possible that COX-2 on the nuclear membrane is mostly responsible for synthesis of PGE$_2$ and PGF$_{2\alpha}$ which have been shown in an osteoblastic cell line to induce COX-2 expression as a positive feedback mechanism (37). The functional significance of this will depend on the cell type and the coupling of COX-2 to phospholipases and the downstream enzymes.

The mechanisms by which the various stimuli induce COX-2 gene transcription have not been entirely elucidated. However, substantial progress has been made due to cloning of the COX-2 gene from mouse, rat, chicken, and human tissues (38–41). The human COX-2 gene spans about 8 kb on the long arm of chromosome 1 (40). It contains 10 exons (Fig. 1). The exon-intron structure of human COX-2 gene is homologous to that of mouse, rat, and chicken COX-2 genes. The exon-intron structure of human COX-2 gene bears resemblance to human COX-1 gene: exons 2–9 of COX-2 gene are almost identical to exons 3–10 of COX-1 gene. The intron sizes of COX-2 gene are generally smaller than these of COX-1 gene. The last exon (exon 10) of COX-2 gene is larger than the last exon of COX-1 gene accounting for a larger COX-2 transcript (~4.5 kb vs. 2.8 kb of COX-1 mRNA). The 5'-flanking region of COX-2 gene bears a canonical TATA box and a number of enhancer elements, typical for an immediate early gene. The sequence of the 5'-flanking region of COX-2 gene from various animal species is homologous within the 250 bp upstream from the transcription start site. In this region, there are cyclic AMP response element (CRE), NF-IL-6, C/EBP, AP2, and NF-κB sites (40).

Further upstream are putative binding sites for Sp1, PEA3, NF-κB, GATA-1, NF-IL-6, and glucocorticoid response element (GRE). A number of studies have shown that CRE and NF-IL-6 sites are involved in activation of COX-2 transcription. Xie et al. have shown that CRE/ATF on the promoter region of murine COX-2 gene is involved in COX-2 gene transcription induced by Src transformation of NIH 3T3 cells (41). Inoue et al. have shown that lipopolysaccharide-induced COX-2 gene transcription in bovine aortic endothelial cells require CRE and NF-IL-6 sites (42). There are two NF-κB sites on the promoter region of COX-2 gene. Yamamoto et al. have indicated that the proximal NF-κB sites and NF-IL-6 sites are involved in COX-2 induction by tumor necrosis factor α in a murine osteogenic MC3T3-E1 cell line (43).

V. Pathophysiological Implications of COX Induction

Constitutive expression of COX-1 is important in maintaining physiological functions of tissues such as gastric mucosa, airway epithelium, arterial endothelium, and renal medulla. Stimulation of COX-1 expressions by physiological agonists fortifies the cytoprotective mechanism (Fig. 3).

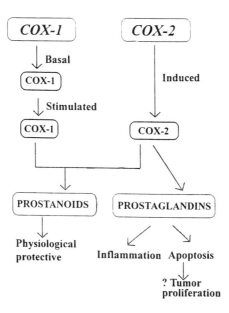

Figure 3 Schematic illustration of the physiological and pathophysiological roles of COX-1 and COX-2 genes.

Physiological and pathophysiological roles of COX-2 are diverse and more complex. They may differ in different tissues and, hence, could not be generalized. COX-2 induction in inflammatory cells including the alveolar macrophages plays an important role in inflammation and tissue injury. COX-2 induction is involved in physiological functions such as ovulation and menstruation. It may be involved in cerebral cortical and spinal functions. COX-2 expression in malignant cells such as colon cancer cells has been considered to be important in reducing apoptosis.

We postulated that in tissues such as vascular endothelium COX-2 induction in response to injurious agents serves as a backup mechanism to synthesize cytoprotective prostanoids. To test this hypothesis we evaluated the effects of lysophosphatidylcholine (lysoPC) on COX-1 and COX-2 expressions in cultured HUVEC. LysoPC is a product of oxidized LDL (oxLDL) and is a major mediator of atherosclerosis (44–46). It has been shown that lysoPC induce mitogenic factor expressions (47,48). We reasoned that it may induce COX expression to augment the synthesis and release of vasoprotective molecules. Cultured HUVEC treated with lysoPC ($100\,\mu$M) in the presence of 5% FBS expressed COX-2 mRNA levels in a time- and concentration-dependent manner (49). Expression of COX-1 mRNA was unaffected in these cells. COX-2 mRNA induction by lysoPC was accompanied by a concordant increase in COX-2 protein expression and PGI_2 synthetic activity. In a separate study, we observed that lysoPC stimulated endothelial nitric oxide synthase mRNA and protein levels, accompanied by increased nitric oxide (NO) production by the treated endothelial cells (50). Concurrent induction of PGI_2 and NO synthesis in endothelial cells by lysoPC is likely to have an impact on defending against lysoPC-induced proinflammatory changes. PGI_2 and NO are potent inhibitors of platelet activation and vasodilators (51,52). NO exerts a potent antiproliferative effect on smooth muscle proliferation and inhibitory effect on monocyte activation and adhesion (53,54). Hence, these two molecules could control the deleterious vascular effects induced by lysoPC. We believe that this serves as a paradigm for the involvement of COX-2 as a defense enzyme against tissue injury. We suspect that COX-2 induction plays a protective role not only in vascular endothelium but also in kidneys and stomach.

VI. COX-1 and COX-2 Gene Deletion in Mice

Physiological and pathophysiological roles of COX-1 and COX-2 genes were evaluated by deletion ("knockout") of either gene by homologous recombination. Langenbach et al. reported COX-1 gene disruption in mice (55). Homozygous COX-1 deletion mutant mice survive normally and have no spontaneous gastric, renal, or vascular abnormalities (55). Paradoxically, these mutant animals were reported to be less prone to indomethacin-induced gastric ul ceration than the wild-type mice despite a marked reduction in gastric PGE_2 synthesis. Homozygous female mutants mated to homozygous male animals produce fewer live offspring, suggesting that COX-1 pathway is essential for normal parturition. COX-2 gene disruption mice were reported by Morham et al. (56) and Dinchuk et al. (57). Homozygous COX-2 disruption mice have a short survival primarily due to renal dysplasia and fibrolysis. Cardiac fibrosis was reported to occur in about 50% of mice by Dinchuk et al. (57). Both studies show that COX-2 deletion mice have a normal inflammatory response. Mor- ham et al. (56) reported that the homozygous mutants are susceptible to peri- tonitis whereas Dinchuk et al. (57) reported that the homozygous mutants are less susceptible to endotoxin-induced hepatocellular cytotoxocity. These ani- mal models provide surprising information regarding the roles of these two isozymes, especially with respect to their contributions to inflammation. These studies imply that both isozymes are involved in inflammation. As inflamma- tory responses involve multiple cells that mount different stages of inflamma- tion, it may be speculated that these two isozymes catalyze the synthesis of inflammatory and/or anti-inflammatory prostaglandins at different stages of inflammation. These gene disruption experiments indicate that both isozymes are important in parturition. COX-2 induction by estrogen in granulosa cells has been shown to correlate with ovulation. COX-2 disruption female mice appear to be defective in ovulation to account for infertility. On the other hand, as suggested by Langenbach et al. (55), COX-1 may be involved in syn- thesizing prostanoids important in maternal or fetal physiology. Interestingly, 50% of COX-2 disrupted mice develop cardiac fibrosis. This observation sup- ports the notion that COX-2 induction in endothelium is cardio- and arterio- protective. A major finding in COX-2 disrupted animals is renal dysplasia and fibrosis postnatally. The mechanism by which this occurs requires further in- vestigation. These COX-1 and COX-2 disrupted mice will serve as useful ani- mals models for further understanding the physiological roles of these two enzymes.

VII. COX Overexpression by Gene Transfer

In a number of human vascular diseases including pulmonary hypertension, administration of PGI_2 or PGE_1 has been shown to have a beneficial effect. However, systemic administration of these compounds has considerable side effects. Since they act as an autacoid, it will be desirable to increase their levels locally. One approach is to transfer the synthetic enzyme gene(s) locally. We have recently shown that COX-1 gene transfer into cultured EC using replication-defective retroviral or adenoviral vectors achieved a high level of

PGI$_2$ synthesis in response to stimulation with physiological agonists (58). Kinetic analysis indicates that increased COX-1 protein expression is accompanied by a more sustained PGI$_2$ synthesis despite COX-1 autoinactivation during catalysis (14). We have further shown that COX-1 gene can be effectively transferred into damaged carotid arteries in pigs using replication-defective adenoviruses as vectors and COX-1 gene transfer significantly reduces thrombus formation (59). COX-1 gene transfer has also been shown to reduce pulmonary hypertension in experimental animals (60). The experimental work suggests that COX-1 gene transfer may have important therapeutical potential for systemic and pulmonary arterial disorders.

References

1. Smith WL, Marnett LJ. Prostaglandin endoperoxide synthase: structure and catalysis. Biochim Biophys Acta 1990; 1083:1–17.
2. Hemler M, Lands WEM, Smith WL. Purification of cyclooxygenase that forms prostaglandins. J Biol Chem 1976; 251:5575–5579.
3. Miyamoto T, Ogino N, Yamamoto S, Hayaishi O. Purification of prostaglandin endoperoxide synthase from bovine vascular gland microsomes. J Biol Chem 1976; 251:2629–2636.
4. Merlie JP, Fagan D, Mudd J, Needleman P. Isolation and characterization of the complementary DNA for sheep seminal vesicle prostaglandin endoperoxide synthase (cyclooxygenase). J Biol Chem 1988; 263:3550–3553.
5. DeWitt DL, Smith WL. Primary structure of prostaglandin G/H synthase from sheep vesicular gland determined from the complementary DNA sequence. Proc Natl Acad Sci USA 1988; 85:1412–1416.
6. Yokoyama C, Takai T, Tanabe T. Primary structure of sheep prostaglandin endoperoxide synthase deduced from cDNA sequence. FEBS Lett 1988; 231:347–351.
7. Funk CD, Funk LB, Kennedy ME, Pong AS, Fitzgerald GA. Human platelet erythroleukemia cell prostaglandin G/H synthase: cDNA cloning, expression, and gene chromosomal assignment. FASEB J 1991; 5:2304–2312.
8. Shimokawa T, Kulmacz RJ, DeWitt DL, Smith WL. Tyrosine 385 of prostaglandin endoperoxide synthase is required for cyclooxygenase catalysis. J Biol Chem 1990; 265:20073–20076.
9. Shimokawa T, Smith WL. Essential histidines of prostaglandin endoperoxide synthase. J Biol Chem 1991; 266:6168–6173.
10. Shimokawa T, Smith WL. Prostaglandin endoperoxide synthase; the aspirin acetylation region. J Biol Chem 1992; 267:12387–12392.
11. Picot D, Loll PJ, Garavito RM. The X-ray crystal structure of the membrane protein prostaglandin H$_2$ synthase-1. Nature 1994; 367:243–249.
12. Egan RW, Praxton J, Kuehl FA, Jr. Mechanism of irreversible self-deactivation of prostaglandin synthase. J Biol Chem 1976; 251:7329–7335.

13. Fagan JM, Goldberg AL. Inhibitors of protein and RNA synthesis cause a rapid block in prostaglandin production at the prostaglandin synthase step. Proc Natl Acad Sci USA 1986; 83:2771–2775.

14. Sanduja SK, Tsai A-L, Matijevic-Aleksic N, Wu KK. Kinetics of prostacyclin synthesis in a PGHS-1 overexpressed endothelial cells. Am J Physiol 1994; 267: C1459–C1466.

15. Kujubu DA, Herschmann HR. Dexamethasone inhibits mitogen induction of the TIS10 prostaglandin synthase/cyclooxygenase gene. J Biol Chem 1992; 267:7991–7994.

16. Xie W, Chipman JG, Robertson DL, Erickson RL, Simmons DL. Expression of a mitogen-responsive gene encoding prostaglandin synthase is regulated by mRNA splicing. Proc Natl Acad Sci USA 1991; 88:2692–2696.

17. Hla T, Nielson K. Human cyclooxygenase-2 cDNA. Proc Natl Acad Sci USA 1992; 89:7384–7388.

18. Jones DA, Carlton DP, McIntyre TM, Zimmerman GA, Prescott SM. Molecular cloning of human prostaglandin endoperoxide synthase type II and demonstration of expression in response to cytokines. 1993.

19. Meade EA, Smith WL, DeWitt DL. Differential inhibition of prostaglandin endoperoxide synthase (cyclooxygenase) isozymes by aspirin and other non-steroidal anti-inflammatory drugs. J Biol Chem 1993; 268:6610–6614.

20. Mitchell JA, Akarasereenont P, Thiemermann C, Flower RJ, Vane JR. Selectivity of nonsteroidal anti-inflammatory drugs as inhibitors of constitutive and inducible cyclooxygenase. Proc Natl Acad Sci USA 1994; 90:11693–11697.

21. Futaki N, Takahashi S, Yokoyama M, Arai I, Higuchi S, Otomo S. NS-398, a novel anti-inflammatory agent, selectively inhibits prostaglandin G/H synthase-2. Prostaglandins 1994; 47:55–59.

22. Futaki N, Yoshikawa K, Hamasaka Y, Arai I, Higushi S, Iizuka H, Otomo S. NS-398 a novel non-steroidal anti-inflammatory drug with potent analgesic and anti-pyretic effects, which causes mini mal stomach lesions. Gen Pharmacol 1993; 24: 105–110.

23. Yokoyama C, Tanabe T. Cloning of human gene encoding prostaglandin endoperoxide synthase and primary structure of the enzyme. Biochem Biophys Res Commun 1989; 165:888–894.

24. Wang L-H, Hajibeigi A, Xu X-M, Loose-Mitchell D, Wu KK. Characterization of the promoter of human prostaglandin H synthase-1 gene. Biochem Biophys Res Commun 1993; 190:406–411.

25. Xu X M, Tang J-L, Hajibeigi A, Loose-Mitchell DS, Wu KK. Transcriptional regulation of endothelial constitutive PGHS-1 expression by phorbol ester. Am J Physiol 1996; 207:C259–C264.

26. Samet JM, Fasano MB, Fonteh AN, Chilton FH. Selective induction of prostaglandin G/H synthase 1 by stem cell factor and dexamethasone in mast cells. J Biol Chem 1995; 270:8044–8049.

27. Kitzler J, Hill E, Hardman R, Reddy N, Philpot R, Eling TE. Analysis and quantitation of splicing variants of the TPA-inducible PGHS-1 mRNA in rat trachael epithelial cells. Arch Biochem Biophys 1995; 316:856–863.

28. Pilbeam CC, Kawaguchi H, Hakeda Y, Voznesensky O, Alander C, Raiss LG. Differential regulation of inducible and constitutive prostaglandin endoperoxide synthase in osteoblastic MC 3T3-E1 cells. J Biol Chem 1993; 268:25643–25649.

29. Yamagata K, Andreasson KI, Kaufman WE, Barnes CA, Worley PF. Expression of a mitogen inducible cyclooxygenase in brain neurons: regulation by synaptic activity and glucocorticoids. Neuron II 1993; 371–386.

30. Iseki S. Immunochemical localization of cyclooxygenase-1 and -2 in the rat stomach. Histochem J 1995; 27:323–328.

31. Wu KK. Inducible cyclooxygenase and nitric oxide synthase. Adv Pharmacol 1995; 33:179–207.

32. Vane JR, Mitchell JA, Appleton I, Tomlinson A, Bishop-Bailey D, Croxtall J, Willoughby DA. Inducible isoforms of cyclooxygenase and nitric oxide synthase in inflammation. Proc Natl Acad Sci USA 1994; 91:2046–2050.

33. Seibert K, Zhang Y, Leahy K, Hauser S, Masferrer J, Perkins W, Lee L, Isakson P. Pharmacological and biochemical demonstration of the role of cyclooxygenase 2 in inflammation and pain. Proc Natl Acad Sci USA 1994; 91:12013–12017.

34. Sirois J, Simmon DL, Richard JS. Hormonal regulation of messenger ribonucleic acid encoding a novel isoform of prostaglandin endoperoxide synthase in rat preovulatory follicles. J Biol Chem 1992; 267:11586–11592.

35. Tsujii M, DuBois RN. Alteractions in cellular adhesion and apoptosis in epithelial cells overexpressing prostaglandin endoperoxide synthase 2. Cell 1995; 83:493–501.

36. Morita I, Schindler M, Regier MK, Oho JC, Hori T, DeWitt DL, Smith WL. Different intracellular locations for prostaglandin endoperoxide H synthase-1 and -2. J Biol Chem 1995; 270:10902–10908.

37. Takahashi Y, Taketani Y, Endo T, Yamamoto S, Kumegawa M. Studies on the induction of cyclooxygenase isozymes by various prostaglandins in mouse osteoblastic cell line with reference to signal transduction pathways. Biochim Biophys Acta 1994; 1212:217–224.

38. Fletcher BS, Kujubu DA, Perrin DM, Herschman HR. Structure of the mitogen-inducible TIS10 gene and demonstration that the TIS10-encoded protein is a functional prostaglandin G/H synthase. J Biol Chem 1992; 267:4338–4344.

39. Kraemer SA, Meade EA, DeWitt DL. Prostaglandin endoperoxide synthase gene structure: identification of the transcriptional start site and 5'-flanking regulatory sequences. Arch Biochem Biophys 1992.

40. Tazawa R, Xu X-M, Wang L-H, Wu KK. Characterization of genomic structure, chromosome location and promoter of human prostaglandin H synthase-2 gene. Biochem Biophys Res Commun 1994; 203:190–199.

41. Xie W, Fletcher BS, Anderson RD, Herschman WR. V-Src induction of the TIS10/PGS2 prostaglandin synthase gene is mediated by an AFT/CRE transcription response element. Mol Cell Biol 1994; 14:6531–6539.

42. Inoue H, Yokoyama C, Hara S, Tone Y, Tanabe T. Transcriptional regulation of human prostaglandin-endoperoxide synthase-2 gene by lipopolysaccharide and phorbol ester in vascular endothelial cells. 1995.

43. Yamamoto K, Arakawa T, Ueda N, Yamamoto S. Transcriptional roles of nuclear factor NF-κB and NF-IL6 in the tumor necrosis factor α-dependent induction of cyclooxygenase-2 in MC3T3E1 cells. J Biol Chem 1995; 270:31315–31320.

44. Portman OW, Alexander M. Lysophosphatidylcholine concentrations and meta bolism in aortic intima plus inner media: effect of nutrionally induced atherosclerosis. J Lipid Res 1969; 10:158–165.
45. Quinn MT, Parthasarathy S, Steinberg D. Lysophosphatidylcholine: a chemotactic factor for human monocytes and its potential role in atherogenesis. Proc Natl Acad Sci USA 1988; 85:2805–2809.
46. Parthasarathy S, Quinn MT, Schwenke DC, Carew TE, Steinberg D. Oxidative modification of beta-very low density lipoprotein. Potential role in monocyte recruitment and foam cell formation. Arteriosclerosis 1989; 9:398–404.
47. Kume N, Cybulsky MI, Gimbrone Jr MA. Lysophosphatidylcholine, a component of atherogenic lipoproteins, induces mononuclear leukocyte adhesion molecules in cultured human and rabbit arterial endothelial cells. J Clin Invest 1992; 90:1138–1144.
48. Kume N, Gimbrone Jr MA. Lysophosphatidylcholine transcriptionally induces growth factor gene expression in cultured human endothelial cells. J Clin Invest 1994; 93:907–911.
49. Zembowicz A, Jones SL, Wu KK. Induction of cyclooxygenase-2 in human umbilical vein endothelial cells by lysophosphatidylcholine. J Clin Invest 1995; 96:1688–1692.
50. Zembowicz A, Tang J-L, Wu KK. Transcriptional induction of endothelial nitric oxide synthase type-III by lysophosphatidylcholine. J Biol Chem 1995; 270:17006–17010.
51. Vane JR, Botting RM. Pharmacodynamic profile of prostacyclin. Am J Cardiol 1995; 73:3A–10A.
52. Moncada S, Palmer RMJ, Higgs EA. Nitricoxide: physiology, pathophysiology and pharmacology. Pharmacol Rev 1991; 43:109–142.
53. Numokawa Y, Tanaka S. Interferon-α inhibits proliferation of rat vascular smooth muscle cells by nitric oxide generation. Biochem Biophys Res Commun 1992; 188:409–415.
54. Kubes P, Suzuki M, Granger DN. Nitricoxide an endogenous modulator of leukocyte adhesion. Proc Natl Acad Sci USA 1991; 88:4651–4655.
55. Langenbach R, Morham SG, Tiano HF, Loftin CD, Ghahayem BI, Chulada PC, Mahler JF, Lee CA, Goulding EH, Kluckman KD, Kim HS, Smithies O. Prostaglandin synthase 1 gene disruption in mice reduces arachidonic acid-induced inflammation and indomethacin-induced gastric ulceration. Cell 1995; 83:483–492.
56. Morham SG, Langenbach R, Loftin CD, Tiano HF, Vouloumanos N, Jennette JC, Mahler JF, Kluckman KD, Ledford A, Lee CA, Smithies O. Prostaglandin synthase 2 gene disruption causes severe renal pathology in the mouse. Cell 1995; 83:473–482.
57. Dinchuk JE, Car BD, Focht RJ, Johnston JJ, Jaffee BD, Covington MB, Contel NR, Eng VM, Cooins RJ, Czerniak PM, Gorry SA, Trzaskos JM. Renal abnormalities and an altered inflammatory response in mice lacking cyclooxygenase II. Nature 1995; 378:406–409.
58. Xu X-M, Ohashi K, Sanduja SK, Ruan K-H, Wang L-H, Wu KK. Enhanced prostacyclin synthesis in endothelial cell by retrovirus-mediated transfer of prostaglandin H synthase. J Clin Invest 1993; 91:1843–1849.

59. Zoldhelyi P, McNatt J, Xu X-M, Loose-Mitchell D, Meidell RS, Clubb FJ, Buja LM, Willerson JT, Wu KK. Prevention of arterial thrombosis by adenovirus-mediated transfer of cyclooxygenase gene. Circulation 1996; 93:10–17.
60. Conary JT, Parker RE, Christman BW, Faulks RD, King GA, Meyrick BO, Brigham KL. Protection of rabbit lungs from endotoxin injury by in vivo hyperexpression of the prostaglandin G/H synthase gene. J Clin Invest 1994; 93:1834–1840.

8

NSAID-Induced Apoptosis
A New Therapeutic Activity of Competitive
Cyclooxygenase Inhibitors?

DANIEL L. SIMMONS

Brigham Young University
Provo, Utah

I. Introduction

A. Eicosanoids and Cyclooxygenases

As described in Chapter 1, prostaglandins and thromboxanes are well-established, arachidonic acid–derived biomediators that affect or modulate a large number of pathological and physiological processes. These eicosanoids are synthesized through the action of two known microsomal cyclooxygenases (COXs), also known as prostaglandin G/H synthases, which cyclize and oxygenate arachidonate to prostaglandin (PG) G_2. A separate peroxidase active site of COXs reduces a hydroperoxyl moiety of PGG_2 to produce PGH_2, the prostaglandin from which all other prostaglandins and thromboxane A_2 are made.

The two COX isoenzymes, COX-1 and COX-2, are both homodimers consisting of 72-kDa, heme-containing, glycosylated subunits (1). COX-1 has been found to be expressed at low to moderate levels in most mammalian tissues, and many cells in culture constitutively express significant amounts of this enzyme (2). Similar to housekeeping proteins, COX-1 expression does not typically fluctuate as a function of the cell cycle in dividing cells. However, some compounds have been shown to evoke long-term induction of COX-1 in cultured cells (3–6). In these cases, induction of COX-1 occurs upon differentiation of the cells, suggesting the COX-1 may play a role in maintaining terminally differentiated homeostasis.

In contrast to COX-1, the hallmark of COX-2 is its high susceptibility to induction by a wide variety of cell stimuli. This induction almost always correlates with increased eicosanoid production in the stimulated cell. In the brief period since its discovery in 1991, COX-2 has been implicated in neoplastic transformation (7–9), neuronal signaling (10), nociception (11), macrophage activation (12), bone resorption (13), mast cell activation (14), ovulation (15–17), parturition (18), lipopolysaccharide (LPS)-induced cell death (18), regulation of salt, volume, and blood pressure homeostasis (19), and inflammation (11). The effects of COX-2 in pulmonary function and in asthma are described elsewhere in this volume. As stated by Vane (20), strong evidence suggests that COX-2 is the inflammatory form of COX, and is involved in transitory intra- or intercell signaling accompanying cellular activation by external mediators. From a developmental viewpoint, COX-2 is also critical to kidney development during the neonatal period, as shown in mice genetically deficient for COX-2, which exhibit profound renal dysplasia (21,22). COX-1-deficient mice, on the other hand, exhibit no known anatomical defects but do experience prolonged labor during parturition (23). This suggests that whatever role COX-1 plays in differentiation, as suggested by the cell studies described above, it is either not essential or is not uniquely required for this function in vivo.

B. NSAID Inhibition of COXs

Aspirin, the prototypical nonsteroidal anti-inflammatory drug (NSAID), inhibits COX-1 and COX-2 activity and an IC_{50} of 1–300 μM (24–29). Acetylation of Ser-530 by aspirin results in this inhibition although the deacetylated derivative of aspirin, salicylate, acts as a very weak competitive inhibitor of the enzyme. Other competitively acting NSAIDs, such as indomethacin and diclofenac, are typically much more potent than aspirin when tested in comparable assays, and often have IC_{50} values ≤ 1 μM (27). COX-1 has now been cocrystallized withh flurbiprofen, brominated aspirin, iodosuprofen, and iodoindomethacin (30). Cocrystallization of COX-2 has recently been achieved for flurbiprofen, indomethacin, and the COX-2-selective drug SC-558 (31). A phenylsulfonamide moiety in the latter drug accesses a "side pocket" present in the cyclooxygenation site of COX-2 that is not present in COX-1, thus conferring its isoenzyme specificity. In contrast, flurbiprofen and indomethacin, which are nonselective COX inhibitors, appear to bind COX-1 and COX-2 with the similar stereospecificity (30,31).

Both COX-1 and COX-2 have very similar three-dimensional structures, although they possess only 60% sequence identity. For both isoenzymes, catalysis begins with the entrance of arachidonic acid substrate from the membrane into the hydrophobic channel of the cyclooxygenation site, where it is cyclized and oxygenated to PGG_2. Each NSAID cocrystallized with COX appears to block substrate entry into this site. In the case of aspirin and its metabolite salicylate, binding in this narrow channel is very weak, thus accounting for their inability to act as competitive COX inhibitors. However, this weak binding is postulated to be important because it positions aspirin to transacetylate Ser-530 near the active site (30). Transacetylation introduces a permanent, covalently linked block to substrate entry; however, this blockage is physically smaller than that provided by mono-, bi-, or tricyclic competitive NSAIDs, which essentially lodge in the cyclooxygenation channel and occlude it. Aspirin acetylation only partially blocks the cyclooxygenation site as evidenced by the fact that aspirin-acetylated COX-2 is still capable of making 15R-HETE, whereas competitive inhibitors completely block this activity (29,32,33). Claria and Serhan have recently demonstrated that 15R-HETE made by cyclooxygenases can be metabolized by 5-lipoxygenase to form 15R-epilipoxins, which are bioactive (34).

Extensive data accumulated by in situ immunohistochemistry and protease sensitivity studies show that COX-1 and -2 are both in the lumen of the endoplasic reticulum (ER) and nuclear envelope, although COX-2 has been found to be more perinuclearly localized than COX-1 (35,36). This has led to the hypothesis that COX-2 may signal intracellularly to the nucleus as well as to neighboring cells in a paracrine fashion through the production of prostaglandins. An isomer of PGJ_2 has recently been found to bind the PPARγ transcription factor, which substantiates the nucleus-signaling aspects of this model (37). Because COX-1 and COX-2 have overlapping subcellular distributions, the question remains as to how these enzymes recognize arachidonate substrate differently as shown by others (38) and how they would promulgate separate eicosanoid signals.

C. COX Isoenzymes and Cell Division

Our past studies and those of others have shown a clear association between COX-2 induction and cell proliferation (7–9,39). Although we now know that COX-2 induction is responsible for the rise in PGE_2 synthesis accompanying mitosis, the role of COX-1 in cell division is unknown. The potential importance of cyclooxygenases in growth control is underscored by epidemiological studies of human cancers of the digestive tract. The majority of these studies have shown that high to moderate use of NSAIDs such as aspirin, piroxicam, ibuprofen, indomethacin, and sulindac reduces the incidence of both adenoma and adenocarcinoma of the colon in human populations (40–42). Further-more, treatment with sulindac or piroxicam of patients suffering from familial adenomatous polyposis causes partial to complete regression of benign ade-nomas, and in combination with 5-fluorouracil and levamisole may show effi-cacy in the treatment of adenocarcinomas of the colon (43–48). The antineo-plastic effect of COX inhibitors also extends to other gastrointestinal tumors, including neoplasms of the esophagus and stomach (41). Also consistent with the notion that COX is involved in tumorigenesis is the fact that many human tumors have been found to overexpress prostaglandins (49).

It is now clear from multiple histological studies that 80–90% of human colon carcinomas show markedly increased levels of COX-2, and that this elevated expression is primarily in the neoplastic cells of the tumor rather than in associated inflammatory cells or adjacent tissue (50–53). Induction of COX-2 during tumorigenesis is due to a transcriptional mechanism that has not yet been defined (54). Similarly, we have found that transforming onco-genes frequently up-regulate COX-1 and COX-2, with *fos* and *fes* being the most frequent up-regulators of COX-2 (55).

Many animal models show an antineoplastic effect of NSAIDs (56–58). Two-stage models of skin carcinogenesis in mice have shown phorbol ester–promoter papilloma formation to be completely blocked by treatment of animals with indomethacin (56). Similarly, NNK-induced pulmonary and gastric tumorigenesis in mice was reduced by sulindac (57). The COX isoen-zyme(s) responsible for these phenomena is (are) unknown, although the find-ing that COX-2 is induced in chemically induced neoplasms of the colon in rats indicates that this isoenzyme is involved in carcinogenesis in this organ (59). Mating of a COX-2 null mutant mouse with one carrying an $APC^{\Delta716}$ mutation, which confers hereditary intestinal polyposis, produces offspring with dramatically reduced polyp number and size compared to mice carrying only the $APC^{\Delta716}$ allele (60). This finding demonstrates an apparent require-ment for COX-2 in this familial form of colon cancer. Therefore, the data are becoming increasingly compelling that COX isoenzymes, and COX-2 in par-ticular, play a significant role in carcinomas of the gastrointestinal (GI) tract, skin, and possibly other tumors.

II. The Role(s) of COXs in Apoptosis

A. Prostaglandins Can Cause Apoptosis

Initiators of apoptosis are varied and include drugs, hormones, and a number of secreted cellular factors such as TNFα and TGFβ. Dexamethasone (DEX), a potent down-regulator of COX-2, is one of the best-studied of all apoptotic agents and initiates apoptosis in a wide variety of cell types but most potently in T cells. Several investigators have shown that PGE_2 and PGJ_2 potently induce apoptosis in lymphoid cells and their relationship to programmed cell death caused by HIV is under active consideration (61,62). An undefined prostaglandin apparently is also involved in programmed cell death of epithelial cells of the basement membrane of the uterus during implantation and of ovarian epithelial cells that cover the surface of the preovulatory follicle (63, 64). As described later, our laboratory has found that all prostaglandin isomers are apoptotic in certain model cell lines. Moreover, we have recently determined that COX-1 and COX-2 can physically associate with nucleobindin, an intralumenal protein of the ER and nuclear envelope (65). Nucleobindin has been implicated in apoptosis of T cells in MRL/lpr mice, which exhibit a systemic lupus erythematosus–like syndrome. Taken together, these data provide circumstantial evidence that COXs should be considered as regulators of apoptosis through prostaglandin synthesis, particularly in cells of lymphoid lineage, and perhaps through other nonprostaglandin mechanisms such as nucleobindin.

B. Apoptosis: Is It the Basis for the Antineoplastic Effect of NSAIDs?

Our laboratory found that, just as prostaglandins cause apoptosis, the converse is true: blocking the cyclooxygenation site with competitive NSAID inhibitors has a marked effect on v-*src* transformation and causes programmed cell death that is dose- and time-dependent. The cellular and biochemical properties of this NSAID-induced apoptosis (NIA) that we have defined are described more fully below. Within the past 12 months, several important studies have shown NSAIDs to cause apoptosis in transformed and nontransformed colonic epithelial cells from rats and humans (66–70). Tsujii and DuBois demonstrated that rat intestinal epithelial (RIE) cells undergo spontaneous apoptosis when cultured in vitro (68). However, upon COX-2 overexpression these cells do not die but proliferate. Treatment with sulindac sulfide in the presence of a coinducer of apoptosis (sodium butyrate) causes the cells to undergo apoptosis.

It is important to note that in all cases, including our own work reported below, that NSAID doses needed to cause apoptosis range from 10 to $800\,\mu M$, concentrations that are typically higher than those needed for significant (i.e., >50%) inhibition of COX-1 or COX-2 in most cell types. Also significant is that the dose and time needed to cause apoptosis are highly dependent on the biochemical test used to measure death. Trypan blue staining, nucleosomal DNA fragmentation, MTT assays, and morphological analyses measure only the late events of apoptosis and are relatively insensitive. With these tests used to measure cell death, it is not uncommon to require dose levels of $>100\,\mu M$

to cause 100% death at 24–48 hr. However, sensitive DNA cleavage assays detect death within 6 hr of treatment and at doses that are five- to 10-fold lower than in the other assays (71). Finally, aspirin is much less effective as an inducer of NIA than are competitively acting NSAIDs. There is at present no evidence that the acetylating property of aspirin is needed for its very weak apoptosis-inducing activity, which probably is due to the ability of salicylate to act as a weak competitive inhibitor of COX. Confirmative of a role for salicylate in apoptosis are the studies of Elder et al. that show salicylate to cause NIA at concentrations above 1 mM in some colorectal cell lines (69).

Doses that most effectively cause NIA are physiologically relevant to NSAID levels that occur in the GI tract, although in some cases they approximate venous levels of the drugs (66,71). In this regard a question remains as to why such high levels of NSAIDs are needed to affect cell death. We hypothesize that competitive NSAIDs evoke apoptosis by preventing synthesis of a COX-generated biomediator that is needed by the cell in only very small concentrations. We speculate, therefore, that the dose needed to trigger the extensive cellular programming leading to cell death may occur only at NSAID levels at which synthesis of this putative biomediator has been stopped (i.e., at IC_{100}). This complete inhibition also may need to be of a sufficient duration to affect a critical part of the cell cycle in dividing cells.

In addition to causing apoptosis, lower NSAID doses also have been reported to be antiproliferative by lengthening the cell cycle, probably through inducing arrest in either G1 or G2 phases of the cell cycle (66). This multifactorial nature of NSAID action in preventing neoplastic disease may be the reason why aspirin apparently reduces the incidence of human colorectal tumors, even though it is ineffective at causing apoptosis. Alternatively, cells in vivo may be more sensitive to the apoptosis-inducing activity of NSAIDs than are cell lines that have been selected for long-term culture in vitro.

C. Cellular and Biochemical Properties of NIA

Our laboratory has focused on NIA in chicken embryo fibroblast cells transformed by Rous sarcoma virus, which carries the v-*src* oncogene (72). In this cell system, temperature-sensitive mutants of the virus are used to neoplastically transform CEF through the action of $pp60^{v-src}$. CEF are refractory to apoptosis initiated by many common apoptosis initiators. However, when neoplastically transformed by v-*src*, CEF show modest apoptosis when cultured in low serum (71). Not surprisingly, NSAIDs are ineffective at causing apoptosis in CEF, but are effective in *src*-transformed CEF, particularly if they are cultured in low serum. This activity is confined only to competitive inhibitors of COX and is not shared with aspirin (Table 1; Ref. 72). In this regard it is similar to results obtained by us in mammalian colorectal cells, where aspirin

Table 1 Morphological Inhibition of Transformation in Response to NSAID Treatment

NSAID	Effect 100 μM	Effect 10 μM
Oxicam		
Isoxicam	—	—
Piroxicam	\	—
Salicylate		
Aspirin	—	—
Diflunisal	×	—
Acetamindophenol	—	—
Acetaphenetidin	—	—
Salicylamide	—	—
Acetic acid		
Indomethacin	×	×
Acemetacin	×	\
Tolmetin	\	—
Sulindac	—	—
Diclofenac	×	\
Zomepirac	\	—
Fenamate		
Mefenamic acid	×	\
Flufenamic acid	×	\
Niflumic acid	×	\
Propionic acid		
Ketoprofen	\	—
Naproxen	\	—
Indoprofen	\	—
Ibuprofen	×	—
Flurbiprofin	\	—
Suprofen	\	—
Fenbufen	\	—
Carprofen	×	—
Pyrazole		
Phenylbutazone	—	—
Oxyphenbutazone	—	—

X, complete inhibition of focus formation by RSV; \, partial inhibition that was characterized by cell rounding and formation of small clumps of cells; —, no effect. (From Ref. 72.)

is ineffective at causing NIA except at very high doses (>4 mM; unpublished data). As in colorectal cells, this effect could be due to competitive inhibition of COX by salicylate. Alternatively, it has been postulated that high-dose effects of aspirin and salicylate may not be through COX inhibition, but through prevention of activation of NF-κB (73,74).

NIA induced in CEF produces all of the morphological and biological features of apoptosis seen in other systems including nucleosomal DNA laddering, the appearance of apoptotic bodies, cell shrinking, nuclear anomalies, and the induction of tissue transglutaminase (Fig. 1, Ref. 72). Other biochemical events that parallel induction of NIA in CEF are: (1) induction of COX-2 mRNA and protein; (2) alteration of splicing of the COX-2 mRNA; (3) induction of c-*myc* mRNA, and suppression of the cellular quiescence-specific protein, p20 (72).

D. Signal Transduction Mechanisms Important to NIA

Bcl-2 inhibits apoptosis in a number of cell-types and also potently inhibits NIA (71). With antisense oligonucleotides used to down-regulate the c-*myc* mRNA, induction of this proto-oncogene by NSAIDs was also found to be essential for the induction of NIA. Our studies thus far have not implicated

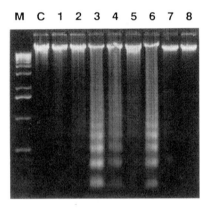

Figure 1   Induction of DNA fragmentation in RSV-transformed CEFs by NSAIDs. Lanes: M, 1-kb molecular size marker (GIBCO/BRL); C, control (serum-starved) RSV-transformed cells without drug treatment); 1–8, serum-starved RSV-transformed cells treated, respectively, with diflunisal, indomethacin, acemetacin, diclofenac, mefenamic acid, flufenamic acid, niflumic acid, and carprofen. Genomic DNA was isolated from cultures after 30 hr of exposure to 100 μM drug and analyzed on a 1% agarose gel.

p53 as a positive effector of NIA. We have found that p53 is not induced during NIA and that immortalized cell lines, where p53 is inactive, undergo NIA, suggesting that p53 is not involved in the NIA pathway. The proto-oncogene *c-rel*, which induces *c-myc* in other apoptosis pathways, is also not induced during NIA and may not be involved in NIA (71,75,76).

The causation of cell death is intrinsically linked with induction of COX-2 and *c-myc*. It is, therefore, tantalizing to speculate that the COX-2-generated product responsible for inhibiting NIA also regulates these two genes.

E. The Role of Prostaglandins in NIA

If NSAIDs initiate NIA by physically blocking the cyclooxygenation site of COX, does this mean that COXs act by inhibiting prostaglandin synthesis? If this is the case, why doesn't aspirin affect NIA? We have methodically tested a wide range of common COX metabolites and substrates and have been unable to find a prostaglandin that rescues CEF or other cells from NAI (Table 2). In these experiments, eicosanoids or related compounds were applied to cells at physiological and superphysiological concentrations, and were applied either as a single dose or repeatedly (every 4 hr) during the course of the 48-hr incubation with NSAID. One striking result we observed was that prostaglandin

Table 2 Prostaglandins and Related Compounds Tested as Rescuers of NIA[a]

Compound	Protection against NIA	Concentration
Arachidonic acid[b]	None	0.01–100 μM
Prostaglandins A$_2$, D$_2$, E$_2$, F$_{2\alpha}$, G$_2$, H$_2$, I$_2$, J$_2$, and 15-deoxy-$\Delta^{12,14}$J$_2$	None	0.01 nM–10 μM
15R-epilipoxins[d]	None	30 ng/ml
12S HTT[e]	None	0.04–30 ng/ml

[a]To evoke apoptosis, CEF were exposed to diclofenac (100 μM) for 48 hr. Protection against NIA is defined as the ability to significantly decrease the amount of cell death observed at the end of this period. The tested compounds were coadministered with the NSAID at the beginning of the assay, or were coadministered with the NSAID followed by additional "boosting" applications being administered every 4 hr during the 48-hr period.

[b]Arachidonic acid was nonapoptotic by itself when administered to cells at the concentrations shown.

[c]At concentrations > 10 ng/ml most prostaglandin isomers induced apoptosis in the absence of NSAIDs.

[d]Six isomers were tested that were kindly provided by C. N. Serhan and described in Ref. 34.

[e]HHT = 12-(S)-hydroxy 5,8,10 heptadecatrienoic acid, which is a breakdown product of PGG$_2$ and PGH$_2$.

concentrations > 10 ng/ml often not only did not inhibit NIA, but by themselves caused apoptosis. Parallel with this induction of apoptosis was the induction of COX-2. Thus, the putative COX-generated product that rescues from NIA is apparently not a common prostaglandin. This is consistent with the notion that aspirin, which potently inhibits prostaglandin synthesis, does not prevent NIA.

The exclusion of common prostaglandins as inhibitors of NIA suggests other intriguing possibilities by which competitive COX inhibitors, but not aspirin, cause this effect. For example, the putative COX-generated metabolite that blocks NIA may not be blocked by aspirin treatment, as is the case with 15R-HETE. Alternatively, the critical COX-generated product may act at the nucleus of the cell to prevent NIA, rather than on cell surface receptors like the common prostaglandins. This putative product may also be made from non–arachidonic acid substrates like linolenic or linoleic acids. The eventual finding of this COX-generated product potentially will reveal a new, vitally important biomediator synthesized by one or more of the COX isoenzymes.

Recently it has been proposed that competitively acting NSAIDs may cause NIA in cells that lack COX, which suggests that these NSAIDs have an additional site of action besides inhibiting the COX isoenzymes (66). This conclusion was based on the finding that HCT-15 cells undergo NIA even though they appeared by PCR analysis to lack COX-1 and COX-2. Our laboratory has recently reevaluated this cell system and has found that it expresses COX-2 mRNA, although at lower amounts than the colorectal-derived HT-29 cells used as a positive control in the original study. Significantly, this cell line does not appear to express COX-1, suggesting that COX-2 and not COX-1 is the isoenzyme responsible for NIA. This supposition is further strengthened by the finding that COX-2 overexpression in RIE cells inhibits apoptosis, an effect that can be relieved by treatment with sulindac sulfide.

Another important recent observation is that sulindac sulfone effectively causes apoptosis even though it is a rather inactive inhibitor of COX activity. If this apoptotic effect is through COX-2, it suggests that the COX-2 target for apoptosis-inducing NSAIDs is conformationally different than the purified or induced enzyme that is studied pharmacologically in NSAID inhibition studies. The finding of nucleobindin as being associated with COX enzymes in the yeast two-hybrid system and in vitro as well as cell assays could provide a mechanism by which different conformations of COX isoenzymes occur. Empirical evidence from epitope mapping studies suggest that different COX-1 conformations exist in cells overexpressing this isoenzyme (77). Therefore, it is possible that subpopulations of COX isoenzymes, possibly present as complexes with other proteins such as nucleobindin, provide unique loci for specialized COX functions within the cell.

F. Pharmacological Implications of NIA

In addition to inhibiting prostaglandin production with its attendant proinflammatory activity, competitively acting NSAIDs initiate intracellular signaling pathways leading to cell death. It can be demonstrated in vitro that cells exhibit varying degrees of sensitivity toward apoptosis initiated by NSAIDs, and the cause of this differential sensitivity is presently unknown. Likewise, the tissues and cells most susceptible to this phenomenon in vivo are unknown, although circumstantial evidence implicates the cells of the GI tract as being sensitive. In the case of cancers of the GI tract, NIA may be beneficial in preventing or treating neoplastic disease. Yet unknown is whether NIA or its signal transduction elements are responsible for any of the negative side effects of NSAIDs such as gastric and intestinal ulceration or asthma.

The fact that aspirin is an ineffective inducer of NIA is mirrored in other syndromes where there is a dichotomy between the effects of competitive versus noncompetitive COX inhibitors. Further research is needed to determine the precise mechanism of NIA, but through such study new facets of COX function may be revealed.

Acknowledgments

The authors thanks Philip Robertson for providing some of the data used in constructing Table 2. This work was supported by NIH Grant CA55585, a Fogarty Senior International Fellowship (FO6 TW02180), and funds from the William Harvey Research Institute.

References

1. Picot D, Loll PJ, Garavito RM. The X-ray crystal structure of the membrane protein prostaglandin H_2 synthase. Nature 1994; 367:243–249.
2. Simmons DL, Xie W, Chipman JG, Evett GE. Multiple cyclooxygenases: cloning of a mitogen-inducible form. In: Bailey JM, ed. Prostaglandins, Leukotrienes, Lipoxins, and PAF. New York: Plenum Press, 1991:67–78.
3. Hoff T, DeWitt D, Kaever V, Resch K, Gappett-Struebe M. Differentiation-associated expression of prostaglandin G/H synthase in monocytic cells. FEBS Lett 1993; 320:38–42.
4. Inase N, Levine TM, Lazarus SC. Mitogen-inducible prostaglandin G/H synthase is expressed in canine mastocytoma cells. Am J Respir Cell Mol Biol 1993; 9:526–532.
5. Nusing RW, Mohr S, Ullrich V. Activin A and retinoic acid synergize in cyclooxygenase-1 and thromboxane synthase induction during differentiation of J774.1 macrophages. Eur J Biochem 1995; 227:130–136.

6. Smith CJ, Morrow JD, Roberts LJ, Marnett LJ. Differentiation of monocytoid THP-1 cells with phorbol ester induces expression of prostaglandin endoperoxide synthase-1 (COX-1). Biochem Biophys Res Commun 1993; 192:787–793.

7. Xie W, Chipman JG, Robertson DL, Erikson RI, Simmons DL. Expression of a mitogen-responsive gene encoding prostaglandin synthase is regulated by mRNA splicing. Proc Natl Acad Sci USA 1991; 88:2692–2696.

8. Kujubu DA, Fletcher BS, Varnum BC, Lim RW, Herschman HR. TIS10, a phorbol ester tumor promoter-inducible mRNA from Swiss 3T3 cells, encodes a novel prostaglandin synthase/cyclooxygenase homologue. J Biol Chem 1991; 2CC:12866–12872.

9. O'Banion MK, Sadowski JB, Winn V, Young DA. A serum- and glucocorticoid-regulated 4-kilobase mRNA encodes a cyclooxygenase-related protein. J Biol Chem 1991; 266:23261–23267.

10. Yamagata K, Andreasson KI, Kaufmann WE, Barnes CA, Worley PF. Expression of a mitogen-inducible cyclooxygenase in brain neurons: regulation by synaptic activity and glucocorticoids. Neuron 1993; 11:371–386.

11. Seibert K, Zhang Y, Leahy K, Hauser S, Masferrer J, Perkins W, Lee L, Isakson P. Pharmacological and biochemical demonstration of the role of cyclooxygenase 2 in inflammation and pain. Proc Natl Acad Sci USA 1994; 91:12013–12017.

12. Lee SH, Soyoola E, Chanmugam P, Sun W, Zhong H, Liou S, Simmons D, Hwang D. Selective expression of mitogen-inducible cyclooxygenase in macrophages stimulated with lipopolysaccharide. J Biol Chem 1992; 267:25934–25938.

13. Pilbeam CC, Kawaguchi H, Hakeda Y, Vosnesensky O, Alander DB, Raisz LG. Differential regulation of inducible and constitutive prostaglandin endoperoxide synthase in osteoblastic MC3T3-E1 cells. J Biol Chem 1993; 268:25643–25649.

14. Wilborn J, DeWitt DL, Peters-Golden M. Expression and role of cyclooxygenase isoforms in alveolar and peritoneal macrophages. Am J Physiol 1995; 268:L294–L303.

15. Sirois J, Simmons DL, Richards JS. Hormonal regulation of messenger ribonucleic acid encoding a novel isoform of prostaglandin endoperoxide H synthase in rat preovulatory follicles: induction in vivo and in vitro. J Biol Chem 1994; 267:11586–11592.

16. Sirous J, Levy LO, Simmons DL, Richards JS. Characterization and hormonal regulation of the promoter of the rat prostaglandin endoperoxide synthase 2 gene in granulosa cells. Identification and functional and protein-binding regions. J Biol Chem 1993; 268:12199–12206.

17. Li J, Simmons DL, Tsang BK. Regulation of hen granulosa cell prostaglandin production by transforming growth factors during follicular development: involvement of cyclooxygenase II. Endocrinology 1996; 137:2522–2529.

18. Silver RM, Edwin SS, Trantman MS, Simmons DL, Branch DW, Dudley DJ, Mitchell MD. Bacterial lipopolysaccharide-mediated fetal death. Production of a newly recognized form of inducible cyclooxygenase (COX-2) in murine decidua in response to lipopolysaccharide. J Clin Invest 1994; 95:725–731.

19. Harris RC, McKanna JA, Akai Y, Jacobson HR, Dubois RN. Cyclooxygenase-2 is associated with the macula densa of rat kidney and increases with salt restriction. J Clin Invest 1994; 94:2504–2510.

20. Vane J. Towards a better aspirin. Nature 1994; 367:215–2165.
21. Dinchuk JE, Car BD, Focht RJ, Johnston JJ, Jaffee BD, Covington MB, Contel NR, Eng VM, Collins RJ, Czerniak PM. Renal abnormalities and an altered inflammatory response in mice lacking cyclooygenase II. Nature 1995; 378: 406–409.
22. Morham SG, Langenbach R, Loftin CD, Tiano HF, Vouloumanos N, Jennette JC, Mahler JF, Kluckman KD, Ledford A, Lee CA. Prostaglandin synthase 2 gene disruption causes severe renal pathaology in the mouse. Cell 1995; 83:473–482.
23. Langenbach R, Morham SG, Tiano HF, Loftin CD, Ghanayem BI. Chulada PC, Mahler JF, Lee CA, Goulding EH, Kluckman KD. Prostaglandin synthase 1 gene disruption in mice reduces arachidonic acid-induced inflammation and indomethacin-induced gastric ulceration. Cell 1995; 83:483–492.
24. Gierse JK, Hauser SD, Creely DP, Koboldt C, Rhangwala SH, Isakson PC. Expression and selective inhibition of the constitutive and inducible forms of human cyclooxygenases. Biochem J 1995; 305:479–484.
25. Laneuville O, Breuer DK, DeWitt DL, Hla T, Funk CD, Smith WL. Differential inhibition of human prostaglandin endoperoxide H synthases-1 and -3 by nonsteroidal anti-inflammatory drugs. J Pharmacol Exp Ther 1994; 271:927–934.
26. Lecomte M, Laneuville O, Ji C, DeWitt DL, Smith WL. Acetylation of human prostaglandin endoperoxide synthase-2 (cyclooxygenase-2) by aspirin. J Biol Chem 1994; 269:13207–13215.
27. Mitchell JA, Akaraserenont P, Thiemerman C, Flower RJ, Vane JR. Selectivity of nonsteroidal antiinflammatory drugs as inhibitors of constitutive and inducible cyclooxygenase. Proc Natl Acad Sci USA 1993; 90:11693–11697.
28. Barnett J, Chow J, Ives D, Chiou M, Mackenzie R, Osen E, Nguyen B, Tsing S, Bach C, Freire J. Purification, characterization and selective inhibition of human prostaglandin G/H synthases-1 and -2 expressed in the baculovirus system. Biochim Biophys Acta 1994; 1209:130–139.
29. O'Neill GP, Mancini JA, Kargman S, Yergey J, Kwan MY, Falgueyret JP, Abramovitz M, Kennedy BP, Ouellet M. Overexpression of human prostaglandin G/H synthase-1 and -2 by recombinant vaccinia virus: Inhibition by nonsteroidal anti-inflammatory drugs and biosynthesis of 15-hydroxyeicosatetraenoic acid. Mol Pharmacol 1994; 45:245–254.
30. Garavito RM. The three-dimensional structure of cyclooxygenases. In: Vane J, Botting J, Botting R, eds. Improved Non-steroid Anti-inflammatory Drugs: COX-2 Enzyme Inhibitors. Amsterdam: Kluwer Academic Press, 1996:29–49
31. Kurumball RG, Stevens AM, Gierse JK, McDonald JJ, Stegeman RA, Pak JY, Gildehaus D, Miyashiro JM, Penning TD, Seibert K, Isakson PC, Stallings WC. Structural basis for selective inhibition of cyclooxygenase-2 by anti-inflammatory agents. Nature 1996; 384:644–648.
32. Holtzman MJ, Turk J, Shornick LP. Identification of a pharmacologically distinct prostaglandin H synthase in cultured epithelial cells. J Biol Chem 1992; 267:21438–21445.
33. Meade EA, Smith WL, DeWitt DL. Differential inhibition of prostaglandin endoperoxide synthase (cyclooxygenase) isozymes by aspirin and other non-steroidal anti-inflammatory drugs. J Biol Chem 1993; 268:6610–6614.

34. Claria J, Serhan CN. Aspirin triggers previously undescribed bioactive eicosanoids by human endothelial cell-leukocyte interactions. Proc Natl Acad Sci USA 1995; 92:9475–9679.

35. Morita I, Schindler M, Regier MK, Ho JC, Hori T, DeWitt DL, Smith WL. Different intracellular locations for prostaglandin endoperoxide H synthase-1 and -2. J Biol Chem 1995; 270:10902–10908.

36. Otto J, DeWitt D, Smith W. N-glycosylation of prostaglandin endoperoxide synthase of cyclooxygenases-1 and -2 and their orientation in the endoplasmic reticulum membrane. J Biol Chem 1993; 268:18234–18242.

37. Forman BM, Tontonoz P, Chen J, Brun RP, Spiegelman BM, Evans RM. 15-deoxy-$\Delta^{12,14}$-prostaglandin J_2 is a ligand for the adipocyte determination factor PPAR$_\gamma$. Cell 1995; 83:803–812.

38. Reddy ST, Herschman HR. Ligand-induced prostaglandin synthesis requires expression of the TIS10-PCS-2 prostaglandin synthase gene in urine fibroblasts and macrophages. J Biol Chem 1994; 269:15473–15480.

39. Simmons DL, Levy DB, Yannoni Y, Erikson RL. Identification of a phorbol ester-repressible v-src-inducible gene. Proc Natl Acad Sci USA 1989; 86:1178–1182.

40. Rosenberg L, Palmer J, Zanber AG, Warshauer ME, Stolley PD, Shapiro S. A hypothesis: nonsteroidal anti-inflammatory drugs reduce the incidence of large-bowel cancer. J Natl Cancer Inst 1991; 83:355–358.

41. Thun MJ, Namboodri MM, Calle EE, Flanders WD, Heath CW. Aspirin use and risk of fatal cancer. Cancer Res 1993; 53:1322–1327.

42. Thun M, Namboodiri M, Heath CW. Aspirin use and reduced risk of fatal colon cancer. N Engl J Med 1991; 325:1593–1596.

43. Marcus A. Aspirin as a prophylaxis against colorectal cancer. N Engl J Med 1995; 333:636–638.

44. Sinicrope FA, Pazdur R, Levin B. Phase I trial of sulindac plus 5-fluorouracil and levamisole: potential adjuvant therapy for colon carcinoma. Clin Cancer Res 1996; 2:37–41.

45. Marnett LJ. Aspirin and the potential role of prostaglandins in colon cancer. Cancer Res 1992; 52:5575–5589.

46. Labayle D, Fischer D, Vielh P, Drouhin F, Pariente A, Bories C, Duhamel O, Trousset M, Attali P. Sulindac causes regression of rectal polyps in familial adenomatous polyposis. Gastroenterology 1991; 101:635–639.

47. Giardiello FM, Offerhaus GJA, DuBois RN. The role of nonsteroidal anti-inflammatory drugs in colorectal cancer prevention. Eur J Cancer 1995; 31A:1071–1076.

48. Lupulescu A. Prostaglandins, their inhibitors and cancer. Prostaglandins, Leukotrienes Essential Fatty Acids 1996; 54:83–94.

49. Xie W, Robertson DL, Simmons DL. Mitogen-inducible prostaglandin G/H synthase: a new target for nonsteroidal antiinflammatory drugs. Drug Dev Res 1992; 25:249–265.

50. Eberhart CE, Coffey RJ, Radhika A, Giardello GM, Ferrenbach S, DuBois RN. Up-regulation of cyclooxygenase 2 gene expression in human colorectal adenomas and adenocarcinomas. Gastroenterology 1994; 107:1183–1188.

51. Gustafson-Svard C, Lilja I, Hallbook O, Sjodahl R. Cyclooxygenase-1 and cyclo-oxygenase-2 gene expression in human colorectal adenocarcinomas and in azoxy-methane induced colonic tumours in rats. Gut 1996; 38:79–84.
52. Kargman SL, O'Neill GP, Vickers PJ, Evans JF, Mancini JA, Jothy S. Expression of prostaglandin G/H synthase-1 and -2 protein in human colon cancer. Cancer Res 1995; 55:2556–2559.
53. Sano H, Kawahito Y, Wilder RL, Hashiramoto A, Mukai S, Asai K, Kimura S, Kato H, Kondo M, Hla T. Expression of cyclooxygenase-1 and -2 in human colorectal cancer. Cancer Res 1995; 55:3785–3789.
54. Kutchera W, Jones DA, Matsunami N, Groden J, McIntyre TM, Zimmerman GA, White RL, Prescott SM. Prostaglandin H synthase 2 is expressed abnormally in human colon cancer: evidence for a transcriptional effect. Proc Natl Acad Sci USA 1996; 93:4816–4820.
55. Evett GE, Xie W, Chipman JG, Robertson DL, Simmons DI. Prostaglandin G/H synthase isoenzyme 2 expression in fibroblasts: regulation by dexamethasone, mitogens and oncogenes. Arch Biochem Biophys 1993; 306:169–177.
56. Verma AK, Rice HM, Boutwell RK. Prostaglandins and skin tumor promotion: inhibition of tumor promoter-induced ornithine decarboxylase activity in epidermis by inhibitors of prostaglandin synthesis. Biochem Biophys Res Commun 1977; 79:1160–1166.
57. Jalbert G, Castonguay A. Effects of NSAIDs on NNK-induced pulmonary and gastric tumorigenesis in A/J mice. Cancer Lett 1992; 66:21–28.
58. Rao CV, Rivenson A, Simi B, Zang E, Kelloff G, Steele V, Reddy BS. Chemoprevention of colon carcinogenesis by sulindac, a nonsteroidal anti-inflammatory agent. Cancer Res 1995; 55:1464–1472.
59. DuBois RN, Radhika A, Reddy BS, Entingh AJ. Increased cyclooxygenase-2 levels in carcinogen-induced rat colonic tumors. Gastroenterology 1996; 110:1259–1262.
60. Oshima M, Dinchuk JE, Kargman SL, Oshima H, Hancock B, Kwong E, Trzaskos JM, Evans JF, Taketo MM. Suppression of intestinal polyposis in APC$^{\Delta716}$ knockout mice by inhibition of cyclooxygenase 2 (COX-2). Cell 1996; 87:803–809.
61. Mastino A, Piacentini M, Grelli S, Favalli C, Autuori F, Tentori L, Oliverio S, Garaci E. Induction of apoptosis in thymocytes by prostaglandin E_2 in vivo. Dev Immunol 1992; 2:263–271.
62. Brown DM, Warner GL, Ale-Martinez JE, Scott DW, Phipps RP. Prostaglandin E_2 induces apoptosis in immature normal and malignant B lymphocytes. Clin Immunol Immunopathol 1992; 63:221–229.
63. Abrahamsohn PA, Zorn TM. Implantation and decidualization in rodents. J Exp Zool 1993; 266:603–628.
64. Ackerman RC, Murdoch WJ. Prostaglandin-induced apoptosis of ovarian surface epithelial cells. Prostaglandins 1993; 45:475–485.
65. Ballif BA, Mincek NV, Barratt JT, Wilson MJ, Simmons DL. Interaction of cyclooxygenases with an apoptosis- and autoimmunity-associated protein. Proc Natl Acad Sci USA 1996; 93:5544–5549.
66. Hanif R, Pittas A, Feng Y, Koutsos MI, Qiao L, Staiano-Coico L, Shiff SI, Rigas B. Effects of nonsteroidal anti-inflammatory drugs on proliferation and on induc-

tion of apoptosis in colon cancer cells by a prostaglandin-independent pathway. Biochem Pharmacol 1996; 52:237–245.

67. Piazza GA, Rahm ALK, Krutzch M, Sperl G, Paranka NS, Gross PH, Brendel K, Burt RW, Alberts DS. Pamukcu R, Ahnen DJ. Antineoplastic drugs sulindac sulfide and sulfone inhibit cell growth by inducing apoptosis. Cancer Res 1995; 55:3110–3116.

68. Tsujii M, DuBois RN. Alterations in cellular adhesion and apoptosis in epithelial cells overexpressing prostaglandin endoperoxide synthase 2. Cell 1995; 83:493–501.

69. Elder DJE, Hague A, Hicks DJ, Paraskeva C. Differential growth inhibition by the aspirin metabolite salicylate in human colorectal tumor cell lines: enhanced apoptosis in carcinoma and in vitro–transformed adenoma relative to adenoma cell lines.Cancer Res 1996; 56:2273–2276.

70. Piazza GA, Kulchak AL, Rahm K, Krutzsch M, Sperl G, Paranka NS, Gross PH, Brendel K, Burt RW, Alberts DS, Pamukcu R, Ahnen DJ. Antineoplastic drugs sulindac sulfide and sulfone inhibit cell growth by inducing apoptosis. Cancer Res 1995; 55:3110–3116.

71. Lu X, Fairbairn DW, Bradshaw WS, O'Neill KL, Ewert DL, Simmons DL. NSAID-induced apoptosis in Rous sarcoma virus-transformed chicken embryo fibroblasts is dependent on v-*src* and c-*myc* and is inhibited by bcl-2. Prostaglandins 1996; 54:549–568.

72. Lu X, Xie W, Reed D, Bradshaw WS, Simmons DL. Nonsteroidal antiinflammatory drugs cause apoptosis and induce cyclooxygenases in chicken embryo fibroblasts. Proc Natl Acad Sci USA 1995; 92:7961–7965.

73. Grilli M, Pizzi M, Memo M, PierFranco S. Neuroprotection by aspirin and sodium salicylate through blockade of NF-κB activation. Science 1996; 274:1383–1385.

74. Kopp E, Ghosh S. Inhibition of NF-kappa B by sodium salicylate and aspirin. Science 1994; 265:956–960.

75. Abbadie C, Kabrun N, Bouali F, Smardova J, Stehelin D, Vandenbunder B, Enrietto PJ. High levels of c-rel expression are associated with programmed cell death in the developing avian embryo and in bone marrow cells in vitro. Cell 1993; 75: 899–912.

76. Lee H, Arsura M, Wu M, Duyao M, Buckler AJ, Sonenshein GE. Role of rel-related factors in controled of c-*myc* gene transcription in receptor-mediated apoptosis of the murine B cell WEHI 231 line. J Exp Med 1995; 181:1169–1177.

77. Ren Y, Walker C, Loose-Mitchell DS, Ruan K-H, Kulmacz RJ. Topology of prostaglandin H synthase-1 in the endoplasmic reticulum membrane. Arch Biochem Biophys 1995; 323:205–214.

9

The Three-Dimensional Structure of Cyclooxygenases

DANIEL PICOT

Institut de Biologie Physico-Chimique
Centre National de la Recherche Scientifique
Paris, France

I. Introduction

The discovery that aspirin blocks prostaglandin biosynthesis and that this inhibition is sufficient to explain the therapeutic and side effects of this drug
opened up a new path in the study of pathophysiological and pharmacological
processes at the molecular level (1). The fact that other NSAIDs act on the
same target lends more general significance to this model (2). Since then, prostaglandin H synthase (PGHS), the target of aspirin, has been purified and
extensively characterized (3–5) (for a recent review see Ref. 6). PGHS is the
first enzyme of the prostanoid pathway of the arachidonate cascade (6). It
catalyzes the synthesis of prostaglandin H_2 (PGH_2) from arachidonic acid (see
Chapter 1). The reaction occurs in two different catalytic sites: the first one,
the cyclooxygenase, converts the arachidonic acid into the peroxide prostaglandin G_2 (PGG_2) through the insertion of two molecules of oxygen; the second one, the peroxidase, reduces PGG_2 to yield PGH_2. PGH_2 is then transformed in a cell-specific manner into the other prostanoid hormones (6).
Aspirin and most NSAIDs inhibit the cyclooxygenase activity of PGHS. More
recently, it has been shown that two isoenzymes exist: one, called PGHS-I, is

constitutively expressed, while the other, PGHS-II, is induced during inflammatory processes in specific cellular systems (7,8) (see Chapter 2). Most currently used NSAIDs inhibit both isoenzymes. However, the inhibition of PGHS-I has been more particularly linked to the inhibition of platelet aggregation and to side effects such as gastric lesions; this stimulates the investigation of more specific inhibition of PGHS-II (9). Therefore, we are facing a unique model system, in which the selectivity between several effects (anti-inflammatory, ulcerogenic, antiplatelet) can be largely inferred from the drug selectivity between two nearly identical and well-characterized targets (9). In other words, a large part of the problem can now be translated into a problem of physical chemistry concerning the specificity of the interaction between one ligand and two receptors.

The aim of this chapter is to describe the recently determined structure of PGHS-I and PGHS-II and to connect this knowledge with functional properties. Special emphasis will be given to the structural basis necessary to understand the specificity of the inhibition of the two cyclooxygenases.

II. Structure Determination

Since 1971 it has been obvious that fundamental and applied research would gain from structural knowledge of the target of aspirin. However, PGHS is a membrane-bound enzyme and this sole fact is sufficient to explain the long delay in the structure determination. Indeed, the methodology to study this type of protein by X-ray crystallography was not implemented until the eighties, when Michel and Garavito independently succeeded in developing means to crystallize membrane-bound proteins (10,11). Since then for only a few proteins have investigators overcome the difficulties of obtaining a large amount of pure and active material and good-quality crystals. The fact that the first structure of PGHS needed about 1 g of protein and about 15,000 crystallization experiments to solve the structure illustrates the problem (12). The prostaglandin H synthase is the first eukaryotic membrane protein whose structure has been solved. Therefore, it offers a unique opportunity to discuss the relationship between the structure and the mechanism of a membrane-bound enzyme at the atomic level. Other membrane proteins play important roles in numerous pathophysiological processes and a better understanding of these proteins would be a great help in designing new therapeutic approaches. The method used here is applicable to other membrane proteins and their structure determination is now possible.

The following descriptions are based on structural determinations by X-ray crystallography, using purified protein solubilized with detergent and then crystallized (see Table 1). The first structure was obtained by the group

Table 1 Inhibitors Used in Published PGHS Structures and Described in the Text

Inhibitor	Enzyme	Source	Resolution Å	IC_{50} PGHS-I μM	IC_{50} PGHS-II μM	Ref.
None	PGHS-II	Murine	3.0	—	—	16
Flurbiprofen	PGHS-I	Ovine	3.1	—	—	13
Flurbiprofen	PGHS-II	Murine	2.5	0.29	2.56	16
Iodosuprofen	PGHS-I	Ovine	3.5	1.0	n.a.	48
Iodoindomethacin	PGHS-I	Ovine	4.5	0.029	n.a.	48
Indomethacin	PGHS-II	Murine	2.9	0.08	0.96	16
Bromo-aspirin	PGHS-I	Ovine	3.4	126	n.a.	49
SC-558	PGHS-II	Murine	3.0	17.7	0.0093	16
SC-558	PGHS-II	Murine	2.8	—	—	16
RS-104897	PGHS-II	Human	3.3	242	0.9	15
RS-57067	PGHS-II	Murine	2.9	>1000	0.7	15

of Garavito at the University of Chicago with ovine PGHS-I cocrystallized with the NSAID flurbiprofen. The protein was purified from ram seminal vesicles and the structure solved first at 3.5 Å resolution (13), and then later extended to 3.1 Å (14). The phase information for this structure was obtained with the method of multiple isomorphous replacement using three heavy atoms (13). This structure was then used for phase determination of the other PGHS-I and PGHS-II structures. The structure of PGHS-I has also been obtained with other inhibitors: bromynated aspirin, iodoindomethacin, and iodosuprofen (see Table 1). The structures of the human and murine PGHS-II have been elucidated by two different groups at Roche Bioscience (15) and at Searle (16). These structures have been determined with the following inhibitors: flurbiprofen, indomethacin, SC-558, RS-104897, and RS-57067 (see Table 1). The structure of murine PGHS-II is also available without inhibitor (16). Both PGHS-II were purified after overexpression in cultured insect cells transfected with a baculovirus transfer vector (17,18). Several crystal forms were obtained using different detergents, which, nevertheless, provide very similar structures, showing thus that these folds are not an artifact induced by a particular crystallization condition. Before embarking on a detailed description of the structure it is important to remember that these structures have been determined at low or medium resolution and that, therefore, information like hydrogen bonds must be considered as an interpretation from the currently available structure, and not as a direct observable. The amino acid numbering used here follows that used for PGHS-I and the naming of helices is based on the structure of myeloperoxidase (19) adapted to PGHS (13). Both conventions have been used consistently within the three published structures (13,15,16).

III. The Structure of PGHS-I and PGHS-II

The overall structures of both isoenzymes are very similar and can be considered as nearly identical at the present resolution. Such similarity can be expected from the amino acid sequences of these enzymes. Indeed, one can observe about 60% identity between the amino acid sequences of PGHS-I and PGHS-II. The two known structures of PGHS-II—the murine and the human—share 87% identical residues. Small but highly significant structural differences between PGHS-I and PGHS-II are, however, seen especially after the binding of specific inhibitors. Those will be mentioned upon the study of the cyclooxygenase inhibition (see below). A further difference is also present at the C-terminal, which is 18 amino acids longer in PGHS-II. However, the N- and C-termini have still not been seen in the electron density of PGHS-I and PGHS-II. The following paragraphs concern general features that are valid for both isoenzymes.

The mature protein is formed by a polypeptide chain of 576 and 587 amino acids for ovine PGHS-I and for murine PGHS-II, respectively, after cleavage of an N-terminal signal sequence. It is a heme protein. PGHS-I has three glycosylation sites; PGHS-II has a fourth partially glycosylated site (20). The protein fold can be subdivided into three main structural entities (Fig. 1): the polypeptide chain begins with an epidermal growth factor (EGF)-like module (residues 34–72) followed by the membrane-binding domain (residues 73–116) and ending with the catalytic domain (from residue 117 to the end).

The major part of the protein is formed by the catalytic domain, which comprises both the cyclooxygenase and the peroxidase active site. The localization of two distinct active sites on a single large domain is quite unusual for bifunctional enzymes, which usually have their active sites on separate folded domains (21). The fold of the catalytic domain, mainly made up of α-helices, has a high structural homology with myeloperoxidase (19), although sequence comparison between the two proteins shows only 19% sequence identity. This peroxidase belongs to a family of mammalian peroxidases, to which the thyroid and the eosinophil peroxidases also belong. Hence, we are in the presence of an interesting evolutionary case, where a second active site, the cyclooxygenase, has been formed within an existing peroxidase domain. Indeed, structural comparison of PGHS with the myeloperoxidase shows that features of the cyclooxygenase cavity are already outlined in myeloperoxidase, but with the channel blocked by a helix (helix 7 of myeloperoxidase) that will disappear in the PGHS structure thus creating favorable conditions for the new active site

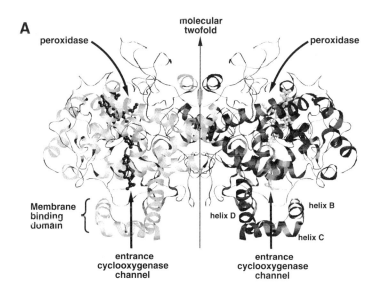

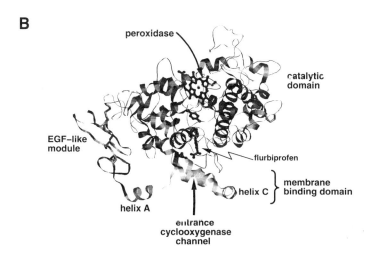

Figure 1 Overall structure of PGHS. (A) The structure of the dimer is outlined with the molecular twofold axis in the plane of the paper (thin arrow separating the two subunits). The cyclooxygenase channel begins in the lower portion of the molecule (thick arrow). (B) Side view relative to (A) of a single subunit (view toward the dimer interface): the EGF-like module is clearly seen here. The cyclooxygenase channel is outlined by the membrane-binding domain, Arg-120, flurbiprofen, and Tyr-385. The peroxidase active site is depicted by its heme.

(21). These observations show that not only the peroxidase, but also the cyclooxygenase active site has evolved from an ancestor peroxidase (22). Nevertheless, it is quite astonishing to see that the most conserved amino acid segment of this family (residues 303–312), which provides the most significant signature to identify proteins of this family, does not belong to the active site and that mutation of a conserved histidine in that region produces an inactive enzyme. Since it does not have an obvious functional significance, this region should be important in maintaining a proper fold in these peroxidases. There is also a more distant but still remarkable similarity with the other known structures of heme peroxidases, such as cytochrome *c* peroxidase. Thus, when viewed in a broader evolutionary context, cyclooxygenase may have arisen from the conversion of an electron donor site into a catalyst.

The *cyclooxygenase active site* (Fig. 2), buried at the center of the catalytic domain, is connected to the protein surface by a long and narrow channel that can be compared to a funnel: The large mouth of the funnel is built up by the membrane-binding domain and is directed toward the protein surface; the other end of the funnel reaches the active site. Its narrow portion begins with a constriction formed around Arg-120 and Glu-524. As discussed later, conformational changes are necessary in this region to let the ligand penetrate deeper into the channel. The narrow portion of the funnel ends near Ser-530, whose side chain can be acetylated by aspirin. The apex of the channel is again wider and contains Tyr-385, which is probably the most important catalytic residue of the cyclooxygenase active site, it is surrounded by an antenna of phenylalanines, Tyr-348, and Trp-387. Two prominent side pockets or alcoves extend to either side of Tyr-385, leaving enough space to accommodate a substrate next to Tyr-385. One of these pockets ends in a thin side channel extending toward the dimer interface. Tyr-385 is at van der Waals distance from the edge of the heme, which lies in the peroxidase active site, although no direct path is visible between the two active sites.

The *peroxidase active site* has characteristics substantially different from those of the cyclooxygenase active site: It is facing not the membrane but the lumen, it is not formed by a narrow channel, but is wide open toward solvent. The main characteristics are a high-spin ferric heme and His-388 as its proximal ligand. On the distal side His-207 occupies a position equivalent to His-52 in cytochrome *c* peroxidase and His-95 of myeloperoxidase, but as in myeloperoxidase, the distal arginine present in other peroxidases is replaced by a glutamine (Gln-203).

The *membrane binding domain* (Fig. 3) of PGHS has no equivalent in myeloperoxidase. The x-ray structure determination provides a model for the interaction of PGHS with the membrane. The large but compact catalytic domain has a hydrophilic surface similar to the other known soluble proteins. Therefore, this part of the protein should not be buried in the membrane. The

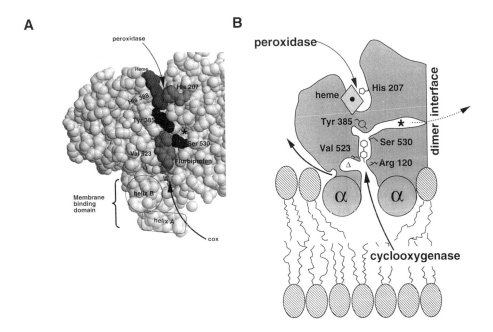

Figure 2 The general spatial organization of the main structural features is represented (A) as a vertical cut through the left subunit of Figure 1A with a space-filling representation and (B) in a more schematic manner. This shows that the cyclooxygenase active site is deeply buried in the protein. The heme, His-207 (distal histidine), Tyr-385, Ser-530, and flurbiprofen are in dark shading. *, the small side channel; Δ, the pocket used by SC-558; W, the larger side window. The thick arrow in (B) [W and Δ in (A)] indicates that side channels exist between the catalytic domain and the membrane-binding domain. The largest one above helix A [W in (A)] could be used as a side window to allow the product PGG_2 to escape from the active site without reentering the membrane bilayer; another smaller one above helix B [Δ in (A)] is used by inhibitors (cf. SC-558) to enhance the selectivity between the two isoenzymes.

protein interacts with the membrane through a set of four α-helices with hydrophobic surfaces, which should be in contact with the hydrophobic core of the bilayer (23). The axes of the first three helices lie approximately parallel to the plane of the membrane, and they surround the entrance of the cyclooxygenase channel, building the large mouth of the funnel mentioned earlier. The fourth helix connects these first three helices with the catalytic domain. The diameter of an α-helix is too small to allow the protein to cross the lipid bilayer; therefore, the protein should interact with only a single leaflet of the membrane. We are therefore in the presence of a monotopic protein (24). This type of protein had been proposed long ago in the fluid mosaic model of the mem-

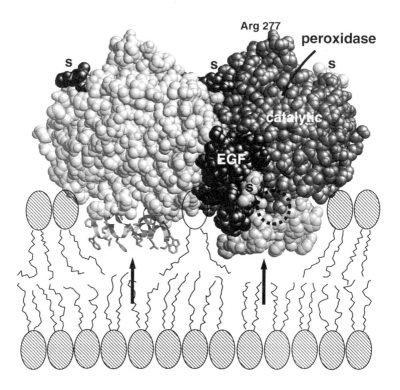

Figure 3 Interaction of PGHS with the membrane. The dimer is represented in the same orientation as in Figure 1A. The whole structure is represented with a space-filling representation up to the membrane-binding domain of the left subunit. In the right subunit, the different structural elements are coded with various gray scales: At the center, as part of the dimer interface, the EGF-like module is in black, the membrane-binding domain in white, and the catalytic domain in gray. The glycosylation site(s) are depicted in either black or white. A schematic representation of the membrane is given, which shows the approximate size of the membrane relative to the protein. It is not known how deep the protein penetrates in the membrane, and how the protein locally modifies the bilayer structure. Indeed, the portion under the membrane-binding domain could as well be filled with lipid tails from a layer in front of the drawing or the protein could induce a local reduction of the membrane thickness. The dotted circle shows a side window (W in Fig. 2A) located between the membrane-binding and the catalytic domain. Arg-277, which is cleaved during limited proteolysis experiments, is shown at the top of the molecule.

brane (25), but had often been forgotten in recent years, since candidates for this type of interaction have been thought to be extremely rare. It is worth mentioning that today a protein is most often classified as a membrane protein from the presence of continuous hydrophobic stretches in the amino acid sequence, and that such pattern are not necessarily seen in a monotopic protein. Thus, monotopic membrane proteins may be overlooked and could be more frequent than expected. Photolabeling with an activable hydrophobic reagent is in good agreement with this model (26).

The membrane binding domain is the least conserved domain between PGHS-I and PGHS-II with only about 33% sequence identity. Nevertheless, the superposition of the atoms of the backbone shows a deviation of only 0.7 Å (15). Furthermore, the insertion in PGHS-II of a proline residue at position 106 between helices C and D has only local effects and does not affect the general structure of this domain (15).

One consequence of this model for PGHS membrane interaction is that it places the whole protein on one face of the membrane. Since the protein has several glycosylation sites and five disulfide bridges, it should not lie in the cytoplasm but on the luminal side of the membrane. This orientation has been confirmed by immunocytofluorescence (27). The same technique has been used to identify the cell compartment as the endoplasmic reticulum and the nuclear envelope for PGHS-I and PGHS-II, but with a preference of the latter for PGHS-II (28).

The *EGF-like module* (Figs. 1 and 3) holds in place the membrane binding domain at its amino-terminal end. This module has the characteristic fold encountered in the other known structures of EGF-like modules (29): It contains two small β-sheets and three intradomain disulfide bridges. However, it has the particularity of being further connected with the catalytic domain through an additional disulfide bridge (connecting Cys-37 to Cys-159). It is also glycosylated. EGF-like modules are encountered in a large number of extracellular and cell-surface proteins; their exact functional or structural role is often unknown. In PGHS, the role of the module is also unclear; however, it most likely plays an important role in keeping the membrane binding domain in a proper conformation, since, as discussed later, the other anchor of this domain, helix D, is somewhat flexible. In addition, the EGF module takes part in the dimer interface and should play a role in stabilizing the dimer. Finally, but in more speculative tone, it could play a role for a proper insertion of the protein in the membrane. The presence of an EGF-like module next to a membrane-interacting segment is not uncommon; thyroid peroxidase is another example.

PGHS forms a *dimer* built up by two identical subunits of about 70 kDa in the crystal structure; this is probably the physiological aggregation state of the protein. This raises the question of the existence of heterodimers of PGHS-

I and PGHS-II. Luong et al. (15) have pointed out that the structures of the two interfaces are well conserved (with 73% sequence identity), but with two important differences at position 137 and 543: these are Ile and Glu in PGHS-I, but Lys and Ala in PGHS-II. These differences may prevent the formation of heterodimers. Another question concerns the functional significance of the dimer. The two active sites are well separated from each other as well as from the dimer interface; they are therefore structurally independent. Furthermore, no experimental evidence exists for cooperative behavior between the active sites. Nevertheless, it has not been possible to isolate active monomeric PGHS (30); this suggests that dimer formation is necessary to preserve the structural, hence functional, integrity of the active sites. The hydrophobic faces of the membrane binding domain of each subunit have the same orientation, thus giving more credit to the membrane binding model described above and further suggesting that this double anchoring of the dimer increases its binding to the membrane.

IV. Catalytic Mechanism

The mechanisms of cyclooxygenase and peroxidase are independent, and it is possible to inhibit each active site independently. However, cyclooxygenase needs to be activated by peroxidase. Not all details of the catalytic mechanism are known, but a general consensus is slowly emerging, with a good correlation between the functional and the structural studies.

The catalytic mechanism of the peroxidase has to be very similar to the one known for the other heme peroxidases (31). The peroxidase active site of PGHS is widely open toward the solvent, in contrast with other peroxidases, which explains the poorer specificity of the PGHS peroxidase. The physiological electron donor is not known, but has to come from the lumen of the endoplasmic reticulum.

Earlier studies on the mechanism of the cyclooxygenase utilized substrate analogs (32). A more recent step toward the understanding of the mechanism was obtained by the detection of the EPR signal of a tyrosyl radical, which has been proposed to play a central role in the mechanism of action of cyclooxygenase and in its activation by the peroxidase (33) (Fig. 4). Mutagenesis studies have identified the residue responsible for this signal as Tyr-385 (34, 35). The role of this Tyr radical has been quite controversial due in part to the complexity of the EPR signal: a wide doublet is assumed to correspond to the catalytic tyrosine radical. But narrow singlets are also observed either after enzyme inactivation, after treatment by indomethacin, or even after mutagenesis of Tyr-385 by Phe. Furthermore, a wide singlet is also observed, which has

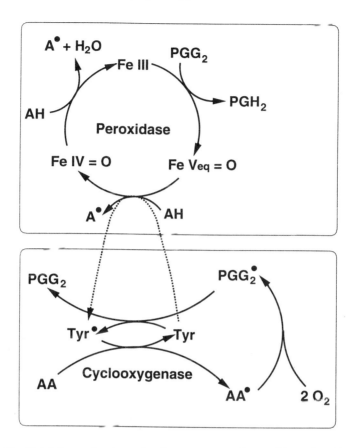

Figure 4 Catalytic mechanism of cyclooxygenase and peroxidase after Karthein et al. (33). The dotted line represents the activation path of cyclooxygenase by peroxidase. AA, arachidonic acid; AH, the reducing compound; $A^•$, its oxidized state. Fe III, Fe Veq = O, and Fe IV = O are, respectively, the resting state, intermediary I, and intermediary II of peroxidase. The inactivation paths are not depicted here.

been assigned to a superposition of one of the narrow singlet with the wide doublet (36). Similar EPR signals are observed with PGHS-II (37,38).

The connection of these functional studies with the structure provides the following tentative picture of the cyclooxygenase reaction. Cyclooxygenase needs first to be activated: a single turnover from peroxidase that uses Tyr-385 as a reducing agent provides the activation by generating the tyrosyl radical. Since peroxidase has only a poor substrate specificity due to the wide opening of its active site, there is no strict requirement for an activator peroxide molecule; i.e., it does not need to be PGG$_2$. The cyclooxygenase is now activated. An arachidonate molecule liberated by a specific phospholipase diffuses in the membrane. The membrane binding domain of PGHS, which acts as a funnel, whose large mouth dips into the membrane, assists the arachidonate to diffuse directly from the membrane into the cyclooxygenase channel (the protonation state of arachidonic acid is not known). Thus, this direct access from the membrane to the active site avoids solvation and desolvation steps. A slight conformational change around the constriction located near Arg-120 is necessary to let the substrate diffuse into the active site (see below). The active site cavity is then able to accommodate an arachidonate in a bent conformation with its carboxylate group interacting with Arg-120 and with its C-13 pro-S hydrogen in a favorable position to be abstracted by the radical sitting on Tyr-385. Insertion of a diffused molecular oxygen at position C-11 can occur. The resulting 11-peroxyl radical initiates a cyclization event that will allow the insertion of a second molecule of oxygen at position C-15, thus producing the peroxide PGG$_2$. This event also regenerates the Tyr-385 radical, which is now able to catalyze further cyclooxygenase reactions without the need of new activation by the peroxidase. The next step is the diffusion of PGG$_2$ out of the cyclooxygenase active site: PGG$_2$ will then be reduced by the peroxidase active site. Several paths that may be used by PGG$_2$ can be envisioned: (1) PGG$_2$ could diffuse directly from the cyclooxygenase to the peroxidase active site. This path raises two problems: First, no channel can be seen connecting the two active sites, meaning that a large conformational change in the core of the protein would be necessary to allow this bulky molecule to pass. Second, PGG$_2$ is able to diffuse at the beginning of a catalytic reaction in vitro to activate other cyclooxygenases; this suggests, but does not necessarily imply, that PGG$_2$ diffuses to a peroxidase other than the one coupled with the cyclooxygenase. (2) PGG could simply take the same path that arachidonic acid uses to reach the cyclooxygenase, i.e., go back into the membrane and then into the luminal space and diffuse to the peroxidase. This should involve a high-energy barrier for what is now a more hydrophilic compound. (3) There is a third, more plausible path: the cyclooxygenase is not completely closed at the interface between the membrane binding and catalytic domain, and there is a small window that could be used by PGG$_2$ to escape from the mouth of the cyclooxygenase channel without the need to go back into the membrane (Figs. 2 and 3). The correct path will influence the mode of activation of the enzyme, and also the design of potential inhibitors: for example if path (1) were the only (but rather unlikely) possibility, it would be possible to design a competitive peroxidase inhibitor that would be also a cyclooxygenase inhibitor.

All experiments indicate that no basic difference exists between the mechanism of PGHS-I and PGHS-II. Both isoenzymes show the same substrate preference: arachidonate > dihomo-γ-linolenate > linoleate > α-linolenate (39).

However, the PGHS-II active site has a broader specificity than PGHS-I (39), which can be related to a larger active site (see below). A further difference is the 10 times lower concentration of hydroperoxide necessary to activate the cyclooxygenase activity of PGHS-II in vitro (40). The physiological consequences are unclear.

V. Structural Basis of the Mechanism of Inhibition of the Cyclooxygenases

The two previous paragraphs provided the structural and functional basis to understand the mechanism of inhibition of the cyclooxygenases by NSAIDs. Potential inhibitors are compounds that will interfere with one of the catalytic steps of cyclooxygenase. Each step can thus be explored to find and assess means to inhibit the activity. For example, an inhibitor of the peroxidase can inhibit cyclooxygenase only if it blocks completely the peroxidase activity, since we have seen that a remaining single peroxidase turnover is probably sufficient to activate cyclooxygenase. It is, however, not easy to deduce the characteristics of NSAIDs from the above mechanistic and structural descriptions: the acetylation of Ser-530 by aspirin would not obviously be shown from such a discussion. On the other hand, this mechanistic scheme will be useful to analyze the mode of action of inhibitors.

The mode of action of NSAIDs is usually divided into three categories: (1) NSAIDs like aspirin inhibit the protein in an irreversible manner. (2) NSAIDs like flurbiprofen or indomethacin inhibit the protein in a time-dependent but reversible manner. (3) NSAIDs like ibuprofen are competitive, reversible inhibitors. This classification is useful in setting up schemes of inhibition, which will provide the basis to ask how the measured inhibition is translated at the structural level. Nevertheless, it is important to realize that these functional differences between the various mode of action of inhibitors will not necessarily be translated into three clearly defined structural classifications of inhibitor-protein complexes. Three examples give a clear illustration of the problem: (1) Flurbiprofen is a time-dependent inhibitor, whereas its methyl ester derivative is a reversible competitive inhibitor (41). (2) Some inhibitors like NS-398, DUP-697 are reversible competitive inhibitors of PGHS-I, whereas they are time-dependent inhibitors of PGHS-II (42). (3) Mutagenesis of Arg-120 to Gln in PGHS-I can transform the time-dependent inhibition of flurbiprofen into a reversible inhibition (43). Therefore, we have to expect that only minor structural differences will decide the type of inhibition. Furthermore, if we are interested in distinguishing between PGHS-I and PGHS-II, we will have to focus on minor differences between the two active sites. Moreover, an important difference between PGHS-I and PGHS-II seems to be correlated with the time-dependent component of the inhibition; this means that we will have to address the question of the dynamics of the structure.

A more comprehensive study of inhibition is given elsewhere in this book (see Chapter 1). In the following paragraphs, we will concentrate our analysis on inhibitors, whose three-dimensional structure has been elucidated as complex with either PGHS-I or PGHS-II (see Table 1 and Fig. 5). The structure of these complexes will teach two main lessons: First, inhibitors are used as structural probes of the active site of the cyclooxygenase providing insight into its catalytic mechanism and the overall flexibility of the protein. Second, we are learning how an inhibitor uses structural features of the protein to obtain a more specific or a more potent inhibition.

We will see from the structural and functional analysis that we can consider most cyclooxygenase inhibitors as compounds that block the narrow channel in a reversible, time-dependent, or covalent manner. However, study of the cyclooxygenase mechanism has shown that there are other potential modes of action of inhibitors. Indeed, PGHS is prone to suicide inactivation. An inhibitor could induce such inactivation by interacting directly or indirectly with Tyr-385. This inhibition does not have to induce a covalent change of the inhibitor itself, since it could simply promote an inactivation reaction on the protein. Indeed, changes in the EPR signal have been observed upon inhibitor binding (44). This potential mode of inhibition could still play a role with some inhibitors, although it will not be discussed here in detail.

VI. Flurbiprofen

The flurbiprofen PGHS complex will be our reference structure for several reasons: It is the only structure that has been determined with both isoforms. Furthermore, both complexes yielded structures with the highest resolution for each isoenzyme (3.1 Å for PGHS-I and 2.5 Å for PGHS-II). The first structure solved of PGHS-I was described in the presence of the time-dependent inhibitor flurbiprofen (13). Indeed, these facts may not be fortuitous, but are rather a consequence of the higher stability of the protein induced upon binding with flurbiprofen as has been shown by limited proteolysis experiments (45). Therefore, it is not only the best available structure from a practical point of view, but also a good model of a tight structure for a time-dependent inhibition with a low IC_{50} value (46). There are no important differences between the structure of PGHS-I and murine PGHS-II [the rms difference is only 0.9 Å for the Cα atoms (16)]. These structures show that flurbiprofen is locked in the narrow cyclooxygenase channel, thus blocking access to the active site. More specifically, one can see potential hydrogen bonds between the carboxylic group of flurbiprofen, which is directed toward the mouth of the channel,

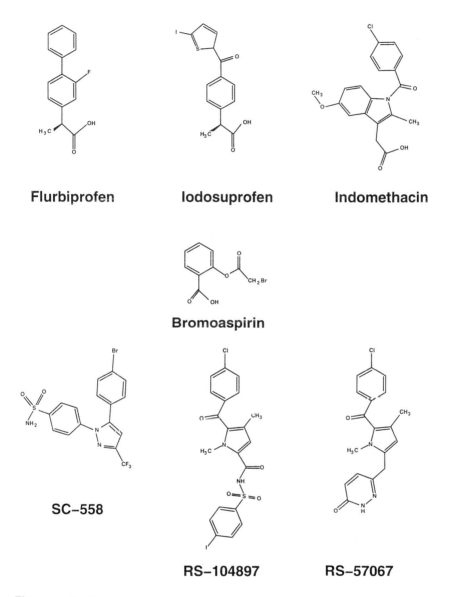

Figure 5 Inhibitors of peroxidase, which have been used for structural determination as complexed with PGHS-I and PGHS-II. The chemical formulas have been oriented in such a way that the groups that are in the vicinity of Tyr-385 are at the top. Groups directed toward or protruding in the lower side pockets are on the left.

and the guanidinium group of Arg-120. Arg-120 forms a salt bridge with Glu-524 in a largely apolar channel. One minor difference between the two isoforms is that the van der Waals contact of flurbiprofen with Ile-523 in PGHS-I is not seen with Val-523 in PGHS-II. The structure suggests that the stereospecificity for S-flurbiprofen is due to a potential steric clash of the R-stereoisomer with Tyr-355 (13). Mutation of that residue to Phe confirms this prediction (43). Therefore, this example shows that a precise structure function relationship is possible and that the position of flurbiprofen observed in the X-ray structure has to be related to its mode of action. Furthermore, the fact that the inhibitor is tightly packed into a narrow channel, and that a conformational change of the protein is necessary to bury flurbiprofen in the active site, is in good agreement with hypotheses describing how slow-binding inhibitors causes time-dependent inhibition. Indeed, a kinetic description of the inhibition has been made with the following scheme of slow-binding inhibitors (47):

$$E + I \underset{k_{-1}}{\overset{k_1}{\Leftrightarrow}} EI \underset{k_{-2}}{\overset{k_2}{\Leftrightarrow}} EI^*$$

with the assumption that EI is in rapid equilibrium with E + I and that the transition EI to EI* and the reverse reaction are slow ($k_{\pm2} \ll k_{\pm1}$). This scheme provides a satisfactory description of the time course of inhibition for PGHS-I and PGHS-II (47). Accordingly, the observed X-ray structure has to correspond to the EI* conformation of this scheme (Fig. 6). No direct observation exists for the EI state. Formally, the EI state could be either a distinct binding site from the EI* or, more likely, the same site but with a conformational change that locks the substrate into place (see below). We will first assess the generality of this closed conformation and try to get more information on the structure of the EI* complex, by looking at other inhibitors.

VII. Iodosuprofen

The structure of iodosuprofen has been obtained with ovine PGHS-I. It occupies the same position as flurbiprofen (48). The structure does not exhibit conformational changes relative to the flurbiprofen structure. An H-bond is present between the carbonyl oxygen and the hydroxyl of Ser-530. The same stereospecificity requirement and justification as for flurbiprofen exists. This provides the first step in showing that the flurbiprofen structural interpretation has a more general validity.

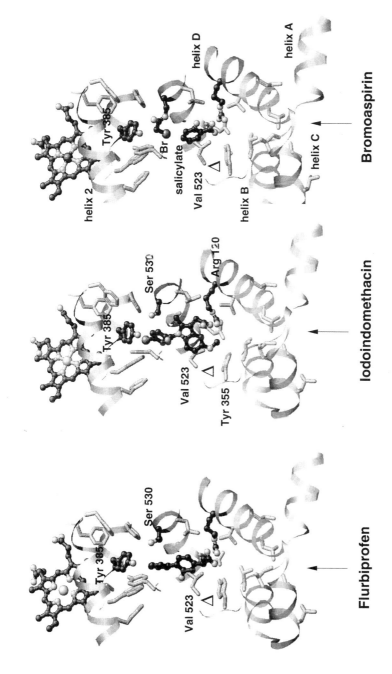

Figure 6 Three PGHS inhibitors, flurbiprofen, indomethacin, and bromoaspirin, in the cyclooxygenase channel. The same orientation is used in the three cases. On the left, the Δ shows the position of the side pocket used by SC-558 in PGHS-II; this access is restricted in PGHS-I by Ile-523 (Val in PGHS-II).

VIII. Indomethacin

The structure of iodoindomethacin complexed with ovine PGHS-I has been determined at low resolution (48) (Fig. 6). Since then, the structure of indomethacin complexed with murine PGHS-II have been obtained at higher resolution (16). Indomethacin occupies the same position in both isoforms. This inhibitor is bulkier than flurbiprofen, but still manages to be buried deeply in the protein. The main features occupies the same binding pocket as flurbiprofen. Nevertheless, the murine PGHS-II structure allows us to observe some small conformational changes of the protein relative to the flurbiprofen structure: the peptide segment 353–356 moves by 0.7 Å. This suggests a mode of action similar to that of flurbiprofen. Furthermore, the same scheme of slow-binding inhibition that was discussed with flurbiprofen can be applied (47).

IX. RS-104897

RS-104897 is formed by a Zomepirac core but with the carboxylic group replaced with an acyl-sulfonamide group; it is 100-fold selective toward PGHS-II (17). Structure comparison between RS-104897/PGHS-II and flurbiprofen/PGHS-I shows a rms deviation of the main chain atoms of 0.9 Å for the overall structure and of 0.4 Å for the core of the catalytic domain, which is at the level of the positional uncertainty at the present resolution; i.e., they are practically identical. Furthermore, RS-104897 binds at the same position as flurbiprofen in PGHS-I and PGHS-II with the Zomepirac core compound binding at the same place with the chlorine atom 3.2 Å from the Tyr-385 oxygen (15). The nitrogen and oxygen of the acyl sulfonamide group interact with Arg-120 and Tyr-355. Arg-120, Glu-524, and Tyr-355 participate in a hydrogen bond network as in the flurbiprofen complex. The sulfonamide group of Rs-104897 does not occupy the same position as the sulfonamide of SC-558 and the iodophenyl group also does not occupy the same pocket as the phenyl group of SC-558 (see below).

X. Aspirin

Aspirin is unique among the NSAIDs: it inhibits PGHS through acetylation of Ser-530. Biochemical and mutagenesis studies have provided a strong basis for the understanding of its mode of action, and these studies are fully supported by crystallographic studies (49) (Fig. 6). The structure determination used a brominated form of aspirin, which is roughly equipotent to aspirin. This compound was initially chosen to overcome the difficulty of working with weakly diffracting crystals. Fortunately, the crystal diffracted better than expected; i.e., it would not have been necessary to use this brominated form. This technical trick provided an unexpected benefit, however, revealing the presence of an additional weaker electron density that suggests the existence of a second rotameric state of the acetyl-serine side chain: The major rotameric component fully blocks access to Tyr-385, while the minor component still allows partial access to Tyr-385. The structure of PGHS-II with aspirin has still not been determined. Nevertheless, a more general interpretation is possible in the light of mutagenesis and inhibition studies done on the two isoforms of PGHS. Indeed, Ser-530 is not necessary for the catalytic activity since the mutant having Ser-530 replaced by Ala is still active (50). On the other hand, aspirin has different effects on PGHS-I and PGHS-II: In PGHS I it inhibits all activity, whereas in PGHS-II the enzyme is still able to function as an oxygenase producing 15R-HETE (51). Lecointe et al. (51) have probed the acetylation site by mutagenesis: The mutation of Ser-530 to Asn removes activity for PGHS-I but not PGHS-II; PGHS-II, however, loses activity when Ser-530 is mutated to Gln. Interestingly, mutation of Ser-530 to Met provides the same result as an acetylated Ser-530 for PGHS-II with the production of 15R-HETE. These results brought together with the structure suggest that the equilibrium between the two rotameric states is different in the two isoenzymes. This means that just minimal changes in the environment of Ser-530 are sufficient to explain this difference (49). This result is supported by the structure of PGHS-II with the RS-104897: Luong et al. (15) have compared the central part of the channel in both isoforms and found the volume to be increased by 17% in PGHS-II. This implies the acetyl serine's conformation in PGHS-II differs from the most populated conformation in PGHS-I, since it allows interaction of arachidonic acid with Tyr-385, in agreement with the two conformations hypothesis of Loll et al. (49). The X-ray structure provides a further result, by showing that the released salicylate still binds to the channel at a position occupied in the flurbiprofen structure by the fluorphenyl ring, with the carboxylate also interacting with Arg-120. Salicylate is a poor inhibitor of PGHS in vitro, but is able to inhibit the acetylation of Ser-530 by aspirin (52). The overall structure is otherwise identical to the structure determined with flurbiprofen, although limited proteolysis experiments show no stabilization of aspirin-treated protein relative to the free holoenzyme (45). This suggests a somewhat limited flexibility of the channel; this aspect will be discussed in more detail with the structure in the absence of inhibitors (see below).

Other salicylates are able to inhibit the cyclooxygenase through acylation of Ser-530: Valeryl(pentanoyl)salicylates inhibit PGHS-1 more effectively than PGHS-2 (53).

XI. SC-558

SC-558 is a diaryl heterocyclic inhibitor with a central pyrazole ring and a sulfonamide substituent attached to one of the aryl ring. It is highly selective for COX-2 (1900-fold). Two different crystal forms have been obtained, which provide identical structures (16). The bromophenyl ring and the trifluoromethyl group occupy a position in murine PGHS-II similar to flurbiprofen in PGHS-II and PGHS-I: the bromophenyl occupies the position of the distal phenyl ring in the flurbiprofen structure and the pyrazole the equivalent position of the flurophenyl ring of flurbiprofen. The trifluoromethyl group of SC-558 and the carboxylate group of flurbiprofen bind at the same position. The phenylsulfonamide group, on the other hand, branches out into a side pocket, unused by flurbiprofen, that provides hydrophobic contacts for the phenyl group. The sulfonamide group reaches a more polar region at the surface of the protein. This same pocket exists also in PGHS-I but Ile-523 limits access to the pocket. This residue is a less bulky valine in PGHS-II. An elegant verification of this hypothesis has been made by the mutation of Val-523 to Ile in PGHS-II (54). The mutant exhibits a selectivity now similar to PGHS-I for inhibitors like NS-398, SC-58125, and SC-236. Therefore, it underlines the critical role for the selectivity of the only residue that is different in the central part of the channel. However, this observation is not sufficient to explain the specificity observed for all inhibitors, implying that other factors influence drug selectivity. Some more subtle effects have to be taken into consideration: Kurumbail et al. (16) have noticed in their structure that Val-434 (Ile-434 in PGHS-I) packs against Phe-518, which interacts with the phenyl group of SC-558. The additional methyl group in the PGHS-I structure restricts the conformation of Phe-518 and thus reduces the size of the pocket used by the phenylsulfonamide group. This shows that residues that are not in direct contact with the inhibitor of the channel surface but are one layer removed and this may play an important role in determining position and flexibility of interacting residues. Other substitutions are also present in the environment of the sulfonamide group, but their localization near the surface of the protein make an assessment of these individual contributions more difficult. The binding of SC-558 induces a disruption of the salt bridge between Arg-120 and Glu-524 and an unwinding of the end of the helices D around Arg-120, probably in a similar manner as with RS-57067 (see below).

XII. RS-57067

This compound is similar to RS-104897 but with the acyl-sulfonamide group replaced by a pyridazinone. It is 1000-fold more selective toward PGHS-II

relatively to PGHS-I (17). This inhibitor induces local but important conformational changes relative to PGHS-I and to the RS-104897/PGHS-II complex, which both exhibit the same conformation, as shown previously. This
conformational change can be described as an unwinding of the two last turns
of helix D, which provokes a positional shift of 2.7 Å of the α-carbon of Arg-
120, whose guanidino group cannot interact any more with the carboxylic
group of Glu-524. The latter also reorients to form a salt bridge with Arg-513.
This salt bridge is not possible in PGHS-I since the arginine at position 513 is
replaced by a histidine. The rest of the structure remains very similar and the
rms deviation of the catalytic core is only 0.6 Å for the backbone atoms. In
particular, the membrane-binding domain, which is connected to the catalytic
domain through the helix D, does not move significantly. This structure provides an important lesson: As Luong et al. (15) pointed out, this conformation
reduces the constriction of the funnel and may thus also provide an approximate picture of an intermediate state formed upon binding a substrate or another inhibitor. It provides another example that the design of inhibitors has
to take into account conformational changes and thus must probe the multiple
possible conformations of a protein.

XIII. PGHS-II Without Inhibitor

We have seen several structures of PGHS-1 and PGHS-2 with bound inhibitors. The structure of murine PGHS-II in the unliganded form has been determined (16). The structure of this unliganded form has been a bit more difficult to obtain, since the difficulty in crystallizing a particular form of the
protein seems to correlates roughly with the susceptibility of that form of the
enzyme to limited proteolysis of PGHS-1, and hence to the overall flexibility
of the protein. Nevertheless, the overall structure of the unliganded enzyme
seems roughly the same as in the liganded forms. The only noticeable difference lies in the region of Arg-120 on helix D. Even there, the conformation
seems to be the same as in the liganded structure with flurbiprofen; i.e., the
salt bridge between Arg-120 and Glu-524 is present; however, the electron
density in this region is poorly defined suggesting a high flexibility in the end
of helix D, the region that has already been shown to exhibit relatively large
conformational changes with RS-57067. This is the region that builds the narrow part of the channel and that needs to undergo a conformational changes
to allow entry of the substrate or the inhibitor into the channel. This, along
with other smaller and more subtle conformational changes, may be the
structural equivalent of the observed time-dependent inhibition. However,
the most important result is that there are no other important conformational
changes, i.e., that the channel stay roughly the same whether liganded or un-

liganded. This feature raises some important questions: the active site of the cyclooxygenase is formed, as already mentioned, by a narrow, mainly hydrophobic channel. This feature fits well with the hydrophobic nature of the substrate and with the continuity between the entry of the active site and the hydrophobic membrane, which avoids the solvation and desolvation steps of the substrate. However, formation of a completely dehydrated Michaelis complex should imply that no water molecule is present in the channel of the unliganded form. In other words, the space occupied by the substrate or the inhibitor should be replaced by the protein in the unliganded form. This is obviously not the case, since the channel cannot be empty, but is likely to be filled with water. It may seem that the ingenious connection between the membrane and the substrate is notable only for its proximity, but not the hydrophobic continuity. This is probably not the case, and the unliganded structure may offer an explanation for a structural feature whose function has hitherto been unclear. Indeed, one can observe a long, narrow channel that begins at the top of the cyclooxygenase channel and goes toward the dimer interface, running in the vicinity of the peroxidase active site. This channel could be used to expel the water from the channel; the substrate would not need to undergo a solvation step, but would have to push a water column. The narrow side channel or vent would thus hinder the formation of hydrostatic pressure inside the channel. This water-expelling mechanism could be energetically more favorable than a conformational change of the protein to induce a constriction of the empty channel. Indeed, most catalytic mechanisms associated with large conformational changes are usually associated with domain movements, but this is not possible here since we are not at the interface between two domains, but rather at the center of a large domain (Fig. 2). Therefore, more complex conformational changes would be needed to cause constriction of the channel within a domain, and might require reorganization of the domain and therefore be energetically more expensive. This function of a water channel has to be distinguished from other water channels that have been postulated for the transfer of protons in the photosynthetic reaction center (55) or cytochrome *f* (56); the water in our case should be weakly bound, in order to be easily expelled.

XIV. Conclusions

We have seen here that the methodology developed for ovine PGHS-I could quickly, if not easily, be applied to human and murine PGHS-II and then be used to study specific inhibition by NSAIDs, thus providing the first example of a membrane protein used as a target in structure-based drug design.

The specificity determinants for the inhibition of PGHS-I and PGHS-II are complex and a simple lock-and-key mechanism is not sufficient to explain the mode of action of inhibitors. Nevertheless, the combined approach of mutagenesis of the protein and the inhibitor combined with structural determinations of both isoforms with various inhibitors allows taking into consideration conformational changes associated with the binding of a time-dependent inhibitor.

Acknowledgments

The author thanks Patrick J. Loll for a critical reading of the manuscript, R. Michael Garavito, who created the proper conditions to solve the PGHS-I structure, and Jean-Luc Popot for allowing a monotopic intrusion in the UPR 9052 of the CNRS.

References

1. Vane JR. Inhibition of prostaglandin synthesis as a mechanism of action for aspirin-like drugs. Nature New Biol 1971; 231:232–235.
2. Flower RJ. Drugs which inhibit prostaglandin biosynthesis. Pharmacol Rev 1974; 26:33–67.
3. Hemler M, Lands WE. Purification of the cyclooxygenase that forms prostaglandins. Demonstration of two forms of iron in the holoenzyme. J Biol Chem 1976; 251:5575–5579.
4. Miyamoto T, Ogino N, Yamamoto S, Hayaishi O. Purification of prostaglandin endoperoxide synthetase from bovine vesicular gland microsomes. J Biol Chem 1976; 251:2629–2636.
5. Van der Ouderaa FJ, Buytenhek M, Nugteren DH, Van Dorp DA. Purification and characterisation of prostaglandin endoperoxide synthetase from sheep vesicular glands. Biochim Biophys Acta 1977; 487:315–331.
6. Smith WL, Dewitt DL. Prostaglandin endoperoxide H synthase-1 and -2. Adv Immunol 1996; 62:167–215.
7. Xie WL, Chipman JG, Robertson DL, Erikson RL, Simmons DL. Expression of a mitogen-responsive gene encoding prostaglandin synthase is regulated by mRNA splicing. Proc Natl Acad Sci USA 1991; 88:2692–2696.
8. Kujubu DA, Fletcher BS, Varnum BC, Lim RW, Herschman HR. TIS10, a phorbol ester tumor promoter-inducible mRNA from Swiss 3T3 cells, encodes a novel prostaglandin synthase/cyclooxygenase homologue. J Biol Chem 1991; 266:12866–12872.
9. Seibert K, Zhang Y, Leahy K, et al. Pharmacological and biochemical demonstration of the role of cyclooxygenase 2 in inflammation and pain. Proc Natl Acad Sci USA 1994; 91:12013–12017.

10. Garavito RM, Rosenbusch JP. Three-dimensional crystals of an integral membrane protein: an initial X-ray analysis. J Cell Biol 1980; 86:327–329.
11. Michel H, Oesterhelt D. Three-dimensional crystals of membrane proteins: bacteriorhodopsin. Proc Natl Acad Sci USA 1980; 77:1283–1285.
12. Garavito RM, Picot D, Loll PJ. Strategies for crystallizing membrane proteins. J Bioenerg Biomembr 1996; 28:13–27.
13. Picot D, Loll PJ, Garavito RM. The X-ray crystal structure of the membrane protein prostaglandin H$_2$ synthase-1. Nature 1994; 367:243–249.
14. Garavito RM, Picot D, Loll PJ. The 3.1 A X-ray crystal structure of the integral membrane enzyme prostaglandin H$_2$ synthase-1. Adv Prostaglandin Thromboxane Leukot Res 1995; 23:99–103.
15. Luong C, Miller A, Barnett J, Chow J, Ramesha C, Browner MF. Flexibility of the NSAID binding site in the structure of human cyclooxygenase-2. Nature Struct Biol 1996; 3:927–933.
16. Kurumbail R, Stevens AM, Gierse JK, et al. Structural basis for selective inhibition of cyclooxygenase-2 by anti-inflammatory agents. Nature 1996; 384:644–648.
17. Barnett J, Chow J, Ives D, et al. Purification, characterization and selective inhibition of human prostaglandin G/H synthase 1 and 2 expressed in the baculovirus system. Biochim Biophys Acta 1994; 1209:130–139.
18. Gierse JK, Hauser SD, Creely DP, et al. Expression and selective inhibition of the constitutive and inducible forms of human cyclo-oxygenase. Biochem J 1995; 305 (Pt 2):479–484.
19. Zeng J, Fenna RE. X-ray crystal structure of canine myeloperoxidase at 3 Å resolution. J Mol Biol 1992; 226:185–207.
20. Otto JC, DeWitt DL, Smith WL. N-glycosylation of prostaglandin endoperoxide synthases-1 and -2 and their orientations in the endoplasmic reticulum. J Biol Chem 1993; 268:18234–18242.
21. Garavito RM, Picot D, Loll PJ. Prostaglandin H synthase. Curr Opin Struct Biol 1994; 4:529–535.
22. Toh H, Yokoyama C, Tanabe T, Yoshimoto T, Yamamoto S. Molecular evolution of cyclooxygenase and lipoxygenase. Prostaglandins 1992; 44:291–315.
23. Picot D, Garavito RM. Prostaglandin H synthase: implications for membrane structure. FEBS Lett 1994; 346:21–25.
24. Blobel G. Intracellular protein topogenesis. Proc Natl Acad Sci USA 1980; 77: 1496–1500.
25. Singer SJ, Nicolson GL. The fluid mosaic model of the structure of cell membranes. Science 1972; 175:720–731.
26. Otto JC, Smith WL. Photolabeling of prostaglandin endoperoxide H synthase-1 with 3-trifluoro-3-(m-[125I]iodophenyl)diazirine as a probe of membrane association and the cyclooxygenase active site. J Biol Chem 1996; 271:9906–9910.
27. Otto JC, Smith WL. The orientation of prostaglandin endoperoxide synthases-1 and -2 in the endoplasmic reticulum. J Biol Chem 1994; 269:19868–19875.
28. Morita I, Schindler M, Regier MK, et al. Different intracellular locations for prostaglandin endoperoxide H synthase-1 and -2. J Biol Chem 1995; 270:10902–10908.

29. Campbell ID, Bork P. Epidermal growth factor–like modules. Curr Opin Struct Biol 1993; 3:385–392.
30. Harlan JE. Solution Structure and Function of Ligand Interactions with Prostaglandin H_2 Synthase. PhD thesis, The University of Chicago, 1993.
31. Smith WL, Marnett LJ. Prostaglandin endoperoxide synthases. In: Sigel H, Sigel A, eds. Metalloenzymes Involving Amino Acid-Residue and Related Radicals. New York: Marcel Dekker, 1994:163–169.
32. Hamberg M, Samuelsson B. On the mechanism of the biosynthesis of prostaglandins E_1 and $F_{1\alpha}$. J Biol Chem 1967; 242:5336–5343.
33. Karthein R, Dietz R, Nastainczyk W, Ruf HH. Higher oxidation states of prostaglandin H synthase. An EPR study of a transient tyrosyl radical in the enzyme during the peroxidase reaction. Eur J Biochem 1988; 171:313–320.
34. Shimokawa T, Kulmacz RJ, DeWitt DL, Smith WL. Tyrosine 385 of prostaglandin endoperoxide synthase is required for cyclooxygenase catalysis. J Biol Chem 1990; 265:20073–20076.
35. Tsai A, Hsi LC, Kulmacz RJ, Palmer G, Smith WL. Characterization of the tyrosyl radicals in ovine prostaglandin H synthase-1 by isotope replacement and site-directed mutagenesis. J Biol Chem 1994; 269:5085–5091.
36. Tsai A, Kulmacz RJ, Palmer G. Spectroscopic evidence for reaction of prostaglandin H synthase-1 tyrosyl radical with arachidonic acid. J Biol Chem 1995; 270: 10503–10508.
37. Hsi LC, Hoganson CW, Babcock GT, Smith WL. Characterization of a tyrosyl radical in prostaglandin endoperoxide synthase-2. Biochem Biophys Res Commun 1994; 202:1592–1598.
38. Xiao G, Tsai A-L, Palmer G, Boyer WC, Marshall PJ, Kulmacz RJ. Analysis of hydroperoxide-induced tyrosyl radicals and lipoxygenase activity in aspirin treated human prostaglandin H synthase-2. Biochemistry 1997; 36:1836–1845.
39. Laneuville O, Breuer DK, Xu N, et al. Fatty acid substrate specificities of human prostaglandin-endoperoxide H synthase-1 and -2. Formation of 12-hydroxy-(9Z, 13E/Z, 15Z)-octadecatrienoic acids from alpha-linolenic acid. J Biol Chem 1995; 270:19330–19336.
40. Kulmacz RJ, Wang LH. Comparison of hydroperoxide initiator requirements for the cyclooxygenase activities of prostaglandin H synthase-1 and -2. J Biol Chem 1995; 270:24019–24023.
41. Rome LH, Lands WE. Structural requirements for time-dependent inhibition of prostaglandin biosynthesis by anti-inflammatory drugs. Proc Natl Acad Sci USA 1975; 72:4863–4865.
42. Copeland RA, Williams JM, Giannaras J, et al. Mechanism of selective inhibition of the inducible isoform of prostaglandin G/H synthase. Proc Natl Acad Sci USA 1994; 91:11202–11206.
43. Bhattacharyya DK, Lecomte M, Rieke CJ, Garavito M, Smith WL. Involvement of arginine 120, glutamate 524, and tyrosine 355 in the binding of arachidonate and 2-phenylpropionic acid inhibitors to the cyclooxygenase active site of ovine prostaglandin endoperoxide H synthase-1. J Biol Chem 1996; 271:2179–2184.
44. Kulmacz RJ, Palmer G, Tsai AL. Prostaglandin H synthase: perturbation of the tyrosyl radical as a probe of anticyclooxygenase agents. Mol Pharmacol 1991; 40:833–837.

45. Kulmacz RJ. Topography of prostaglandin H synthase. Antiinflammatory agents and the protease-sensitive arginine 253 region. J Biol Chem 1989; 264:14136–14144.
46. Laneuville O, Breuer DK, Dewitt DL, Hla T, Funk CD, Smith WL. Differential inhibition of human prostaglandin endoperoxide H synthases-1 and -2 by non-steroidal anti-inflammatory drugs. J Pharmacol Exp Ther 1994; 271:927–934.
47. Callan OH, So OY, Swinney DC. The kinetic factors that determine the affinity and selectivity for slow binding inhibition of human prostaglandin H synthase 1 and 2 by indomethacin and flurbiprofen. J Biol Chem 1996; 271:3548–3554.
48. Loll PJ, Picot D, Ekabo Ok Garavito RM. Synthesis and use of iodinated non-steroidal antiinflammatory drug analogs as crystallographic probes of the prostaglandin H_2 synthase cyclooxygenase active site. Biochemistry 1996; 35:7330–7340.
49. Loll PJ, Picot D, Garavito RM. The structural basis of aspirin activity inferred from the cyrstal structure of inactivated prostaglandin H_2 synthase. Nat Struct Biol 1995; 2:637–643.
50. Shimokawa T, Smith WL. Prostaglandin endoperoxide synthase. The aspirin acetylation region. J Biol Chem 1992; 267:12387–12392.
51. Lecomte M, Laneuville O, Ji C, DeWitt DL, Smith WL. Acetylation of human prostaglandin endoperoxidase synthase-2 (cyclooxygenase-2) by aspirin. J Biol Chem 1994; 269:13207–13215.
52. Vargaftig BB. The inhibition of cyclooxygenase in rabbit platelets by aspirin is prevented by salicylic acid and by phenanthrolines. Eur J Pharmacol 1978; 50:231–241.
53. Bhattacharyya DK, Lecomte M, Dunn J, Morgans DJ, Smith WL. Selective inhibition of prostaglandin endoperoxide synthase-1 (cyclooxygenase-1) by valeryl-salicylic acid. Arch Biochem Biophys 1995; 317:19–24.
54. Gierse JK, McDonald JJ, Hauser SD, Rangwala SH, Koboldt CM, Seibert K. A single amino acid difference between cycloxygenase-1 (COX-1) and -2 (COX-2) reverses the selectivity of COX-2 specific inhibitors. J Biol Chem 1996; 271:15810–41581.
55. Ermler U, Fritzsch G, Buchanan SK, Michel H. Structure of the photosynthetic reaction centre from *Rhodobacter sphaeroides* at 2.65 Å resolution: cofactor and protein-cofactor interactions. Structure 1994; 2:925–936.
56. Martinez S, Huang D, Ponomarev M, Cramer W, Smith J. The heme redox center of chloroplast cytochrome *f* is linked to a buried five-water chain. Protein Sci 1996; 5:1081–1092.

10

The Role of 5-Lipoxygenase Products in a Mouse Model of Allergic Airway Inflammation

COLIN D. FUNK and
XIN-SHENG CHEN

University of Pennsylvania
Philadelphia, Pennsylvania

YUAN-PO TU

Everett Clinic
Everett, Washington

CHARLES G. IRVIN

National Jewish Center for Immunology
  and Respiratory Medicine
Denver, Colorado

JAMES R. SHELLER

Vanderbilt University School of Medicine
Vanderbilt Medical Center
Nashville, Tennessee

I. Introduction

Asthma is a complex disorder that displays hallmark signs of an exaggerated response of the airways to nonspecific stimuli, inflammation and reversible, intermittent airway obstruction. Although the present animal models of asthma are not ideal, some of the major features of the disease can be recapitulated in mice sensitized with ovalbumin (OVA) intraperitoneally injected and challenged with OVA inhalation. The leukotrienes, derived by initial oxygenation of arachidonic acid via 5-lipoxygenase (5LO), have been implicated in the pathophysiology of asthma. We have exploited the murine model of OVA-induced allergic airway inflammation and the availability of 5LO-deficient mice to explore further the role of leukotrienes.

II. Asthma, Airways Hyperresponsiveness, and Leukotrienes

The pathogenesis of airways hyperresponsiveness (AHR) is unclear, although in asthma it is linked with inflammation (1). It is evident, however, that it is a complex functional disorder that can be dissociated from inflammation in some settings and has both smooth-muscle-dependent and nonmuscular components (1–3; Fig. 1).

Atopic asthmatics display a dual inflammatory response in the lungs post–bronchial challenge with allergen (4). The early-phase response that results from IgE-mediated mast cell degranulation is followed several hours later by a late-phase bronchospastic response characterized by infiltration of the airways by eosinophils, interstitial edema, and mucus glycoprotein release. To understand the mechanism of enhanced AHR, in particular as it pertains to asthma, animal models have been developed, including mouse models that can be used in conjunction with gene knockout technology to dissect the contributions of individual gene products (5,6). Genetic components to AHR have been defined in mice and humans (7–9). One genetic linkage study (7) found loci on mouse chromosomes 2, 15, and 17, and another study (8) implicated an interval on chromosome 6 with acetylcholine-induced AHR. The latter locus contains the genes for the interleukin-5 receptor, as well as 5LO. The locus on chromosome 17 maps close to the gene for mouse mast cell protease-7 (7). In the murine system developed by several investigators, progressive airflow limitation and AHR are features of chronic antigen exposure (10–12). The airway inflammation observed in allergic asthma is thought to be orchestrated by an antigen-driven T-helper-2 (Th2) lymphocyte response (13–15; see Fig. 2). Pulmonary levels of mRNA and protein for the Th2 cytokines IL-4 and IL-5 are elevated after antigen challenge and this leads to the functional response of eosinophil migration into the airways (4). IL-12 suppresses the expression of Th2 cytokines and their associated responses, including eosinophilia, increased serum IgE, mucosal mastocytosis, and antigen-induced AHR (16).

The cysteinyl leukotrienes are known bronchoactive agonists with diverse proinflammatory effects (17,18). Their proinflammatory actions include the ability to increase microvascular permeability in airways, to promote eosinophil migration and recruitment, and to stimulate mucus release and decrease mucus transport (see Fig. 2 box). Zileuton, an orally active 5LO inhibitor, when administered chronically to moderate asthmatics decreased AHR as determined by reactivity to cold, dry air (19). Its effect persisted well after the enzyme inhibitory action should have dissipated, based on the short half-life of zileuton, suggesting that 5LO products can mediate AHR separately from their acute bronchospastic actions. Leukotriene D_4 receptor ($CysLT_1$) antagonists have shown equal, if not better, efficacy in various trials with mild-moderate asthmatic patients (20,21). Thus, clinical trials now support significant improvement in several objective and subjective measures of asthma with $CysLT_1$ blockers like pranlukast, montelukast (MK-476), and zafirlukast (ICI-204,219). Airway smooth muscle hyperplasia is another feature of chronic severe asthma. Some data suggest that the cysteinyl leukotrienes play

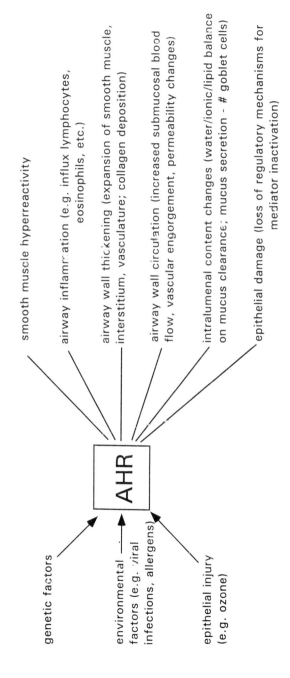

Figure 1 The development of airway hyperresponsiveness (AHR). AHR is a complex response to diverse factors (left) resulting in an array of pathophysiological endpoints (right).

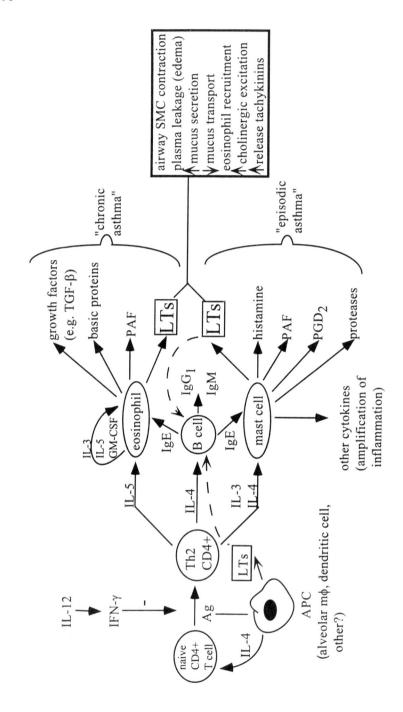

a role in the regulation of airway smooth muscle cell proliferation from studies in ovalbumin-sensitized Brown Norway rats, but it is not known if they are acting directly or indirectly to potentiate the effects by other substances (22). Evidence is mounting that cysteinyl leukotrienes can alter airway function by modulating the activity of the afferent nervous system (23). Studies with guinea pigs suggest that when synthesized by airway mast cells (or other cell types) leukotrienes interact with sensory fibers leading to changes in their excitability as well as enhancement of the release of tachykinins (24). The model presented in Figure 2 depicts the various components in the development of asthma and allergic airway inflammation and the resultant AHR to agents such as methacholine. The long-anticipated arrival of 5LO inhibitors and $CysLT_1$ receptor antagonists for use in clinical medicine and the treatment of asthma has now occurred without a complete understanding of the biology of their actions (25). A solid understanding of the role 5LO products play in the development of AHR is important for understanding the therapeutic basis of antileukotriene drugs.

III. 5LO Products, B Lymphocytes, and the Immune Response

IL-4 is the key cytokine that induces major pleiotropic effects on B lymphocytes (26). These effects include: acting as a growth and differentiation factor for preactivated cells, modulation of expression of FcεRII/CD23 (low-affinity IgE receptor), and Ig isotype switching. B cells express 5LO and are capable of leukotriene biosynthesis under certain conditions (27,28). T cells, on the other hand, do not express 5LO and are unable to make leukotrienes from

---

Figure 2 Pathways in asthma pathogenesis. In the mouse model, allergen antigen (Ag = ovalbumin) interacting with an antigen-presenting cell (APC) sets in motion a series of events leading to a Th2 lymphocyte response. Interleukin-12 and interferon γ can suppress the ensuing events. Committed Th2 cells undergo expansion and the secretion of characteristic cytokines like IL-4 and IL-5 follows. IL-4 leads to immunoglobulin isotype switching in B cells and IgE release. IgE can elicit mast cell degranulation. IL-5 promotes eosinophilia and the survival and activation of eosinophils. Leukotrienes (LTs) released from mast cells and eosinophils contribute to a host of "proasthmatic" events (box on right). An involvement of LTs, released possibly from macrophages, mast cells, and/or B lymphocytes, at an early stage in the cascade is suggested by the ability of leukotrienes to enhance IL-4-induced IgE production. For sake of clarity, the scheme does not depict all potential molecular and cellular interrelationships.

endogenous arachidonic acid (28,29). However, a number of immunomodulatory actions of leukotrienes on T cells have been ascribed (30). Leukotriene B$_4$ (LTB$_4$) enhances activation, proliferation, and differentiation of human B lymphocytes in vitro (31). LTB$_4$, but not LTC$_4$, potentiates both FcεRII/CD23 and class II MHC antigen expression and release of soluble CD23 when resting human B lymphocytes are challenged with a suboptimal dose of IL-4 (32). LTB$_4$ also potentiates the IL-4-induced production of IgE from peripheral blood mononuclear cells, an effect that was dependent on the presence of a monocyte/macrophage population (33). Its mode(s) of action appeared to be through an increase of IL-4 receptor–positive cells and release of soluble CD23.

IV. A Murine System of Antigen-Driven Hyperresponsiveness: Model Characterization

An antigen-driven murine system that is characterized by an immune response (IgE) shows dependence on a Th2 lymphocyte response and exhibits signs of eosinophil infiltration has been developed (6,10). Mice have been shown to mount an IgE response after intraperitoneal sensitization with ovalbumin (OVA) (10). In the studies presented here, mice were immunized and chronically exposed (8 days) to aerosolized antigen (see Fig. 3). In vivo pulmonary function measurements of airway resistance (R$_L$) and dynamic compliance (C$_L$) were measured by the methods of Martin et al. (34). Briefly, mice are anesthetized with pentobarbital, tracheotomized with a cannula, placed in a plethysmograph, and mechanically ventilated. Transpulmonary pressure is measured as the pressure difference between the airway opening and the body plethysmograph; volume is the volume-calibrated pressure change in the body plethysmograph; and flow is the digital differentiation of the volume signal.

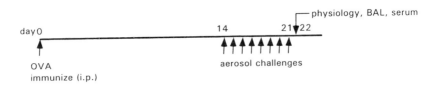

Figure 3 Standard mouse allergic airway inflammation model. Two weeks after an intraperitoneal injection of ovalbumin, mice are exposed to aerosolized antigen for 20 min each day during 8 consecutive days. Twenty-four hours later, airway physiology measurements and bronchoalveolar lavage are performed and serum sampled for immunoglobulin production.

R_L and C_L are obtained as the linear regression of the pressure flow and pressure-volume relationship using a digital solution of the equation of motion with a computer program (Labview). The dose-response curve to methacholine ($5-3700\,\mu g/kg$) is established by i.v. injection 24 hr after the last aerosol challenge.

Airway responsiveness to methacholine in wild-type mice is shifted several logs to the left, and the magnitude of maximal resistance generated at the highest dose is increased well over 20 times the baseline values indicating excessive airways narrowing. Baseline resistance is not elevated and animals that were only immunized but not challenged were similar to control nonimmune animals. These shifts in methacholine responsiveness and $R_L$max are similar in magnitude to changes seen in human asthmatics (35). This hyperresponsiveness is antigen-specific because if mice are immunized to OVA and challenged with an irrelevant antigen (ragweed), they do not produce a similar response.

V. Diminished Airway Responsiveness and Eosinophilia in 5LO-Deficient Mice Using a Mouse Model of Allergic Airway Inflammation

To determine the role of 5LO products in the development of airway reactivity following antigen exposure, we sensitized and serially exposed mice to aerosols of OVA. 5LO-deficient mice and their wild-type controls had measurements of R_L made in response to intravenous methacholine. Wild-type mice developed striking increases in cholinergic responsiveness; 5LO-deficient mice manifested a small increase in methacholine responsiveness (R_L at the highest methacholine dose was 9.9 ± 2.4 cmH$_2$O/ml/sec at baseline vs. 27.6 ± 4.6 after OVA in wild-type mice; 5.9 ± 0.9 vs. 7.01 ± 2.2 in 5LO-deficient mice) (Fig. 4).

To establish that this system is germane to current concepts of asthma pathogenesis, we performed measurements of total serum IgE and OVA-specific IgG levels and examined the influx of eosinophils. Ovalbumin provoked airway eosinophilia (performed by whole-lung bronchoalveolar lavage) and increased immunoglobulins in wild-type mice (Figs. 5–7). Total cells and eosinophils recovered by BAL in 5LO-deficient mice were markedly lower (Fig. 5 and 6). OVA-specific IgG and total IgE levels in the knockout mice did not increase to the same extent as in wild-type mice (Fig. 7), suggesting a potential action of 5LO products directly on the immune response, as mentioned earlier. The model used here elicits a Th2-type response that fits the current understanding of asthma pathogenesis (13–15). All of our initial studies were performed with mice of the hybrid strains C57BL/6 and 129 Sv

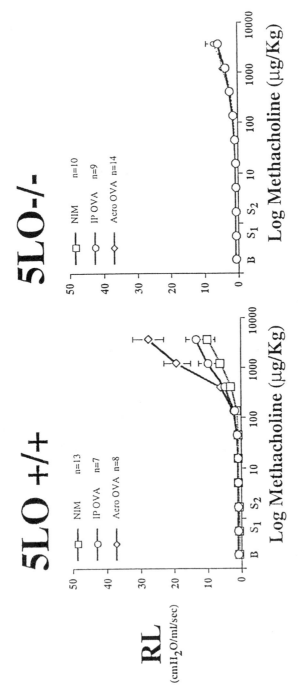

Figure 4 Effect of intravenous methacholine on lung resistance (R_L) in NIM (nonimmune), IP OVA (ovalbumin intraperitoneal, saline aerosol), and Aero OVA (ovalbumin intraperitoneal and ovalbumin aerosol)-treated wild-type (left) and 5LO-deficient (right) mice. R_L increased in a dose-dependent fashion in response to methacholine. The increase in responsiveness after Aero OVA was significantly greater in wild-type mice than in 5LO-deficient mice. B, baseline; S_1, S_2, saline injections.

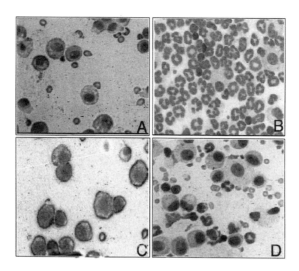

Figure 5 Bronchoalveolar lavage cells recovered from wild-type (A,B) and 5LO-deficient (C,D) mice. The cells recovered in A and C were from a mouse that received i.p. OVA and subsequent saline inhalation (IP OVA). The cells recovered in B and D were from a mouse that received i.p. OVA and subsequent OVA inhalation (Aero OVA). The lavaged cells from IP OVA mice contain almost exclusively alveolar macrophages. The lavaged cells in B consist primarily of eosinophils (characteristic doughnut-shaped nucleus) with some lymphocytes and macrophages. In contrast, the lavaged cells from a 5LO-deficient mouse contained fewer cells consisting of primarily macrophages and some eosinophils.

(B6/129). The C57BL/6 strain exhibits less hyperresponsiveness in vivo than the 129 Sv strain, but both strains can accumulate eosinophils (11,12). These findings are consistent with a preferred Th1 response in C57BL/6 mice and Th2 response in the 129 Sv strain. Recently, we have performed measurements with genetically pure 5LO-deficient mice of the 129 Sv strain and have observed the same phenotype as with the hybrid B6/129 genetic background. In fact, in terms of eosinophil recruitment, in the 129 Sv 5LO-deficient mice there was an even more pronounced reduction than with the hybrid strain mice (Fig. 6 top).

VI. Conclusions

In summary, a well-characterized murine model of ovalbumin-induced allergic airway inflammation was used to study the role of 5LO products on pulmonary

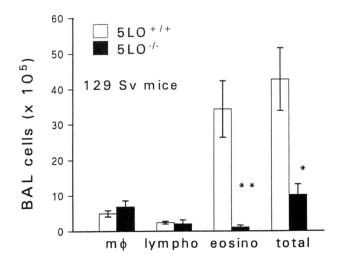

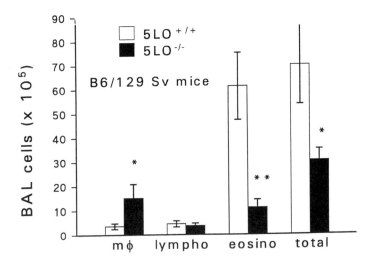

Figure 6 Comparison of bronchoalveolar lavage cell populations isolated from wild-type and 5LO-deficient mice subjected to OVA sensitization and subsequent aerosolized challenge for 8 days in the standard airway inflammation model. (Bottom) Results from mice of the hybrid B6/129 Sv genetic background. (Top) Results from mice of the 129 Sv genetic background. $n = 5\text{--}6$ for all groups. $*p < 0.05$; $**p < 0.01$.

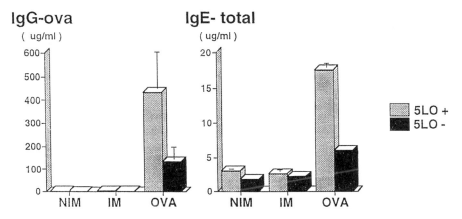

Figure 7 Serum OVA-specific IgG (left) and total serum IgE (right) in NIM, IM, and Aero OVA wild-type (stippled bars) and 5LO-deficient mice (solid bars). Data are presented as mean ± SEM, $n = 16$–32. There was a statistically significant lesser increase in the immune response in 5LO-deficient Aero OVA treated mice compared to wild-type mice.

eosinophil infiltration and airway hyperresponsiveness. 5LO-deficient mice showed a dramatically reduced cholinergic responsiveness when compared to normal 5LO-containing mice. The knockout mice also manifested a significantly lesser influx of eosinophils into the airways and a reduced serum immunoglobulin response. These results support the crucial role of 5LO products in mediating allergic pulmonary inflammation and nonspecific airway reactivity in mice. Similar results were achieved recently with the use of specific 5LO and 5LO-activating protein (FLAP) inhibitors in terms of eosinophil recruitment by Henderson et al. (36) in an essentially identical mouse model. These investigators also indicated a key role for leukotrienes in modulating mucus release; however, they could not establish a role for leukotrienes or eosinophils in mediating the airway hyperresponsiveness to antigen. The reasons for the discrepancy between our results and those of Henderson et al. (36) in terms of AHR are not clear at present. The models used were somewhat different in terms of antigen delivery (nebulized aerosol in conscious mice vs. intranasal instillation in anesthetized mice) and timing of the delivered antigen (eight consecutive days 14–21 vs. days 14, 25, 26, and 27) and the strains of mice were not the same (B6/129 vs. Balb/c). Differences in the murine model in terms of cytokine and cellular involvement have been observed previously (11,12,37). Mast cell versus eosinophil-dependent roles have been invoked to explain the differences between mouse strains (37). What is certain, though, is that 5LO products are very important in the process of eosinophil infiltration. The exact 5LO product important in this model has yet to be conclusively proved. LTB₄, the cysteinyl leukotrienes LTC_4/LTD_4, or possibly, 5-oxo-ETE (38) could be important in this respect. The latter compound appears to be a more potent eosinophilic chemoattractant than the other compounds for human cells but it is not known with certainty if it is generated in vivo in sufficient quantities to exert this action.

The sequence of events for eosinophil recruitment in this model appears to involve an initial role of $CD4^+$ T-lymphocytes (39). The presence of these cells is necessary for the subsequent enhancement of adhesion molecule expression during allergic inflammation thus enabling the cells to extravasate (39). Other eosinophil chemoattractants like eotaxin, RANTES, and MIP-1α are also implicated in playing a role in this model (39). Future studies will involve examining the precise timing of the role of 5LO products in the development of AHR, eosinophil recruitment, and the immune response by adding back the enzyme (via adenoviral delivery) or 5LO products at different time points in the development of the allergic inflammation in this model. These studies and similar ones should enhance our understanding of the mechanisms of action of 5LO products in airway inflammation and the development of AHR.

References

1. Sterk PJ. The place of airway hyperresponsiveness in the asthma phenotype. Clin Exp Allergy 1995; 25(Suppl 2):8–11.
2. Boucher RC, Gilbert IA, Hogg JC, King M, Knowles MR, Nadel J. Nonmuscular airway obstruction and asthma. Am J Respir Crit Care Med 1995; 152:408–410.
3. Coyle AJ, Uchida D, Ackerman SJ, Mitzner W, Irvin CG. Role of cationic proteins in the airway. Hyperresponsiveness due to airway inflammation. Am J Respir Crit Care Med 1994; 150:S63–71.
4. Goldstein RA, Paul WE, Metcalfe DD, Busse WW, Reece ER. Asthma. Ann Intern Med 1994; 121:698–708.
5. Djukanovic R. Asthma "of mice and men"—how do animal models help us understand human asthma? Clin Exp Allergy 1994; 24:6–9.
6. Tu Y-P, Larsen GL, Irvin CG. Utility of murine systems to study asthma pathogenesis. Eur Respir Rev 1995; 5:29, 224–230.
7. De Sanctis GT, Merchant M, Beier DR, Dredge DR, Grobholz JK, Martin TR, Lander ES, Drazen JM. Quantitative locus analysis of airway hyperresponsiveness in A/J and C57BL/6J mice. Nature Genet 1995; 11:150–154.
8. Ewart SL, Mitzner W, DiSilvestre DA, Meyers DA, Levitt RC. Airway hyperresponsiveness to acetylcholine: segregation analysis and evidence for linkage to murine chromosome 6. Am J Respir Cell Mol Biol 1996; 14:487–495.
9. Doull IL, Lawrence S, Watson M, Begishvili T, Beasley RW, Lampe F, Holgate T, Morton NE. Allelic association of gene markers on chromosomes 5q and 11q with

atopy and bronchial hyperresponsivness. Am J Respir Crit Care Med 1996; 153: 1280–1284.

10. Renz H, Smith HR, Henson JE, Ray BS, Irvin CG, Gelfand EW. Aerosolized antigen exposure without adjuvant causes increased IgE production and increased airway responsiveness in the mouse. J Allergy Clin Immunol 1992; 89:1127–1138.

11. Corry DB, Folkesson HG, Warnock ML, Erle DJ, Matthay MA, Wiener-Kronish JP, Locksley RM. Interleukin 4, but not interleukin 5 or eosinophils, is required in a murine model of acute airway hyperreactivity. J Exp Med 1996; 183:109–117.

12. Foster PS, Hogan SP, Ransay AJ, Matthaei KI, Young IG. Interleukin 5 deficiency abolishes eosinophilia, airways hyperreactivity, and lung damage in a mouse asthma model. J Exp Med 1996; 183:195–201.

13. Anderson GP, Coyle AJ. TH2 and "TH2-like" cells in allergy and asthma: pharmacological perspectives. Trends Pharm Sci 1994; 15:324–332.

14. Gavett SH, Chen X, Finkelman F, Wills-Karp M. Depletion of murine CD4⁺ T lymphocytes prevents antigen-induced airway hyperreactivity and pulmonary eosinophilia. Am J Respir Cell Mol Biol 1994; 10:587–593.

15. Busse WW, Coffman RL, Gelfand EW, Kay AB, Rosenwasser LJ. Mechanisms of persistent airway inflammation in asthma. A role for T cells and T-cell products. Am J Respir Crit Care Med 1995; 152:388–393.

16. Gavett SH, O'Hearn DJ, Li X, Huang SK, Finkelman FD, Wills-Karp M. Interleukin 12 inhibits antigen-induced airway hyperresponsiveness, inflammation, and Th2 cytokine expression in mice. J Exp Med 1995; 182:1527–1536.

17. Samuelsson B. Leukotrienes: mediators of immediate hypersensitivity reactions and inflammation. Science 1983; 220:568–575.

18. Lewis RA, Austen KF, Soberman RJ. Leukotrienes and other products of the 5-lipoxygenase pathway. Biochemistry and relation to pathobiology in human diseases. N Engl J Med 1990; 323:645–655.

19. Fischer AR, McFadden CA, Frantz R, Awni WM, Cohn J, Drazen JM, Israel E. Effect of chronic 5-lipoxygenase inhibition on airway hyperresponsiveness in asthmatic subjects. Am J Respir Crit Care Med 1995; 152:1203–1207.

20. Hay DW, Torphy TJ, Undem BJ. Cysteinyl leukotrienes in asthma: old mediators up to new tricks. Trends Pharm Sci 1995; 16:304–309.

21. Spector SL, Smith LJ, Glass M. Effects of 6 weeks of therapy with oral doses of ICI 204,219, a leukotriene D_4 receptor antagonist, in subjects with bronchial asthma. ACCOLATE Asthma Trialists Group. Am J Respir Crit Care Med 1994; 150:618–623.

22. Du T, Xu LJ, Lei M, Wang NS, Eidelman DH, Ghezzo H, Martin JG. Morphometric changes during the early airway response to allergen challenge in the rat. Am Rev Respir Dis 1992; 146:1037–1041.

23. Stewart AG, Thompson DC, Fennessy MR. Involvement of capsaicin-sensitive afferent neurones in a vagal-dependent interaction between leukotriene D4 and histamine on bronchomotor tone. Agents Actions 1984; 15:500–508.

24. Ellis JL, Undem BJ. Role of peptidoleukotrienes in capsaicin-sensitive sensory fibre-mediated responses in guinea-pig airways. J Physiol 1991; 436:469–484.

25. McGill KA, Busse WW. Zileuton (Drug profile). Lancet 1996; 348:519–524.

26. Snapper CM, Finkelman FD, Paul WE. Regulation of IgG1 and IgE production by interleukin 4. Immunol Rev 1988; 102:51–75.
27. Jakobsson PJ, Shaskin P, Larsson P, Feltenmark S, Odlander B, Aguilar-Santelises M, Jondal M, Biberfeld P, Claesson HE. Studies on the regulation and localization of 5-lipoxygenase in human B-lymphocytes. Eur J Biochem 1995; 232:37–46.
28. Jakobsson PJ, Steinhilber D, Odlander B, Radmark O, Claesson HE, Samuelsson B. On the expression and regulation of 5-lipoxygenase in human lymphocytes. Proc Natl Acad Sci USA 1992; 89:3521–3525.
29. Fu JY, Medina JF, Funk CD, Wetterholm A, Radmark O. Leukotriene A$_4$, conversion to leukotriene B$_4$ in human T-cell lines. Prostaglandins 1988; 36:241–248.
30. Rola-Pleszczynski M. Differential effects of leukotriene B4 on T4$^+$ and T8$^+$ lymphocyte phenotype and immunoregulatory functions. J Immunol 1985; 135:1357–1360.
31. Yamaoka KA, Claesson HE, Rosen A. Leukotriene B$_4$ enhances activation, proliferation, and differentiation of human B lymphocytes. J Immunol 1989; 143:1996–2000.
32. Dugas B, Paul-Eugene N, Cairns J, Gordon J, Calenda A, Mencia-Huerta JM, Braquet P. Leukotriene B$_4$ potentiates the expression and release of Fc epsilon RII/CD23, and proliferation and differentiation of human B lymphocytes induced by IL-4. J Immunol 1990; 145:3406–3411.
33. Yamaoka KA, Dugas B, Paul-Eugene N, Mencia-Huerta JM, Braquet P, Kolb JP. Leukotriene B$_4$ enhances IL-4-induced IgE production from normal human lymphocytes. Cell Immunol 1994; 156:124–34.
34. Martin TR, Gerard NP, Galli SJ, Drazen JM. Pulmonary responses to bronchoconstrictor agonists in the mouse. J Appl Physiol 1988; 64:2318–2323.
35. Cockcroft DW, Killian DN, Mellon JJ, Hargreave FE. Bronchial reactivity to inhaled histamine: a method and clinical survey. Clin Allergy 1977; 7:235–243.
36. Henderson WR, Lewis DB, Albert RK, Zhang Y, Lamm WJE, Chiang GKS, Jones F, Eriksen P, Tien Y, Jonas M, Chi EY. The importance of leukotrienes in airway inflammation in a mouse model of asthma. J Exp Med 1996; 184:1483–1494.
37. Drazen JM, Arm JP, Austen KF. Sorting out the cytokines of asthma. J Exp Med 1996; 183:1–5.
38. Powell WS, Chung D, Gravel S. 5-Oxo-6,8,11,14-eicosatetraenoic acid is a potent stimulator of eosinophil migration. J Immunol 1995; 154:4123–4132.
39. Gonzalo J-A, Lloyd CM, Kremer L, Finger E, Martinez-A C, Siegelman MH, Cybulsky M, Gutierrez-Ramos J-C. Eosinophil recruitment to the lung in a murine model of allergic inflammation. The role of T cells, chemokines, and adhesion receptors. J Clin Invest 1996; 98:2332–2345.

11

Genetic Influences on Asthma

WILLIAM O. C. M. COOKSON

John Radcliffe Hospital
Oxford, England

I. Introduction

Because asthma runs in families, it is likely to be due at least in part to genetic facxtors. Defining these factors will improve the understanding of the etiology and pathophysiololgy of the disease. The involvement of particular genes will identify distinct clinical courses and responses to therapy. The early identification of children at genetic risk of asthma will be possible. Although the estimate of risk may be relatively imprecise, the prevention of illness by environmental or other intervention in susceptible children is both feasible and desirable. Genetic discoveries will in the long run lead to new pharmacological treatments for asthma.

In contrast to single-gene disorders such as cystic fibrosis or muscular dystrophy, genes predisposing to asthma will not usually contain mutations. Rather they will be variants of normal genes ("polymorphisms"), whose evolutionary advantage has been lost in the current Western environment. It is also important to recognize that the environmental component to asthma and atopy is at least as strong as the genetic component.

Asthma is not one disease but many. In children 95% of asthma is allergic, or atopic. Of the various types of asthma, atopic asthma is clinically most easily recognized and defined, and has the most obvious familial clustering. Although aspirin-sensitive asthma (ASA) is neither familial nor atopic, it is still likely to result from the interaction between genetic and environmental factors.

II. Finding Genes

Genes causing disease may be found either by the process known as "positional cloning" or by examining candidate genes.

Positional cloning relies on the phenomenon of genetic linkage. Genes are arranged in a linear array of DNA known as the genome. The genome of an individual is divided into a brace of 23 chromosomes. The mechanism to pass on the genetic material to a subsequent generation is called reduction division, or meiosis. During meiosis chromosomes pair up in the cell, break at certain points, form a link (crossover) to the other member of the pair, and recombine to form two entirely novel chromosomes, containing elements of each of the original chromosome brace. After crossover and recombination, a single copy of the 23 chromosomes remains in the gamete (the ovum or sperm), and the full compliment of 46 chromosomes is only recreated at fertilization.

The number of crossovers occurring along a given chromosome is small, often numbering only one or two. Because of this, large segments of DNA remain intact during meiosis, and genes or segments of DNA that are close together will tend to be passed on to the next generation together. If they are very close they will remain together through many generations. This process, the coinheritance of stretches of adjacent genes, is known as genetic linkage.

Positional cloning relies on the demonstration of genetic linkage (coinheritance) of disease and genetic markers of known chromosomal localization. Once linkage is established, the linked region can be dissected by further genetic mapping with a dense array of closely linked markers. Genetic mapping is followed by "physical mapping," the assembly of overlapping DNA clones covering the linked regions, and the eventual identification and sequencing of genes from the DNA.

The positional cloning approach has the advantage of not requiring any preexisting knowledge of the pathophysiology of the disease. However, the power to detect linkage in complex genetic diseases is very limited, so several thousand two-generation families may be necessary to detect linkage to a gene affecting 10% of subjects with disease. Genetic linkage has traditionally been assessed with a statistic known as the lod score. This elegant statistic was the main tool for localization of single-gene disorders such as cystic fibrosis. It has not functioned well in complex disorders because it requires that the "model" of inheritance (i.e., the gene frequency of the disorder, the Mendelian type, and its penetrance at different ages) is known with some precision. For this reason, "nonparametric" statistics, based on the phenotypes of siblings and ignoring parental phenotypes, are now to be preferred. Genetic linkage in complex disorders, however assessed, often replicates poorly, at least in the early stages (1). This is because linkage to a heterogeneous trait will normally only be found fortuitously, in samples that contain an exceptional proportion of individuals or families influenced by that particular gene. Simulation experiments have shown that, in these circumstances, many studies may be necessary before replication occurs.

Candidate genes are genes that are already known to have a role in the pathophysiology of disease. For a candidate, or any gene, to be responsible for the difference between asthmatic and nonasthmatic subjects, it must come in at least two varieties: normal ("wild type") and abnormal. The abnormal gene may be nonfunctional, or it may be a variant that functions slightly differently from the wild type.

The role of candidate genes may be assessed by defining polymorphisms within the respective genes, and testing for associations with disease. Associations may be found even if the polymorphisms do not alter the function of a gene. This is because when a new mutation or variant first arises in a gene, it will be physically associated or linked with polymorphisms (alleles) of other sequences on the same chromosome. This association of alleles on a chromosome is somewhat clumsily named "linkage disequilibrium." Within a gene, linkage disequilibrium of alleles persists for hundreds of generations, so nonfunctional alleles will serve as surrogates for the functional sequence nearby. The testing of candidate genes can be difficult, because of uncertainty whether a polymorphism is functional or not, if, for example, it occurs in the promoter region of a gene, or within the introns.

The enormous increase in understanding of the complex cytokine networks that influence atopy and inflammation means that a plausible case could be put for as many as 30 different candidates. Successful identification of genes predisposing to asthma is therefore likely to depend on a combination of positional cloning and candidate gene strategies.

III. Genes Influencing Asthma

Many different kind of genes may be involved in atopy and asthma. These can be divided into four classes: (1) genes predisposing in general to IgE-mediated inflammation, (2) genes influencing the specific IgE response, (3) genes influencing bronchial hyperresponsiveness independently of atopy, and (4) genes influencing non-IgE-mediated inflammation.

A. Class 1 Asthma Genes: Genes Influencing Generalized IgE Responses

Genetic loci predisposing to generalized atopy have been identified on chromosome 11 and chromosome 5, by a combination of genetic linkage and candidate gene approaches.

Chromosome 11q12-13

The first suggested linkage of atopy was to the marker D11S97 on chromosome 11q13 (2). Following some controversy (3), linkage has been replicated consistently (4–8). It is now obvious that the early difficulty replicating the linkage to chromosome 11 was due to inappropriate use of the lod statistic and the testing of very small sample sizes. This linkage was also confounded by the high prevalence of atopy, and because the linkage was predominantly seen in maternal meioses (9,10). In the largest study described, linkage was exclusively maternal (9). The reasons for the maternal linkage are not known, and it is not clear that this maternal phenomenon corresponds to the phenotypic maternal inheritance of atopy previously noted.

Recognition of the maternal linkage allowed fine mapping of the atopy locus, to within a 7-centiMorgan, 1-lod-unit support interval (10,11). This interval was centromeric to and excluded the original D11S97 marker to which linkage was first observed. A lymphocyte surface marker, *CD20*, was noted to be within the interval. *CD20* shows sequence homology to the beta chain of the high-affinity receptor for IgE (FcεRIβ), and has been localized close to that gene on mouse chromosome 19 (12). The human FcεRIβ was subsequently found to be on chromosome 11q13, in close genetic linkage to atopy (10).

Two coding polymorphisms were initially identified within the gene, FcεRIβ Leu-181 and FcεRIβ Leu-181/Leu-183 (13). These variants, situated at the beginning of exon 6, both showed strong associations with atopy when maternally inherited, and seemed quite common (13). However, a study of 1000 subjects found the population prevalence of FcεRIβ Leu-181/Leu-183 to be only 4%, and FcεRIβ Leu-181 was not found at all (14). Subsequently, both variants have been difficult to assay reliably, and their status is currently uncertain. The detection of a third homologous gene, *Htm4*, in close proximity to FcεRIβ and *CD20* (15), suggests the possibility of homologous sequences in unknown genes or pseudogenes confouding the detection of these variants.

A further variant in the receptor, FcεRIβ E237G, has recently been described. It also is associated with atopy and bronchial hyperresponsiveness (16). It is present in approximately 5% of the U.K. and other European populations. It has also been found in 20% of Japanese asthmatics (17). The glutamine-to-glycine change coded by this variant makes a substantial polarity change in the intracellular part of the protein, which is likely to have functional implications. Functional studies are still ongoing.

Chromosome 5

Linkage of the total serum IgE to markers near the cytokine cluster on chromosome 5q31–33 has been demonstrated by Marsh et al. (18). Marsh and his colleagues studied Amish pedigrees, selected to contain members with positive skin prick tests. Linkage was, however, strongest in families with the lowest serum IgE. The result was replicated by Myers et al. (19) in Dutch asthmatic families.

The region contains a number of cytokines, the most important of which, from the point of view of atopy, are IL-4, IL-13, the p40 subunit of IL-12, and IL-5. Other cytokines include IL-9 and granulocyte-colony stimulating factor (G-CSF). A substantial amount of work is now required to establish which of these various candidates accounts for the linkage.

B. Class 2 Asthma Genes: Genes Influencing Specific IgE Responses to Particular Allergens

Atopic individuals differ in the particular allergens to which they react. This difference is of clinical significance, as asthma and bronchial hyperresponsiveness are associated with allergy to house dust mite (HDM) but not grass pollens (20,21). It is therefore of interest to examine whether particular genes influence the IgE response to specific allergens. In addition, study of these genes may give an insight into the inheritance of normal variation within the immune system, and the functional consequences of such variation.

Two classes of genes are likely candidates for constraining specific IgE reactions. These are the genes encoding the human leukocyte antigen (HLA) proteins, and the genes for the T-cell receptor (TCR). These molecules are central to the handling and recognition of foreign antigen.

Inhaled allergen sources such as HDM are complex mixtures of many proteins. A number of "major allergens," to which IgE responses are consistently found in most individuals, have been identified from each allergen source. It is likely that genetic associations will be better detected with reactions to purified major allergens, rather than with complex allergen sources. Major allergens include *Der p* I (25.4 kDa) and *Der p* II (14.1 kDa) from the house dust mite *Dermatophagoides pteronyssinus*, *Alt a* I (28 kDa) from the mould *Alternaria alternata*, *Can f* I (25 kDa) from the dog *Canis familiaris*, *Fel d* I (18 kDa) from the cat *Felis domesticus*, and *Phl p* V (30 kDa) from Timothy grass, *Phleum pratense*.

IV. HLA

The human major histocompatibility complex (MHC) includes genes coding for HLA class II molecules (HLA-DR, DQ, and DP), which are involved in the recognition and presentation of exogenous peptides.

An HLA influence on the IgE response was first noted by Levine et al. (22), who found an association between HLA class I haplotypes and IgE responses to antigen E derived from ragweed allergen (*Ambrosia artemisifolia*). This association has been subsequently found to be due to restriction of the response to a minor component of ragweed antigen (*Amb a* V) by HLA-DR2 (23). To date the association of *Amb a* V (molecular weight 5000) and HLA-DR2 is the only HLA association to have been consistently confirmed (22–24). Other suggested associations are of the rye grass antigens *Lol p* I, *Lol p* II, and *Lol p* III with HLA-DR3 (in the same 53 allergic subjects) (25,26), American feverfew (*Parthenium hysterophorus*) and HLA-DR3 in 22 subjects from the Indian subcontinent (27), the IgE response to *Bet v* I, the major allergen of birch pollen, HLA-DR3 in 37 European subjects (28), and an HLA-DR5 association with another ragweed antigen *Amb a* VI in 38 subjects (29).

Other authors have reported negative associations with particular allergens. These include HLA-DR4 and IgE responses to moutain cedar pollen (37 subjects) (30) and HLA-DR4 and melittin (from bee venom) (22 subjects) (31). Nonresponsiveness to Japanese cedar pollen may be associated with HLA-DQw8 (32).

There is to date no confirmation of many of these results, and the number of subjects has generally not approached that required to establish an unequivocal HLA association. In addition, there has not been recognition of the problems of reactivity to multiple allergens: significant relationships between HLA-DR alleles and five antigens (*Amb a* V, *Lol p* I, *Lol p* II, *Lol p* III, and *Amb a* VI) have been claimed from the same pool of approximately 200 subjects (23,25,26,29).

To test more definitively if HLA class II gene products have a general influence on the ability to react to common allergens, we have genotyped for HLA-DR and HLA-DP in a large sample of atopic subjects from the British population (33). The subjects were tested for IgE responses to the most common British major allergens.

A total of 431 subjects from 83 families were genotyped at the HLA-DR and HLA-DP loci and serotyped for IgE responses to six major allergens from common aeroallergen sources. Three hundred subjects were used as controls. The subjects and the controls have come from the same relatively homogeneous population. In the United Kingdom and Europe, allergens other than *Bet v* I and those tested for in our study are uncommon causes of sensitization and IgE-mediated allergy.

The results showed only weak associations between HLA-DR allele frequencies and IgE responses to common allergens. A possible excess of HLA-DR1 was found in subjects who were responsive to *Fel d* I compared to those who were not [odds ratio (OR) = 2, p = 0.002], and a possible excess of HLA-DR4 was found in subjects responsive to *Alt a* I (OR = 1.9, p = 0.006). Increased sharing of HLA-DR/DP haplotypes was seen in sibling pairs responding to both allergens. *Der p* I, *Der p* II, *Phl p* V, and *Can f* I were not associated with any definite excess of HLA-DR alleles. No significant correlations were seen with HLA-DP genotype and reactivity to any of the allergens.

Of the possible associations, that of *Alt a* I with HLA-DR4 and of *Fel d* I with HLA-DR1 were supported by a finding of excess sharing of a HLA haplotype in affected sibling pairs. Regression analysis shows the apparent association of *Phl p* V with HLA-DR4 is due to the presence of many individuals who have reacted with an IgE response to both *Alt a* I and *Phl p* V. The association of HLA-DR1 and *Fel d* I is the strongest statistically, and is significant even taking the multiple comparisons into account.

The study was the first to investigate HLA-DP alleles and reactivity to common allergens. As no definite correlation was found between any antigen response and HLA-DP genotypes in a large data set, HLA-DP genes are unlikely to have a major role in restricting IgE responses to these allergens.

Aspirin-induced asthma (AIA) affects one in 10 individuals with adult-onset asthma. It does not seem more common in individuals with atopy. It is not known if aspirin sensitivity is due to immune mechanisms or to interference with biochemical pathways. Possible involvement of the genes MHC in AIA has been tested by HLA-DPB1 and HLA DRB1 genotyping in 59 patients with positive challenge tests for AIA and in 48 normal and 57 asthmatic controls (34). The DPB1*0301 frequency was increased in AIA patients when compared to normal controls [19.5% vs. 5.2%, OR = 4.4, 95% confidence interval (CI) 1.6–12.1, p = 0.002], and compared to asthmatic controls (4.4%, OR = 5.3, 95% CI = 1.9–14.4, p = 0.0001). The frequency of DPB1*0401 in AIA subjects was decreased when compared to normal controls (28.8% vs. 49.0%, OR = 0.42, 95% CI = 0.24–0.74, p = 0.003) and asthmatic controls (45.6%, OR = 0.48, 95% CI = 0.28–0.83, p = 0.008). The results remained significant when corrected for multiple comparisons. There were no significant HLA-DRB1 associations with AIA. The presence of an HLA association suggests that immune recognition of an unknown antigen may be part of the etiology of AIA. The relative role of HLA-DP in antigen presentation, compared to HLA-DR and HLA-DQ, is unknown.

The results from the various studies therefore show that HLA-DR alleles do modify the ability to mount an IgE response to particular antigens. However, the OR for the association is usually 2.0 or less. Thus class II HLA restriction seems insufficient to account for individual differences in reactivity to common allergens. It is therefore likely that environmental factors or other loci such as T-cell receptor (TCR) genes may be of greater relevance in determining an individual's susceptibility to specific allergens.

V. The T-Cell Receptor

The TCR is usually made up of α and β chains, although 5% of receptors consist of γ and δ chains. The β-chain locus is on chromosome 7, and the α-chain locus is on chromosome 14. The δ-chain genes are found within the α-chain locus.

An enormous potential for TCR variety follows from the presence of many variable (V) and junctional (J) segments within the TCR loci. However, the usage of the TCR Vα and Vβ segments by lymphocytes is not random, and may be under genetic control (35–38).

To examine if the TCR genes influence susceptibility to particular allergens, we have therefore tested for genetic linkage between IgE responses and microsatellites from the TCR-α/δ and TCR-β regions (39). Two independent sets of families, one British and one Australian, were investigated. Because the mode of inheritance was unknown, and because of interactions from the environment and other loci, affected sibling pair methods were used to test for linkage.

No linkage of IgE serotypes to TCR-β was detected, but significant linkage of IgE responses to the house dust mite allergens *Der p* I and *Der p* II, the cat allergen *Fel d* I, and the total serum IgE to TCR-α was seen in both family groups. The results show that a locus in the TCR α/δ region is modulating IgE responses. The close correlation between total and specific IgE makes it difficult to determine if the locus controls specific IgE reactions to particular allergens or confers generalized IgE responsiveness. Nevertheless, linkage was strongest with highly purified allergens, suggesting that the locus primarily influences specific responses.

Replication of positive results of linkage in a second set of subjects is important in interpreting this study. Differences between the populations for the serotypes showing TCR-α allele sharing may be due to different allergen exposures, as grass pollen responses were much more common in Australian subjects. In addition, British subjects were recruited through clinics, whereas Australian subjects were not selected by symptoms.

No association was seen between particular IgE responses and specific TCR-α microsatellite alleles, implying that the microsatellite is not in immediate proximity to the IgE-modulating elements. The degree of linkage disequilibrium across the TCR-α/δ locus seems low (40), and the microsatellite has only been localized within a 900-kb yeast artificial chromosome (41). The observed linkage may therefore be with any elements of TCR-α or TCR-δ, or with other genes in the locality.

Several Vα genes have been recognized to be polymorphic (42), and limitation of the response to an allergen may correspond to these polymorphisms. Particular TCR-Vα usage may induce IL-4-dominant (Th2) helper T cells, which enhance IgE production (43). A reported nonrandom usage of Vα13 usage in *Lol p* I–specific T-cell clones supports independently the possibility of Vα genes controlling IgE responses (44).

The TCR-δ locus is also a candidate for this linkage. The function of TCR-γ/δ cells is not known, but their location on mucosal surfaces, where allergens initiate IgE responses, could suggest a role in IgE regulation (45).

The genetic restriction of specific IgE responses by TCR-α/δ may be of clinical significance, and may be of general interest in understanding the control of humoral immunity. Further localization of this genetic effect requires the identification of TCR α/δ elements showing allelic associations with specific IgE responses. Studies are also needed to investigate the interactions between this chromosome 14 linkage, and the HLA class II genes.

A. Class 3 Asthma Genes: Genes Influencing Bronchial Responsiveness

No genes have yet been identified that predispose to bronchial hyperresponsiveness independently of atopy. Variants in the beta-adrenergic receptor have however been identified, and it has been suggested that these may be associated with nocturnal asthma or other subdivisions of the asthma phenotype (46).

B. Class 4 Asthma Genes: Genes Influencing Non-IgE-Mediated Inflammation

Airway inflammation is a characteristic of asthma that may be independent of mechanisms controlling atopy. Tumour necrosis factor alpha (TNFα) is a potent proinflammatory cytokine that shows constitutional variations in the level of secretion which are linked to polymorphisms in the TNF gene complex (47–49). We have therefore investigated TNF polymorphisms for association with asthma in 800 normal and abnormal subjects from general population and asthma clinic samples. We found that asthma was significantly increased in subjects with alleles associated with increased secretion of TNFα, most notably the TNFα promoter polymorphism TNFα-308. Considering unrelated subjects only (the parents) from both populations, the OR for asthma in individuals homozygous for the high-secretor allele was 3.9 compared to homozygotes for the low-secretor alleles (95% CI 1.4–11.0, $p = 0.007$) (50).

VI. Whole Genome Screens for Atopy and Asthma

The genes and genetic linkages described above do not account for all asthma or atopy. The chromosome 5 locus would appear not to have major effects on the population as a whole, and HLA and TCR-α loci modify the specific response rather than endowing any general predisposition to atopy. Segregation analysis is unable to predict with any accuracy the number and nature of genes contributing to atopy and asthma. To discover if asthma is a genuine polygenic disorder, my group have carried out a complete genome screen in 80 nuclear families, with 300 markers spaced at approximately 10% recombination (51). We searched for linkage to one qualitative and four quantitative traits associated with asthma: namely atopy, a skin prick test index, the total serum IgE, the peripheral eosinophil count, and bronchial responsiveness. Six potential linkages ($p < 0.001$) were identified on chromosomes 4, 6, 7, 11, 13, and 16, five of which were to quantitative traits. Monte Carlo simulations showed that 1.6 false positive linkages at this level of significance would be expected from the data. Two linkages, one to chromosome 11q13 and the other to chromosome 6 near the MHC, had been established previously. Three of the new loci (on chromosome 4, 13, and 16) showed evidence of linkage to a second panel of families, in which maternal effects and pleiotropy of linked phenotypes were seen.

The results show the extent and the complexity of the genetic predisposition to asthma. Similar large-scale genome scans are to be carried out in the United States and Canada, so it is likely general agreement will soon be reached on the number and nature of the most important loci underlying asthma and the allergic disorders. There remains a formidable amount of work to move from genetic linkage to the identification of the relevant genes.

VII. Conclusions

The genetic basis for asthma is gradually becoming more certain; the methodological tools for finding genetic linkage and association are now established, and it is likely that all the important genes and their variants will be found in the next 10 years. It should not be forgotten, however, that the environment strongly influences asthma, and that the rising prevalence of asthma in recent decades is probably due to environmental factors. The increase in prevalence has an important corollary: asthma is preventable. Recognition of children or infants genetically predisposed to asthma is likely to be the first step in strategies for prevention by environmental or other manipulations in the first year of life.

References

1. Suarez BK, Hampe CL, Van Eerdewegh P. Problems of replicating linkage claims in psychiatry. In: Gershon ES, Cloninger CR, eds. Genetic Approaches to Mental Disorders. Washington, DC: American Psychiatric Press, 1994:23–46.
2. Cookson WOCM, Sharp PA, Faux JA, Hopkin JM. Linkage between immunoglobulin E responses underlying asthma and rhinitis and chromosome 11q. Lancet 1989; 1:1292–1295.
3. Marsh DG, Myers DA. A major gene for allergy—fact or fancy? Nature Genet 1992; 2:252–254.
4. Young RP, Lynch J, Sharp PA, Faux JA, Cookson WOCM, Hopkin JM. Confirmation of genetic linkage between atopic IgE responses and chromosome 11q13. J Med Genet 1992; 29:236–238.
5. Shirakawa T, Morimoto K, Hashimoto T, Furuyama J, Yamamoto M, Takai S. Linkage between severe atopy and chromosome 11q in Japanese families. Clin Genet 1994; 46:125–129.
6. Collée JM, ten Kate LP, de Vries HG, Kliphuis JW, Bouman K, Scheffer H, Gerritsen J. Allele sharing on chromosome 11q13 in sibs with asthma and atopy. Lancet 1993; 342:936.
7. Herwerden L, Harrap SB, Wong ZYH, Abramson MJ, Kutin JJ, Forbes AB, Raven J, Lanigan A, Walters EH. Linkage of high affinity receptor gene with bronchial hyperreactivity, even in absence of atopy. Lancet 1995; 346:1262–1265.
8. Fölster-Holst R, Moises H-W, Fritsch W, Lang L, Weissenbach J, Christophers E. Linkage between atopy and the high-affinity receptor gene at 11q13 in atopic dermatitis families. Hum Genet 1996 (in press).
9. Cookson WOCM, Young RP, Sandford AJ, et al. Maternal inheritance of atopic IgE responsiveness on chromosome 11q. Lancet 1992; 340:381–384.
10. Sandford AJ, Shirakawa T, Moffatt MF, Daniels SE, Ra C, Faux JA, Young RP, Nakamura Y, Lathrop GM, Cookson WOCM, Hopkin JM. Localisation of atopy and the β subunit of the high affinity IgE receptor (FcεRI) on chromosome 11q. Lancet 1993; 341:332–334.
11. Sandford AJ, Moffatt MF, Daniels SE, Nakamura Y, Lathrop GM, Hopkin JM, Cookson WOCM. A genetic map of chromosome 11q, including the atopy locus. Eur J Hum Genet 1995; 3:188–194.
12. Hupp K, Siwarski D, Mock BA, Kinet JP. Gene mapping of the three subunits of the high affinity FcR for IgE to mouse chromosomes 1 and 19. J Immunol 1989; 143:3787–3791.
13. Shirakawa TS, Li A, Dubowitz M, Dekker JW, Shaw AE, Faux JA, Ra C, Cookson WOCM, Hopkin JM. Association between atopy and variants of the β subunit of the high-affinity immunoglobulin E receptor. Nature Genet 1994; 7:125–129.
14. Hill MR, James AL, Faux JA, Ryan G, Hopkin JM, le Souef P, Musk AW, Cookson WOCM. FcεRI-β polymorphism and risk of atopy in a general population sample. Br Med J 1995; 311:776–779.
15. Adra CN, Lelias J-M, Kobayashi H, Kaghad M, Morrison P, Rowley JD, Lim B. Cloning of the cDNA for a haemopoietic cell-specific protein related to CD20 and

the beta subunit of the high-affinity IgE receptor: evidence for a family of proteins with four membrane spanning regions. Proc Natl Acad Sci USA 1994; 91:10178–10182.

16. Hill MR, Cookson WOCM. A new variant of the β subunit of the high-affinity receptor for Immunoglobulin E (FcεRI-β E237G): associations with measures of atopy and bronchial hyper-responsiveness. Hum Mol Genet 1996 (in press).

17. Shirakawa TS, Mao XQ, Sasaki S, Nomoto TE, Kawai M, Morimoto K, Hopkin JM. Association between atopic asthma and a coding variant of FcεRI-β in a Japanese population. Hum Mol Genet 1996 (in press).

18. Marsh DG, Neely JD, Breazeale DR, Ghosh B, Freidhoff LR, Erlich-Kautzky E, Schou C, Krishnaswamy G, Beaty TH. Linkage analysis of IL4 and other chromosome 5q31.1 markers and total serum IgE concentrations. Science 1994; 264:1152–1155.

19. Myers DA, Postma DS, Panhuysen CIM, Xu J, Amelung PJ, Levitt RC, Bleeker ER. Evidence for a locus regulating total serum IgE levels mapping to chromosome 5. Genomics 1994; 23:464–470.

20. Cookson WOCM, De Klerk NH, Ryan GR, James AL, Musk AW. Relative risks of bronchial hyper-responsiveness associated with skin-prick test responses to common antigens in young adults. Clin Exp Allergy 1991; 21:473–479.

21. Sears MR, et al. The relative risks of sensitivity to grass pollen, house dust mite and cat dander in the development of childhood asthma. Clin Allergy 1989; 18:419.

22. Levine BB, Stember RH, Fontino M. Ragweed hayfever: genetic control and linkage to HL-A haplotypes. Science 1972; 178:1201–1203.

23. Marsh DG, Meyers DA, Bias WB. The epidemiology and genetics of atopic allergy. N Engl J Med 1981; 305:1551–1559.

24. Blumenthal MN, Awdeh Z, Alper C, Yunis E. Ra5 immune responses, HLA antigens and complotypes. J Allergy Clin Immunol 1985; 75:155 (abstract).

25. Freidhoff LR, Ehrlich-Kautzky E, Meyers DA, Ansari AA, Bias WB, Marsh DG. Association of HLA-DR3 with human immune response to *Lol p* I and *Lol p* II allergens in allergic subjects. Tissue Antigens 1988; 31:211–219.

26. Ansari AA, Freidhoff LR, Meyers DA, Bias WB, Marsh DG. Human immune responsiveness to Lolium perenne pollen allergen *Lol p* III (rye III) is associated with HLA-DR3 and DR5 [published erratum appears in Hum Immunol 1989; 26:149]. Hum Immunol 1989; 25:59–71.

27. Sriramarao P, Selvakumar B, Damodaran C, Rao BS, Prakash O, Rao PV. Immediate hypersensitivity to *Parthenium hysterophorus*. I. Association of HLA antigens and *Parthenium* rhinitis. Clin Exp Allergy 1990; 20:555–560.

28. Fischer GF, Pickl WF, Fae I, Ebner C, Ferreira F, Breiteneder H, Vikoukal E, Scheiner O, Kraft D. Association between IgE response against *Bet v* I, the major allergen of birch pollen, and HLA-DRB alleles. Hum Immunol 1992; 33:259–265.

29. Marsh DG, Friedhoff LR, Ehrlich-Kautzky E, Bias WB, Roebber M. Immune responsiveness to *Ambrosia artemisiifolia* (short ragweed) pollen allergen *Amb a* VI (Ra6) is associated with HLA-DR5 in allergic humans. Immunogenetics 1987; 26(4–5):230–236.

30. Reid MJ, Nish WA, Whisman BA, Goetz DW, Hylander RD, Parker WA Jr, Freeman TM. HLA-DR4-associated nonresponsiveness to mountain cedar allergen. J Allergy Clin Immunol 1992; 89:593–598.

31. Lympany P, Kemeny DM, Welsh KI, Lee TH. An HLA-associated nonresponsiveness to mellitin: a component of bee venom. J Allergy Clin Immunol 1990; 86:160–170.
32. Sasazuki T, Nishimura Y, Muto M, Ohta N. HLA-linked genes controlling immune response and disease susceptibility. Immunol Rev 1983; 70:51–75.
33. Young RP, Dekker JW, Wordsworth BP, Schou C, Pike KD, Matthiesen F, Rosenberg WMC, Bell JI, Hopkin JM, Cookson WOCM. HLA-DR and HLA-DP genotypes and immunoglobulin E responses to common major allergens. Clin Exp Allergy 1994; 24:431–439.
34. Dekker JW, Nizankowska E, Schmitz-Schumann M, Pile K, Bochenek G, Dyczek A, Cookson WOCM, Szczeklik A. Aspirin-induced asthma and HLA-DRB1 and HLA-DPB1 genotypes. Clin Exp Allergy 1997 (in press).
35. Loveridge JA, Rosenberg WMC, Kirkwood TBL, Bell JI. The genetic contribution to human T-cell receptor repertoire. Immunology 1991; 74:246–250.
36. Moss PAH, Rosenberg WMC, Zintzaras E, Bell JI. Characterization of the human T cell receptor α-chain repertoire and demonstration of a genetic influence on Vα usage. Eur J Immunol 1993; 23:1153–1159.
37. Gulwani-Akolar B, Posnett DN, Janson CH, Grunewald J, Wigzell H, Akolkar P, Gregersen PK, Silver J. T cell receptor V-segment frequencies in peripheral blood T cells correlate with human leukocyte antigen type. J Exp Med 1991; 174:1139–1146.
38. Robinson MA. Usage of human T-cell receptor V beta, J beta C beta and V alpha gene segments is not proportional to gene number. Hum Immunol 1992; 35:60–67.
39. Moffatt MF, Hill MR, Cornélis F, Schou C, Faux JA, Young RP, James AL, Ryan G, le Souef P, Musk AW, Hopkin JM, Cookson WOCM. Genetic linkage of the TCR-α/δ region to specific immunoglobulin E responses. Lancet 1994; 343:1597–1600.
40. Robinson MA, Kindt TJ. Genetic recombination within the human T-cell receptor alpha-chain complex. Proc Natl Acad Sci USA 1987; 84:9089–9093.
41. Cornélis F, Hashimoto L, Loveridge J, MacCarthy A, Buckle V, Julier C, Bell J. Identification of a CA repeat at the TCRA locus using yeast artificial chromosomes: a general method for generating highly polymorphic markers at chosen loci. Genomics 1992; 13:820–825.
42. Cornélis F, Pile K, Loveridge J, Moss P, Harding C, Julier C, Bell JI. Systematic study of human αβ T-cell receptor V segments shows allelic variations resulting in a large number of distinct TCR haplotypes. Eur J Immunol 1993; 23:1277–1283.
43. Heinzel FP, Sadick MD, Mutha SS, Locksley RM. Production of interferon gamma, interleukin 2, interleukin 4, and interleukin 10 by CD4+ lymphocytes in vivo during healing and progressive murine leishmaniasis. Proc Natl Acad Sci USA 1991; 88:7011–7015.
44. Mohapatra SS, Mohapatra S, Yang M, Ansari AA, Parronchi P, Maggi E, Romagnani S. Molecular basis of cross-reactivity among allergen-specific human T cells. T-cell receptor Vα gene usage and epitope structure. Immunology 1994; 81:15–20.
45. Holt PG, McMenamin C. IgE and mucosal immunity: studies on the role of intraepithelial Ia+ dendritic cells and δ/γ T-lymphocytes in regulation of T-cell activation in the lung. Clin Exp Allergy 1991; 21(Suppl):148–152.

46. Turki J, Pak J, Green SA, Martin RJ, Liggett SB. Genetic polymorphisms of the beta-2 adrenergic receptor in nocturnal and non-nocturnal asthma. J Clin Invest 1995; 95:1635–1641.

47. Jacob CO, Fronek Z, Lewis GD, Koo M, Hansen JA, McDevitt HO. Heritable major histocompatibility complex class II–associated differences in production of tumor necrosis factor α: relevance to genetic predisposition to systemic lupus erythematosis. Proc Natl Acad Sci USA 1990; 87:1233–1237.

48. Messer G, Spengler U, Jung MC, Honold G, Blömer K, Pape GR, Riethmüller G, Weiss EH. Polymorphic structure of the tumor necrosis factor (TNF) locus: an NcoI polymorphism in the first intron of the human TNF-β gene correlates with a variant amino acid in position 26 and a reduced level of TNF-β production. J Exp Med 1991; 173:209–219.

49. Wilson AG, Symons JA, McDowell TL, di Giovine FS, Duff GW. Effects of a tumour necrosis factor (TNF-α) promotor base transition on transcriptional activity. Br J Rheumatol 1994; 33:89 (abstract).

50. Moffatt MF, Cookson WOCM. Asthma and tumour necrosis factor polymorphism. Hum Immunol 1996; 47:160.

51. Daniels SE, Bhattacharyya S, James A, Leaves NI, Young A, Hill MR, Faux JA, Ryan GE, le Söuef PN, Lathrop GM, Musk AW, Cookson WOCM. A genome-wide search for quantitative trait loci underlying asthma. Nature 1996; 383:247–250.

12

Intrinsic Asthma

**LEONARDO M. FABBRI,
GAETANO CARAMORI,
and BIANCA BEGHÉ**

University of Ferrara
Ferrara, Italy

CRISTINA MAPP

University of Padua
Padua, Italy

I. Introduction

In the past, asthma was defined in terms of symptoms and lung function abnormalities, i.e., reversible airflow limitation and nonspecific airway hyperresponsiveness (1). Advances in the knowledge of the airway pathology and of the mechanisms involved in asthma have made this definition unsatisfactory. The *Global Initiative for Asthma*, a document prepared by a panel convened by the National Heart, Lung, and Blood Institute and the World Health Organization (2), has recently proposed a definition of asthma based on pathology and its clinical and functional consequences, recognizing that asthma is associated with chronic inflammation of the airways, and that asthma exacerbations are associated with acute inflammatory changes of the airway mucosa. Asthma is now defined as

> a chronic inflammatory disorder of the airways, in which many cells play a role, in particular eosinophils, mast cells, and T lymphocytes. In susceptible individuals, this inflammation causes recurrent episodes of wheezing, breathlessness, chest tightness, and cough, particularly at night and in the early morning. These symptoms are usually associated with widespread but variable airflow limitation

that is at least partly reversible, either spontaneously or with treatment. The airway inflammation also causes an associated increase in airway responsiveness to a variety of stimuli.

If one accepts this definition, any bronchopulmonary disease that manifests itself with asthma symptoms and is associated with (1) airway inflammation, (2) reversible airflow limitation, and (3) airway hyperresponsiveness may be labeled asthma. However, airway inflammation is not easy to measure noninvasively, and nonspecific airway hyperresponsiveness, which can be measured with standardized methods (3), is not specific for asthma, as it may be present in other chronic obstructive diseases of the airways, e.g., cystic fibrosis, bronchiectasis, and chronic bronchitis (3–5). In addition, airway hyperresponsiveness may be present in asymptomatic subjects (6), and may not be present at all times in all asthmatics (7), and in many asthmatic subjects it does not reflect the severity of the disease (4).

Thus, from a clinical standpoint, the only reliable, simple objective method to confirm the diagnosis of asthma in a subject with symptoms of asthma (vide infra) is still the assessment of reversible airflow limitation. While the spontaneous reversibility of airflow limitation may be assessed by monitoring the peak expiratory flow (PEF), the reversibility of airflow limitation induced by treatment may be assessed by measuring either PEF or forced expiratory volume in one second (FEV_1) before and after a single dose of a bronchodilator, or before and after a short course of full antiasthma treatment including systemic steroids.

II. Classification of Asthma

Asthma may be classified according to its severity or etiology. Asthma may differ greatly in terms of overall severity and of severity of its exacerbations. No single test is able to precisely classify the severity of the disorder. The characterization of the severity of asthma and of its exacerbations is based on the combination of symptom scores, repeated measurements of spirometry and/or PEF, and the amount of medication required to keep asthma under control. In clinical practice, it is important to define the severity of asthma, as the physician's decisions on short- and long-term management depend almost entirely on severity (2). In addition, a classification of a patient's asthma based on disease severity over the preceding year (8) has been shown to relate to pathological indices of airway inflammation. The descriptions of scores of disease severity based on a combination of symptoms and treatment requirements, as well as objective measurements of lung function, differ little between the guidelines produced in various countries, and include the categories of intermittent asthma, and mild, moderate, and severe persistent asthma.

Special consideration is paid in some guidelines to brittle asthma because it may be life-threatening (9,10).

In addition to a classification of asthma in terms of severity, a classification based on etiology is frequently reported in textbooks, guidelines, and review articles (2,11–14). According to its etiology, asthma may be defined as extrinsic, also called atopic or allergic, and intrinsic, also called nonatopic asthma (15–17).

Although the term *extrinsic* refers to a well-recognized environmental agent, extrinsic asthma is usually defined as asthma that occurs in atopic subjects, i.e., in subjects predisposed to develop an increased amount of IgE antibodies in response to environmental allergens. Atopic subjects are usually recognized through their familial and clinical history. Positive skin prick tests against common environmental allergens are the most frequently used objective diagnostic tests for atopy. Sometimes it is possible to identify the allergen(s) associated with the development and maintenance of asthma in an atopic asthmatic, but it is almost impossible to establish the cause-effect relationship between allergen(s) and asthma because atopic asthmatics develop symptoms and exacerbations after exposure to the allergens they are sensitized to, but also to a variety of other different stimuli.

The existence of a group of patients in whom no environmental causal agent can be identified has limited the classification of asthma according to etiology. Asthma induced by unknown causes in a nonatopic subject is defined as *intrinsic*. Usually intrinsic asthma develops at an older age, is more severe at diagnosis, and has a more severe course (17). Asthma induced by pharmacological agents (e.g., aspirin) or occupational small-molecular-weight sensitizing agents present in the workplace (e.g., isocyanates, plicatic acid) may occur in nonatopic subjects. In these subjects asthma is difficult to classify because the subjects are nonatopic and the agents are not allergens. Thus, on one hand asthma may be considered extrinsic, as it is induced by a clearly identifiable extrinsic agent, but it occurs in a nonatopic subject, and thus it should be considered intrinsic.

Apart from differences in age of onset, severity, and possibly some aspects of immunopathology (18–24), extrinsic and intrinsic asthma share similar clinical manifestations, abnormalities of respiratory function, and response to pharmacological treatment.

III. Epidemiology of Intrinsic Asthma

Although in some studies up to one-third of children with asthma are nonatopic and might be classified as intrinsic (25), asthma in nonatopic subjects usually has a late onset (over 30 years), with an increased prevalence in women

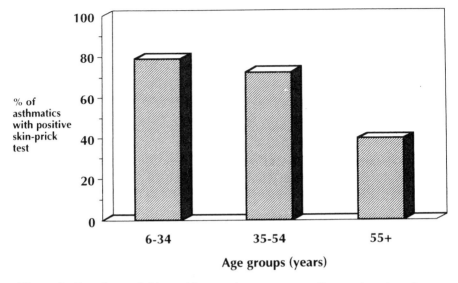

Figure 1 Prevalence of skin-positive reaction to common allergens in asthmatics re-cruited in a large population study. (Adapted from Ref. 30. By courtesy of the authors and the *New England Journal of Medicine*.)

(26,27). Although the prevalence of atopy is higher in asthmatics compared to the general population, still 30–50% of the asthmatics examined in large stud-ies are nonatopic (28,29).

The few epidemiological studies available that included children and elderly subjects show that the prevalence of atopy decreases with age in asth-matics (Fig. 1) (30). While young asthmatics have a prevalence of atopy that ranges from 75% (31) to as high as 90% (32,33), asthma that develops after the age of 40 may be associated with atopy in less than 40% of the subjects (30).

IV. Pathogenesis and Pathology of Intrinsic Asthma

A. Is Intrinsic Asthma a Distinct Immunopathological Entity?

This question has been extensively and elegantly discussed in a recent editorial by Kroegel et al. (17). Intrinsic asthma is indeed a distinct phenotypic variant of asthma (18,19) since, unlike atopic asthma, patients with intrinsic asthma have no familial or personal history of allergic diseases, are skin-test-negative to common aeroallergens, and have total serum IgE concentrations within the normal range (17–19).

However, the airway pathology of atopic and nonatopic asthma is similar. Bronchial biopsies from both atopic and nonatopic asthmatics show an increased number of activated T lymphocytes, eosinophils, and mast cells, and some degree of epithelial damage. Also, both atopic and nonatopic asthmatics exhibit a thicker subepithelial reticular layer of the basement membrane (8, 20–22,34–38). Interestingly, sputum cell counts also show no significant difference between atopic and nonatopic asthmatics (39).

Most of the studies on asthma death reported in the literature do not differentiate atopic or nonatopic asthmatics; thus it is not clear whether the pathology of asthma death is similar or different in atopic and nonatopic asthmatics. However, in some studies of sudden asthma death, a history of rapidly progressing asthma exacerbations seems more frequent in atopic as compared to nonatopic asthmatics (40,41).

Some recent pivotal studies have shed light on the pathology and possibly in the pathogenesis of instrinsic asthma (20–22; Fig. 2). Humbert et al. have elegantly described an increased number of cells expressing the high-affinity IgE receptor (FcεRI) in bronchial biopsies from atopic and nonatopic asthmatic patients (20; Fig. 2). Interestingly, the majority of FcεRI-bearing cells were mast cells and macrophages, with a much smaller percentage of eosinophils (20).

Interleukin-4 (IL-4) is an essential cofactor for IgE synthesis (42), and there is strong evidence that interleukin-5 (IL-5) plays a major role in eosinophil accumulation in asthmatic inflammation (43). As compared with controls, bronchial biopsies from both atopic and nonatopic asthmatic subjects have increased numbers of IL-4 mRNA and IL-5 mRNA copies and an increased number of cells expressing IL-4 and IL-5 mRNA and protein (Th2-type cytokines) (21; Fig. 2). Using double immunohistochemistry and in situ hybridization, these authors elegantly showed that 70% of IL-4 and IL-5 mRNA+ve signals colocalized to CD3+ve T cells, the majority (>70%) of which were CD4+ve, although CD8+ve cells also expressed IL-4 and IL-5 mRNA. The remaining 30% of IL-4 and IL-5 mRNA signals colocalized to mast cells and eosinophils (44). Interestingly, the cellular distribution of these mRNA species did not differ between atopic and nonatopic asthmatic patients (44). IL-4 and IL-5 protein immunoreactivity was predominantly associated with eosinophils and mast cells, with few IL-4 and IL-5 immunoreactive CD3+ve T cells detectable (44), however, total IL-4 or IL-5 positive cells detected by double immunohistochemistry were <40% of the total mRNA+ve cells (44). This discrepancy may be partly attributable to technical problems (44). Both atopic and nonatopic asthmatics were characterized by elevated numbers of bronchial mucosal cells expressing mRNAs encoding interleukin-3 (IL-3), interleukin-5 (IL-5), granulocyte-macrophage colony-stimulating factor (GM-CSF), RANTES, and monocyte chemotactic protein 3 (MCP-3), providing further

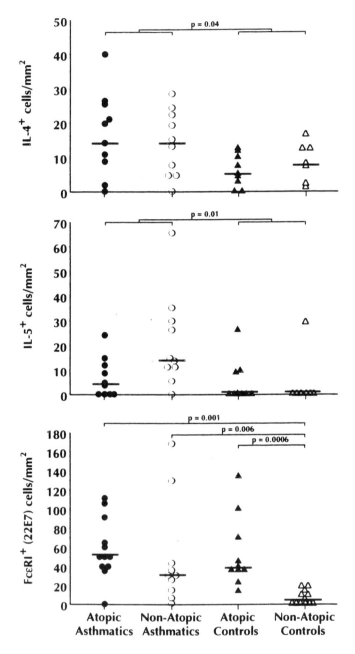

Figure 2 Number of high-affinity IgE receptor (FcεRI), interleukin-4 and interleukin-5 immunoreactive cells in the bronchial mucosa of patients with atopic and nonatopic asthma, and in atopic and nonatopic controls. (Adapted from Refs. 20,21. By courtesy of the authors and the *American Journal of Respiratory and Critical Care Medicine*.)

evidence for similarities in the immunopathogenesis of these clinically distinct forms of asthma (22).

Thus, in conclusion, according to these recent data produced by Kay's group (20–22,44), it appears that both atopic and nonatopic asthmatics have very similar immunopathological abnormalities in the bronchial mucosa. These results, taken together with the epidemiological evidence indicating that serum IgE concentrations are closely related to asthma prevalence independently from the atopic status (30,45), suggest that IgE-mediated mechanisms may participate in the pathogenesis of both atopic and nonatopic asthma.

The results of Humbert et al. (21) are in contrast with those of Walker and colleagues, who found that IL-4 and IL-5 protein concentration is increased in bronchoalveolar lavage (BAL) fluid and in the supernatant of peripheral blood and bronchoalveolar lavage T cells from atopic, but not from nonatopic, asthmatics, who instead have increased concentrations of interleukin-2 (IL-2) and IL-5 protein but not of IL-4 protein (19). The reasons for the discrepancy between the results of the two studies remain unclear, and more studies are required to clarify the difference (if any) in immunopathology between intrinsic and extrinsic asthma.

Occupational asthma induced by high-molecular-weight sensitizers and some low-molecular-weight sensitizers that are believed to act as haptens (e.g., trymellitic anhydrides) occurs more frequently in atopic subjects and resembles extrinsic asthma. By contrast, occupational asthma induced by some low-molecular-weight sensitizers (e.g., isocyanates, plicatic acid) occurs more frequently in nonatopic subjects. However, there is little difference in the pathological findings of occupational asthma induced by high or low molecular weight. Activated T lymphocytes CD25+ve (i.e., T lymphocytes expressing IL-2R), activated eosinophils, and mast cells are increased in the bronchial mucosa of patients with occupational asthma induced by isocyanates and plicatic acid (34,38,46,47), suggesting that similar immunological mechanisms may be involved in asthma of occupational as well as nonoccupational origin. Although an immunological mechanism has never been firmly established, occupational asthma induced by toluene diisocyanate (TDI) shares several features with nonatopic asthma. However, at variance with atopic asthma in which the majority of T-cell clones derived from the atopic patients are CD4+ve, with a Th2 pattern of cytokines (producing IL-4 and IL-5 but not IFN-γ), the majority of T-cell clones derived from patients with isocyanates induced asthma are CD8+ve, and these CD8+ve T cells produce IL-5, a cytokine that attracts, activates, and increases survival of eosinophils, and IFN-γ (a cytokine that inhibits the synthesis of IgE), but not IL-4. Thus, while CD4+ve Th2-like T cells, because of their pattern of cytokine production, may play a central role in determining the nature of inflammatory response seen in bronchial mucosa of atopic (extrinsic) asthmatics through the induction of both allergen-specific IgE (via

IL-4) and eosinophilia (via IL-5), CD8+ve T cells may play a similar role in nonatopic subjects with TDI asthma, by directly causing bronchial eosinophilia via local production of IL-5. Interestingly, these results are similar to the results obtained in intrinsic nonatopic asthmatic subjects (vide supra; 19).

B. Etiology of Intrinsic Asthma

The term *intrinsic* implies lack of knowledge of the cause of the disease. However, there are now recent studies comparing nonatopic with atopic asthma that allow some speculation about the potential causes or contributing factors of intrinsic asthma. The current hypothesis on the etiology of asthma is that the onset of asthma is dependent on (1) genetic factors that predispose individuals to asthma (48), and (2) environmental exposure to sensitizing agents, particularly allergens (14,49–53), and occupational agents (54,55).

C. Genes in the Etiology of Intrinsic Asthma

First-degree relatives of asthmatic subjects have a prevalence of asthma of 20–25%, i.e., a risk ratio of 5–6 compared to the general population, suggesting a significant genetic predisposition to develop asthma (48). Atopy is the strongest identifiable predisposing factor for asthma, and thus most studies on the genetics of asthma have utilized surrogate markers of atopy, e.g., total IgE, specific IgE, and/or the response to skin-prick tests. However, some studies have also examined the genetic predisposition of clinical asthma, or of bronchial hyperresponsiveness or severity of asthma as surrogate markers of clinical asthma (56–59). Interestingly, some genetic loci that have been found to be associated with atopy, like the FcεRIβ locus on chromosome 11q (60) and the region 5q (61,62), have been subsequently found to be associated also with the predisposition to develop asthma or its surrogate markers independently from atopy (57–59). These observations suggest (1) that the predisposition to develop atopy and asthma may be inherited independently (63), (2) that the same gene (59) or genes from the same region (64) may influence both asthma and atopy (58,59), and (3) that some genes like the ones encoding for the β2-adrenergic receptor (65) or platelet-activating factor acetylhydrolase (66) may be more relevant for asthma or its clinical manifestation than for atopy. Indeed, similarly to atopic asthma, nonatopic intrinsic asthma has also been shown to have a strong genetic predisposition, even if the risk ratio appears to be lower (67,68).

D. Role of IgE in the Etiology of Intrinsic Asthma

The demonstration of increased numbers of cells expressing the high-affinity IgE receptor (FcεRI) in bronchial biopsies from atopic and nonatopic asthmatic patients (20), together with the epidemiological evidence indicating that serum IgE concentrations are closely related to asthma prevalence regardless of atopic status (30,45), suggest that allergy and allergens may participate in the etiology of both atopic and nonatopic asthma (20). However, the bronchial mucosal expression of FcεRI receptors and of IL-4 mRNA is increased in both atopic asthmatic and atopic nonasthmatic subjects, and the degree of expression does not correlate with the severity of asthma (20,21). These observations suggest that the increased expression of FcεRI receptors and Il-4 mRNA, i.e., the expression of the atopic trait, is necessary but not sufficient for the manifestation of asthma in adults. It is conceivable the additional presence in atopic subjects of an increased amount of IgE specific to some allergens may increase the risk of these subjects (and not of nonatopic subjects) to develop asthma exacerbations upon exposure to the allergens they are sensitized to.

E. Is Intrinsic Asthma an Autoimmune Disease?

It has been suggested that intrinsic asthma might be an autoimmune disease (17,69). This hypothesis derived from some immunological and pathological data. In the serum of a significant number of patients with intrinsic asthma, an autoantibody directed against a 55-kDa epithelial antigen is present (70). In addition, patients with intrinsic or nonatopic occupational asthma (23,24,47) have increased number of CD8+ve cells in bronchial biopsies and/or bronchoalveolar lavage. Because, unlike CD4+ve cells, most CD8+ve T-lymphocytes recognize endogenous antigens, and are mainly involved in the response to intracellular infectious agents, tumors, and autoimmune diseases, it has been suggested that also some forms of occupational asthma occurring in nonatopic subjects (intrinsic occupational asthma) might result from autoimmune mechanisms (17,69). This hypothesis is attractive, but highly speculative, and remains to be confirmed experimentally both in occupational and in nonoccupational asthma (17,71).

F. Clinical Features of Intrinsic Asthma

There is no clinical feature that is characteristic of intrinsic asthma. By definition, patients with intrinsic asthma are subjects with skin-prick test negative against common environmental aeroallergens.

In the past it was believed that aspirin-induced asthma, in addition to some specific characteristics (e.g., developing in adults, often preceded by rhinitis, and associated with nasal polyposis), occurred more frequently in nonatopic asthma (72–78). However, recent studies have demonstrated that it occurs with similar frequency both in atopic and nonatopic asthmatics (79). Also, it seems that nonatopic aspirin-sensitive asthmatics develop a more severe disease (72–78), but this remains to be confirmed in larger populations.

There is no evidence that the response to pharmacological treatment is different in intrinsic and extrinsic asthma, but most of the studies have included atopic asthmatics and no real comparative study between intrinsic and extrinsic asthma has been conducted.

In some, but not all (80), epidemiological studies, adults with intrinsic asthma have been reported to have an accelerated decline of lung function compared with the decline of lung function of atopic asthmatics (81). More recent studies have shown that the rate of decline of forced expiratory volume in one second (FEV_1) is increased only in patients with new-onset asthma, and not in patients with ongoing asthma (82), and that atopy is a significant independent predictor of subsequent decline of lung function among nonasthmatics (83,84).

V. Conclusions

In conclusion, although intrinsic asthma is indeed a distinct entity, with some different epidemiological and clinical characteristics, it shares several features with atopic extrinsic asthma. Extrinsic asthma definitely requires a different management, as prevention of environmental exposure and in some cases immunotherapy are treatment options obviously not available for intrinsic asthmatics. Further studies are required to determine whether intrinsic asthma indeed has different mechanisms of development as compared to extrinsic asthma, or whether the combination of asthma and atopy makes extrinsic asthma only an apparently different clinical entity, having in common with intrinsic asthma all the mechanisms of development of the pathological, functional, and clinical manifestations of asthma. Atopy, then, defined in terms of production of specific IgE, might just play an aggravating factor of asthma present in atopic extrinsic asthmatics and not in nonatopic intrinsic asthmatics.

References

1. American Thoracic Society Committee on Diagnostic Standards for Nontuberculous Respiratory Diseases. Definitions and classification of chronic bronchitis, asthma, and pulmonary emphysema. Am Rev Respir Dis 1962; 85:762–768.
2. Sheffer AL, ed. Global Initiative for Asthma. NHLBI/WHO Workshop Report. National Institutes of Health, National Heart, Lung and Blood Institute, Publication No. 95-3659, January 1995.
3. Sterk PJ, Fabbri LM, Quanjer Ph, Cockcroft DW, O'Byrne PM, Anderson SD, Juniper EF, Malo JL. Airway responsiveness: standardized challenge testing with pharmacological, physiological, and sensitizing stimuli. Eur Respir J 1993; 6(Suppl 16):53–83.

4. Josephs LK, Gregg I, Mullee MA, Holgate ST. Nonspecific bronchial reactivity and its relationship to the clinical expression of asthma: a longitudinal study. Am Rev Respir Dis 1989; 140:350–357.

5. Perin PV, Weldon D, McGeady SJ. Objective indicators of severity of asthma. J Allergy Clin Immunol 1994; 94:517–522.

6. Cockcroft DW, Hargreave FE. Airway hyperresponsiveness: relevance of random population data to clinical usefulness. Am Rev Respir Dis 1990; 142:497–500.

7. Mapp CE, Dal Vecchio L, Boschetto P, De Marzo N, Fabbri LM. Toluene diisocyanate-induced asthma without airway hyperresponsiveness. Eur J Respir Dis 1986; 68:89–95.

8. Bousquet J, Chanez P, Lacoste JY, Barnèon G, Ghavanian N, Enander I, Venge P, Ahlstedt S, Simony-Lafontaine J, Godard P, Michel FB. Eisonophilic inflammation in asthma. N Engl J Med 1990; 323:1033–1039.

9. The British Thoracic Society, the National Asthma Campaign, the Royal College of Physicians of London in association with the General Practitioner in Asthma Group, the British Association of Accident and Emergency Medicine, the British Paediatric Respiratory Society and the Royal College of Paediatrics and Child Health. The British guidelines on asthma management: 1995 review and position statement. Thorax 1997; 52(Suppl 1):S1–S21.

10. Expert Panel report II: Guidelines for the Diagnosis and Management of Asthma (EPR-II). National Heart, Lung, and Blood Institute. NIH Publication No. 97-4051, July 1997.

11. Barnes PJ, Djukanovic R, Holgate ST. Pathogenesis. In: Brewis RAL, Corrin B, Geddes DM, Gibson GJ, eds. Respiratory Medicine, 2nd ed. London: WB Saunders, 1995:1108–1153.

12. Hoover GE, Platts-Mills TAE. What the pulmonologist needs to know about allergy. In: Martin RJ, ed. Asthma. Clin Chest Med 1995; 16:603–620.

13. Woolcock AJ. Asthma. In: Murray JF, Nadel JA, eds. Textbook of Respiratory Medicine, 2nd ed. Philadelphia: WB Saunders, 1994:1288–1330.

14. Platts-Mills TAE, Wheatley LM. The role of allergy and atopy in asthma. Curr Opin Pulm Med 1996; 2:29–34.

15. Rackemann FM. Intrinsic asthma. J Allergy 1940; 11:147–162.

16. Rackemann FM. A working classification of asthma. Am J Med 1947; 3:601–606.

17. Kroegel C, Jager L, Walker C. Is there a place for intrinsic asthma as a distinct immunopathological entity? Eur Respir J 1997; 10:513–515.

18. Virchow JC Jr, Kroegel C, Walker C, Matthys H. Cellular and immunological markers of allergic and intrinsic bronchial asthma. Lung 1994; 172:313–334.

19. Walker C, Bode E, Boer L, Hansel TT, Blaser K, Virchow JC Jr. Allergic and non-allergic asthmatics have distinct patterns of T-cell activation and cytokine production in peripheral blood and bronchoalveolar lavage. Am Rev Respir Dis 1992; 146:109–115.

20. Humbert M, Grant JA, Taborda-Barata L, Durham SR, Pfister R, Menz G, Barkans J, Ying S, Kay AB. High affinity IgE receptor (FcεRI)-bearing cells in bronchial biopsies from atopic and nonatopic asthma. Am J Respir Crit Care Med 1996; 153:1931–1937.

21. Humbert M, Durham SR, Ying S, Kimmitt P, Barkans J, Assoufi B, Pfister R, Menz G, Robinson DS, Kay AB, Corrigan CJ. IL-4 and IL-5 mRNA and protein in bronchial biopsies from patients with atopic and nonatopic asthma: evidence against "intrinsic" asthma being a distinct immunopathologic entity. Am J Respir Crit Care Med 1996; 154:1497–1504.
22. Humbert M, Ying S, Corrigan CJ, Menz G, Barkans J, Pfister R, Meng Q, Van Damme J, Opdenakker G, Robinson DS, Durham SR, Kay AB. Bronchial mucosa expression of the genes encoding chemokines RANTES and MCP-3 in symptomatic atopic and nonatopic asthmatics. Relationship to the eosinophil-active cytokines interleukin (IL)-5, granulocyte macrophage-colony-stimulating factor, and IL-3. Am J Respir Cell Mol Biol 1997; 16:1–8.
23. Maestrelli P, Del Prete GF, De Carli M, D'Elios M, Saetta M, Di Stefano A, Mapp CE, Romagnani S, Fabbri LM. CD8 T-cell clones producing interleukin-5 and interferon-gamma in bronchial mucosa of patients with asthma induced by toluene diisocyanate. Scand J Work Environ Health 1994; 20:376–381.
24. Del Prete GF, De Carli M, D'Elios MM, Maestrelli P, Ricci M, Rabbri L, Romagnani S. Allergen exposure induces the activation of allergen-specific Th2 cells in the airway mucosa of patients with allergic respiratory disorders. Eur J Immunol 1993; 23:1445–1449.
25. Ulrik CS, Backer V, Dirksen A, Pedersen M, Koch C. Extrinsic and intrinsic asthma from childhood to adult age: a 10-yr follow-up. Respir Med 1995; 89:547–554.
26. Hendrick DJ, Davies RJ, D'Souza MF, Pepys J. An analysis of skin prick test reactions in 656 asthmatic patients. Thorax 1975; 30:2–8.
27. Molina C, Brun J, Coulet M, Betail M, Delage C. Immunopathology of the bronchial mucosa in "late onset asthma." Clin Allergy 1977; 7:137–145.
28. Herbert FA, Weimer N, Salkine ML. RAST and skin test in the investigation of asthma. Ann Allergy 1982; 49:311–314.
29. Kalliel JN, Goldstein BM, Braman SS, Settipane GA. High frequency of atopic asthma in a pulmonary clinic population. Chest 1989; 96:1336–1340.
30. Burrows B, Martinez FD, Halonen M, Barbee RA, Cline MG. Association of asthma with serum IgE levels and skin test reactivity to allergens. N Engl J Med 1989; 320:271–277.
31. Martin AJ, Landau LT, Phelan PD. Natural history of allergy in asthmatic children followed to adult life. Med J Aust 1981; 2:470–474.
32. Kelly W, Hudson I, Phelan P, Pain M, Olinsky A. Atopy in subjects with asthma followed to the age of 28 years. J Allergy Clin Immunol 1990; 85:548–557.
33. Corne JM, Smith S, Schreiber J, Holgate ST. Prevalence of atopy in asthma. Lancet 1994; 344:344–345.
34. Bentley AM, Menz G, Storz Chr, Robinson DS, Bradley B, Jeffery PK, Durham SR, Kay AB. Identification of T lymphocytes, macrophages, and activated eosinophils in the bronchial mucosa in intrinsic asthma: relationship to symptoms and bronchial responsiveness. Am Rev Respir Dis 1992; 146:500–506.
35. Bentley AM, Durham SR, Kay AB. Comparison of the immunopathology of extrinsic, intrinsic and occupational asthma. J Invest Allergol Clin Immunol 1994; 4:222–232.

36. Djukanovic R. Bronchial biopsies. In: Busse WW, Holgate ST, eds. Asthma and Rhinitis. London: Blackwell Scientific Publications, 1995:118–129.

37. Holgate ST. The immunopharmacology of mild asthma. J Allergy Clin Immunol 1996; 98(Suppl):S7–S16.

38. Saetta M, Di Stefano A, Maestrelli P, De Marzo N, Milani GF, Pivirotto F, Mapp CE, Fabbri LM. Airway mucosal inflammation in occupational asthma induced by toluene diisocyanate. Am Rev Respir Dis 1992; 145:160–168.

39. Radermecker M, Kayembe JM, Weber Th, Duysinx B, Louis R. Induced sputum cell counts in intrinsic asthma. Am J Respir Crit Care Med 1996; 153(Suppl): A290.

40. Tough SC, Green FHY, Paul JE, Wigle DT, Butt JC. Sudden death from asthma in 108 children and young adults. J Asthma 1996; 33:179–188.

41. British Thoracic Society. Comparison of atopic and non-atopic patients dying of asthma. Br J Dis Chest 1987; 81:30–34.

42. Ricci M. IL-4: a key cytokine in atopy. Clin Exp Allergy 1994; 24:801–812.

43. Egan RW, Umland SP, Cuss FM, Chapman RW. Biology of interleukin-5 and its relevance to allergic disease. Allergy 1996; 51:71–81.

44. Ying S, Humbert M, Barkans J, Corrigan CJ, Pfister R, Menz G, Larchè M, Robinson DS, Durham SR, Kay AB. Expression of IL-4 and IL-5 mRNA and protein product by CD4+ve and CD8+ve T cells, eosinophils, and mast cells in bronchial biopsies obtained from atopic and nonatopic (intrinsic) asthmatics. J Immunol 1997; 158:3539–3544.

45. Sears MR, Burrows B, Flannery EM, Herbison GP, Hewitt CJ, Holdaway MD. Relation between airway responsiveness and serum IgE in children with asthma and in apparently normal children. N Engl J Med 1991; 325:1067–1071.

46. Fabbri LM, Ciaccia A, Maestrelli P, Saetta M, Mapp CE. Pathophysiology of occupational asthma. In: Holgate ST, Austen KF, Lichetenstein LM, Kay AB, eds. Asthma. New York: Marcel Dekker, 1993:301–322.

47. Frew AJ, Chan H, Lam S, Chan-Yeung M. Bronchial inflammation in occupational asthma due to western red cedar. Am J Respir Crit Care Med 1995; 151:340–344.

48. Sandford A, Weir T, Parè P. The genetics of asthma. Am J Respir Crit Care Med 1996; 153:1749–1765.

49. Arruda LK, Vailes LD, Platts-Mills TAE, Fernandez-Caldas E, Montealegre F, Lin K-L, Chua K-Y, Rizzo MC, Naspitz CK, Chapman MD. Sensitization to Blomia tropicalis in patients with asthma and identification of allergen *Blo t 5*. Am J Respir Crit Care Med 1997; 155:343–350.

50. Chan-Yeung M, Quirce S. Aeroallergens and asthma. Can Respir J 1994; 1:248–256.

51. Peat JK, Tovey E, Toelle BG, Haby MM, Gray EJ, Mahmic A, Woolcock AJ. House dust mite allergens: a major risk factor for childhood asthma in Australia. Am J Respir Crit Care Med 1996; 153:141–146.

52. Platts-Mills TAE, Sporik RB, Chapman MD, Heymann PW. The role of indoor allergens in asthma. Allergy 1995; 50(Suppl 22):5–12.

53. Platts-Mills TAE, Carter MC. Asthma and indoor exposure to allergens. N Engl J Med 1997; 336:1382–1384.

54. Chan-Yeung M, Malo J-L. Occupational asthma. N Engl J Med 1995; 332:107–112.

55. Fabbri L, Caramori G, Maestrelli P. Etiology of occupational asthma. In: Sipes G, McQueen CA, Gandolfi AJ, eds. Comprehensive Toxicology. 1997: vol. 8:425–435.
56. Townley RG, Bewtra AK, Nair NM, Brodkey FD, Watt GD, Burke KM. Methacholine inhalation challenge studies. J Allergy Clin Immunol 1979; 64:569–574.
57. Liggett SB, Meyers DA. The Genetics of Asthma. New York: Marcel Dekker, 1997.
58. Postma DS, Bleeker ER, Amelung PJ, Holroyd KJ, Xu J, Panjuysen CIM, Meyers DA, Levitt RC. Genetic susceptibility to asthma—bronchial hyperresponsiveness coinherited with a major gene for atopy. N Engl J Med 1995; 333:894–900.
59. van Herderweden L, Harrap SB, Wong ZYH, Abramson MJ, Kutin JJ, Forbes AB, Raven J, Laningan A, Walters EH. Linkage of high-affinity IgE receptor gene with bronchial hyper-reactivity, even in the absence of atopy. Lancet 1995; 346:1262–1265.
60. Cookson WOCM. Genetics, atopy and asthma. Allergol Int 1996; 45:3–11.
61. Marsh DG, Neely JD, Breazeale DR, Freidhoff LR, Ehrlich-Kautzky E, Schou C, Krihnasway, and Beaty TH. Linkage analysis of IL4 and other chromosome 5q31.1 markers and total serum immunoglobulin E concentrations. Science 1994; 264: 1152–1156.
62. Doull IJ, Lawrence S, Watson M, Begishvili T, Beasley RW, Lampe F, Holgate T, Morton NE. Allelic association of gene markers on chromosome 5q and 11q with atopy and bronchial hyperresponsiveness. Am J Respir Crit Care Med 1996; 153: 1280–1284.
63. Sibbald B, Horn MEC, Brain EA, Gregg I. Genetic factors in childhood asthma. Thorax 1980; 35:671–674.
64. Levitt RC, Holroyd KJ. Fine-structure mapping of genes providing susceptibility to asthma on chromosome 5q31-q33. Clin Exp Allergy 1995; 25(Suppl 2): 119–123.
65. Turki J, Pak J, Green SA, Martin RJ, Liggett SB. Genetic polymorphisms of the β2-adrenergic receptor in nocturnal and nonnocturnal asthma. J Clin Invest 1995; 95:1635–1641.
66. Stafforini DM, Satoh K, Atkinson DL, Tjoelker LW, Eberhardt C, Yoshida H, Imaizumi T, Takamatsu S, Zimmerman GA, McIntyre TM, Gray PW, Prescott SM. Platelet-activating factor acetylhydrolase deficiency: a missense mutation near the active site of an anti-inflammatory phospholipase. J Clin Invest 1996; 97:2784–2791.
67. Pirson F, Charpin D, Sansonetti M, Lanteaume A, Kulling G, Charpin J, Vervloet D. Is intrinsic asthma a hereditary disease? Allergy 1991; 46:367–371.
68. Sibbald B, Turner-Warwick M. Factors influencing the prevalence of asthma among first degree relatives of extrinsic and intrinsic asthmatics. Thorax 1979; 34:332–337.
69. Kroegel C, Virchow JC Jr, Walker C. T lymphocyte activation in bronchial asthma. N Engl J Med 1993; 328:1639–1640.
70. Lassale P, Delneste Y, Gosset P, Gras-Masse H, Wallaert B, Tonnel AB. T and B-cell immune response to a 55 kDa endothelial cell-derived antigen in severe asthma. Eur J Immunol 1993; 23:796–803.
71. Szczeklik A, Nizankowska E, Serafin A, Dyczek A, Duplaga M, Musial J. Autoimmune phenomena in bronchial asthma with special reference to aspirin intolerance. Am J Respir Crit Care Med 1995; 152:1753–1756.

72. Chafee FH, Settipane Ga. Aspirin intolerance. I. Frequency in an allergic population. J Allergy Clin Immunol 1974; 3:193–199.
73. Delaney JC, Kay AB. Complement components and IgE in patients with asthma and aspirin idiosyncrasy. Thorax 1976; 31:425–427.
74. McDonald JR, Mathison DA, Stevenson DD. Aspirin intolerance in asthma: detection by oral challenge. J Allergy Clin Immunol 1972; 50:198–207.
75. Samter M, Beers RF Jr. Intolerance to aspirin: clinical studies and consideration of its pathogenesis. Ann Intern Med 1968; 68:975–983.
76. Schlumberger HD, Lobbecke EA, Kallos P. Acetylsalicylic acid intolerance: lack of *N*-acetylsalicyclic acid specific, skin-sensitizing antibodies in the serum of intolerant individuals. Acta Med Scand 1974; 196:451–458.
77. Smith AP. Response of aspirin-allergic patients to challenge by some analgesics in common use. Br Med J 1971; 2:494–496.
78. Spector SL, Wangaard CH, Farr RS. Aspirin and concomitant idiosyncrasies in adult asthmatic patients. J Allergy Clin Immunol 1979; 64:500–506.
79. Bochenek G, Nizankowska G, Szczeklik A. The atopy trait in hypersensitivity to nonsteroidal anti-inflammatory drugs. Allergy 1996; 51:16–23.
80. Peat JK, Woolcock AJ, Cullen K. Rate of decline of lung function in subjects with asthma. Eur J Respir Dis 1987; 70:171–179.
81. Ulrik CS, Backer V, Dirksen A. A 10 year follow up of 180 adults with bronchial asthma: factors important for the decline in lung function. Thorax 1992; 47:14–18. See also the comments of Quanjer PH. Thorax 1992; 47:484.
82. Ulrik CS, Lange P. Decline of lung function in adults with bronchial asthma. Am J Respir Crit Care Med 1994; 150:629–634.
83. Gottlieb DJ, Sparrow D, O'Connor GT, Weiss ST. Skin test reactivity to common aeroallergens and decline of lung function: the normative aging study. Am J Respir Crit Care Med 1996; 153:561–566.
84. Tracey M, Villar A, Dow L, Coggon D, Lampe FC, Holgate ST. The influence of increased bronchial responsiveness, atopy and serum IgE on decline in FEV_1: a longitudinal study in the elderly. Am J Respir Crit Care Med 1995; 151:656–662.

13

Viral Infection and Asthma
The Modulatory Role of Nitric Oxide on Prostaglandin H Synthase

GERT FOLKERTS and FRANS P. NIJKAMP

Utrecht University
Utrecht, The Netherlands

I. Introduction

A characteristic feature of most asthmatic patients is that their airways have an increased tendency to narrow on exposure to a variety of chemical, pharmacological, or physical stimuli, a phenomenon called "airway hyperresponsiveness." Although its etiology is still unclear, it is well known that viral respiratory infections also can induce or aggravate airway hyperresponsiveness (1–6). Interestingly airway hyperresponsiveness, airway inflammation, and epithelial damage are observed in *both* persons with a viral respiratory tract infection or with asthma. One hypothesis is that the inflammatory cells release mediators that can induce epithelial damage and accordingly, airway hyperresponsiveness (7). Indeed, relationships have been described between the degree of epithelial damage and the degree of airway hyperresponsiveness (8). The epithelial layer releases a number of mediators that may interfere with the reactivity of the underlying smooth muscle. Two of these epithelium-derived relaxing factors are nitric oxide (NO) and prostaglandin (PG) E_2. NO, first identified as an endothelium-derived relaxing factor, is now known to be an intra- and extracellular mediator of cell function. NO formed by the constitutive nitric oxide synthase (cNOS) is a key regulator of homeostasis, while NO formed by inducible NO synthase (iNOS) plays an important role in inflammation, host-defense responses, and tissue repair. Recent studies have shown that NO can modulate the activity of prostaglandin H synthase (PGHS). This is the enzyme responsible for prostanoid production from arachidonic acid, which needs to be released from cell membranes by phospholipase A_2. Like NO, prostaglandins are potent mediators of intra- and intercellular communications in diverse physiological and pathophysiological processes. Like NO synthase, PGHS consists of two isomers: a constitutive (PGHS-1, containing COX-1) and an inducible one (PGHS-2, containing COX-2). The main role of PGHS-1 is to maintain homeostasis and PGHS-2 induces the pathological effects. In this review the interaction of nitric oxide on arachidonic acid metabolism will be discussed with special reference to the development of airway hyperresponsiveness.

II. Overview of the Release and Interaction of NO on Prostaglandin H Synthase

A. Corelease of NO and Prostaglandins

Many stimulators of NO production lead to the simultaneous release of mediators from the PGHS pathway (such as PGE_2 and PGI_2) (9–11), or other mediators, such as tissue plasminogen activator (11). This is true for the rapidly acting agonists acting on cNOS and PGHS-1, such as acetylcholine (12), adenosine diphosphate, bradykinin (13,14), and substance P (15), and for the longer-acting agents acting on iNOS and PGHS-2, such as endotoxins, cytokines, and mitogens (10,13,16–18).

B. Synergism Between NO and Prostaglandins

Increasing the level of cyclic nucleotides (i.e., cAMP and cGMP) (10,11,13) may be one mechanism through which the NOS and PGHS paracrine systems operate to reach a synergistic effect (10,11,19), to amplify a physiological or pathological response (10,19). However, it does not necessarily mean that the coreleased prostanoids and NO always interact with each other and have synergistic effects (12). Nor does it necessarily mean that they are always coreleased.

Interleukin (IL)-1β can activate both PGHS and phospholipase A_2 in vascular smooth muscle cells, independent of NO, with a consequent production of prostaglandins via an increased level of arachidonic acid. Since phospholipase A_2 does not contain a heme component, it is unlikely that NO stimulates phospholipase A_2 activity (20). However, Davidge et al. (21) showed a non-receptor-mediated coactivation of cNOS and phospholipase A_2 by an increase in intracellular calcium, leading to an increased production of NO and prostanoids. This increased level of NO would lead to a coactivation of phospholipase A_2 and PGHS. Endothelial cells contain cNOS and PGHS-1, which can be coactivated by receptor-stimulating factors (14,17,19). This receptor-mediated release of PGI_2 and NO is coupled most probably at the level of phospholipase C and diacylglycerol, which, like phospholipase A_2, modulate arachidonic acid metabolism (15). Similarly, iNOS and PGHS-2 may coexist in the cell and thus NO and PGI_2 may be coreleased after a lag phase in response to cytokines, endotoxin, or mitogen stimulation (14), which has been shown to occur in several cell types (10–12,14,20–23). The differential regulation of iNOS and PGHS-2 may be attributed to the changing profile of cytokines as the inflammatory process progresses. Tumor necrosis factor (TNF) α increases PGHS mRNA in fibroblasts and synergizes with IL-1β to stimulate prostaglandin production. Similarly, iNOS activity is induced by several cytokines, such as IL-1β and TNFα (24). IL-1β induces both iNOS and PGHS-2 mRNA by transcriptional activation and/or stabilizing mRNA and these mRNAs are translated into proteins (11). Although exogenous NO is capable of directly stimulating PGE_2 release, the amount of PGE_2 is much smaller than that induced by IL-1β. Therefore, other, NO-independent, second-messenger systems may be involved in the full activation of the NO-dependent mechanism for PGE_2 release (20).

C. Activation of PGHS by NO

It is not likely that NO participates in basal PGE_2 synthesis (9,25,26). However, the endogenous release of NO from cNOS after receptor stimulation results in an optimal PGE_2 release (9,27). In addition, under pathological conditions, NO release from iNOS activates PGHS-2 resulting in a markedly increased release of proinflammatory prostaglandins (20–22,28). It cannot be excluded that PGHS-2 and iNOS are nonendothelially localized, since endothelial removal failed to block the time-dependent release of NO_2^- and PGE_2 release (9).

PGHS is thought to have an intrinsic self-inactivation mechanism (21) for which the activator possibly is an oxygen radical $(O)_x$, formed by the peroxidase domain of PGHS (29). Indeed, incubation of PGHS with agents that initially stimulate this enzyme results finally in an inhibition 24 hr after incubation with these agents.

It is not likely that NO induces the synthesis of PGHS, but rather activates the COX component of preexisting PGHS (21). This is supported by the finding that acetylation of preexisting PGHS with acetylsalicylic acid, which results in inactivation of the enzyme, prevents the NO-stimulated 6-keto $PGF_{1\alpha}$ production (21). On the other hand, many transcription factors are regulated by oxygen radicals. PGHS is the product of an immediate early gene that has characteristics similar to transcription factors that may be activated by NO, acting as an oxidizing radical, leading to new synthesis of PGHS (21,23).

Stimulation of PGHS Through NO Radical Effects

1. NO can interact with oxygen-derived free radicals and as such be considered a radical scavenger. Free radicals are known to be capable of modulating the PGHS pathway (21,23,29), leading to a modulatory role for NO in PGHS activation.
2. NO could potentially activate PGHS through oxidizing the COX component of the enzyme. Activation of the heme group in the COX domain of PGHS requires oxidative conversion from the ferrous to the ferric form (21).
3. Possible mechanisms of activation of PGHS by means of superoxide anions:

   NO reacts with superoxide anions to form peroxynitrite along with hydroxyl radicals. The results may be an increase in lipid peroxidation, which would enhance PGHS activity (30–32).

   Superoxide anions and NO may be simultaneously formed by NOS, depending on the amount of L-arginine and tetrahydrobiopterin present in the medium (33). These superoxide anions may act as modulators of cyclooxygenase activity.

D. Stimulation of PGHS Through Heme Binding

NO could activate PGHS through its heme-binding properties in a manner similar to its activation of other heme-containing enzymes, such as guanylate cyclase. However, depending on the heme protein itself, the consequence of the heme-binding effect of NO may vary and may not be associated with a catalytic function (13,21).

NO has a relatively weak affinity for heme in ferric PGHS (the active form), the resting oxidation state of this heme protein. NO reacts strongly and completely with ferrous PGHS (the inactive form) under anaerobic conditions, displacing the proximal ligand, through a slow dissociation, forming a complex and consequently an activated enzyme. The ferric PGHS-NO complex, however, is not entirely reversible (34). The complete reaction of NO with ferrous PGHS results in disruption of the bond between PGHS and heme. Loss of the proximal ligand by this conversion of free PGHS to the NO complex, probably does not result in complete dissociation of the heme. PGHS has a considerable capacity for nonspecific heme binding, leading to a nonspecific binding of heme

NO to PGHS (34). On the other hand, Hajjar et al. (35) reported that under aerobic conditions, NO stimulates the conversion of arachidonic acid to PGE_2 and PGD_2 in a dose- and time-dependent manner, independent of heme.

E. Modulation of Substrate Amount

The finding that L-arginine increased NO_2^- and PGE_2 release in inflammation suggests that in inflammation there is an alteration in the synthesis or a more efficient conversion of L-arginine into NO, resulting in a decreased level of this substrate necessary for NO synthesis under these circumstances (27). Salvemini et al. (10) have reported earlier that L-arginine depletion did not affect PGHS-2 activity in human fibroblasts, but did reduce PGE_2 release. Therefore, it can be concluded that this reduction is the result of decreased PGHS induction due to inhibition of NO.

III. Prostaglandin E_2 as an Epithelium-Derived Relaxing Factor

For many years it has been suggested that the epithelial layer of the respiratory tract acts as a barrier and can release relaxing factors that may protect the airways from excessive constriction. This idea was based on the fact that tracheal smooth muscle responsiveness to contractile drugs could be enhanced after removal of the epithelial layer (36–38). Prostaglandins may have a modulating role in the induction of airway smooth muscle hyperresponsiveness. Prostaglandin E_2 (PGE_2), in particular, is released during contractions of animal and human tracheal preparations (39–41), and can be synthesized by animal and human epithelial cells (42–46). This prostaglandin relaxes respiratory airway smooth muscle and inhibits, in the nanomolar range, contractile responses evoked in intact and epithelium-denuded tracheal preparations (47–49), whereas prostaglandin synthesis inhibitors augment the responses of trachea to contractile agents (50).

In a number of studies we found a relationship between PGE_2 release and airway responsiveness (51–53). Arachidonic acid induced a relaxation of intact tracheal tissues with an obvious prostaglandin E_2 production, and a contraction in epithelium-denuded preparations with significant less synthesis of this prostanoid (51). Moreover, epithelium removal induced a similar degree of tracheal hyperresponsiveness to histamine, as incubation of intact tissues incubated with the cyclooxygenase inhibitor indomethacin (52). Addition of indomethacin to epithelium-denuded tissues did not result in an additional increase in tracheal responsiveness. Interestingly, histamine increased the PGE_2 production in intact tissues but this increase was significantly diminished in epithelium-denuded preparations (52). These results together strengthen the concept that PGE_2 released by the epithelial layer can modulate the reactivity of the underlying smooth muscle.

IV. PGE_2 in Animal Models of Airway Hyperresponsiveness

Bronchial hyperresponsiveness is induced in guinea pigs by intraperitoneal administration of the gram-negative bacterium *Hemophilus influenzae* or the active cell constituent endotoxin. These animals show an altered responsiveness of the respiratory airways in vitro and in vivo (54–56). Tracheal spirals obtained from endotoxin-pretreated animals display increased maximal contractions and decreased EC_{50} values to histamine compared to controls. Interestingly, these effects were associated with decreased PGE_2 concentrations in the organ bath compared to controls (52). Moreover, tissues from endotoxin-pretreated animals, incubated with indomethacin, demonstrated a similar degree of airway hyperresponsiveness as control preparations incubated with indomethacin alone. These results again point to a role of PGE_2 in modulating airway responsiveness in this animal model.

Guinea pigs intratracheally inoculated with parainfluenza (PI)-3 virus demonstrated a long-lasting airway hyperresponsiveness in vitro and in vivo (57,58). In PI-3 virus–infected animals, epithelial damage with loss of cilia and mucus-depleted goblet cells was observed (59). Further, a relationship was found between airway inflammation and the development of airway hyperresponsiveness (60). Despite the inflammatory reaction and the mild degree of epithelial damage, no differences were observed in the spontaneous or histamine-induced release of PGE_2 by the tracheal spirals obtained from virus-infected animals compared to controls (59). Moreover, the PGE_2 concentration in the bronchoalveolar lavage fluid was not different between the experimental groups (59). Pretreatment of the animals in vivo with a cyclooxygenase inhibitor also did not modulate the virus induced airway inflammation or hyperresponsiveness (60). From these studies it must be concluded the prostaglandins are not per definition involved in the modulation of airway function.

V. NO as an Epithelium-Derived Relaxing Factor

It has been known for more than half a century that nitrates induce bronchial relaxation (61). NO-containing vasodilatators such as glyceryl trinitrate and sodium nitroprusside induce relaxation of isolated airway smooth muscle, activate guanylate cyclase, and raise cGMP levels (62–64). The cGMP-mediated relaxation may involve decreased formation of inositol metabolites, reduced concentration of cytosolic Ca^{2+}, and inhibition of contractile proteins. NO and

NO donors also relax human airway smooth muscle in vitro via activation of guanylyl cyclase and an increase in cyclic GMP (65,66). Sadeghi-Hashjin et al. (67) showed, in a perfused organ bath system, that a number of substances increasing cGMP such as Zaprinast (an inhibitor of cGMP phosphodiesterase) and 8-bromo-cGMP caused a concentration-dependent relaxation of guinea pig trachea. Inactivation of guanylate cyclase induced an airway hyperresponsiveness in vivo and in vitro (67).

Under physiological conditions NO can react with reduced thiols, which lead to the production of *S*-nitrosothiols, that have a substantially greater half-life than NO (68,69). It is possible that these thiols can be produced in the airway lining fluid (70). *S*-nitrosothiols cause relaxation of human and guinea pig airway tissue in vitro (70,71). In vivo inhalation of nitric oxide diminishes the airways contractions induced by cholinergic receptor agonists in guinea pigs, rabbits, and humans (72–74).

Contractile agents, including histamine, stimulate the constitutive nitric oxide synthase (75). Endothelial NOS is expressed in cultured human bronchial epithelium (76). A cultured human epithelial cell line produces nitrite spontaneously, which can be suppressed by a nitric oxide synthesis inhibitor and restored by L-arginine, suggesting the constitutive production of NO (77). The constitutive and inducible NOS is present in rat and human epithelial cells (78–80). Immunoreactivity for NOS has been demonstrated in epithelium of both large and small airways (78,81). Rengasamy et al. (82) showed NOS immunoreactivity within rat respiratory epithelium but not in the bronchial smooth muscle. In contrast, guanylate cyclase activity was shown in respiratory smooth muscle but not in the epithelium pointing to a paracrine role of NO in bronchial function. Clara cells in the small airways contain NADPH diaphorase, which has been suggested to be identical with NOS (83,84). Robbins et al. (85) clearly substantiated the role of inducible NOS in a murine epithelial cell line. Stimulation with a mixture of cytokines (IL-1, TNFα, and IFN-γ) elevated nitrite levels by 873%, increased NOS activity, and increased inducible NOS mRNA. Dexamethasone decreased these cytokine-induced increases. Also in primary cultured human airway epithelial cells, a mixture of cytokines increased inducible NOS (85). Cytokines released by mononuclear cells could, therefore, induce airway epithelial cells to express inducible NOS and to release NO. Guo et al. (86), on the other hand, showed through molecular cloning that NO synthesis in normal human airways is due to a continuous expression of the inducible NOS in airway epithelial cells.

We provided pharmacological evidence that one of the epithelium-derived relaxing factors might be NO (87). In a perfused tracheal tube set up according to Pavlovic et al. (88), in which selectively the serosal (out)side or the mucosal (in)side of the trachea can be stimulated with drugs, it was demonstrated that luminal perfusion of guinea pig tracheal tubes in vitro with NO

synthesis inhibitors shifted the maximum effect of the histamine concentration-response curve upward by 335%. This effect was mimicked by removal of
airway epithelium, suggesting that the airway epithelial layer releases NO,
which counteracts the bronchoconstrictor effect of spasmogens (87). Addition
of L-NAME to epithelium-denuded tissues did not further increase the responsiveness to histamine. Furthermore, the effect of L-NAME was concentration-dependently inhibited by coincubation with L-arginine. In additional
experiments it was investigated whether these effects were species specific.
When fourth- and fifth-generation airways of the horse were incubated with
L-NAME, the maximal contraction in response to histamine was increased by
250%. Similar findings were observed in bronchi of humans (89). This means
that the effect with the NO synthesis inhibitors is not species specific.

Interestingly, bradykinin induces a concentration-dependent relaxation
when applied on the inside of intact tracheal tubes, which could be reversed
into a contraction by either preincubation with NO synthesis inhibitors or
epithelium removal (90). The bradykinin-induced relaxations were associated
with an increase in cGMP and blocked by the kinin B_2-receptor antagonist
HOE 140, but not influenced by indomethacin (90).

The release of NO by the epithelial layer was further confirmed in a
non-receptor-mediated study (38). Potassium applied to the mucosal side induced a concentration-dependent relaxation in intact tissues and a potent mo-
nophasic contractions in skinned preparations. Addition of potassium on the
outside induced an identical contraction. Preincubations of the tracheal tubes
on the inside with L-NAME prevented the potassium-induced relaxation, but
did not reverse the relaxation into a contraction (38). This means that the
epithelial layer acts as a firm barrier, which does not allow even a simple
molecule such as potassium to penetrate to the smooth muscle layer. It is likely
that potassium induces a depolarization of epithelial cells, which causes the
release of NO and a subsequent relaxation, and in epithelium-denuded preparations, potassium induces depolarization of smooth muscle cells, which causes
a contraction.

VI. NO and Virus-Induced Airway Hyperresponsiveness

As mentioned above, epithelial damage, airway inflammation, and an enhanced
release of reactive oxygen species by inflammatory cells are observed during
both viral respiratory infections and asthma (7,8,91,92). We showed that intratracheal inoculation of parainfluenza type 3 virus to guinea pigs induces a
marked increase in airway responsiveness to histamine in vivo and in vitro
(59,60,93,94). Interestingly, after inhalation of low doses of L-arginine this hyperresponsiveness is completely blocked (95). In addition, preincubation of

L-arginine concentration-dependently inhibited the virus-induced tracheal hyperresponsiveness to histamine in vitro. Indeed, in control tissues the mild contractions induced by histamine were associated with a significant NO release. In contrast, the release of NO from virus-inoculated tracheal tubes was diminished by 75% and associated with a significantly enhanced contraction. The decreased production of NO could, like the increased contraction, be restored by preincubation of L-arginine (95). Moreover, the virus-induced tracheal hyperresponsiveness could not be further enhanced by preincubation of the tissues with the NOS inhibitor with L-NAME. Therefore, it is likely that a deficiency in endogenous NO after a viral infection is due to a dysfunction of the constitutive NOS. Interestingly, Saiboku-to, a traditional Chinese herbal medicine that has been widely used in the treatment of asthma in Asian countries, stimulates the epithelial NO generation (96).

Among others, four possible mechanisms may account for the NO deficiency in virally infected airways. First, the decreased nitric oxide production can be explained by substrate limitation, e.g., a decreased concentration of L-arginine in virus-treated animals. However, intracellular levels of arginine are already high and the supply of arginine is normally not rate-limiting for the constitutive enzyme (97). On the other hand, the possibility cannot be excluded that the activity of arginase, the enzyme that breaks down arginine, is increased. Arginase is widely distributed in the body including the lungs (98) and is elevated during growth of tissues and tumors (99). Whether the arginase activity is increased in the lungs during viral respiratory infections needs to be investigated.

The epithelial layer is damaged in virus-infected animals (57,59). Therefore, a second explanation for the lack in NO production in virus-treated animals is a diminished activity or availability of the constitutive NOS, which might be due to epithelial damage. In biopsies of human airways, immunoreactivity to inducible NOS was seen in the epithelium in 22 of 23 asthmatic cases, but in only 2 of 14 nonasthmatic controls (100). Although in normal subjects during symptomatic upper respiratory tract infections the concentration of NO in exhaled air is markedly increased (101), it cannot be excluded that the NO released by the activity of the constitutive enzyme is diminished during bronchoconstriction.

Third, during viral infections interferon-γ is produced (102–104). This might stimulate inducible NOS and the high amount of NO could inactivate the constitutive NOS (105–107).

The last mechanism by which the concentration of NO can be decreased is the following. Nitric oxide is inactivated by products released from inflammatory cells, i.e., superoxide anions (62,75). Parainfluenza type 3 virus activates inflammatory cells (57,58) and the number of inflammatory cells is increased in lungs of virus-infected guinea pigs (58,60). Naïve guinea pig tracheas incubated with inflammatory cells obtained from lungs of virus-treated animals become hyperresponsive to histamine (108). Besides decreasing the nitric oxide concentration, the reactive peroxynitrite (ONOO-) is produced by the interaction of superoxide anions with nitric oxide (69,75), which accordingly may lead to "additional" epithelial damage. Interestingly, Akaike et al. (109) demonstrated a role for peroxynitrite in the pathogenesis of influenza virus–induced pneumonia in mice. By means of an immunohistochemical study, they showed formation of peroxynitrite by inflammatory cells, including macrophages and neutrophils, and of intraalveolar exudate. Their results suggest formation of peroxynitrite in the lung through the reaction of NO with superoxide, which is generated by alveolar phagocytic cells and xanthine oxidase. We recently demonstrated that incubation of tracheal tubes with peoxynitrite induces airway hyperresponsiveness and epithelial damage (110). Moreover, harmful effects to eosinophils and an increase in major basic protein levels were observed after peroxynitrite exposure. Whether the epithelial damage is due to a direct effect of peroxynitrite or is due to the release of mediators from eosinophils is not clear. Further, intratracheal inoculation of peroxynitrite (100 nmol) in vivo induces, like viruses, a long-lasting airway hyperresponsiveness (>20 days) as measured by the increase in pulmonary resistance after intravenously administered histamine (110).

Therefore, a number of processes may act additive or synergistically during the development of virus-induced airway hyperresponsiveness.

VII. Functional Effects of NO Acting on Prostaglandin H Synthase

The epithelial layer of the bovine trachea releases a basal amount of NO, which can be increased by L-arginine incubation or histamine stimulation (111). These effects can be inhibited by the nitric oxide synthase inhibitor L-NMMA (111). Histamine also increased the release of PGE_2. Surprisingly, this increase was inhibited by L-NMMA (Fig. 1). Similar results were obtained in a functional study using the guinea pig tracheal tube. The arachidonic acid concentration-response curve was shifted to the right in tracheal tubes incubated with L-NAME, which points to a diminished PGE_2 and/or enhanced leukotriene production (Fig. 2). Further, preincubation of the tracheas with L-NAME resulted in a significant upward shift of the histamine concentration-response curve with a concomitant inhibition of prostaglandin E_2 production compared to controls (51). Interestingly, preincubation of the preparations with a 5-lipoxygenase inhibitor (AA-861) or a leukotriene C_4,D_4,E_4-receptor antagonist (FPL 55712) totally blocked the L-NAME-

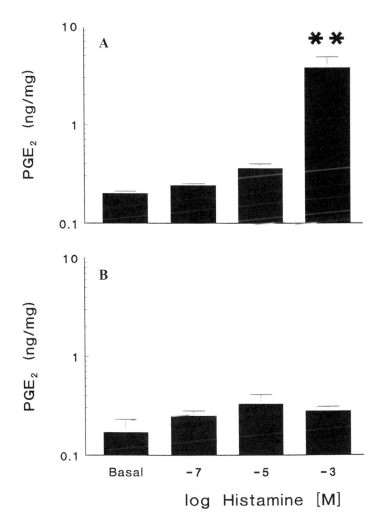

Figure 1 The release of PGE$_2$ from the epithelial layer of bovine isolated trachea is increased by histamine (A). Preincubation of the nitric oxide synthase inhibitor L-NMMA (120 μM) for 25 min completely prevented the histamine-induced increase in PGE$_2$ by the epithelial layer (B). $^{**}p < 0.01, n = 4$.

induced tracheal hyperresponsiveness. These data are in line with the findings of Adcock and Garland (112), who demonstrated that guinea pig tracheal hyperresponsiveness to histamine, after cyclooxygenase inhibition, was attributable to an augmenting effect of lipoxygenase products. Now, abundant evidence has been obtained that leukotrienes are involved in airway

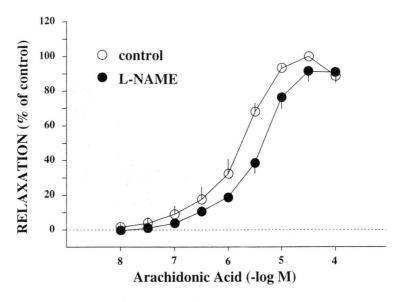

Figure 2 Arachidonic acid–induced relaxations of the perfused guinea pig tracheal tube. The concentration-response curve is shifted rightward in tissues preincubated with the nitric oxide synthase inhibitor L-NAME (120 μM, 25 min). $pD_2 = 5.81 \pm 0.13$ for the control group and $pD_2 = 5.34 \pm 0.08$ for the L-NAME group ($p < 0.02, n = 5$).

hyperresponsiveness (113). Biochemical data support the interaction between NO and cyclooxygenase. As predicted, indomethacin prevents the increase in PGE_2 production by tracheal tubes after histamine stimulation (Fig. 3). Surprisingly, indomethacin doubled the NO production after histamine stimulation. In contrast, L-NAME decreased both the NO and PGE_2 production after histamine stimulation (Fig. 3). These results point to an interaction between NO and prostaglandin H synthase.

VIII. Hypothesis on the Interaction of NO on PGHS in the Respiratory Airways

From the biochemical data provided above it is clear that NO can stimulate PGHS via many different ways. In our airway reactivity measurements it was also concluded that there was an interaction between NO and PGE_2 release. Since receptor stimulation was involved in this process, it is very likely that

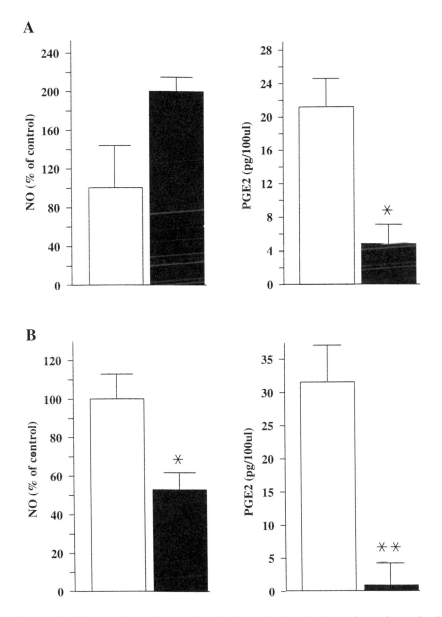

Figure 3 Nitric oxide and prostaglandin E_2 production by the guinea pig tracheal tube after incubation with (A) indomethacin (1 μM, 25 min) or (B) L-NAME (120 μM, 25 min) and stimulation with histamine (1 mM). After indomethacin incubation the histamine-induced NO release was doubled and the prostaglandin E_2 production was significantly decreased (*$p < 0.02$, A). Incubation of L-NAME decreased the nitric oxide production by 50% (*$p < 0.05$, B) and completely inhibited the prostaglandin E_2 synthesis (*$p < 0.001$, B). $n = 3$.

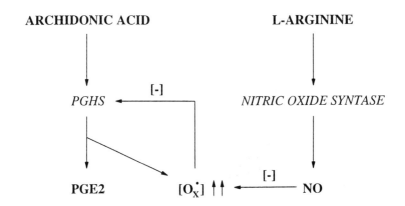

Figure 4 PGHS converts arachidonic acid into prostaglandins by which reactive oxygen species are formed. Via a negative feedback system, reactive oxygen species inhibit the activity of PGHS by which less prostaglandins are formed. Nitric oxide synthase forms nitric oxide from L-arginine. Nitric oxide can interfere with reactive oxygen species formed by the metabolism of arachidonic acid. This leads to less inhibition of the reactive oxygen species on PGHS and hence more prostaglandins will be formed.

cNOS and PGHS-1, and not iNOS and PGHS-2, contributed to the observed effects.

Stimulation of PGHS leads to the formation of prostaglandins and oxygen free radicals. These oxygen free radicals can turn off COX activity by which less prostaglandins are formed (negative feedback system, Fig. 4). However, receptor stimulation also leads to activation of cNOS and the release of NO. Part of this NO may interact with the oxygen free radicals released by activation of PGHS. When the concentration of oxygen free radicals is decreased, less inhibition takes place on PGHS and more prostaglandins will be formed (Fig. 4).

Inhibition of NO production by NOS inhibitors will lead to less interaction with oxygen free radicals and accordingly to inhibition of PGHS and less PGE$_2$ production. This may explain why in the bovine epithelial layer and guinea pig trachea the increased PGE$_2$ production after stimulation with histamine or arachidonic acid is decreased after NOS inhibition. NO and histamine can stimulate phospholipase A$_2$ and/or C. The activity of either enzyme causes the metabolism of arachidonic acid. Therefore, it is likely that enough arachidonic is available for conversion. If PGHS is inhibited, more free arachidonic acid is available for the lipoxygenase enzyme and hence more leukotrienes will be formed. It is likely that these leukotrienes are involved in the development of airway hyperresponsiveness.

References

1. Busse WW. Respiratory infections and bronchial hyperreactivity. J Allergy Clin Immunol 1988; 81:770–775.
2. Busse WW. Respiratory infections: their role in airway responsiveness and the pathogenesis of asthma. J Allergy Clin Immunol 1990; 85:671–683.
3. Bardin PG, Johnston SL, Pattemore PK. Viruses as precipitants of asthma symptoms. II. Physiology and mechanisms. Clin Exp Allergy 1992; 22:809–822.
4. Pattemore PK, Johnston SL, Bardin PG. Viruses as precipitants of asthma symptoms. Clin Exp Allergy 1992; 22:325–336.
5. Sterk PJ. Virus-induced airway hyperresponsiveness in man. Eur Respir J 1993; 6:894–902.
6. Folkerts G, Nijkamp FP. Virus-induced airway hyperresponsiveness: role of inflammatory cells and mediators. Am J Respir Crit Care Med 1995; 151:1666–1674.
7. Folkerts G, Nijkamp FP. Cells and mediators involved in airway hyperresponsiveness. In: Tarayre JP, Vergaftig B, Carilla E, eds. New Concepts in Asthma. London: Macmillan, 1993:224–244.
8. Laitinen LA, Heino M, Laitinen A, Kava T, Haahtela T. Damage of the airway epithelium and bronchial reactivity in patients with asthma. Am Rev Respir Dis 1985; 131:599–606.
9. Kelner MJ, Uglik SF. Mechanism of prostaglandin E_2 release and increase in PGH2/PGE2 isomerase activity by PDGF: involvement of nitric oxide. Arch Biochem Biophys 1994; 312:240–243.
10. Salvemini D, Misko TP, Masferrer JL, Seibert K, Currie MG, Needleman P. Nitric oxide activates cyclooxygenase enzymes. Proc Natl Acad Sci USA 1993; 90:7240–7244.
11. Tetsuka T, Daphna-Iken D, Baier LD, DuMaine J, Morrison A. Cross-talk between cyclo-oxygenase and nitric oxide pathways: Prostaglandin E_2 negatively modulates induction of nitric oxide synthase by interleukin-1. Proc Natl Acad Sci USA 1994; 91:12168–12172.
12. Gryglewski RJ. Interactions between endothelial mediators (minireview). Pharmacol Toxicol 1995; 77:1–9.
13. Milano S, Arcoleo E, Dieli M, D'Agostino P, DeNucci G, Cillari E. Prostaglandin E_2 regulates inducible nitric oxide synthase in the murine macrophage cell line J774. Prostaglandins 1995; 49:105–115.
14. Swierkosz TA, Mitchell JA, Warner TD, Botting RM, Vane JR. Co-induction of nitric oxide synthase and cyclo-oxygenase: interactions between nitric oxide and prostanoids. Br J Pharmacol 1995; 114:1335–1342.
15. Mitchell JA, DeNucci G, Warner TD, Vane JR. Different patterns of release of endothelium-derived relaxing factor and prostacyclin. Br J Pharmacol 1992; 105:485–489.
16. Amin AR, Vyas P, Atuur M, Leszczynska-Piziak J, Patel IR, Weissmann G, et al. The mode of action of aspirin-like drugs: effect on inducible nitric oxide synthase. Proc Natl Acad Sci USA 1995; 92:7926–7930.

17. Mitchell JA, Swierkosz TA, Warner TD, Gross S, Thiemermann C, Vane JR. Regulation of prostacyclin synthesis by the release of endogenous nitric oxide in response to bacterial lipopolysaccharide. Br J Pharmacol 1993; 109:4P.

18. Akarasereenont P, Mitchell JA, Bahkle YS, Thiemermann C, Vane JR. Comparison of the induction of cyclooxygenase and nitric oxide synthase by endotoxin in endothelial cells and macrophages. Eur J Pharmacol 1995; 273:121–128.

19. Xu XP, Tanner MA, Myers PR. Prostaglandin-mediated inhibition of nitric oxide production by bovine aortic endothelium during hypoxia. Cardiovasc Res 1995; 30:345–350.

20. Inoue T, Fukuo K, Morimoto S, Koh E, Ogihara T. Nitric oxide mediates interleukin-1 induced prostaglandin E_2 production by vascular smooth muscle cells. Biochem Biophys Res Commun 1993; 194:420–424.

21. Davidge ST, Baker PN, McLaughlin MK, Roberts JM. Nitric oxide produced by endothelial cells increases production of eicosanoids through activation of prostaglandin H synthase. Circ Res 1995; 77:274–283.

22. Misko TP, Trotter JL, Cross AH. Mediation of inflammation by encephalitogenic cells: interferon g induction of nitric oxide synthase and cyclooxygenase 2. J Neuroimmunol 1995; 61:195–204.

23. Mitchell JA, Larkin S, Williams TJ. Cyclooxygenase-2: regulation and relevance in inflammation. Biochem Pharmacol 1995; 50:1535–1542.

24. Vane JR, Mitchell JA, Appleton I, Tomlinson A, Bishop-Bailey D, Croxtall J, et al. Inducible isoforms of cyclooxygenase and nitric-oxide synthase in inflammation. Proc Natl Acad Sci USA 1994; 91:2046–2050.

25. Franchi AM, Chaud M, Rettori V, Suburo A, McCann SM, Gimeno M. Role of nitric oxide in eocosanoid synthesis and uterine motility in estrogen-treated rat uteri. Proc Natl Acad Sci USA 1994; 91:539–543.

26. Keen M, Pickering SAW, Hunt JA. Modulation of the bradykinin-stimulated release of prostaglandin from endothelial cells. Br J Pharmacol 1990; 101:524P.

27. Salvemini D, Deibert K, Masferrer JL, Misko TP, Currie MG, Needleman P. Endogenous nitric oxide enhances prostaglandin production in a model of renal inflammation. J Clin Invest 1994; 93:1940–1947.

28. Sautebin L, Ialenti A, Ianaro A, Di Rosa M. Modulation by nitric oxide of prostaglandin biosynthesis in the rat. Br J Pharmacol 1995; 114:323–328.

29. Rainsford KD, Swann BP. The biochemistry and pharmacology of oxygen radical involvement in eicosanoid production. In: Bannister JV, Bannister WH, eds. The Biology and Chemistry of Active Oxygen. New York: Elsevier, 1984:105–127.

30. Muijsers RBR, Folkerts G, Henricks PAJ, Sadeghi-Hashjin G, Nijkamp FP. Peroxynitrite: a two faced metabolite of nitric oxide. Life Sci 1997; 60:1833–1845.

31. Beckman JS, Koppenol WH. Nitric oxide, superoxide, and peroxynitrite: the good, the bad, and the ugly. Am J Physiol 1996; 271:C1424–1437.

32. Landino LM, Crews BC, Timmons MD, Morrow JD, Marnett LJ. Peroxynitrite, the coupling product of nitric oxide and superoxide, activates prostaglandin biosynthesis. Proc Natl Acad Sci USA 1996; 93:15069–15074.

33. Schmidt HHHW, Hofmann H, Schindler U, Shutenko ZS, Cunningham DD, Feelisch M. No NO from NO synthase. Proc Natl Acad Sci USA 1996; 93:14492–14497.

34. Tsai A, Wei C, Kulmacz RJ. Interaction between nitric oxide and prostaglandin H synthase. Arch Biochem Biophys 1994; 313:367–372.

35. Hajjar DP, Lander HM, Pearce SFA, Upmacis RK, Pomerantz KB. Nitric oxide enhances prostaglandin-H synthase-1 activity by a heme-independent mechanism: evidence implicating nitrosothiols. J Am Chem Soc 1995; 117:3340–3346.

36. Barnes PJ, Cuss FM, Palmer JB. The effect of airway epithelium on smooth muscle contractility in bovine trachea. Br J Pharmacol 1985; 86:685–691.

37. Vanhoutte PM. Epithelium-derived relaxing factor(s) and bronchial reactivity. Am Rev Respir Dis 1988; 138:S24–30.

38. Folkerts G, Linde van der H, Verheyen AKCP, Nijkamp FP. Endogenous nitric oxide modulation of potassium-induced changes in guinea pig airway tone. Br J Pharmacol 1995; 115:1194–1198.

39. Orehek J, Douglas JS, Lewis AJ, Bouhuys A. Prostaglandin regulation of airway smooth muscle tone. Nature New Biol 1973; 245:84–85.

40. Steel L, Kaliner M. Prostaglandin-generating factor of anaphylaxis. J Biol Chem 1981; 256:12692–12698.

41. Grodzinska L, Panczenko B, Gryglewski RJ. Generation of prostaglandin-E like material by the guinea pig trachea contracted by histamine. J Pharm Pharmacol 1975; 27:88–91.

42. Churchill L. Resau JH, Bascom R, Hubbard WC, Proud D. Production of prostaglandins (PGs) by human tracheal epithelial cells in culture. FASEB J 1988; 2:A959.

43. Butler GB, Adler KB, Evans JN, Morgan DW, Szarek JL. Modulation of rabbit airway smooth muscle responsiveness by respiratory epithelium. Am Rev Respir Dis 1987; 135:1099–1104.

44. Asano K, Lilly CM, Drazen JM. Prostaglandin G/H synthase-2 is the constitutive and dominant isoform in cultured human lung epithelial cells. Am J Physiol 1996; 271:L126–131.

45. Campbell AM, Chanez P, Vignola AM, Bousquet J, Couret I, Michel FB, et al. Functional characteristics of bronchial epithelium obtained by brusing from asthmatic and normal subjects. Am Rev Respir Dis 1993; 147:529–534.

46. Noah TL, Paradiso AM, Madden MC, McKinnon K, Devlin RB. The response of a human bronchial epithelial cell line to histamine: intracellular calcium changes and extracellular release of inflammatory mediators. Am J Respir Cell Mol Biol 1991; 5:484–492.

47. Mathe AA, Hedqvist P, Strandberg K, Leslie CA. Aspects of prostaglandin function in the lung. N Engl J Med 1977; 296:850–910.

48. Anderson WH, Krzanowski JJ, Polson JB, Szentivanyi A. The effect of prostaglandin E_2 on histamine-stimulated calcium mobilization as a possible explanation for histamine tachyphylaxis in canine tracheal smooth muscle. Naunyn Schmiedebergs Arch Pharmacol 1983; 322:72–77.

49. Braunstein G, Labat C, Brunelleschi S, Benveniste J, Marsac J, Brink C. Evidence that the histamine sensitivity and responsiveness of guinea-pig isolated trachea are modulated by epithelial prostaglandin E_2 production. Br J Pharmacol 1988; 95: 300–308.

50. Orehek J, Douglas JS, Bouhuys A. Contractile responses of the guinea-pig trachea in vitro: modification by prostaglandin synthesis-inhibiting drugs. J Pharmacol Exp Ther 1975; 194:554–564.

51. Nijkamp FP, Folkerts G. Reversal of arachidonic acid-induced guinea-pig tracheal relaxation into contraction after epithelium removal. Eur J Pharmacol 1987; 131: 315–316.

52. Folkerts G, Engels F, Nijkamp FP. Endotoxin-induced hyperreactivity of the guinea pig isolated trachea coincides with decreased prostaglandin E_2 production by the epithelial layer. Br J Pharmacol 1989; 96:388–394.

53. Folkerts G, Van der Linde H, Van de Loo PGF, Engels F, Nijkamp FP. Leukotrienes mediate tracheal hyperresponsiveness after nitric oxide synthesis inhibition. Eur J Pharmacol 1995; 285:R1–2.

54. Engels F, Folkerts G, Van Heuven-Nolsen D, Nijkamp FP. Haemophilus influenzae-induced decreases in lung β-adrenoceptor function and number coincide with decreases in spleen noradrenaline. Naunyn Schmiedebergs Arch Pharmacol 1987; 336:274–279.

55. Van Heuven-Nolsen D, Folkerts G, De Wildt DJ, Nijkamp FP. The influence of Bordetella pertussis and its constituents on the beta-adrenergic receptor in the guinea pig respiratory system. Life Sci 1986; 38:677–685.

56. Folkerts G, Nijkamp FP. Haemophilus influenzae induces a potential increase in guinea pig pulmonary resistance to histamine. Eur J Pharmacol 1985; 119: 117–120.

57. Folkerts G, Verheyen A, Nijkamp FP. Viral infection in guinea pigs induces a sustained non-specific airway hyperresponsiveness and morphological changes of the respiratory tract. Eur J Pharmacol 1992; 228:121–130.

58. Folkerts G, Esch B van, Janssen M, Nijkamp FP. Virus-induced airway hyperresponsiveness in guinea pigs in vivo: study of broncho-alveolar cell number and activity. Eur J Pharmacol 1992; 228(4):219–227.

59. Folkerts G, Verheyen AKCP. Geuens GMA, Folkerts HF, Nijkamp FP. Virus-induced changes in airway responsiveness, morphology, and histamine levels in guinea pigs. Am Rev Respir Dis 1993; 147:1569–1577.

60. Folkerts G, De Clerck F, Reijnart I, Span P, Nijkamp FP. Virus-induced airway hyperresponsiveness in the guinea-pig: possible involvement of histamine and inflammatory cells. Br J Pharmacol 1993; 108:1083–1093.

61. Goodman LS, Gilman A. The Pharmacological Basis of Therapeutics. Philadelphia: Lea & Febiger, 1936.

62. Nijkamp FP, Folkerts G. Nitric oxide and bronchial reactivity. Clin Exp Allergy 1994; 24:905–914.

63. Gruetter GA, Childers CE, Bosserman MK, Lemke SM, Ball JG, Valentovic MA. Comparison of relaxation induced by glyceryl trinitrate, isosorbide dinitrate, and sodium nitroprusside in bovine airways. Am Rev Respir Dis 1989; 139:1192–1197.

64. Sadeghi-Hashjin G, Folkerts G, Henricks PAJ, Van de Loo PGF, Dik IEM, Nijkamp FP. Relaxation of guinea pig trachea by sodium nitroprusside: cyclic GMP and nitric oxide not involved. Br J Pharmacol 1996; 118:466–470.

65. Ward JK, Barnes PJ, Springall DR, Abelli L, Tadjkarimi S, Yacoub MH, et al. Distribution of human i-NANC bronchodilator and nitric oxide-immunoreactive nerves. Am J Respir Cell Mol Biol 1995; 13:175–184.
66. Gaston B, Fackler JC, Drazen JM, Singel DJ, Reilly J, Mullin M, et al. Nitrogen oxides in normal and abnormal tracheal secretions. Am Rev Respir Dis 1993; 147:A455.
67. Sadeghi-Hashjin G, Folkerts G, Henricks PAJ, Van de Loo PGF, Van der Linde HJ, Dik IEM. Induction of guinea pig airway hyperresponsiveness by inactivation of guanylate cyclase. Eur J Pharmacol 1996; 302:109–115.
68. Oae S, Shinhama K. Organic thionitrites and related substances. Org Prep Proc Int 1983, 15:165–198.
69. Nijkamp FP, Folkerts G. Nitric oxide and bronchial hyperresponsiveness. Arch Int Pharmacodyn Ther 1995; 329:81–96.
70. Gaston B, Reilly J, Drazen JM, Fackler J, Ramden P, Arnelle D, et al. Endogenous nitrogen oxides and bronchodilator S-nitrosolthiols in human airways. Proc Natl Acad Sci USA 1993; 90:10957–10961.
71. Bynoe TC, Stuart-Smith K, Hirshman CA. Porcine bronchial smooth muscle exhibits functional antagonism to relaxation to sodium nitroprusside and SIN-1. Am Rev Respir Dis 1992; 145:A399.
72. Dupuy PM, Shore SA, Drazen JM, Frostell C, Hill WA, Zapol WM. Bronchodilator action of inhaled nitric oxide in guinea pigs. J Clin Invest 1992; 90:421–428.
73. Högman M, Frostell C, Arnberg H, Hedenstierna G. Inhalation of nitric oxide modulates methacholine-induced bronchoconstriction in the rabbit. Eur Respir J 1993; 6:177–180.
74. Högman M, Frostell CG, Hedenstrom H, Hedenstrierna G. Inhalation of nitric oxide modulates adult human bronchial tone. Am Rev Respir Dis 1993; 148:1474–1478.
75. Barnes PJ, Belvisi MG. Nitric oxide and lung disease. Thorax 1993; 48:1034–1043.
76. Shaul P, North AJ, Wu LC, Wells LB, Brannon TS, Lau S, et al. Endothelial nitric oxide synthase is expressed in cultured human bronchial epithelium. J Clin Invest 1994; 94:2231–2236.
77. Chee C, Gaston B, Gerard C, Loscalzo J, Kobzik L, Drazen JM, et al. Nitric oxide is produced by human epithelial cell line. Am Rev Respir Dis 1993; 147:A433.
78. Schmidt HHHW, Gagne GD, Nakane M, Pollock JS, Miller MF, Murad F. Mapping of neural nitric oxide synthase in the rat suggests frequent co-localization with NADPH diaphorase but not with soluble guanylyl cyclase, and novel paraneural functions for nitrinergic signal transduction. J Histochem Cytochem 1992; 40: 1439–1456.
79. Hamid Q, Springall DR, Riveros-Moreno V, Chanez P, Howarth P, Redington A, et al. Induction of nitric oxide synthase in asthma. Lancet 1993; 342:1510–1513.
80. Kobzik L, Bredt DS, Lowenstein CJ, Drazen J, Gaston B, Sugarbaker D, et al. Nitric oxide synthase in human and rat lung: immunocytochemical and histochemical localization. Am J Respir Cell Mol Biol 1993; 9:371–377.
81. Fischer A, Mundel P, Mayer B, Preissler U, Phillipin B, Kummer W. Nitric oxide synthase in guinea pig lower airway innervation. Neurosci Lett 1992; 149:157–160.

82. Rengasamy A, Xue C, Johns RA. Immunohistochemical demonstration of a paracrine role of nitric oxide in bronchial function. Am J Physiol 1994; 267:L704–711.
83. Dawson TM, Bredt DS, Fotuhi M, Hwang PM, Snyder SH. Nitric oxide synthase and neuronal NADPh diaphorase are identical in brain and peripheral tissues. Proc Natl Acad Sci USA 1991; 88:7797–7801.
84. Hope BT, Micheal GJ, Knigge KM, Vincent SR. Neuronal NADPH diaphorase is a nitric oxide synthase. Proc Natl Acad Sci USA 1991; 88:2811–2814.
85. Robbins RA, Springall DR, Warren JB, Kwon OJ, Buttery LDK, Wilson AJ, et al. Inducible nitric oxide synthase is increased in murine lung epithelial cells by cytokine stimulation. Biochem Biophys Res Commun 1994; 198:835–843.
86. Guo FH, De Raeve HR, Rice TW, Stuehr DJ, Thunissen FBJM, Erzurum SC. Continuous nitric oxide synthesis by inducible nitric oxide synthase in normal human airway epithelium in vivo. Proc Natl Acad Sci USA 1995; 92:7809–7813.
87. Nijkamp FP, Van der Linde HJ, Folkerts G. Nitric oxide synthesis inhibitors induce airway hyperresponsiveness in the guinea pig in vivo and in vitro. Am Rev Respir Dis 1993; 148:727–734.
88. Pavlovic D, Fournier M, Aubier M, Pariente R. Epithelial vs. serosal stimulation of tracheal muscle: role of epithelium. J Appl Physiol 1989; 67:2522–2526.
89. Folkerts G, Van der Linde H, Schreuers AJM, Verheyen FKCP, Blomjous FJ, Nijkamp FP. Hyperresponsiveness of human bronchi after nitric oxide synthesis inhibition. Am J Respir Crit Care Med 1995; 151:A832.
90. Figini M, Ricciardolo FLM, Javdan P, Nijkamp FP, Emanueli C, Pradelles P, et al. Evidence that epithelium-derived relaxing factor released by bradykinin in the guinea pig trachea is nitric oxide. Am J Respir Crit Care Med 1996; 153:918–923.
91. Djukanovic R, Roche WR, Wilson JW, Beasley CRW, Twentyman OP, Howart PH, et al. Mucosal inflammation in asthma. Am Rev Respir Dis 1990; 142:434–4357.
92. Calhoun WJ, Reed HE, Moest DR, Stevens CA. Enhanced superoxide production by alveolar macrophages and air-space cells, airway inflammation, and alveolar macrophage density changes after segmental antigen bronchoprovocation in allergic subjects. Am Rev Respir Dis 1992; 145:317–325.
93. Oosterhout AJM, Ark van I, Folkerts G, Linde van der HJ, Savelkoul HFJ, Verheyen AKCP, et al. Antibody to interleukin-5 inhibits virus-induced airway hyperresponsiveness to histamine in guinea pigs. Am J Respir Crit Care Med 1995; 151:177–183.
94. Ladenius ARC, Folkerts G, Linde van der HJ, Nijkamp FP. Potentiation by viral respiratory infection of ovalbumin-induced guinea pig tracheal hyperresponsiveness: role for tachykinins. Br J Pharmacol 1995; 115:1048–1052.
95. Folkerts G, Linde van der HJ, Nijkamp FP. Virus-induced airway hyperresponsiveness in guinea pigs is related to a deficiency in nitric oxide. J Clin Invest 1995; 95:26–30.
96. Tamaoki J, Kondo M, Ciyotani A, Takemura H, Konno K. Effect of Saiboku-to, an antiasthmatic herbal medicine, on nitric oxide generation from cultured canine airway epithelial cells. Jpn J Pharmacol 1995; 69:29–35.
97. McCall T, Vallance P. Nitric oxide takes centre-stage with newly defined roles. TIPS 1992; 13:1–6.

98. Aminlari M, Vaseghi T. Arginase distribution in tissues of domestic animals. Comp Biochem Physiol 1992; 103B:385–389.

99. Taylor AA, Stewart GR. Tissue and subcellular localization of enzymes of arginine metabolism in pisum sativum. Biochem Biophys Res Commun 1981; 101: 1281–1289.

100. Springall DR, Hamid OA, Buttery LKD, Chanez P, Howart P, Bousquet J, et al. Nitric oxide synthase induction in airways of asthmatic subjects. Am Rev Respir Dis 1993; 147:A515.

101. Kharitonov SA, Yates D, Barnes PJ. Increased nitric oxide in exhaled air of normal human subjects with upper respiratory tract infections. Eur Respir J 1995; 8:295–297.

102. Hall CB, Douglas RG, Simons RL, Geiman JM. Interferon production in children with respiratory syncytial, influenza, and parainfluenza virus infections. J Pediatr 1978; 93:28–33.

103. Harmon AT, Harmon MW, Glezen WP. Evidence of interferon production in the hamster lung after primary or secondary exposure to parainfluenza virus type 3. Am Rev Respir Dis 1982; 125:706–711.

104. Vacheron F, Rudent A, Perin S, Labarre C, Quero AM, Guenounou M. Production of interleukin 1 and tumour necrosis factor activities in bronchoalveolar washings following infection of mice by influenza virus. J Gen Vir 1990; 71:477–479.

105. Lu J-L, Schmiege LM, Kuo L, Liao JC. Downregulation of endothelial constitutive nitric oxide synthase expression by lipopolysaccharide. Biochem Biophys Res Commun 1996; 225:1–5.

106. De Kimpe SJ, Tielemans W, Van Heuven-Nolsen D, Nijkamp FP. Reversal of bradykinin-induced relaxation to contractiion after interferon-gamma bovine isolated mesenteric arteries. Eur J Pharmacol 1994; 261:111–120.

107. Rengasamy A, Johns RA. Regulation of nitric oxide synthase by nitric oxide. Mol Pharmacol 1993; 44:124–128.

108. Folkerts G, Verheyen A, Janssen M, Nijkamp FP. Virus-induced airway hyperresponsiveness in the guinea pig can be transferred by bronchoalveolar cells. J Allergy Clin Immunol 1992; 90:364–372.

109. Akaike T, Noguchi Y, Ijiri S, Setoguchi K, Suga M, Zheng YM, et al. Pathogenesis of influenza virus-induced pneumonia: involvement of both nitric oxide and oxygen radicals. Proc Natl Acad Sci USA 1996; 93:2448–2453.

110. Sadeghi-Hashjin G, Folkerts G, Henricks PAJ, Verheyen AKCP, Van der Linde IIJ, Van Ark I, et al. Peroxynitrite induces airway hyperresponsiveness in guinea pigs in vitro and in vivo. Am J Respir Crit Care Med 1996; 153:1697–1701.

111. Sadeghi-Hashjin G, Folkerts G, Henricks PAJ, Verheyen AKCP, Van der Linde HJ, Nijkamp FP. Bovine tracheal responsiveness in vitro: role of epithelium and nitric oxide. Eur Respir J 1996; 9:2286–2293.

112. Adcock JJ, Garland LG. A possible role for lipoxygenase products as regulators of airway smooth muscle reactivity. Br J Pharmacol 1980; 69:167–169.

113. O'Byrne PM. Eicosanoids and Asthma. Ann NY Acad Sci 1994; 744:251–261.

14

The Pharmacology of Prostaglandin E₂
Actions in Human Diseases Involving the Mast Cell

JOHN A. OATES,
JOHN J. MURRAY,
JAMES R. SHELLER,
RYSZARD DWORSKI,
and L. JACKSON ROBERTS II

Vanderbilt University School of Medicine
Vanderbilt Medical Center
Nashville, Tennessee

DAVID D. HAGAMAN

St. Thomas Hospital
Nashville, Tennessee

HOWARD R. KNAPP

University of Iowa School of Medicine
Iowa City, Iowa

I. Introduction

Prostaglandin E₂ (PGE₂) is known to inhibit activation-initiated responses of a number of bone marrow–derived inflammatory cells including the neutrophils (1–4), peritoneal and alveolar macrophages (5–7), some T lymphocytes (8; see 9–11), and mast cells (12,13). These inhibitory effects are associated with an elevation of intracellular cyclic AMP. The actions of PGE₂ on neutrophils and mast cells appear to be mediated through the EP2 subtype of the PGE₂ receptors. The present studies address the effect of PGE₂ and the PGE analog misoprostol on the function of mast cells in human diseases.

Episodes of aspirin-induced systemic mast cell activation (aspirin-induced anaphylactoid attacks) are manifested clinically by marked vasodilatation with flushing, hypotension, tachycardia, and in some cases syncope. The systemic release of mast cell mediators also causes pruritus, urticaria, dyspnea, hypoxia, and gastrointestinal symptoms that include abdominal cramping, nausea, vomiting, and diarrhea. Although dyspnea, cough, and bronchorrhea can be severe, asthma is not a feature of this syndrome.

These attacks can be triggered by aspirin, even in doses as low as 20 mg, and by all cyclooxygenase inhibitors. The attacks may be severe and even

253

fatal. Aspirin-induced systemic mast cell activation may occur in patients with systemic mastocytosis or in those without this disease of mast cell hyperproliferation.

During aspirin-induced anaphylactoid attacks, it is possible to measure massive release of mast cell mediators. Urinary histamine and methylhistamine are increased, often by more than an order of magnitude. In some patients, a urinary metabolite of prostaglandin D_2 also is elevated.

We hypothesized that inhibition of the cyclooxygenase enzyme causes these anaphylactoid attacks because a product of that enzyme acts constitutively to restrain mast cell activation. Inasmuch as PGD_2 was actually increased during some attacks, it was thought unlikely that PGD_2 was acting to inhibit mast cell activation. Because of this and the known action of PGE_2 to inhibit mast cell activation in vitro, the effects of PGE_2 on aspirin-induced anaphylactoid attacks were investigated. PGE_2 was administered by infusion in a double-blinded study in which PGE_2 and vehicle were given in randomized sequence before and for 4 hr following the administration of a dose of aspirin previously shown to evoke systemic mast cell activation. It was demonstrated that PGE_2 infusion prevented the aspirin-induced attacks and totally blocked the histamine release caused by cyclooxygenase inhibition.

Many patients whose anaphylactoid attacks can be induced by cyclooxygenase inhibitors also have spontaneous episodes of systemic mast cell activation that occur in the absence of exposure to an inhibitor of cyclooxygenase. These range from mild to severe and, in some cases, require frequent therapeutic injections of epinephrine and visits to hospital emergency departments. Therefore, an unblinded pilot study was conducted to ascertain whether the orally bioavailable PGE analog misoprostol could prevent spontaneous attacks in patients with aspirin-induced anaphylactoid attacks as well as in patients whose anaphylactoid attacks were idiopathic. Although the dose of 200 μg misoprostol 4 times daily has been recommended for its therapeutic effect on the gastrointestinal tract, which is presumed to be a local action, the dose of misoprostol required to produce a systemic effect on mast cells was unknown. Therefore, the relationship of the dose to this systemic response was examined initially. It was found that doses in the range of 400 μg four times daily to 600 μg five times daily were required to maintain suppression of symptoms resulting from mast cell mediator release throughout the dosage interval. Doses of this magnitude usually could be obtained only through gradual escalation of dose to produce a tolerance to the gastrointestinal and uterine side effects.

II. Pilot Study

To provide further evidence on the dose-response curve, the effect of misoprostol in vivo on basophil histamine release studied ex vivo was examined. It was found that whereas 200-μg and 600-μg doses both would inhibit basophil histamine release at the 2-hr time point, only the 600-μg dose continued to inhibit histamine release at 6 hr (14).

In this pilot study, one patient with aspirin-induced anaphylactoid attacks was completely relieved of his spontaneous attacks by misoprostol, with a striking increase in general well-being. A patient who had idiopathic anaphylactoid attacks (not related to aspirin) who required frequent epinephrine injections and emergency department visits despite being on prednisone 35 mg/day experienced total prevention of these major attacks on misoprostol. Whereas some side effects were noted, they were considered by the patients to be acceptable in comparison with the morbidity associated with the attacks of systemic mast cell activation.

III. Misoprostol Trial in Idiopathic Anaphylactoid Attacks

Based on these pilot studies and evaluation of the dose-response curve, a double-blinded, placebo-controlled trial of misoprostol was conducted to evaluate its effects in patients with spontaneously occurring anaphylactoid attacks. Included were patients who had a history or demonstration of attacks evoked by aspirin or nonsteroidal anti-inflammatory drugs as well as patients who were tolerant to these cyclooxygenase inhibitors. This study was conducted at doses of 300–600 μg every 6 hr, the dose being dependent on the level of side effects that each individual patient deemed to be tolerable as ascertained in an open-label component of the study.

Thirteen patients participated in the study, seven with idiopathic anaphylactoid attacks, three with idiopathic anaphylactoid attacks that could be induced with aspirin, and three that were categorized as "other" (two with atopy and one with the hyperimmunoglobulin E syndrome). Misoprostol or placebo was administered for periods of 10 weeks each in randomized sequence. The severity of the attacks was assessed with an analog scale. Misoprostol significantly reduced the frequency/severity of attacks ($p = 0.0086$).

IV. Misoprostol Effect on Late-Phase Allergic Bronchoconstriction

Mast cell activation in the airway is known to contribute to the acute bronchoconstriction that results from allergen inhalation. Pavord and colleagues demonstrated that acute bronchoconstriction could be completely blocked by inhalation of prostaglandin E$_2$. Surprisingly, late bronchoconstriction, occurring 5–7 hr after allergen, also was inhibited by PGE$_2$ inhalation (15). To understand the mechanism whereby PGE$_2$ blocks late-phase bronchoconstriction,

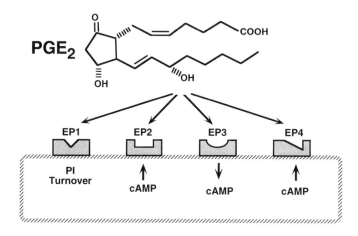

Figure 1   There are at least four subtypes of the prostaglandin E_2 (EP) receptors. The effects of PGE_2 on the EP1 receptor are transduced via phosphatidyl inositol hydrolysis. The EP2 and EP4 subtypes are G_s-coupled receptors that elevate cyclic AMP whereas the EP3 subtype is a G_i-coupled receptor that lowers cyclic AMP.

we initiated a study to determine the effects of misoprostol on the cells, mediators, and cytokines that participate in the late bronchoconstrictor response, as measured in bronchoalveolar lavage fluid obtained from a lung segment 24 hr after allergen challenge in that segment. The study is currently underway. Preliminary data demonstrate that when compared with placebo, misoprostol 600 μg four times daily for 1 week reduces the levels of interleukin-5 and LTC-4 in the bronchoalveolar lavage fluid 24 hr after allergen challenge.

V. Conclusion

The above studies have been designed to provide proof of the concept that a prostaglandin E agonist can inhibit the activation of mast cells and the release of important cytokines and mediators that determine airway inflammation and hyperreactivity. The side effects of administering misoprostol orally and the cough induced by inhaling PGE_2 limit the potential utility of these particular agents for treatment. However, it is now known that PGE_2 transduces its cellular effects through at least four major subtypes of EP receptors (Fig. 1) (16–20). Of those, EP2 and EP4 signal the elevation of cyclic AMP, and EP2 is considered to be the receptor subtype that mediates inhibition of mast cell activation. Misoprostol, which acts through the EP2 receptor, also activates the EP3 receptor, which probably accounts for the gastrointestinal and uterine side effects of this drug. Clearly, a drug that is more selective for the EP2 receptor, more potent than the current EP2 agonists, and metabolically protected would have potential for use as an orally available inhibitor of mast cell activation.

References

1. Ham EA, Soderman DD, Zanetti ME, Dougherty HW, McCauley E, Kuehl FA Jr. Inhibition by prostaglandins of leukotriene B$_4$ release from activated neutrophils. Proc Natl Acad Sci USA 1983; 80:4349–4353.
2. Fantone JC, Kinnes DA. Prostaglandin E$_1$ and prostaglandin I$_2$ modulation of superoxide production by human neutrophils. Biochem Biophys Res Commun 1983; 113:506–512.
3. Hecker G, Ney P, Schrör K. Cytotoxic enzyme release and oxygen centered radical formation in human neutrophils are selectively inhibited by E-type prostaglandins but not by PGI$_2$. Arch Pharmacol 1990; 341:308–315.
4. Wheeldon A, Vardey CJ. Characterization of the inhibitory prostanoid receptors on human neutrophils. Br J Pharmacol 1993; 108:1051–1054.
5. Kunkel SL, Spengler M, May MA, Spengler R, Larrick J, Remick D. Prostaglandin E$_2$ regulates macrophage-derived tumor necrosis factor gene expression. J Biol Chem 1988; 263(11):5380–5384.
6. Zimmer T, Jones PP. Combined effects of tumor necrosis factor-α, prostaglandin E$_2$, and corticosterone on induced Ia expression on murine macrophages. J Immunol 1990; 145(4):1167–1175.
7. Christman BW, Christman JW, Dworski R, Blair IA, Prakash C. Prostaglandin E$_2$ limits arachidonic acid availability and inhibits leukotriene B$_4$ synthesis in rat alveolar macrophages by a nonphospholipase A$_2$ mechanism. J Immunol 1993; 151:2096–2104.
8. Henney CS, Bourne HR, Lichtenstein LM. The role of cyclic 3′, 5′ adenosine monophosphate in the specific cytolytic activity of lymphocytes against mast cells. J Immunol 1972; 108:1526–1534.
9. Goodwin JS, Ceuppens J. Regulation of the immune response by prostaglandins. J Immunol 1983; 3:295–299.
10. Kunkel SL, Chensue SW. Prostaglandins and the regulation of the immune response. Adv Inflam Res 1984; 7:93–102.
11. Phipps RP, Stein SH, Roper RL. A new view of prostaglandin E regulation of the immune response. Immunol Today 1991; 12:349–352.
12. Tauber A, Kaliner M, Stechschulte DJ, Austen KF. Immunologic release of histamine and slow reacting substance of anaphylaxis from human lung. J Immunol 1973; 111(1):27–32.
13. Nials AT, Vardey CJ, Denyer LH, Thomas M, Sparrow, Shepherd GC, Coleman RA. AH13205, a selective prostanoid EP$_2$-receptor agonist. Cardiovasc Drug Rev 1993; 11:165–179.
14. Murray JJ, Mullins MD, Knapp KR, Keller SL, Serafin WE, Roberts LJ II, Struthers BJ, Oates JA. Regulation of the immune response by eicosanoids: pharmacol-

ogy and clinical effects of prostaglandin E in aspirin-sensitive syndromes. Am J Ther 1996; 140–149.

15. Pavord ID, Wong CS, Williams J, Tattersfield AE. Effect of inhaled prostaglandin E_2 on allergen-induced asthma. Am Rev Respir Dis 1993; 148:87–90.

16. Coleman RA, Smith WL, Narumiya S. International Union of Pharmacology classification of prostanoid receptors: properties, distribution, and structure of the receptors and their subtypes. Pharmacol Rev 1994; 46:205–229.

17. Breyer RM, Breyer MD. Renal prostanoid receptors. In: Schlondorff D, Bonventre J, eds. Molecular Biology of the Kidney in Health and Disease. New York: Marcel Dekker, 1995:201–213.

18. Regan JW, Bailey TJ, Pepperl DJ, Pierce KL, Bogardus AM, Donello JE, Fairbairn CE, Kedzie KM, Woodward DF, Gil DW. Cloning of a novel human prostaglandin receptor with characteristics of the pharmacologically defined EP2 subtype. Mol Pharmacol 1994; 46:213–220.

19. Katsuyama M, Nishigaki N, Sugimoto Y, Morimoto K, Negishi M, Narumiya S, Ichikawa A. The mouse prostaglandin E receptor EP2 subtype: cloning, expression, and Northern blot analysis. FEBS Lett 1995; 372:151–156.

20. Nishigaki N, Negishi M, Honda A, Sugimoto Y, Namba T, Narumiya S, Ichikawa A. Identification of prostaglandin E receptor "EP2" cloned from mastocytoma cells as EP4 subtype. FEBS Lett 1995; 364:339–341.

15

Eicosanoids in the Pathogenesis of Exercise- and Allergen-Induced Asthma

PAUL M. O'BYRNE

McMaster University
Hamilton, Ontario, Canada

I. Introduction

Asthma is a condition characterized by symptoms of wheezing, chest tightness, coughing, and dyspnea, as well as characteristic physiological abnormalities of variable airflow obstruction and airway hyperresponsiveness to bronchoconstrictor stimuli (1). Airway responsiveness is a term that describes the ability of the airways to narrow after exposure to constrictor agonists. Thus, airway hyperresponsiveness is an increased ability to develop this response. Airway hyperresponsiveness consists both of an increased sensitivity of the airways to constrictor agonists, as indicated by a smaller concentration of a constrictor agonist needed to initiate the bronchoconstrictor response (2), and a greater maximal response to the agonist (3).

Asthmatics have airway hyperresponsiveness to a wide variety of bronchoconstrictor agonists. These include inhaled pharmacological agonists, such as histamine (4), acetylcholine (5), methacholine (6), cysteinyl leukotrienes (7), and stimulatory prostaglandins (8,9). In addition, airway hyperresponsiveness is also present to a number of physical stimuli such as exercise (10), and to inhaled allergens (11).

II. Exercise-Induced Bronchoconstriction

Exercise is a common cause of bronchoconstriction in patients with asthma. The term "exercise-induced asthma" has often been used to describe this phenomenon; however, this is a misnomer, as exercise, unlike allergen inhalation (12) or occupational sensitizers (13), is not known to cause asthma, but rather causes bronchoconstriction in patients with asthma. Thus, the term "exercise-induced bronchoconstriction" is to be preferred.

Exercise-induced bronchoconstriction occurs in 70–80% of patients with current symptomatic asthma, and is more likely to occur in patients with moderate to severely increased airway responsiveness. Indeed, for any given exercise challenge, the magnitude of the resulting bronchoconstriction is correlated with the degree of airway hyperresponsiveness (14). This means that in many patients with mild, episodic asthma, who, in general, have mildly increased airway responsiveness, even strenuous exercise does not cause bronchoconstriction. Occasionally, exercise-induced bronchoconstriction can be the only manifestation of asthma, and the management of this clinical entity is different from that of patients in whom exercise-induced bronchoconstriction is only one part of regular daily symptoms.

Exercise-induced bronchoconstriction very occasionally occurs during the exercise itself. Much more commonly, bronchodilation occurs during exercise, and this lasts for 1–3 min following exercise (15). This is followed by the onset of bronchoconstriction, beginning by 3 min, which generally peaks by 10–15 min and has resolved by 60 min. Exercise-induced bronchoconstriction is likely caused by the airways' efforts to condition to body temperature and to fully humidify the increased volumes of air inhaled during exercise (16). This results in the release of bronchoconstrictor mediators (most likely from airway mast cells). The closer to body temperature and fully humidified the inspired air is during exercise, the less likely bronchoconstriction is to occur (17).

III. Exercise Refractoriness

In 1966 McNeill and colleagues (18) identified that, in many asthmatic patients with exercise-induced bronchoconstriction, the episode of bronchoconstriction is followed by a period during which exercise causes less bronchoconstriction, and that with repeated bouts of exercise the bronchoconstriction can be abolished. Subsequently, Edmunds et al. (19) labeled this effect as exercise refractoriness and noted that the refractory period after exercise generally lasts less than 4 hr. Exercise refractoriness is often described by asthmatic patients, who have identified that exercise-induced bronchoconstriction often improves with repeated bouts of exercise, separated by minutes. In the laboratory, the effect is usually demonstrated by repeated exercise challenges followed by periods of recovery during which measurements of airflow are made, most usually by the forced expired volume expired in 1 sec (FEV_1) or peak expired flows (PEF). The recovery periods are usually between 30 and 60 min.

Several mechanisms have been proposed to explain exercise refractoriness. These have included: (1) depletion of preformed mediators from mast cells, (2) a prolonged protection afforded by increases in catecholamines released during the first exercise challenge, and (3) release of inhibitory mediators during exercise bronchoconstriction, which partially protects the airways against repeated episodes of bronchoconstriction.

IV. Allergen-Induced Airway Responses

The inhalation of environmental allergens is overall the most important cause of asthma. Inhalation of allergens by sensitized subjects results in bronchoconstriction, which develops within 10 min of the inhalation, reaches a maximum within 30 min, and generally resolves within 1–3 hr, the early asthmatic response (20). In some subjects who develop an early asthmatic response, the bronchoconstriction persists and either does not return to baseline values or recurs after 3–4 hr and reaches a maximum over the next few hours, the late asthmatic response (20), and may last 24 hr or more. Furthermore, the late asthmatic response need not necessarily be preceded by a clinically evident early response. In a subset of sensitized subjects, the inhaled antigen does not cause an early response, but is followed 3–8 hr later by a late asthmatic response.

Allergen inhalation can also result in a transient increase in airway hyperresponsiveness, which has been described to occur as early as 3 hr after allergen inhalation (21) and which can persist for days or weeks after allergen inhalation (22). In general, however, allergen-induced airway hyperresponsiveness lasts 2–4 days (22). Allergen-induced airway hyperresponsiveness is most marked in subjects who develop late responses (22), although very small and transient changes also occur in individuals with isolated early responses.

Allergen-induced late responses and airway hyperresponsiveness are associated with airway inflammation (23), with numbers of activated airway eosinophils and metachromatic cells being increased at 7–8 hr and eosinophils further increased 24 hr after allergen (24). The appearance of metachromatic cells and activated eosinophils in the airways likely explains the development of late responses.

V. Investigating the Role of a Mediator in Asthma

Identifying a role for any mediator in asthma has relied on the collection of various types of evidence. The initial step has generally been to deliver the mediator, after its structure has been identified and it has been synthesized, usually by inhalation to asthmatics, to identify whether it can mimic some component of the asthmatic response. Subsequently, when assays for its measurement are available, efforts are made to measure it in biological fluids, to determine whether it is released (and excreted) during asthmatic responses. The most direct evidence is obtained when selective antagonists or synthesis inhibitors are available that block components of asthmatic responses in clinical models of asthma. The final, and most difficult, hurdle is to determine whether the mediator antagonists or synthesase inhibitors are useful in treating asthmatic patients, thereby proving that the mediator has an important role in its pathogenesis.

VI. Cysteinyl Leukotrienes and Exercise Bronchoconstriction

The cysteinyl leukotrienes are, overall, the most important mediators causing exercise-induced bronchoconstriction in asthmatics. This was not immediately

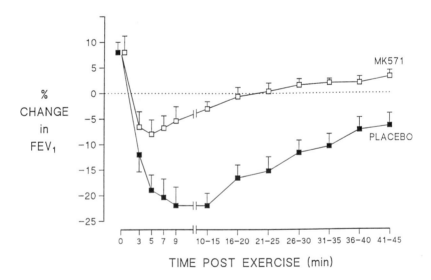

Figure 1   Effect of a selective *CysLT₁* receptor antagonist, MK-571, on the % fall from baseline in the forced expired volume in 1 sec (FEV₁) after exercise in asthmatic subjects. Pretreatment with MK-571 (open squares) markedly attenuates the fall in FEV₁ after exercise. (Reproduced with permission from Ref. 27.)

obvious from the initial studies that attempted to measure mediator release in the airways after exercise by measuring the excretion of urinary LTE$_4$ (25). However, one study in asthmatic children did demonstrate an increase in urinary LTE$_4$ after exercise-induced bronchoconstriction (26). The most compelling evidence for an important role for the cysteinyl leukotrienes comes from a number of studies that have demonstrated marked attenuation of exercise-induced bronchoconstriction after pretreatment with a variety of different *Cys LT$_1$* receptor antagonists, and thereby block the action of the cysteinyl leukotrienes on their receptors in human airways. Receptor antagonists, such as MK-571 (27), or zafirlukast (Accolate), given either orally (28) or by inhalation (29), inhibit the maximal bronchoconstrictor response after exercise by 50–70%, greatly shorten the time to recovery of normal lung function, and thereby markedly reduce the time-response curve (Fig. 1); and indeed, in 30–50% of asthmatic subjects studied, completely inhibit the response. One long-lasting receptor antagonist, cinalukast, inhibited the area under the time-response curve after exercise by >80% in asthmatic subjects, and this effect lasted more than 8 hr after dosing (30) (Fig. 2). There is heterogeneity among subjects, in that in some subjects interruption of the leukotriene cascade results in a complete inhibition of the bronchospastic response to exercise while in others

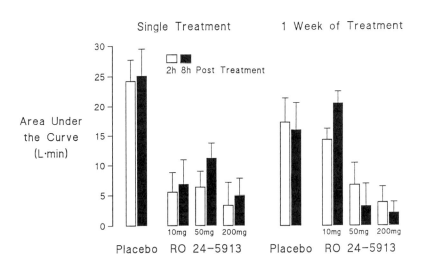

Figure 2 Effect of treatment with three doses of the *CysLT$_1$* receptor antagonist Cinalukast on exercise-induced bronchoconstriction. The degree of exercise-induced bronchoconstriction is measured by the area under the FEV$_1$-time curve. On the first day of treatment, the protective effect at each of the three doses is maintained for at least 8 hr. After 1 week of treatment the protective effect is lost for the lowest (10 mg) dose, but preserved for the two higher doses. (Reproduced with permission from Ref. 30.)

this intervention has no effect. This indicates that the pathways leading to bronchoconstriction after exercise vary in different asthmatics, and that in some, mediators other than the leukotrienes may be more important bronchoconstrictor agonists.

VII. Inhibitory Prostaglandins and Exercise Refractoriness

Prostaglandins are most easily considered in two classes. These are stimulatory prostaglandins, such as PGD_2 and $PGF_{2\alpha}$, which are potent bronchoconstrictors (8,9), and inhibitory prostaglandins, such as PGE_2, which can reduce bronchoconstrictor responses (31) and can attenuate the release of acetylcholine from airway nerves (32). However, differentiation of the prostaglandins into stimulatory and inhibitory classes is somewhat inappropriate. For example, both PGE_2 and $PGF_{2\alpha}$ can have different effects on the airways depending on the time after inhalation at which the response is measured (31). However, the main action of PGE_2 and PGI_2 on airway function is to relax airway smooth muscle, to antagonize the contractile responses of other bronchoconstrictor agonists, and to inhibit the release of acetylcholine from airway cholinergic nerves.

Inhibitory prostaglandins are important in causing histamine tachyphylaxis in a variety of species, but tachyphylaxis to inhaled histamine was not believed to occur in asthmatic subjects (33,34). The studies in asthmatics were conducted in subjects taking a variety of medications to treat asthma, including inhaled corticosteroids. To address this issue more carefully, Manning et al. (35) conducted a study in mild, stable asthmatics, not taking any regular medications for asthma treatment. When histamine inhalation challenges were conducted 1 and 6 hr apart, histamine tachyphylaxis was demonstrated in all subjects, which lasted at least 6 hr. This effect was abolished by pretreatment with the cyclooxygenase inhibitor indomethacin (35), implicating the release of inhibitory prostaglandins in causing this response. Subsequent studies have shown that the development of histamine tachyphylaxis in asthmatics does not occur in subjects who were treated with inhaled corticosteroids (36), which may help explain the descrepancy with the earlier studies. In asthmatics, the effect was initially thought to be specific for histamine, as repeated inhalations of the cholinergic agonists acetylcholine (5) or methacholine (37) did not induce tachyphylaxis; however, once released by histamine, the inhibitory prostaglandins reduced airway responsiveness to acetylcholine (5) or exercise (38). In addition, pretreatment with exogenous oral PGE_1 reduces airway hyperresponsiveness to inhaled histamine and methacholine (39). Interestingly, in normal subjects, who do not have airway hyperresponsiveness, and who can inhale higher concentrations of inhaled bronchoconstrictor agonists, methacholine tachyphylaxis can be demonstrated (37).

Histamine tachyphylaxis is mediated by stimulation of histamine H_2 receptors, as pretreatment with the H_2-receptor antagonist cimetidine prevented histamine tachyphylaxis in asthmatic subjects (40). The cell(s) of origin of this prostanoid is not yet known, but is likely a structural cell in the airway epithelium (41) or airway smooth muscle (42).

As a result of these studies, we postulated that histamine released following exercise (43) causes bronchoconstriction in asthmatic subjects, but also provides partial protection against subsequent allergen- or exercise-induced bronchoconstriction, through inhibitory prostaglandin released by stimulation of histamine H_2 receptors. This was supported by our initial studies that demonstrated that pretreatment with indomethacin prevented the development of exercise refractoriness (44), implicating the release of an inhibitory prostaglandin in mediating this response. This was confirmed in a subsequent study (45). However, several subsequent studies suggested that this hypothesis is incorrect. This is because exercise-induced bronchoconstriction is markedly attenuated, and indeed in some subjects abolished, by pretreatment with *Cys LT₁* receptor antagonist, such as MK-571 (27), Accolate (28), or Cinalukast (46). This indicates that the cysteinyl leukotrienes, rather than histamine, are the main mediator responsible for exercise-induced bronchoconstriction. Also, pretreatment with the H_2-receptor antagonists cimetidine or ranitidine, which effectively prevent histamine tachyphylaxis, did not prevent exercise refractoriness (47). Therefore, *histamine-induced* inhibitory prostaglandin release did not appear to be the cause of exercise refractoriness.

To explain these diverse findings, we speculated that stimulation of the *Cys LT₁* receptor by the cystineyl leukotrienes after exercise may result in inhibitory prostaglandin release and the development of exercise refractoriness. This hypothesis was supported by studies that demonstrated that tachyphylaxis to inhaled LTD_4 occurs in asthmatic subjects, that cross-tachyphylaxis exists between exercise and inhaled LTD_4 and this cross-tachyphylaxis was prevented by pretreatment with the cyclooxygenase inhibitor flurbiprofen (Fig. 3) (48). Also, inhaled PGE_2 markedly attenuates exercise bronchoconstriction (49). Therefore, it appears that cysteinyl leukotrienes are released in response to loss of heat or water from the airways, in an effort to fully condition the increase volumes of inhaled air during exercise. This results in bronchoconstriction, but also in the release of inhibitory prostaglandins, such as PGE_2, which partially attenuates further exercise-induced bronchoconstriction.

VIII. Cysteinyl Leukotrienes and Allergen Responses

The bronchoconstriction that occurs during the early and late responses is in large part caused by allergen-induced release of cysteinyl leukotrienes. This was initially suggested by Brocklehurst (50), who demonstrated the production

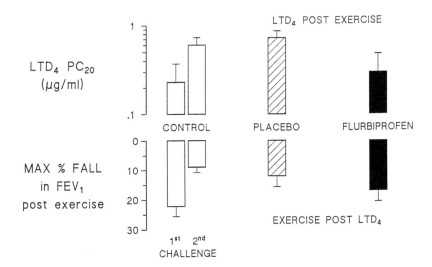

Figure 3 (Top) Mean PC$_{20}$ LTD$_4$ for two LTD$_4$ challenges separated by 1 hr and for an LTD$_4$ challenge 1 hr after exercise during treatment with either placebo or flurbiprofen. LTD$_4$ tachyphylaxis occurred in these subjects (open bars). LTD$_4$ tachyphylaxis also occurred following exercise during placebo treatment (cross-hatched bars), and this effect was significantly attenuated ($p = 0.027$) during flurbiprofen treatment (solid bars). (Botton) Mean (SEM) % fall in FEV$_1$ post exercise for two exercise challenges separated by 1 hr and for an exercise challenge 1 hr after LTD$_4$ during treatment with either placebo or flurbiprofen. Exercise refractoriness occurred in these subjects (open bars). Exercise refractoriness also occurred following LTD$_4$ during placebo treatment (cross-hatched bars), and this effect was significantly attenuated during flurbiprofen treatment (solid bars). (Reproduced with permission from Ref. 48.)

of slow-reacting substance of anaphylaxis (SRS-A) after sensitized lung fragments were challenged by specific allergens. SRS-A is now known to consist of the cysteinyl leukotrienes (LT) C$_4$, D$_4$, and their stable excretory metabolite LTE$_4$ (51).

Several investigators have demonstrated increases in urinary LTE$_4$ after allergen-induced bronchoconstriction (52,53). The increases in urinary LTE$_4$ were significantly correlated, in one study, with the magnitude of the bronchoconstriction (52). Interestingly, no significant increases in urinary LTE$_4$ could be demonstrated during the allergen-induced late asthmatic response, even though the magnitude of the bronchoconstriction was similar to the early response (52). These data suggested that the cysteinyl leukotrienes were released during allergen inhalation and were important causes of bronchoconstriction during the allergen-induced early phase, but not the late-phase bronchoconstrictor responses.

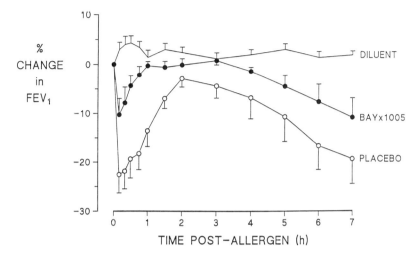

Figure 4   Effect of pretreatment with a leukotriene synthesis inhibitor, BAYx1005 or placebo, on allergen-induced bronchoconstriction. The mean % (± SEM) change in FEV_1 from baseline during the early and late asthmatic response after BAYx1005 (closed circles) and placebo (open circles) pretreatment and after inhaled diluent. (Reproduced with permission from Ref. 55.)

The best evidence for a central role for the cysteinyl leukotrienes in causing allergen-induced bronchoconstriction is suggested by the observations that a number of different LTD_4-receptor antagonists and leukotriene synthesis inhibitors have been demonstrated to markedly attenuate the bronchoconstrictor responses after inhaled allergen (54–57) (Fig. 4). These studies have indicated that LTD_4 antagonists and leukotriene synthesis inhibitors attenuate allergen-induced early responses by up to 80% (54,55), and, surprisingly considering the data on urinary LTE_4 excretion during the late response, also attenuate the late response by up to 50% (55), suggesting that, as inhaled leukotriene D_4 does not itself cause the development of late responses (58), newly generated cysteinyl leukotrienes, possible from inflammatory cells, such as eosinophils recruited into the airways during the late asthmatic response (23,24), are partially responsible for the bronchoconstriction during this response. The component of allergen-induced early responses not influenced by antileukotrienes is caused by thromboxane A_2 (59) and histamine release, while the combination of cysteinyl leukotriene and histamine is mainly responsible for bronchoconstriction during the late response.

Allergen-induced airway inflammation may also be due in part to the release of the cysteinyl leukotrienes. Inhaled LTE_4 has been shown to cause eosinophil infiltration into airway biopsies from asthmatic subjects, an effect not seen with inhaled methacholine (60). Also, a recent study has shown that pretreatment with the *CysLT₁ receptor* antagonist has been shown to attenuate allergen-induced influex into the airways after segmental allergen challenge (61). These studies suggest that the cysteinyl leukotrienes, released as a result of allergen inhalation, may play a role in causing allergen-induced airway inflammation.

IX. Conclusions

The release of the cysteinyl leukotrienes is the most important cause of bronchoconstriction after inhaled environmental allergens in atopic asthmatic subjects and of exercise-induced bronchoconstriction. In addition, the cysteinyl leukotrienes are also important in causing allergen-induced late responses and possibly eosinophil influx into the airways. The cysteinyl leukotrienes also appear to initiate the release of inhibitory prostaglandins that attenuate subsequent bronchoconstrictor responses to themselves, which is responsible for the development of exercise refractoriness with repeated exercise challenges.

References

1. Hargreave FE, Gibson PG, Ramsdale EH. Airway hyperresponsiveness, airway inflammation, and asthma. Immunol Allergy Clin North Am 1990; 10:439–448.
2. Hargreave FE, Ryan G, Thomson NC, et al. Bronchial responsiveness to histamine or methacholine in asthma: measurement and clinical significance. J Allergy Clin Immunol 1981; 68:347–355.
3. Woolcock AJ, Salome CM, Yan K. The shape of the dose-response curve to histamine in asthmatic and normal subjects. Am Rev Respir Dis 1984; 130:71–75.
4. Cockcroft DW, Killian DN, Mellon JJ, Hargreave FE. Bronchial reactivity to inhaled histamine: a method and clinical survey. Clin Allergy 1977; 7:235–243.
5. Manning PJ, O'Byrne PM. Histamine bronchoconstriction reduces airway responsiveness in asthmatic subjects. Am Rev Respir Dis 1988; 137:1323–1325.
6. Juniper EF, Frith PA, Dunnett C, Cockcroft DW, Hargreave FE. Reproducibility and comparison of responses to inhaled histamine and methacholine. Thorax 1978; 33:705–710.
7. Adelroth E, Morris MM, Hargreave FE, O'Byrne PM. Airway responsiveness to leukotrienes C4 and D4 and to methacholine in patients with asthma and normal controls. N Engl J Med 1986; 315:480–484.
8. Thomson NC, Roberts R, Bandouvakis J, Newball H, Hargreave FE. Comparison of bronchial responses to prostaglandin F2 alpha and methacholine. J Allergy Clin Immunol 1981; 68:392–398.

9. Hardy CC, Robinson C, Tattersfield AE, Holgate ST. The bronchoconstrictor effect of inhaled prostaglandin D2 in normal and asthmatic men. N Engl J Med 1984; 311:209–213.
10. Anderson SD. Exercise-induced asthma. The state of the art. Am Rev Respir Dis 1985; 87S:191–195.
11. O'Byrne PM. Allergen-induced airway hyperresponsiveness. J Allergy Clin Immunol 1988; 81:119–127.
12. Cockcroft DW, Ruffin RE, Dolovich J, Hargreave FE. Allergen-induced increase in non-allergic bronchial reactivity. Clin Allergy 1977; 7:503–513.
13. Chan-Yeung M, Lan S. Occupational asthma. Am Rev Respir Dis 1986; 133:686–703.
14. Anderton RC, Cuff MT, Frith PA, et al. Bronchial responsiveness to inhaled histamine and exercise. J Allergy Clin Immunol 1979; 63:315–320.
15. Gelb AF, Tashkin DP, Epstein JD, Gong H Jr, Zamel N. Exercise-induced bronchodilation in asthma. Chest 1985; 87:196–201.
16. McFadden ER Jr, Ingram RH Jr. Exercise-induced asthma: observations on the initiating stimulus. N Engl J Med 1979; 301:763–769.
17. Deal EC, McFadden ER Jr, Ingram RH Jr, Strauss RH, Jaegar JJ. Role of respiratory heat exchange in production of exercise-induced asthma. J Appl Physiol 1979; 46:467–475.
18. McNeill RS, Nairn JR, Millar JS, Ingram CG. Exercise-induced asthma. Q J Med 1966; 137:55–67.
19. Edmunds AT, Tooley M, Godfrey S. The refractory period after exercise-induced asthma: its duration and relation to the severity of exercise. Am Rev Respir Dis 1978; 117:247–254.
20. O'Byrne PM, Dolovich J, Hargreave FE. Late asthmatic responses. Am Rev Respir Dis 1987; 136:740–751.
21. Durham SR, Craddock CF, Cookson WO, Benson MK. Increases in airway responsiveness to histamine precede allergen-induced late asthmatic responses. J Allergy Clin Immunol 1988; 82:764–770.
22. Cartier A, Thomson NC, Frith PA, Roberts R, Hargreave FE. Allergen-induced increase in bronchial responsiveness to histamine: relationship to the late asthmatic response and change in airway caliber. J Allergy Clin Immunol 1982; 70:170–177.
23. de Monchy JG, Kauffman HF, Venge P, et al. Bronchoalveolar eosinophilia during allergen-induced late asthmatic reactions. Am Rev Respir Dis 1985; 131:373–376.
24. Choudry NB, Watson R, Hargreave FE, O'Byrne PM. Time course of inflammatory cells in sputum after allergen inhalation in asthmatic subjects. J Allergy Clin Immunol 1993; 91:64A.
25. Taylor IK, Wellings R, Taylor GW, Fuller RW. Urinary leukotriene E4 excretion in exercise induced bronchoconstriction. J Appl Physiol 1992; 145:743–748.
26. Kikawa Y, Miyanomae T, Inoue Y, et al. Urinary leukotriene E4 after exercise challenge in children with asthma. J Allergy Clin Immunol 1992; 89:1111–1119.
27. Manning PJ, Watson RM, Margolskee DJ, Williams VC, Schwartz JI, O'Byrne PM. Inhibition of exercise-induced bronchoconstriction by MK-571, a potent leukotriene D4-receptor antagonist. N Engl J Med 1990; 323:1736–1739.

28. Finnerty JP, Wood-Baker R, Thomson H, Holgate ST. Role of leukotrienes in exercise-induced asthma. Inhibitory effect of ICI 204219, a potent leukotriene D4 receptor antagonist. Am Rev Respir Dis 1992; 145:746–749.

29. Makker HK, Lau LC, Thomson HW, Binks SM, Holgate ST. The protective effect of inhaled leukotriene D4 receptor antagonist ICI 204,219 against exercise-induced asthma. Am Rev Respir Dis 1993; 147:1413–1418.

30. Adelroth E, Inman M, Summers E, Pace D, Modi M, O'Byrne PM. Prolonged protection against exercise-induced bronchoconstriction by the leukotriene D4-receptor antagonist Cinalukast. J Allergy Clin Immunol 1997; 99:210–215.

31. Walters EH, Davies BH. Dual effect of prostaglandin E2 on normal airways smooth muscle in vivo. Thorax 1982; 37:918–922.

32. Walters EH, O'Byrne PM, Fabbri LM, Graf PD, Holtzman MJ, Nadel JA. Control of neurotransmission by prostaglandins in canine trachealis smooth muscle. J Appl Physiol Respir Env Exc Physiol 1984; 57:129–134.

33. Schoeffel RE, Anderson SD, Gillam I, Lindsay DA. Multiple exercise and histamine challenge in asthmatic patients. Thorax 1980; 35:164–170.

34. Polosa R, Finnerty JP, Holgate ST. Lack of tachyphylaxis to histamine in both moderate and mild asthmatic subjects. Agents Actions 1990; 30:281–283.

35. Manning PJ, Jones GL, O'Byrne PM. Tachyphylaxis to inhaled histamine in asthmatic subjects. J Appl Physiol 1987; 63:1572–1577.

36. Strban M, Manning PJ, Watson RM, O'Byrne PM. Effect of magnitude of airway responsiveness and therapy with inhaled corticosteroid on histamine tachyphylaxis in asthma. Chest 1994; 105:1434–1438.

37. Stevens WH, Manning PJ, Watson RM, O'Byrne PM. Tachyphylaxis to inhaled methacholine in normal but not asthmatic subjects. J Appl Physiol 1990; 69:875–879.

38. Hamielec CM, Manning PJ, O'Byrne PM. Exercise refractoriness after histamine inhalation in asthmatic subjects. Am Rev Respir Dis 1988; 138:794–798.

39. Manning PJ, Lane CG, O'Byrne PM. The effect of oral prostaglandin E1 on airway responsiveness in asthmatic subjects. Pulm Pharmacol 1989; 2:121–124.

40. Henriksen JM, Wenzel A. Effect of an intranasally administered corticosteroid (budesonide) on nasal obstruction, mouth breathing, and asthma. Am Rev Respir Dis 1984; 130:1014–1018.

41. Leikauf GD, Ueki IF, Nadel JA, Widdicombe JH. Bradykinin stimulates C1 secretion and prostaglandin E2 release by canine tracheal epithelium. Am J Physiol 1985; 248:F48–55.

42. Manning PM, Jines GL, Lane CG, O'Byrne PM. Histamine-induced prostaglandin E2 release from canine tracheal smooth muscle is inhibited by H2-receptor blockade. Am Rev Respir Dis 1988; 137:A373.

43. Barnes PJ, Brown MJ. Venous plasma histamine in exercise- and hyperventilation-induced asthma in man. Clin Sci 1981; 61:159–162.

44. O'Byrne PM, Walters EH, Aizawa H, Fabbri LM, Holtzman MJ, Nadel JA. Indomethacin inhibits the airway hyperresponsiveness but not the neutrophil influx induced by ozone in dogs. Am Rev Respir Dis 1984; 130:220–224.

45. Margolskee DJ, Bigby BG, Boushey HA. Indomethacin blocks airway tolerance to repetitive exercise but not to eucapnic hyperpnea in asthmatic subjects. Am Rev Respir Dis 1988; 137:842–846.

46. Adelroth E, Inman MD, Summers E, Pace D, Modi M, O'Byrne PM. Prolonged protection against exercise-induced bronchoconstriction by the leukotriene D4-receptor antagonist Cinalukast. J Allergy Clin Immunol 1977; 99:210–215.
47. Manning PJ, Watson R, O'Byrne PM. The effects of H2-receptor antagonists on exercise refractoriness in asthma. J Allergy Clin Immunol 1992; 90:125–126.
48. Manning PJ, Watson RM, O'Byrne PM. Exercise-induced refractoriness in asthmatic subjects involves leukotriene and prostaglandin interdependent mechanisms. Am Rev Respir Dis 1993; 148:950–954.
49. Melillo E, Woolley KL, Manning PJ, Watson RM, O'Byrne PM. Effect of inhaled PGE_2 on exercise-induced bronchoconstriction in asthmatic subjects. Am J Respir Crit Care Med 1994; 149:1138–1141.
50. Brocklehurst W. The release of histamine and formation of a slow reacting substance (SRS-A) during anaphylatic shock. J Physiol 1960; 151:416–435.
51. Samuelsson B. Leukotrienes: mediators of immediate hypersensitivity reactions and inflammation. Science 1983; 220:568–575.
52. Manning PJ, Rokach J, Malo JL, et al. Urinary leukotriene E4 levels during early and late asthmatic responses. J Allergy Clin Immunol 1990; 86:211–220.
53. Taylor GW, Black P, Turner N, et al. Urinary leukotriene E4 after antigen challenge and in acute asthma and allergic rhinitis. Lancet 1989; 1:585–587.
54. Taylor IK, O'Shaughnessy KM, Fuller RW, Dollery CT. Effect of a cysteinylleukotriene receptor antagonist, ICI 204-219 on allergen-induced bronchoconstriction and airway hyperactivity in atopic subjects. Lancet 1991; 337:690–694.
55. Hamilton AL, Watson RM, Wyile G, O'Byrne PM. A 5-lipoxygenase activating protein antagonist, Bay 1005, attenuates both early and late phase allergen-induced bronchoconstriction in asthmatic subjects. Thorax 1997; 52:348–354.
56. Diamant Z, Timmers MC, van der Veen H, et al. The effect of MK-0591, a novel 5-lipoxygenase activating protein inhibitor, on leukotriene biosynthesis and allergen-induced airway responses in asthmatic subjects in vivo. J Allergy Clin Immunol 1995; 95:42–51.
57. Friedman BS, Bel EH, Buntinx A, et al. Oral leukotriene inhibitor (MK-886) blocks allergen-induced airway responses. Am Rev Respir Dis 1993; 147:839–844.
58. Higgins DA, O'Byrne PM. Inhaled leukotriene D4 does not cause a late response in atopic subjects. Allergy Clin Immunol 1987; 79:141.
59. Manning PJ, Stevens WH, Cockcroft DW, O'Byrne PM. The role of thromboxane in allergen-induced asthmatic responses. Eur Respir J 1991; 4:667–672.
60. Laitinen LA, Laitinen A, Haahtcla T, Vikka V, Spur BW, Lee TH. Leukotriene E4 and granulocytic infiltration into asthmatics airways. Lancet 1993; 341:989–990.
61. Calhoun WJ, Williams KL, Simonson SG, Lavins BJ. Effect of Zalfirlukast (Accolate) on airway inflammation after segmental allergen challenge in patients with mild asthma. Am J Respir Crit Care Med 1997; 155:A662.

16

Endotoxin-Induced Acute Respiratory Distress Syndrome in Nitric Oxide-Deficient Rats

PAWEL P. WOLKOW, EWA JANOWSKA, JOANNA B. BARTUS, WOJCIECH URACZ, and RYSZARD J. GRYGLEWSKI

Jagiellonian University School of Medicine
Krakow, Poland

I. Introduction

In the early 1990s nitric oxide (NO) (1,2) and, later, peroxynitrite (ONOO⁻) (3), a product of interaction of NO with superoxide anion (O_2^-), were recognized as mediators of endotoxic shock. It is widely accepted that the late phase of lipopolysaccharide (LPS)-evoked arterial hypotension and lethal vasoplegia as well as multiple organ failure syndrome (MOFS) are associated with overproduction of NO (4) owing to the induction of NO synthase (iNOS) in macrophages (5), leukocytes (6), cardiac myocytes (7), hepatocytes, pulmonary (8), vascular endothelial (9), and smooth muscle cells (10). Then NO is made by iNOS in sufficiently high concentrations to generate pneumotoxic peroxynitrite in the lung (11), although under special conditions NO by itself may protect the lung against the oxidative insult (12). Inhibition of the excessive NO production seems to be a promising pharmacological approach to the treatment of sepsis (13) especially by selective iNOS inhibitors (14). Synthetic antimetabolites of L-arginine such as N^G-monomethyl-L-arginine (L-NMMA) or N^G-nitro-L-arginine (L-NNA) are nonselective ecNOS/iNOS inhibitors, which are expected not only to attenuate hypotension characteristic for the late phase of acute endotoxemia (4,14) but also to prevent generation of toxic peroxynitrite (3) and, in this way, to become a shield against MOFS. Successful treatment of experimental endotoxemia with L-NMMA was followed by its administration to patients with septic shock, and the results obtained (15) were encouraging.

However, in parallel with clinical trials on L-NMMA in septic shock (15) warnings appeared on possible detrimental effects of nonselective pharmacological iNOS/ecNOS inhibition during experimental endotoxemia. In the LPS-treated animals, L-NMMA, L-NNA, and other NOS inhibitors have been reported to be responsible for enhanced intestinal (16), hepatic (17), renal (18), and cardiac (19) injuries, and increased mortality (20) possibly owing to decreased organ blood flow (21), impaired tissue oxygen delivery (22), and increased plasma cytokine levels (23). In endotoxic shock nonselective NOS inhibitors were accused of precipitating pulmonary hypertension and decreased cardiac output (24). In light of the above beneficial effect of inhalation of NO gas on pulmonary circulation during endotoxic shock (25) as well as the protective effect of NO on superoxide-induced (!) lung injury (12), we may speculate that in endotoxemia NO may also play a desired defensive role.

In the literature we find a pronounced misunderstanding of "early" and "late" phases of endotoxemia. In the rat model described here (LPS 2 mg/kg/min i.v. for 10 min) both phases are clear-cut. The early transient phase of a fall in MABP lasts 30–45 min, and then, the late phase develops, which ends after 4–6 hr with death of animals among symptoms of irreversible deep hypotension and vasoplegia.

II. Methods

A. Animals

Thirty-three male Sprague-Dawley rats (180–250 g) were maintained at constant temperature ($22 \pm 1°C$), with a 12-hr light/dark cycle in our animal facility, where they were allowed water and standard rat chow ad libitum.

B. Reagents

Escherichia coli lipopolysaccharide (LPS, serotype 0127:B8) and N^G-nitro-L-arginine (L-NNA) were purchased from Sigma. LPS was dissolved in saline and administered as an intravenous (i.v.) infusion (2 mg/kg/min for 10 min, total dose 20 mg/kg). L-NNA (10 mg/kg, i.v.) was dissolved in 0.1 M phosphate buffer pH = 7.4 and administered as a bolus injection.

C. Surgery and Instrumentation

Under thiopentone anaesthesia (Thiopental, Vuab 120 mg/kg, i.p.) rats were intubated intratracheally and ventilated with room air (Ugo Basile 7025 rodent ventilator, tidal volume 10 ml/kg, respiratory rate 50 breaths/min). Polyurethane catheters were inserted into left jugular and left femoral veins for administration of drugs. Another catheter was placed in the right carotid artery and connected to the pressure transducer for continuous recording of mean arterial blood pressure (MABP).

D. Experimental Protocol

Rats were assigned into three groups and subjected to one of the following intravenous regimens: (LPS group, $n = 9$)—LPS infusion alone; (LPS + L-NNA group, $n = 6$)—LPS infusion followed 45 min later with injection of L-NNA; (L-NNA + LPS group, $n = 18$)—injection of L-NNA 45 min prior to infusion of LPS.

E. Pathological Examination

Routine pathological examination of internal organs—lung, liver, spleen, kidneys, and hearts of rats—was performed. Then organs were fixed in 10% buffered formalin (pH = 7.5) overnight at room temperature, then washed for 2 hr, dehydrated through a graded series of ethanols (50% 30 min, 60% 60 min, 80% 2 hr, 96% 30 min, and 100% 30 min), xylene (3 × 15 min), embedded in paraffin (58°C, 3 hr), and cast into blocks. Tissue samples were cut into 3–5-μm-thick sections on a microtome and placed on glass slides. Before staining, paraffin slides were heated to 60°C for 30–45 min, paraffin was removed by placing the slides in fresh xylene (3 × 10 min), then slides were rehydrated following standard procedure (ethanol 100% 2 × 5 min, 70% 2 min, and 50% 2 min), and finally they were dipped into phosphate-buffered saline (pH = 7.4). The slides were stained routinely with hematoxylin and eosin (H&E) or by the Weigert technique for fibrin (26). Light-microscopic examination was performed with photographic documentation.

F. Statistical Analysis

MABP (mmHg) was expressed as arithmetic mean ± standard deviation (SD). Differences between the studied groups were evaluated by two-tailed unpaired Student's t-test unless stated otherwise. All calculations, as well as probability of survival, and graphs were done in Sigma Plot 3.03 for Windows package (A00517, Jandel Scientific GmbH, Germany).

III. Results

Fifteen minutes after the surgery had been completed control MABP was measured. Control MABP did not differ significantly between three studied groups: it was 126 ± 17 mmHg in the LPS group, 119 ± 13 mmHg in the LPS + L-NNA group, and 118 ± 18 mmHg in the L-NNA + LPS group. To make the matter clear we have introduced "initial MABP," i.e., MABP measured 5 min before infusion of LPS. In the LPS and LPS + L-NNA groups, initial MABP did not differ from the control values. In L-NNA + LPS the initial MABP rose to 135 ± 19 mmHg from the control value of 118 ± 18 mmHg and this rise was statistically significant ($p < 0.001$) in the paired Student's t-test (Fig. 1). Ten minutes after administration of LPS in the LPS group, MABP fell from 126 ± 17 mmHg to 55 ± 12 mmHg (fall by 56 ± 7%, $p < 0.001$). Forty-five minutes after administration of LPS, MABP partially returned to 83 ± 18 mmHg, to fall again to 68 ± 26 mmHg 3 hr after administration of LPS. In the LPS + L-NNA group, respective values were 119 ± 13 mmHg initially, 65 ± 8 mmHg after 10 min, and 82 ± 9 mmHg 45 min after LPS. At

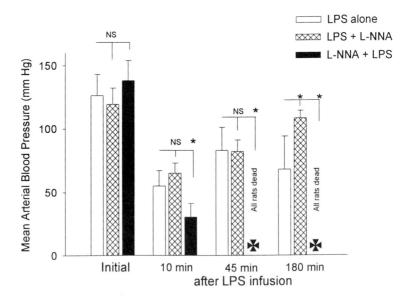

Figure 1   Mean arterial blood pressure in rats of: (1) LPS group (open columns, n = 9), (2) LPS + L-NNA group (cross-hatched columns, n = 6), and (3) L-NNA + LPS group (solid columns, n = 18) before the treatment (initial) and 10, 45, and 180 min after LPS infusion. Bars represent SD. NS, difference nonsignificant between LPS group; *difference significant $p < 0.001$.

that particular moment, the administration of L-NNA caused a significant rise in MABP to 108 ± 8 mmHg after 180 min ($p < 0.001$). In contrast with this hemodynamic improvement, the survival time in the LPS + L-NNA group showed only a nonsignificant tendency to be longer (314 ± 77 min) as compared to the LPS group (288 ± 40 min, Fig. 2). In both groups the animals were dying with symptoms of deep hypotension and vasoplegia.

In L-NNA + LPS group, the administration of L-NNA alone first raised control MABP from 118 ± 18 mmHg to 135 ± 19 mmHg ($p < 0.001$, paired Student's *t*-test). Ten minutes after administration of LPS, a value of initial MABP fell down to 30 ± 11 mmHg, i.e., by 78 ± 8% ($p < 0.001$). None of the rats of the L-NNA + LPS group recovered from this deep hypotension. All animals died 20 ± 5 min after LPS infusion had started ($p < 0.001$, Fig. 2). The death was preceded by an appearance of bloody and foamy exudate pouring out of the respiratory tract. Autopsy revealed that lungs were heavy, firm, red, and boggy. All other examined macroscopically organs such as kidney, liver, spleen, intestine, heart, and brain appeared to be normal. After cutting of removed lungs, a large amount of foamy and blood-stained exudate was seen on the surface of cut organ. Histological changes were distributed almost equally in whole lungs. Widespread edema and marked, diffused hemorrhage were constantly observed (Figs. 3 and 4). Massive congestion was seen in capillaries of the alveoli, and "ring-shaped" hemorrhage in perivascular spaces of

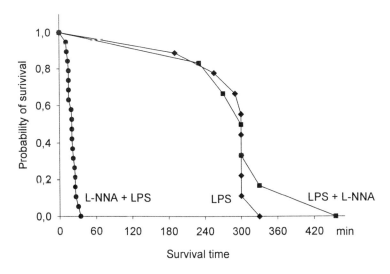

Figure 2 Probability of survival time (abcissa) of rats in three studied groups (ordinate = survival time in minutes).

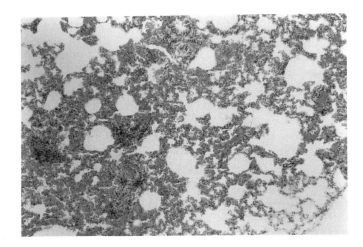

Figure 3 Microscopic picture (hematoxylin-eosin staining) of the lungs of a rat with acute respiratory distress syndrome in the L-NNA + LPS group. Massive hemorrhages distributed almost equally across the whole lung. Marked congestion of alveolar wall was noted (final magnification 165×).

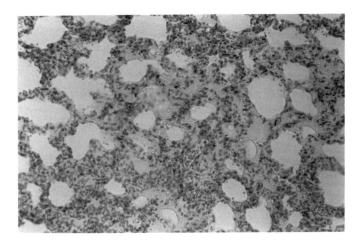

Figure 4 Microscopic picture (hematoxylin-eosin staining) of the lungs of the same rat as in Figure 3 with edema and exudate in alveoli (final magnification ×165).

pulmonary vessels, as well as diffuse hemorrhage into interstitium, subpleural connective tissue, and alveoli, were noted. Additionally, significant accumulation and margination of granulocytes in pulmonary vessels were observed. Capillary plugging by neutrophils was seen in alveolar capillaries, and in both pre- and postcapillary vessels. Intra-alveolar granulocytes and mononuclear cells were scarce. Also the number of alveolar macrophages was not increased. In Weigert-stained lung tissue, fibrin strands were seen in small vessels. Perivascular edema with presence of red blood cells was found in nonmuscular and some muscular vessels, the alveolar walls were thicker than normal, and pale-pink-stained edema was seen in the air-exchange spaces of the lung. Acute lung injury and not subtle changes in other organs appeared to be the cause of death of these rats. The above macroscopic and microscopic features are characteristic for the acute respiratory distress syndrome (ARDS).

IV. Discussion

LPS at a total dose of 10–20 mg/kg given to rats as intravenous injection or infusion is known to produce a biphasic blood pressure response with subsequent multiorgan injury resulting in lethal shock (2,4,27,28). Our attempt to evaluate the contribution of NO to early and late phases of arterial hypotension in endotoxemia was triggered by an unexpected finding of sudden death in NO-deficient rats, i.e., in animals pretreated with L-NNA 45 min prior to administration of LPS. These animals were dying with symptoms of acute lung injury and autopsy revealed that their lungs were heavy, firm, red, and boggy. All other organs appeared macroscopically to be normal. By light microscopy the widespread lung injury was characterized by acute hemorrhages to perivascular tissue, by perivascular, interstitial, and intra-alveolar edema, fibrin deposition in small vessels, and capillary plugging by aggregated neutrophils. In kidney and liver there was evidence of congestion and accumulation of granulocytes but not hemorrhages. An obvious cause of death of these rats was acute lung injury. The above macroscopic and microscopic changes in the lung are characteristic for ARDS.

    An initial, transient fall in arterial blood pressure that occurs immediately after administration of LPS is of unknown origin and it is considered to be an unimportant epiphenomenon (2). However, our data suggest that at this early phase of endotoxic shock, the harmful effect of LPS is opposed by endogenous NO. Pharmacological inhibition of NO biosynthesis by L-NNA prior to administration of LPS exacerbates an "innocent" transient fall of MABP to fulminant injury of the pulmonary circulation. It seems that LPS during the first contact with the lung releases endogenous toxins along with pneumoprotective NO. When generation of NO is inhibited, the unopposed LPS-released toxins evoke ARDS. L-NNA treatment of the preexisting endotoxic shock raises MABP, as has been shown by the others (2,4,13), but it does not prolong survival time. It may well be that an essential sequence of lethal events is triggered in the lung during the first contact of endotoxin with this organ. It explains why later removal of NO by L-NNA, although it offers considerable symptomatic improvement, cannot change the lethal course of endotoxic shock. Indeed, the lung is known to be a prime target organ for LPS (11,12,25,29). In septic shock, the lung is usually the first organ to fail, followed by failure of the liver, intestine, and kidney. The major vascular pulmonary effects of LPS in vivo are: increased vascular resistance (pulmonary hypertension), enhanced vascular permeability (edema), diffused endothelial injury, leukocyte margination, accumulation of platelet- and fibrin-containing microthrombi (29). Some of those might be mediated by peroxynitrite (11).

What is a pneumotoxic mediator in our model of ARDS? Of course, it cannot be peroxynitrite. In our model we suppress generation of one of the substrates (NO) required for production of peroxynitrite. We are rather close to a situation when pulmonary endogenous NO (12) or inhaled NO gas (30) has cytoprotective action. Feasible candidates for pneumotoxins are platelet-activating factor (PAF), thromboxane A_2, or leukotrienes, all of which have also been claimed to mediate lung injury (31). Further studies are required to explain the paradox of ARDS in LPS-treated, NO-deficient rats.

Acknowledgments

This work was supported by a research grant of the State Committee for Scientific Research in Poland (No 559/P05/96/11) and a grant from Yamanouchi Europe Foundation.

References

1. Fleming I, Gray GA, Julou Schaeffer G, Parratt JR, Stoclet JC. Incubation with endotoxin activates the L-arginine pathway in vascular tissue. Biochem Biophys Res Commun 1990; 171:562–568.
2. Parratt JR. Nitric oxide and cardiovascular dysfunction in sepsis and endotoxaemia: an introduction and an overview. In: Schlag G, Redl H, eds. Shock, Sepsis and Organ Failure—Nitric Oxide. Berlin: Springer Verlag, 1995:1–29.
3. Szabó C. The pathophysiological role of peroxynitrite in shock, inflammation, and ischaemia-reperfusion injury. Shock 1996; 6:79–88.
4. Thiemermann C, Vane J. Inhibition of nitric oxide synthesis reduces the hypotension induced by bacterial lipopolysaccharides in the rat in vivo. Eur J Pharmacol 1990; 182:591–595.

5. Hauschildt S, Luckhoff A, Mulsch A, Kohler J, Bessler W, Busse R. Induction and activity of NO synthase in bone-marrow-derived macrophages are independent of Ca^{2+}. Biochem J 1990; 270:351–356.
6. Kolls J, Xie J, LeBlanc R, Malinski T, Nelson S, Summer W, et al. Rapid induction of messenger RNA for nitric oxide synthase II in rat neutrophils in vivo by endotoxin and its suppression by prednisolone. Proc Soc Exp Med 1994; 205:220–229.
7. Schulz R, Nava E, Moncada S. Induction and potential biological relevance of a Ca(2+)-independent nitric oxide synthase in the myocardium. Br J Pharmacol 1992; 105:575–580.
8. Knowles RG, Merrett M, Salter M, Moncada S. Differential induction of brain, lung and liver nitric oxide synthase by endotoxin in the rat. Biochem J 1990; 270: 833–836.
9. Kilbourn RG, Belloni P. Endothelial cell production of nitrogen oxides in response to interferon gamma in combination with tumor necrosis factor, interleukin-1, or endotoxin. J Natl Cancer Inst 1990; 82:772–776.
10. Busse R, Mulsch A Induction of nitric oxide synthase by cytokines in vascular smooth muscle cells. FEBS Lett 1990; 275:87–90.
11. Wizemann TM, Gardner CR, Laskin JD, Quinones S, Durham SK, Goller NL, et al. Production of nitric oxide and peroxynitrite in the lung during acute endotoxemia. J Leukoc Biol 1994; 56:759–768.
12. Gutierrez HH, Nieves B, Chumley P, Rivera A, Freeman BA. Nitric oxide regulation of superoxide-dependent lung injury: oxidant-protective actions of endogenously produced and exogeneously administered nitric oxide. Free Radical Biol Med 1996; 21:43–52.
13. Vallance P, Moncada S. Role of endogenous nitric oxide in septic shock. New Horiz 1993; 1:77–86.
14. Thiemermann C. Selective inhibition of the activity of inducible nitric oxide synthase in septic shock. Prog Clin Biol Res 1995; 392:383–392.
15. Petros A, Lamb G, Leone A, Moncada S, Bennett D, Vallance P. Effects of a nitric oxide synthase inhibitor in humans with septic shock. Cardiovasc Res 1994; 28:34–39.
16. Hutcheson IR, Whittle BJ, Boughton Smith NK. Role of nitric oxide in maintaining vascular integrity in endotoxin-induced acute intestinal damage in the rat. Br J Pharmacol 1990; 101:815–820.
17. Harbrecht BG, Stadler J, Demetris AJ, Simmons RL, Billiar TR. Nitric oxide and prostaglandins interact to prevent hepatic damage during murine endotoxemia. Am J Physiol 1994; 266:G1004–1010.
18. Shultz PJ, Raij L. Endogenously synthesized nitric oxide prevents endotoxin-induced glomerular thrombosis. J Clin Invest 1992; 90:1718–1725.
19. Avontuur JA, Bruining HA, Ince C. Inhibition of nitric oxide synthesis causes myocardial ischemia in endotoxemic rats. Circ Res 1995;76:418–425.
20. Minnard EA, Shou J, Naama H, Cech A, Gallagher H, Daly JM. Inhibition of nitric oxide synthesis is detrimental during endotoxemia. Arch Surg 1994; 129:142–147.
21. Mulder MF, van Lambalgen AA, Huisman E, Visser JJ, van den Bos GC, thijs LG. Protective role of NO in the regional hemodynamic changes during acute endotoxemia in rats. Am J Physiol 1994; 266:H1558–1564.

22. Statman R, Cheng W, Cunningham JN, Henderson JL, Damiani P, Siconolfi A, et al. Nitric oxide inhibition in the treatment of the sepsis syndrome is detrimental to tissue oxygenation. J Surg Res 1994; 57:93–98.

23. Tiao G, Rafferty J, Ogle C, Fischer JE, Hasselgren PO. Detrimental effect of nitric oxide synthase inhibition during endotoxemia may be caused by high levels of tumor necrosis factor and interleukin-6. Surgery 1994; 116:332–337.

24. Pastor C, Teisseire B, Vicaut E, Payen D. Effects of L-arginine and L-nitroarginine treatment on blood pressure and cardiac output in a rabbit endotoxin shock model [see comments]. Crit Care Med 1994; 22:465–469.

25. Weitzberg E, Rudehill A, Lundberg JM. Nitric oxide inhalation attenuates pulmonary hypertension and improves gas exchange in endotoxin shock. Eur J Pharmacol 1993; 233:85–94.

26. Burck WH. Weigert technique. In: Hans-Christian Burck, ed. Histologische Technik. Stuttgart: Georg Thieme Verlag, 1973:166.

27. Casals Stenzel J. Protective effect of WEB 2086, a novel antagonist of platelet activating factor, in endotoxin shock. Eur J Pharmacol 1987; 135:117–122.

28. Kilbourn RG, Jubran A, Gross SS, Griffith OW, Levi R, Adams J, et al. Reversal of endotoxin-mediated shock by N^G-methyl-L-arginine, an inhibitor of nitric oxide synthesis. Biochem Biophys Res Commun 1990; 172:1132–1138.

29. VanderMeer TJ, Menconi MJ, O'Sullivan BP, Larkin VA, Wang H, Sofia M, et al. Acute lung injury in endotoxemic pigs: role of leukotriene B4. J Appl Physiol 1995; 78:1121–1131.

30. Guidot DM, Repine MJ, Hybertson BM, Repine JE. Inhaled nitric oxide prevents neutrophil-mediated, oxygen radical-dependent leak in isolated rat lungs. Am J Physiol 1995; 269:L2–5.

31. Uhlig S, Wollin L, Wendel A. Contributions of thromboxane and leukotrienes to PAF-induced impairment of lung function in the rat. J Appl Physiol 1994; 77:262–269.

17

Eicosanoid Regulation by Glucocorticoids in Asthma

RYSZARD DWORSKI

Vanderbilt University School of Medicine
Vanderbilt Medical Center
Nashville, Tennessee

I. Introduction

Glucocorticoids (GC) are by far the most effective pharmacological agents available for the treatment of asthma. When they are delivered directly to the airways by inhalation, the devastating side effects of prolonged systemic GC therapy are avoided. The use of inhaled steroids has become increasingly popular because of the growing understanding that asthma is an inflammatory disease that should be treated early and ceaselessly with anti-inflammatory agents. GC are superior to any other antiasthmatic drugs in reducing airway hyperresponsiveness, symptoms, use of bronchodilators, and the frequency of exacerbations as well as improving pulmonary function in asthmatics (1–5). GC undoubtably influence the crucial components of the asthmatic inflammatory process, but they do not cure the disease. Therefore, discontinuation of the treatment usually results in worsening of the clinical course of asthma (5,6), indicating that GC do not remove the most basic factor or factors responsible for the pathogenesis of asthma.

Despite the paramount importance of GC in the therapy of asthma, their mechanisms of action is unclear. They do not appear to have direct bronchodilatory effects. In experimental asthma in humans provoked by inhalation of a specific allergen, GC given acutely have no effect on the immediate bronchoconstriction but do inhibit the late-phase reaction and allergen-induced increase in bronchial reactivity (7,8). However, prolonged treatment with steroids may also reduce the acute response to inhaled allergen (9). In addition, pretreatment with GC attenuates aspirin-induced bronchospasm in aspirin-intolerant asthmatics (10).

GC affect many aspects of the immune response. A potential mechanism for immunomodulation involves alteration of arachidonic acid (AA) metabolism, and in this regard an inhibition of eicosanoid production by steroids has frequently been postulated. The hypothesis is predominantly driven by data from in vitro studies demonstrating steroid-dependent reduction of eicosanoid release from many (although not all) cell types potentially involved in the inflammation in asthma. However, it is uncertain to what extent the in vitro findings apply to the natural or acquired immune responses that occur in asthmatics. The purified cell systems utilized for the in vitro studies do not exactly mirror the complexity of the allergic inflammation in vivo, which widely depends on coordinated interactions among many different cell types.

II. Effects of GC on Eicosanoid Metabolism in Cells Relevant to Asthma In Vitro

A. Phospholipase

The phospholipase A_2 (PLA_2) enzymes release AA from the membrane phospholipids, and thus function as the rate-limiting step in the production of eicosanoids. In addition, the activation of PLA_2 results in the production of lysophospholipids, which may themselves be inflammatory mediators or they may be converted by acetylation to a number of 2-acetylated phospholipids, such as platelet-activating factor. There are two major groups of PLA_2, which differ structurally and enzymatically (11). The secretory PLA_2 has been suggested as a potential proinflammatory component of allergy and asthma (12–16). Expression of human group II PLA_2 in transgenic mice resulted in a dermatopathy; however, inflammatory infiltrate was absent. The group II PLA_2 gene was also hyperexpressed in the lungs of those animals, but no lung abnormalities were reported in the study (17). GC deficiency in experimental animals causes up-regulation of PLA_2 (18). On the other hand, high doses of GC may suppress eicosanoid generation via inhibition of PLA_2 (19–21), although the role of this mechanism, particularly in vivo, is uncertain.

B. COX Pathway

Prostaglandin endoperoxide synthase (PGHS, cyclooxygenase, COX) is the enzyme regulating the conversion of AA to PGH_2, the common precursor to all prostaglandins and thromboxane A_2. There are two distinct isozymes for PGHS: PGHS-1, which is constitutively expressed in most cell types and tissues, and is encoded by a 2.8-kb transcript, and a 4.4-kb transcript designated PGHS-2, which is regulated by cytokines, growth factors, tumor promoters, and hormones (22,23).

Although PGHS-1 and PGHS-2 share many catalytic and kinetic properties, a growing body of evidence suggests that the enzymes function independently. For example, the intracellular location (24), coupling to signaling pathways (25), utilization of arachidonate pools (26), and the affinity toward some fatty acid substrates and nonsteroidal anti-inflammatory drugs (27) differ between PGHS-1 and PGHS-2. Recently, the distinctive physiological roles of PGHS-1 and -2 isozymes have been demonstrated in mice in which the genes coding for the enzymes have been selectively deleted (28–30). Nevertheless, our present understanding of the biological functions of the PGHS isozymes is incomplete (31), and therefore, the common notion that PGHS-1 mediates physiological responses and PGHS-2 has predominantly proinflammatory actions is oversimplified, and must be viewed with caution.

In vitro, GC inhibit stimulated release of COX products from many human cell types including alveolar macrophages from normal, atopic, and asthmatic subjects (32–34), normal monocytes (35–38), airway epithelial cells (39), and fibroblasts (40). Inasmuch as GC have been shown to down-regulate PGHS-2 in most of the in vitro studies employing different cell systems as well as in animal models of acute inflammation in vivo, this effect has been linked to the inhibition of PGHS-2 (36–41). In addition, Masferrer and colleagues demonstrated that endogenous GC have a profound inhibitory effect on baseline and endotoxin-primed COX expression in mouse peritoneal macrophages (42). However, there are exceptions to this paradigm and they may have important physiological consequences. For example, dexamethasone (DEX) inhibited the release of 6-keto-$PGF_{1\alpha}$, PGE_2, and $PGF_{2\alpha}$ from human lung fragments stimulated with anti-IgE, but failed to inhibit the anti-IgE-induced production of PGD_2 and TXB_2, suggesting that the regulation of AA metabolism by GC differs in different types of cells (43). Indeed, in mast cells isolated from human airway tissue DEX did not reduce the IgE-dependent release of PGD_2 (44). More detailed experiments on the regulation of the COX pathways in mast cells by GC offer some insights. Murakami and colleagues demonstrated in mouse bone marrow–derived mast cells (BMMC) that the immediate IgE-dependent release of PGD_2 was mediated by PGHS-1, and was not altered by DEX. In cytokine-primed BMMC the immediate phase was followed by the delayed up-regulation of PGHS-2 expression and PGD_2 production, which was diminished by DEX (25,45). Interestingly, the combination of stem cell factor and DEX causes up-regulation of PGHS-1, and a five- to eightfold increase in the capacity of BMMC to produce PGD_2 without affecting PGHS-2 levels. Thus in the murine mast cell in vitro, PGHS-1 can be the regulatable enzyme responsible for PGD_2 formation (46).

C. Lipoxygenase Pathways

The three major enzymes of lipoxygenation are designated 5-, 12-, and 15-lipoxygenase, for the number of the carbon atom of AA at which one molecule of oxygen is introduced. The conversion of AA to leukotrienes, a group of potent mediators of allergic inflammation, is initiated by the enzyme 5-lipoxygenase (5-LO) (47). Recently, significant progress has been made in understanding the intracellular events involved in 5-LO activation (48). The product of 5-LO, leukotriene A_4, is converted by LTA_4 hydrolase in alveolar macrophages, monocytes, and neutrophils to leukotriene B_4 (LTB_4). Mast cells, eosinophils, and basophils, the predominant cells in the inflammatory responses in asthma, generate high amounts of cysteinyl leukotrienes (LTC_4, LTD_4, and LTE_4) through LTC_4 synthase. The regulation of 5-LO levels is less dramatic than for PGHS-2.

In general, GC are not potent inhibitors of leukotriene production in vitro. DEX failed to inhibit either the anti-IgE-induced release of LTC_4 from human lung tissue (43) or the synthesis of LTC_4 in human lung and other types of mast cells stimulated by an IgE-dependent mechanism (44). A relatively weak and somewhat variable inhibition of induced production of LTB_4 and LTC_4 by methylprednisolone or DEX was found in alveolar macrophages from normal, atopic, and asthmatic subjects (32–34).

Unexpectedly, treatment of normal human monocytes with DEX was reported to enhance their 5-LO bioactivity in vitro (49).

III. Eicosanoid Involvement in the Inflammatory Responses in Asthma

Bronchoalveolar lavage (BAL) fluid from atopic asthmatics has detectable levels of eicosanoids at baseline indicating that ongoing chronic ariway inflammation is present even in the airways of mild subjects with asthma, and that the eicosanoid levels are the biochemical markers of that inflammation (50–54). After instillation of specific allergen, the levels of eicosanoids increase still further. PGD_2 is the principal COX product, and LTC_4 the main 5-LO product released following allergen stimulation, but other prostanoids, including $9\alpha,11\beta$-PGF_2, $PGF_{2\alpha}$, TXB_2, and 6-keto-$PGF_{1\alpha}$ as well as LO products, LTB_4, and 5-, 12-, and 15-HETE, are also augmented (50,51,53,54). Twenty-four hours after segmental allergen challenge in human atopics the levels of LTE_4 in BAL fluid remain elevated, while the COX products are only slightly increased compared to baseline (55). In addition to local increases in the airways, elevated eicosanoid levels have been detected in urine of asthmatics undergoing specific inhalation challenges (56–59), and during acute asthma (56,60).

Several types of cells can contribute to the spectrum of lipid mediators present in asthmatic airways. Prostanoids can be generated by mast cells, eosinophils, alveolar macrophages, epithelial cells, and basophils. PGD_2 is the main COX product of mast cells, although macrophages also release PGD_2. Interestingly, no difference in the expression of PGHS-1 and PGHS-2 in alveolar macrophages and blood monocytes (61) or in epithelial cells (62) was found between asthmatic and normal subjects. The 5-LO has a narrow cellular distribution, and the predominant cells with the full enzymatic pathway capable of producing cysteinyl leukotrienes are mast cells, eosinophils, and baso phils. However, a transcellular metabolism resulting in leukotriene synthesis has been described in cells not equipped with 5-LO; e.g., platelets possess the LTC_4 synthase and may generate LTC_4 from LTA_4 synthesized by neutrophils. Interestingly, a greater quantity of immunoreactive 5-LO protein without a corresponding increase in 5-LO bioactivity was found recently in neutrophils from asthmatics compared to those obtained from normals (63). Several polymorphisms have been described in the human 5-LO gene sequence in both normal and asthmatic subjects, but the functional significance of this finding is unknown (64). In addition, macrophages, lymphocytes, and neutrophils have been suggested as sources of 5-HETE. 15-HETE is produced in the lung predominantly by epithelial cells and eosinophils, but macrophages and monocytes are also capable of expressing 15-LO and synthesizing 15-HETE when stimulated with IL-4 or IL-13 (65,66). Both epithelial cells and platelets are sources of 12-HETE.

IV. Regulation of AA Metabolism by GC in Asthmatics In Vivo

In patients with mild atopic asthma, oral prednisone for 1 week in clinically effective doses had no any significant effect on baseline BAL-fluid levels of PGD_2 and LTC_4 nor on other cyclooxygenase and lipoxygenases products of AA. Likewise, prednisone did not affect the early increase of eicosanoids in BAL fluid caused by allergen instillation. Surprisingly, allergen-triggered PGE_2 release might even be increased by treatment with GC (54). Similarly, in a double-blind, placebo-controlled, crossover study in atopic subjects, 2-day pretreatment with prednisone had no effect on either the early or late increase in LTB_4 levels in nasal washing after nasal antigen challenge (67). Further support for the failure of steroids to inhibit global eicosanoid synthesis in asthmatics comes from the systemic production of prostanoids and leukotrienes as reflected by unchanged urinary levels of PGD-M and LTE$_4$ after oral prednisone (54), or urinary LTE$_4$ excretion following allergen challenge after 2-week administration of a highly potent inhaled steroid, fluticasone (9). Similarly, in normal subjects either oral or inhaled GC did not alter the excretion of the dinor metabolites of TXA$_2$ and PGI$_2$ as well as LTE$_4$ (35,68), whereas excretion of PGE-M even slightly increased (68). It is worthwhile mentioning that PMN from subjects with rheumatoid arthritis treated with pulse GC had an increased capacity to produce leukotrienes ex vivo despite the clinical improvement of the patients (69).

The failure to detect a change in eicosanoid levels was not a result of insufficient treatment with GC because the dose of prednisone was adequate to produce measurable levels of its active metabolite, prednisolone, in plasma and BAL fluid. Moreover, after prednisone or fluticasone all patients experienced a decrease in inhaler use and/or an improvement of symptoms and bronchial hyperreactivity (9,54).

GC are not completely impotent where eicosanoids are concerned in human subjects. Sebaldt and colleagues found that 1 week of prednisone treatment in healthy volunteers effectively reduced the resting and stimulated release of COX products as well as LTB$_4$ from macrophage-rich BAL-fluid cells ex vivo (68). Similar inhibition of spontaneous release of prostanoids and LTB$_4$ from BAL cells after prednisone was demonstrated in mild atopic asthmatics (54). After a single dose of prednisone Wenzel and co-workers detected suppression of LTB$_4$ but not TXB$_2$ synthesis by stimulated alveolar macrophages from patients with nocturnal asthma, simultaneously with the decrease in granulocytic cells influx and improvement of pulmonary function (70). These results suggest that inhibition by GC of eicosanoid synthesis in vivo occurs in some, but not all, types of cells.

Little is known about the regulation of eicosanoids by GC on the level of gene expression in asthmatics in vivo. Inasmuch as asthma is a disease associated with elevated levels of prostanoids in BAL fluid, one could expect an increased expression of PGHS-2 in the airways of asthmatic patients. Nonetheless, as mentioned above, at least the baseline expression of PGHS-1 and -2 isozymes in alveolar macrophages and blood monocytes (61) and in epithelial cells (62) does not discriminate asthmatics from normal subjects. It has been hypothesized that GC may act to inhibit PGHS-2 induction in vivo and that this may contribute to their anti-inflammatory effects. However, the common paradigm regarding the role of PGHS-1 and PGHS-2 in normal and pathophysiological conditions, does not appear to be universal, particularly in vivo. Surprisingly, in atopic subjects, treatment with prednisone actually resulted in a significant increase of PGHS-2 mRNA and protein in blood monocytes and alveolar macrophages in vivo. As expected, in normal volunteers prednisone greatly reduced PGHS-2 if the message and protein were present at baseline (61) (Figs. 1 and 2). In vitro, DEX did not increase PGHS-2 levels in monocytes from atopic individuals and effectively blocked the stimulatory effect of endotoxin on PGHS-2 expression, indicating that the dichotomy between the in vitro and in vivo regulation of this enzyme by GC is not imposed by a different response of atopic mononuclear phagocytes to GC but rather results from the effect of prednisone on other cells producing mediators, such as cytokines, capable of regulating PGHS-2. Atopy is characterized by a disturbed equilibrium between the Th1 and Th2 cytokines, in favor of the Th2 response, and the Th2 cytokines, IL-4, and IL-10 inhibit the induction of PGHS-2 by endotoxin and cytokines (71,72). Interestingly, GC have a significant modulatory effect on cytokine gene expression in asthmatics in vivo. Treatment with oral prednisolone causes a reduction in IL-4 and an increase in IFN-γ mRNA in BAL cells and within the bronchial mucosa (73,74). Hence, it is possible that a different profile of cytokines created by prednisone in atopics in vivo, characterized by an elimination of cytokines inhibiting PGHS-2, and increase in cytokines stimulating, or at least promoting, the expression of this enzyme, may explain this surprising observation. Neither the increase in PGHS-2 mRNA and protein in atopics nor the decrease in normal subjects was associated with any significant differences in the spontaneous and AA-stimulated synthesis of prostanoids by purified macrophages and monocytes ex vivo. These results differ from the study utilizing macrophage-rich BAL cells that were not subject to adherence and washing, thereby leaving other airway cells such as lymphocytes, mast cells, and polymorphonuclear leukocytes in the milieu. A similar lack of eicosanoid release inhibition from purified alveolar macrophages ex vivo obtained from normal volunteers after DEX treatment in vivo was reported by Yoss and co-workers (34). While several potential explanations may account for the discrepancy between the increased amount of immunoreactive PGHS-2 protein and unaltered prostanoid synthesis, this failure certainly does not indicate that the new generated enzyme is biologically inactive. Prostaglandin production by phagocytes in vitro does not necessarily reflect the state of activation of these cells in vivo. Moreover, it has been reported that PGHS-2 can be induced in phagocytes without an associated increase in prostaglandin product formation (75)

Does the increase in PGHS-2 in monocytes and alveolar macrophages from atopic patients have functional significance? This is a difficult question to answer, because our understanding of the function of PGHS-2 is incomplete. Certainly, prostanoids, particularly PGE$_2$, have pleiotropic immunoregulatory effects not only on monocytes/macrophages themselves, but also on cells that do not metabolize AA via the COX pathway, such as T lymphocytes. Therefore, it is attractive to speculate that the GC-associated increase in PGHS-2 could allow for an increase in vivo of the synthesis of PGE$_2$, which could amplify the effect of prednisone. As mentioned above, the role of the

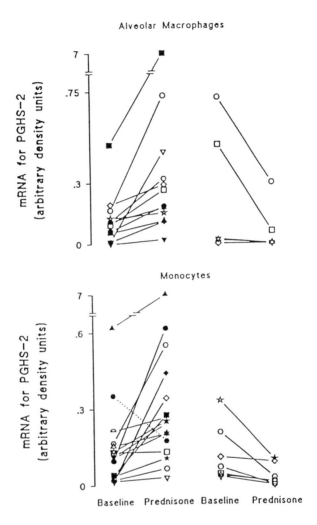

Figure 1 Effect of prednisone on the expression of PGHS-2 mRNA in monocytes from 17 atopic and seven normal subjects and in alveolar macrophages from 12 atopic and five normal subjects. The levels are expressed in arbitrary densitometric units. Prednisone in vivo increased the amount of PGHS-2 mRNA in atopic subjects but decreased it in normal individuals. No difference was found between asthmatic and nonasthamtic atopic subjects, and therefore the results of the atopic subjects have been combined.

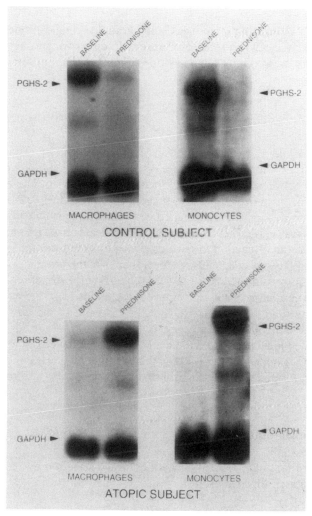

Figure 2 Representative Northern blot for PGHS-2 in macrophages and monocytes at baseline and after prednisone in a control and atopic subject. The characteristic increase in PGHS-2 in the atopic and decrease in the normal subject is evident.

inducible COX in both physiological and pathophysiological conditions needs to be elucidated, and indeed some recent studies strongly suggest that the PGHS-2 enzyme may have not only proinflammatory but important protective functions in vivo (29,30,40,76).

V. Conclusion

GC alter arachidonic acid metabolism in asthmatics in vivo. The response to GC depends on the type of eicosanoid-generating cells. Moreover, there are differences between normal and asthmatic subjects in vivo. There is a dichotomy between the in vitro and in vivo regulation of the inducible PGHS isozyme by GC in atopics and asthmatics, and it is tempting to speculate that more such differences may exist. This observation also indicates that one cannot predict the kind of cellular reaction to steroids in vivo by such potential determinants as suppressibility of eicosanoids by steroids ex vivo, the presence of membrane steroid receptors, or the enzymatic capacity to synthesize arachidonate metabolites. The failure of GC to remove eicosanoids from the asthmatic epithelial lining fluid does not mean that the response of the airway cells and tissue to these mediators is the same in the presence of steroids. Recent advances in the biochemistry and molecular biology of the eicosanoid receptors should provide opportunities to study this exciting but unexplored area. After all, eicosanoids possess not only proinflammatory but also anti-inflammatory properties.

Acknowledgment

The author thanks Dr. J. R. Sheller for helpful discussions and for assistance in preparation of this manuscript.

References

1. Salmeron S, Guerin J-C, Godard P, Renon D, Henry-Amar M, Duroux P, Taytard A. High doses of inhaled corticosteroids in unstable chronic asthma. A multicenter, double-blind, placebo-controlled study. Am Rev Respir Dis 1989; 140:167–171.
2. Juniper EF, Kline PA, Vanzieleghem MA, Ramsdale EH, O'Byrne PM, Hargreave FE. Effect of long-term treatment with an inhaled corticosteroid (Budesonide) on airway hyperresponsiveness and clinical asthma in nonsteroid-dependent asthmatics. Am Rev Respir Dis 1990; 142:832–836.
3. Haahtela T, Järvinen M, Kava T, Kiviranta K, Koskinen S, Lehtonen K, Nikander K, Persson T, Reinikainen K, Selroos O, Sovijärvi A, Stenius-Aarniala B, Svahn

T, Tammivaara R, Laitinen LA. Comparison of a β2-agonist, terbutaline, with an inhaled corticosteroid, budesonide, in newly detected asthma. N Engl J Med 1991; 325:388–392.

4. Dompeling E, van Schayck CP, van Grunsven PM, van Herwaarden CLA, Akermans R, Molema J, Folgering H, van Weel C. Slowing the deterioration of asthma and chronic obstructive pulmonary disease observed during bronchodilator therapy by adding inhaled corticosteroids. A 4-year prospective study. Ann Intern Med 1993; 118:770–778.

5. Haahtela T, Järvinen M, Kava T, Kiviranta K, Koskinen S, Lehtonen K, Nikander K, Persson T, Selroos O, Sovijärvi A, STenius-Aarniala B, Svahn T, Tammivaara R, Laitinen LA. Effects of reducing or discontinuing inhaled budesonide in patients with mild asthma. N Engl J Med 1994; 331:700–705.

6. Waalkens HJ, van Essen-Zandvliet EE, Hughes MD, Gerritsen J, Duiverman F, Knol K, Kerrebijn KF, and the Duch CNSLD Study Group. Cessation of long-term treatment with inhaled corticosteroid (Budesonide) in children with asthma result in deterioration. Am Rev Respir Dis 1993; 148:1252–1257.

7. Cockcroft DW, Murdock KY. Comparative effects of inhaled salbutamol, sodium cromoglycate, and beclomethasone dipropionate on allergen-induced early asthmatic responses, late asthmatic responses, and increased bronchial responsiveness to histamine. J Allergy Clin Immunol 1987; 79:734–740.

8. Cockcroft DW, McParland CP, O'Byrne PM, Manning P, Friend JL, Rutherford BC, Swystun VA. Beclomethasone given after the early asthmatic response inhibits the late response and the increased methacholine responsiveness and cromolyn does not. J Allergy Clin Immunol 1993; 91:1163–1168.

9. O'Shaughnessy KM, Wellings R, Gillies B, Fuller RW. Differential effects of fluticasone propionate on allergen-evoked bronchoconstriction and increased urinary leukotriene E_4 excretion. Am Rev Respir Dis 1993; 147:1472–1476.

10. Nizankowska E, Szczeklik A. Glucocorticosteroids attenuate aspirin-precipitated adverse reactions in aspirin-intolerant patients with asthma. Ann Allergy 1989; 63:159–162.

11. Dennis EA. Diversity of group types, regulation, and function of phospholipase A_2. J Biol Chem 1994; 269:13057–13060.

12. Mehta D, Gupta S, Gaur SN, Gangal SV, Agrawal KP. Increased leukocyte phospholipase A_2 activity and plasma lysophosphatidylcholine levels in asthma and rhinitis and their relationship to airway sensitivity to histamine. Am J Respir Dis 1990; 142:157–161.

13. White SR, Strek ME, Kulp GVP, Spaethe SM, Burch RA, Neeley SP, Leff AR. Regulation of human eosinophil degranulation and activation by endogenous phospholipase A_2. J Clin Invest 1993; 91:2118–2125.

14. Stadel JM, Hoyle K, Naclerio RM, Roshak A, Chilton FH. Characterization of phospholipase A_2 from human nasal lavage. Am J Respir Cell Mol Biol 1994; 11:108–113.

15. Touqui L, Herpin-Richard N, Gene R-M, Jullian E, Aljabi D, Hamberger C, Vargaftig BB, Dessanger J-F. Excretion of platelet activating factor-acetylhydrolase and phospholipase A_2 into nasal fluids after allergenic challenge: possible role in the regulation of platelet activating factor release. J Allergy Clin Immunol 1994; 94:109–119.

16. Chilton FH, Averill FJ, Hubbard WC, Fonteh AN, Triggiani M, Liu MC. Antigen-induced generation of lyso-phospholipids in human airways. J Exp Med 1996; 183: 2235–2245.
17. Grass DS, Felkner RH, Chiang M-Y, Wallace RE, Nevalainen TJ, Bennett CF, Swanson ME. Expression of human group II PLA$_2$ in transgenic mice results in epidermal hyperplasia in the absence of inflammatory infiltrate. J Clin Invest 1996; 97:2233–2241.
18. Vishwanath BS, Frey FJ, Bradbury MJ, Dallman MF, Frey BM. Glucocorticoid deficiency increases phospholipase A$_2$ activity in rats. J Clin Invest 1993; 92: 1974–1980.
19. Gryglewski RJ, Panczenko B, Korbut R, Grodzińska L, Ocetkiewicz A. Corticosteroids inhibit prostaglandin release from perfused mesenteric blood vessels of rabbit and from perfused lungs of sensitized guinea pig. Prostaglandins 1975; 10: 343–355.
20. Hong S-CL, Levine L. Inhibition of arachidonic acid release from cells as the biochemical action of antiinflammatory corticosteroids. J Biol Chem 1976; 73: 1730–1734.
21. Nakano T, Ohara O, Teraoka H, Arita H. Glucocorticoids suppress group II phospholipase A$_2$ production by blocking mRNA synthesis and post-transcriptional expression. J Biol Chem 1990; 265:12745–12748.
22. Xie W, Chipman JG, Robertson DL, Erikson RL, Simmons DL. Expression of a mitogen-responsive gene encoding prostaglandin synthase is regulated by mRNA splicing. Proc Natl Acad Sci USA 1991; 88:2692–2696.
23. Kujubu DA, Fletcher BS, Varnum BC, Lim RW, Herschman HR. TIS10, a phorbol ester tumor promoter-inducible mRNA from Swiss 3T3 cells, encodes a novel prostaglandin synthase-cyclooxygenase homologue. J Biol Chem 1991; 266: 12866–12872.
24. Morita I, Schindler M, Regier MK, Otto JC, Hori T, DeWitt DL, Smith W. Different intracellular locations for prostaglandin endoperoxide H synthase-1, and -2. J Biol Chem 1995; 270:10902–10908.
25. Murakami M, Matsumoto R, Austen KF, Arm JP. Prostaglandin endoperoxide synthase-1 and -2 couple to different transmembrane stimuli to generate prostaglandin D$_2$ in mouse bone marrow-derived mast cells. J Biol Chem 1994; 269:22269–22275.
26. Reddy ST, Herschman HR. Ligand-induced prostaglandin synthesis requires expression of the TIS10/PGS-2 prostaglandin synthase gene in murine fibroblasts and macrophages. J Biol Chem 1994; 269:15473–15480.
27. Meade EA, Smith WL, DeWitt DL. Differential inhibition of prostaglandin endoperoxide synthase (cyclooxygenase) isozymes by aspirin and other non-steroidal antiinflammatory drugs. J Biol Chem 1993; 268:6610–6614.
28. Langenbach R, Morham SG, Tiano HF, Loftin CD, Ghanayem BI, Chulada PC, Mahler JF, Lee CA, Goulding EH, Kluckman KD, Kim HS, Smithies O. Prostaglandin synthase 1 gene disruption in mice reduces arachidonic acid-induced inflammation and indomethacin-induced gastric ulceration. Cell 1995; 83: 483–492.
29. Morham SG, Langenbach R, Liftin CD, Tiano HF, Vouloumanos N, Jennette JC, Mahler JF, Kluckman KD, Ledford A, Lee CA, Smithies O. Prostaglandin syn-

thase 2 gene disruption causes severe renal pathology in the mouse. Cell 1995; 83:473–482.

30. Dinchuk JE, Car BD, Focht RJ, Johnston JJ, Jaffee BD, Covington MB, Contel NR, Engl VM, Collins RJ, Czerniak PM, Gorry SA, Trzaskos JM. Renal abnormalities and an altered inflammatory response in mice lacking cyclooxygenase II. Nature 1995; 378:406–409.

31. Smith WL, DeWitt DL. Biochemistry of prostaglandin endoperoxide H synthase-1 and synthase-2 and their differential susceptibility to nonsteroidal anti-inflammatory drugs. Semin Nephrol 1995; 15:179–194.

32. Fuller RW, Kelsey CR, Cole PJ, Dollery CT, MacDermot J. Dexamethasone inhibits the production of thromboxane B_2 and leukotriene B_4 by human alveolar and peritoneal macrophages in culture. Clin Sci 1984; 67:653–656.

33. Balter MS, Eschenbacher WL, Peters-Golden M. Arachidonic acid metabolism in cultured alveolar macrophages from normal, atopic, and asthmatic subjects. Am Rev Respir Dis 1988; 138:1134–1142.

34. Yoss FD, Spannhake EW, Flynn JT, Fish JE, Peters SP. Arachidonic acid metabolism in normal alveolar macrophages: stimulus specificity for mediator release and phospholipid metabolism, and pharmacologic modulation in vitro and in vivo. Am J Respir Cell Mol Biol 1990p; 2:69–80.

35. Manso G, Baker AJ, Taylor IK, Fuller RW. In vivo and in vitro effects of glucorticoids on arachidonic acid metabolism and monocyte function in nonasthmatic humans. Eur Respir J 1992; 5:712–716.

36. Fu Ji-Yi, Masferrer JL, Seibert K, Raz A, Needleman P. The induction and suppression of prostaglandin H_2 synthase (cyclooxygenase) in human monocytes. J Biol Chem 1990; 265:16737–16740.

37. Kujubu DA, Herschman HR. Dexamethasone inhibits mitogen induction of the TIS10 prostaglandin synthase/cyclooxygenase gene. J Biol Chem 1992; 267: 7991–7994.

38. O'Banion MK, Winn VD, Young DA. cDNA cloning and functional activity of a glucocorticoid-regulated inflammatory cyclooxygenase. Proc Natl Acad Sci USA 1992; 89:4888–4892.

39. Mitchell JA, Belvisi MG, Akarasereenont P, Robbins RA, Kwon OJ, Croxtall J, Barnes PJ, Vane JR. Induction of cyclo-oxygenase-2 by cytokines in human pulmonary epithelial cells: regulation by dexamethasone. Br J Pharmacol 1994; 113: 1008–1014.

40. Wilborn J, Crofford LJ, Burdick MD, Kunkel SL, Strieter RM, Peters-Golden M. Cultured lung fibroblasts isolated from patients with idiopathic pulmonary fibrosis have a diminished capacity to synthesize prostaglandin E_2 and to express cyclooxygenase-2. J Clin Invest 1995; 95:1861–1868.

41. Masferrer JL, Zweifel BS, Manning PT, Hauser SD, Leahy KM, Smith WG, Isakson PC, Seibert K. Selective inhibition of inducible cyclooxygenase 2 in vivo is antiinflammatory and nonulcerogenic. Proc Natl Acad Sci USA 1994; 91: 3228–3232.

42. Masferrer JL, Seibert K, Sweifel B, Needleman P. Endogenous glucocorticoids regulate an inducible cyclooxygenase enzyme. Proc Natl Acad Sci USA 1992; 89: 3917–3921.

43. Schleimer RP, Davidson DA, Lichtenstein LM, Adkinson NF. Selective inhibition of arachidonic acid metabolite release from human lung tissue by antiinflammatory steroids. J Immunol 1986; 136:3006–3011.

44. Cohan VL, Undem BJ, Fox CC, Adkinson NF Jr, Lichtenstein LM, Schleimer RP. Dexamethasone does not inhibit the release of mediators from human mast cells residing in airway, intestine, or skin. Am Rev Respir Dis 1989; 140:951–954.

45. Murakami M, Bingham CO III, Matsumoto R, Austen KF, Arm JP. IgE-dependent activation of cytokine-primed mouse cultured mast cells induces a delayed phase of prostaglandin D_2 generation via prostaglandin endoperoxide synthase-2. J Immunol 1995; 155:4445–4453.

46. Samet JM, Fasano MB, Fonteh AN, Chilton FH. Selective induction of prostaglandin G/H synthase I by stem cell factor and dexamethasone in mast cells. J Biol Chem 1995; 270:8044–8049.

47. Lewis RA, Austen KF, Soberman RJ. Leukotrienes and other products of the 5-lipoxygenase pathway. N Engl J Med 1990; 323:645–655.

48. Woods JW, Coffey MJ, Brock TG, Singer II, Peters-Golden M. 5-lipoxygenase is located in the euchromatin of the nucleus in resting human alveolar macrophages and translocates to the nuclear envelope upon cell activation. J Clin Invest 1995; 95:2035–2046.

49. Riddick CA, Ring WL, Baker JR, Hodulik CR, Bigby TD. Dexamethasone increases expression of 5-lipoxygenase and its activating protein in human monocytes and THP-1 cells. Am J Respir Crit Care Med 1996; 153(4):A216 (abstract).

50. Murray JJ, Tonnel AB, Brash AR, Roberts LJ II, Gosset P, Workman R, Capron A, Oates JA. Release of prostaglandin D_2 into human airways during acute antigen challenge. N Engl J Med 1986; 315:800–804.

51. Wenzel SE, Westcott JY, Smith HR, Larsen GL. Spectrum of prostanoid release after bronchoalveolar lavage allergen challenge in atopic asthmatics and control groups. Am Rev Respir Dis 1989; 139:450–457.

52. Liu MC, Bleecker ER, Lichtenstein LM, Kagey-Sobotka A, Niv Y, McLemore TL, Permutt S, Proud D, Hubbard WC. Evidence for elevated levels of histamine, prostaglandin D_2, and other bronchoconstricting prostaglandins in the airways of subjects with mild asthma. Am Rev Respir Dis 1990; 142:126–132.

53. Wenzel SE, Westcott JY, Larsen GL. Bronchoalveolar lavage fluid mediator levels 5 minutes after allergen challenge in atopic subjects with asthma: relationship to the development of late asthmatic responses. J Allergy Clin Immunol 1991; 87: 540–548.

54. Dworski R, FitzGerald GA, Oates JA, Sheller JR. Effect of oral prednisone on airway inflammatory mediators in atopic asthma. Am Rev Respir Dis 1994; 149: 953–959.

55. Kane GC, Tollino M, Pollice M, Kim C-J, Cohn J, Murray JJ, Dworski R, Sheller JR, Fish JE, Peters SP. Insights into IgE-mediated lung inflammation derived from a study employing a 5-lipoxygenase inhibitor. Prostaglandins 1995; 50:1–18.

56. Taylor GW, Black P, Turner N, Taylor I, Maltby NH, Fuller RW, Dollery CT. Urinary leukotriene E_4 after antigen challenge and in acute asthma and allergic rhinitis. Lancet 1989; 1:584–587.

57. Stadek K, Dworski R, FitzGerald GA, Buitkus KL, Block FJ. Marney SR Jr, Sheller JR. Allergen-stimulated release of thromboxane A_2 and leukotriene E_4 in humans. Am Rev Respir Dis 1990; 141:1441–1445.
58. Stadek K, Sheller JR, FitzGerald GA, Morrow JD, Roberts LJ II. Formation of PGD_2 after allergen inhalation in atopic asthmatics. Adv Prostagl Thromb Leuk Res 1990; 21A:433–436.
59. Knapp HR, Stadek K, FitzGerald GA. Increased excretion of leukotriene E_4 during aspirin-induced asthma. J Lab Clin Med 1992; 119:48–51.
60. Taylor IK, Ward PS, O'Shaughnessy KM, Dollery CT, Black P, Barrow SE, Taylor GW, Fuller RW. Thromboxane A_2 biosynthesis in acute asthma and after antigen challenge. Am Rev Respir Dis 1991; 143:119–125.
61. Dworski RT, Funk CD, Oates JA, Sheller JR. Prednisone increases PGH-synthase in atopic humans in vivo. Am J Respir Crit Care Med 1997; 155:351–357.
62. Demoly P, Jaffuel D, Lequeux N, Weksler B, Créminon C, Michel F-B, Godard P, Bousquet J. Prostaglandin H synthase 1 and 2 immunoreactivities in the bronchial mucosa of asthmatics. Am J Respir Crit Care Med 1997; 155:670–675.
63. Munafo DA, Fu L, Ring WL, Riddick CA, Bigby TD. Increased immunoreactive 5-lipoxygenase in neutrophils of asthmatic patients. Am J Respir Crit Care Med 1996; 153:A416 (abstract).
64. In KH, Asano K, Beier D, et al. Naturally occurring mutations in the human 5-lipoxygenase gene promoter that modify transcription factor binding and reporter gene transcription. J Clin Invest 1997; 1130–1137.
65. Conrad DJ, Kuhn H, Mulkins M, Highland E, Sigal E. Specific inflammatory cytokines regulate the expression of human monocyte 15-lipoxygenase. Proc Natl Acad Sci USA 1992; 89:217–221.
66. Nassar GM, Morrow JD, Roberts LJ III, Lakkis FG, Badr KF. Induction of 15-lipoxygenase by interleukin-13 in human blood monocytes. J Biol Chem 1994; 269:27631–27634.
67. Freeland HS, Pipkorn U, Schleimer RP, Bascom R, Lichtenstein LM, Naclerio RM, Peters SP. Leukotriene B_4 as a mediator of early and late reactions to antigen in humans: the effect of systemic glucocorticoid treatment in vivo. J Allergy Clin Immunol 1989; 83:634–642.
68. Sebaldt RJ, Sheller JR, Oates JA, Roberts LJ II, FitzGerald GA. Inhibition of eicosanoid biosynthesis by glucocorticoids in humans. Proc Natl Acad Sci USA 1990; 87:6974–6978.
69. Thomas E, Leroux JL, Blotman F, Descomps B, Chavis C. Enhancement of leukotriene A_4 biosynthesis in neutrophils from patients with rheumatoid arthritis after a single glucocorticoid dose. Biochem Pharmacol 1995; 49:243–248.
70. Wenzel SE, Trudeau JB, Westcott JY, Beam WR, Martin RJ. Single oral dose of prednisone decreases leukotriene B_4 production by alveolar macrophages from patients with nocturnal asthma but not control subjects: relationship to changes in cellular influx and FEV_1. J Allergy Clin Immunol 1994; 94:870–881.
71. Niiro H, Otsuka T, Tanabe T, Hara S, Kuga S, Nemoto Y, Tanaka Y, Nakashima H, Kitajima S, Abe M, Niho Y. Inhibition by interleukin-10 of inducible cyclooxygenase expression in lipopolysaccharide-stimulated monocytes: its underlying mechanism in comparison with interleukin-4. Blood 1995;85:3736–3745.

72. Dworski RT, Sheller JR. Differential sensitivities of human blood monocytes and alveolar macrophages to the inhibition of prostaglandin endoperoxide synthase-2 by interleukin-4. Prostaglandins 1997; 53:237–251.

73. Robinson D, Hamid Q, Ying S, Bentley A, Assoufi B, Durham S, Kay AB. Prednisolone treatment in asthma is associated with modulation of bronchoalveolar lavage cell interleukin-4, interleukin-5, and interferon-γ cytokine gene expression. Am Rev Respir Dis 1993; 148:401–406.

74. Bentley AM, Hamid Q, Robinson DS, Schotman E, Meng Q, Assoufi B, Kay AB, Durham SR. Prednisolone treatment in asthma. Reduction in the numbers of eosinophils, T cells, tryptase-only positive mast cells, and modulation of IL-4, IL-5 and interferon-gamma cytokine gene expression within the bronchial mucosa. Am J Respir Crit Care Med 1996; 153:551–556.

75. Wilborn J, DeWitt DL, Peters-Golden M. Expression and role of cyclooxygenase isoforms in alveolar and peritoneal macrophages. Am J Physiol (Lung Cell Mol Physiol) 1995; 268:L294–L301.

76. Reuter BK, Asfaha S, Buret A, Sharkey KA, Wallace JL. Exacerbation of inflammation-associated colonic injury in rat through inhibition of cyclooxygenase-2. J Clin Invest 1996; 98:2076–2085.

18

Mechanisms of Aspirin-Induced Asthma

ANDRZEJ SZCZEKLIK

Jagiellonian University School of Medicine
Krakow, Poland

I. Introduction

Shortly after its introduction into therapy, aspirin was implicated as the cause of a violent bronchospasm. The association of aspirin sensitivity, asthma, and nasal polyps was described by Widal and colleagues in 1922. This clinical entity, subsequently named aspirin triad, was popularized by Samter and Beers (1), who, in the late 1960s, presented a perceptive description of the clinical course of the syndrome.

Adverse reactions to aspirin and other nonsteroidal anti-inflammatory drugs (NSAID) may have different clinical presentation and different pathogenesis (2–5). Here we discuss one of them. It affects asthmatics and, indeed, constitutes a special type of asthma, called aspirin-induced asthma (AIA).

II. Clinical Presentation

AIA is a clear-cut clinical syndrome with a distinct clinical picture (6,7). Precipitation of asthma attacks by aspirin and other NSAID is the hallmark of the syndrome. It affects about 10% of adults with asthma, more often women than men, but is rare in asthmatic children. The majority of patients have a negative family history.

In most patients the first symptoms occur during the third decade, as intense rhinitis. Over a period of months, chronic nasal congestion with rhinorrhea develops; physical examination often reveals nasal polyps and anosmia. Bronchial asthma and intolerance to aspirin develop subsequently. The intolerance presents as a unique picture: within an hour after ingestion of aspirin an acute asthma attack occurs, often accompanied by rhinorrhea, conjunctival irritation, and scarlet flushing of head and neck. Aspirin is a common precipitating factor of life-threatening attacks of asthma (8); in a recent large survey, 25% of asthmatic patients requiring emergency mechanical ventilation were found to be aspirin-intolerant (9).

Not only aspirin, but several other NSAID precipitate attacks. Major offenders include: indomethacin, fenamic acid, ibuprofen, fenoprofen, ketoprofen, naproxen, diclofenac, piroxicam, tiaprofenic acid, noramidopyrine, sulfinpyrazone, and phenylbutazone. Not all of these drugs produce adverse symptoms with the same frequency. This depends on the drug's anticyclooxygenase potency, dosage, and on individual sensitivity. If necessary, patients with AIA can take safely sodium salicylate, choline magnesium trisalicylate, dextropropoxyphene, azapropazone, and benzydamine. Most patients also tolerate paracetamol well at a dose not exceeding 1000 mg daily (10). Tartrazine very rarely triggers adverse reactions (11–13).

Asthma runs a protracted course, despite the avoidance of aspirin and cross-reactive drugs. Blood eosinophil count is raised, and eosinophils are present in airways. Skin tests with aspirin are negative. Atopy traits, contrary to early reports (1), are not rare, and, in fact, are somewhat more common than in the general population (14). The asthma is not easy to treat; half of the patients require maintenance therapy with systemic corticosteroids to control the symptoms.

Although a patient's clinical history might raise the suspicion of AIA, the diagnosis can be established with certainty only by aspirin provocation tests. There are three types of the tests, depending on the route of aspirin administration: oral, inhaled, and nasal. Oral challenge tests are most commonly performed. In inhalation tests, aerosol of L-lysine acetylsalicylic acid is administered (15). Inhalation challenge is faster than the oral one, but symptoms are usually restricted only to the bronchopulmonary tract. Nasal provocation testing (16,17) is an attractive research model, and can be also used as a diagnostic procedure on an outpatient basis; its value, however, is limited by lower sensitivity as compared to oral or inhalation provocations. In the majority of patients, once it develops, aspirin intolerance remains for the rest of the patient's life. Repeated aspirin challenges are, therefore, positive although some variability in intensity of symptoms occurs. However, in an occasional patient a positive aspirin challenge might become negative after a few years.

III. Allergic Mechanism

Clinical reactions precipitated by aspirin in the sensitive patients with asthma are reminiscent of immediate-type hypersensitivity reactions. Therefore, an underlying antigen-antibody mechanism has been suggested. However, skin tests with aspirin are negative, and numerous attempts to demonstrate specific antibodies against aspirin or its derivatives were unsuccessful (18). Neither differences in bioavailability of aspirin nor the formation of salicylic acid seems to contribute to aspirin-elicited reactions (19). Furthermore, in patients with AIA asthmatic attacks can be precipitated not only by aspirin, but by several other analgesics with different chemical structures, which makes immunological cross-reactivity most unlikely.

IV. Platelet Mechanism

It has been reported that platelets from patients with aspirin-induced asthma could react abnormally in vitro to aspirin and other cyclooxygenase (COX) inhibitors by generating free oxygen radicals that can kill parasitic larvae (20). This abnormality could be associated with the inhibiting properties of the analgesics on the COX pathway, leading to a defect of the binding of prostaglandin endoperoxide PGH_2 to its receptors on the platelet membrane. Others, however, found that in vitro platelet activation precipitated by aspirin is not a reliable indicator of in vivo sensitivity (21,22).

The ratio of COX to lipoxygenase products was reported to be similar in platelets of patients with AIA as compared to controls (23). Nizankowska et al. (24) measured 12-HETE production by platelets in 10 aspirin-sensitive asthmatics and 10 matched healthy controls before and after administration of the threshold doses of aspirin. Initial levels of 12-HETE did not differ between the two groups. Following aspirin challenge, 12-HETE rose to similar levels in both groups. These data do not support a concept that there is a generalized abnormality in arachidonic acid oxidative pathways in platelets of aspirin-sensitive asthmatics. Lack of protective effect of prostacyclin infusion on aspirin challenge raises doubts about participation of platelets in the discussed reactions (25). Most recent work also (26) tends to refute the pathogenetic role of platelet activation in AIA.

V. The Cyclooxygenase Theory

The COX theory (27) proposes that precipitation of asthma attacks by aspirin is not based on antigen-antibody reaction, but stems from the pharmacological action of the drug (28), namely specific inhibition in the respiratory tract of the enzyme COX. The original observations (2,29) that the drug intolerance can be predicted on the basis of its in vitro inhibition of COX have been consistently reaffirmed during the ensuing years (30,31).

Evidence in favor of the COX theory can be summarized as follows: (1) NSAID with anti-COX activity invariably precipitate bronchoconstriction in aspirin-sensitive patients; (2) NSAID that do not affect COX activity do not provoke bronchospasm; (3) there is a positive correlation between the potency of NSAID to inhibit COX in vitro and their potency to induce asthma attacks in the sensitive patients; (4) after aspirin desensitization, cross-desensitization to other NSAID, which inhibit COX, also occurs.

The enzyme, which appears to be central to the mechanism of aspirin intolerance, recently became the subject of broad interest (32) when its isoforms were discovered. We now know that COX exists in at least two isoforms, COX-1 and COX-2, encoded by distinct genes. The constitutive isoform, COX-1, expressed in most tissues, has clear physiological functions, while the inducible isoform, COX-2, is induced by proinflammatory stimuli in a number of cells, including human pulmonary epithelial cells, fibroblasts, alveolar macrophages, and blood monocytes (33). Cytokine induction of cytosolic phospholipase A2 and COX-2 mRNA is suppressed by glucocorticoids in epithelial cells (34). Both isoforms are expressed in normal human respiratory epithelium and are not quantitatively unregulated in the main bronchi in stable asthma and chronic bronchitis (35). Immunostaining for COX-1 and COX-2 is not different in bronchial biopsies of AIA patients as compared to aspirin-intolerant asthmatics (36,37).

Aspirin, indomethacin, and piroxicam, which at low doses precipitate asthmatic attacks in the sensitive patients, are much more potent inhibitors of COX-1 than COX-2. Salicylate is practically deprived of activity on COX-1 in intact cells, but has half of the potency of aspirin in inhibiting COX-2 in certain cell lines. Nimesulide, a drug known to inhibit COX-2 preferentially, was very well tolerated by AIA patients at a dose of 100 mg, but at a higher dose of 400 mg it induced mild pulmonary obturation (38). New selective COX inhibitors, which are some 1000-fold more potent against COX-2 than against COX-1, have been synthesized (32). In experimental animals they display strong anti-inflammatory activity, with little, if any, side effects on stomach or kidney. Their introduction into the clinic will provide a new interesting tool for probing COX isoforms in AIA.

VI. Involvement of Leukotrienes

In AIA, inhibition of COX is associated with release of cysteinyl-leukotrienes (cys-LTs) which have emerged as important mediators of asthma, and may be particularly prominent in aspirin-induced respiratory reactions. Indeed, their biological effects (39,40) are consistent with most symptoms observed in AIA. Furthermore, eosinophil and mastocyte, two cells that play an essential role in AIA, have the capacity to produce large quantities of cysteinyl leukotrienes.

Some patients with AIA excrete two- to 10-fold higher amounts of LTE_4 in urine than other asthmatics who tolerate aspirin well (41,42). However, when baseline urinary LTE_4 levels in 10 AIA patients were compared to those in 31 aspirin-tolerant asthmatics (43), there was a substantial overlap between the groups and no correlation was found between urinary LTE_4 and histamine PD_{20} or baseline forced expiratory volume in 1 sec (FEV_1). There is no doubt that aspirin challenge results in a temporary, though significant, increase in urinary LTE_4 excretion (44–46), believed to reflect global cys-LTs body production (41,42). Cysteinyl leukotrienes are also released into the nasal cavity following nasal challenge with aspirin (47–50), and into the bronchi following inhalation challenge with lysine-aspirin (51). This is accompanied by inhibition of TXB_2 and PGE_2, while 15-lipoxygenase metabolites remain unaltered (49) (Fig. 1).

Cells expressing the principal enzymes of the 5-lipoxygenase (5-LO) pathway have recently been identified and quantified in bronchial mucosal biopsies of AIA patients, aspirin-tolerant asthmatics, and normal subjects (37).

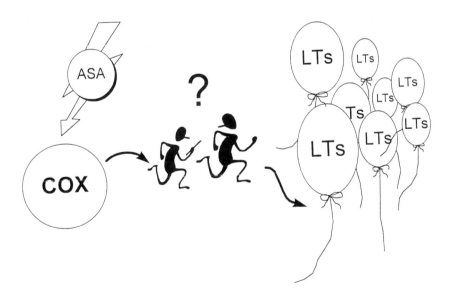

Figure 1 In AIA, inhibition of cyclooxygenase by aspirin leads to release of cysteinyl-leukotrienes. The mechanism linking these two key reactions remains a mystery.

Immunostaining for 5-LO, its activating protein (FLAP), and LTA_4 hydrolase were not different. There was, however, overrepresentation in AIA bronchial biopsies of cells expressing LTC_4 synthase, the essential enzyme for cys-LTs synthesis, compared to significantly fewer cells expressing the enzyme in biopsies from aspirin-tolerant asthmatics and normal subjects. LTC_4 synthase$^+$ cells were predominantly eosinophils ($EG2^+$) and a small number were mast cells ($AA1^+$). The gene for LTC_4 synthase has been localized to chromosome 5q, close to other candidate asthma genes (52), and a polymorphism causing constitutive overexpression of LTC_4 synthase in aspirin-sensitive patients is an attractive hypothesis (37) to explain this highly leukotriene-dependent asthma.

The proof for the critical role of cys-LTs has been provided with the advent of antileukotriene drugs. These compounds either: (1) inhibit leukotriene synthesis by blocking 5-LO or its activator, FLAP, or (2) block specific cys-LTs receptors. Premedication with leukotriene synthesis inhibitors or cys-LTs receptor antagonists has led to marked attenuation of aspirin-precipitated nasal and bronchial reactions (53–56), while histamine antagonists have little effect (57,58). Bronchodilatation has been also observed with antileukotriene agents, indicating that cys-LT have an effect on intrinsic airway tone in AIA (54).

Antileukotriene drugs may soon find a place in chronic treatment of AIA. In a placebo-controlled, crossover, Swedish-Polish study (59), 40 AIA patients received 6 weeks of treatment with the 5-LO inhibitor Zileuton and placebo. Zileuton produced a significant improvement in airway function, decrease in nasal obstruction, return of smell, and reduction in airway responsiveness to histamine. A recently concluded (60), double-blind, placebo-controlled, parallel-group, 4-week study assessed the therapeutic effects of montelukast, a cysteinyl leukotriene receptor antagonist. Eighty aspirin-intolerant asthmatic patients, incompletely controlled with corticosteroids, were randomized to receive montelukast or placebo once daily at bedtime. Patients on montelukast had fewer days with asthma exacerbations, more asthma-free days, and significant improvement in parameters of asthma control, including FEV_1 and PEFR.

Inhaled frusemide, which inhibits the response to a wide range of indirectly acting stimuli including aspirin (61), may interact with leukotriene production in the bronchial mucosa. These interesting bronchoprotective properties of inhaled loop diuretics, discovered by Bianco (62), might open new therapeutic possibilities in asthma.

VII. Release of Mediators at Site of the Reaction

Local instillation of aspirin in the nose or bronchi of sensitive patients, followed by nasal washing or bronchoalveolar lavage, allows investigation of tissue response to aspirin and the course of the reaction. Kowalski et al. (63) reported that intranasal challenge with aspirin led to increased vascular permeability and early influx of eosinophils into nasal secretions of aspirin-intolerant patients. This was accompanied by an increase in concentrations of eosinophil cationic protein and tryptase and development of clinical symptoms, consisting of rhinorrhea, sneezing, and nasal congestion in AIA patients. No changes were detected in nasal washings of the asthmatic patients who tolerated aspirin well. Cysteinyl-LTs were not measured in this study, but their enhanced release has been demonstrated convincingly in previous reports (48–50,55). On the contrary, studies of the response of histamine and PGD_2 yielded inconsistent results. Some authors (55) reported a marked rise in levels of these two mediators in nasal washings following oral aspirin challenge, while others (50) did not confirm these findings. Studies in atopics indicate that PGD_2 measurement in nasal secretion might not be a reliable marker for mast cell activation (64).

Segmental bronchial challenge with aspirin has been recently performed in two well-matched groups of patients: AIA and asthmatics tolerant to aspirin (65). At baseline the two groups did not differ with respect to BAL fluid concentrations of COX products, cys-LTs, histamine, tryptase, interleukin-5 (IL-5), or eosinophil number. Fifteen minutes after intrabronchial instillation of 10 mg L-lysine aspirin, there was a statistically significant rise in cys-LTs, IL-5, and eosinophil number in BAL fluid of AIA, but not of aspirin-tolerant patients (Fig. 2). Mean histamine concentrations rose in response to aspirin, approaching the level of statistical significance. Aspirin significantly depressed PGE_2 and TXB_2 in both groups; however, mean PGD_2, PGF2α, and 9α, 11β-PGF_2 decreased only in aspirin-tolerant patients. In individual AIA subjects, PGD_2 levels showed variability in response to aspirin: from marked increase to depression. Interestingly, Warren et al. (66) reported that segmental bronchial challenge with indomethacin led to a rise in PGD_2 and histamine in BAL fluid of three aspirin-sensitive asthmatics, in contrast to three aspirin-tolerant asthmatics. Thus, bronchial aspirin challenge causes specific eicosanoid response in aspirin-sensitive asthmatics. By removing bronchodilator PGE_2 and leaving unchecked bronchoconstrictor PGD_2 and $PGF_{2\alpha}$, aspirin might further tip the eicosanoid balance toward bronchial obstruction, the balance already disturbed by cys-LT overproduction (Fig. 3).

VIII. PGE₂ and the Switch in Eicosanoid Metabolism

It has been speculated that blocking of the COX pathway would result in increased bioavailability of arachidonic acid and its shunting to leukotrienes, but there is no experimental proof for this. Perhaps, in AIA aspirin promotes re-

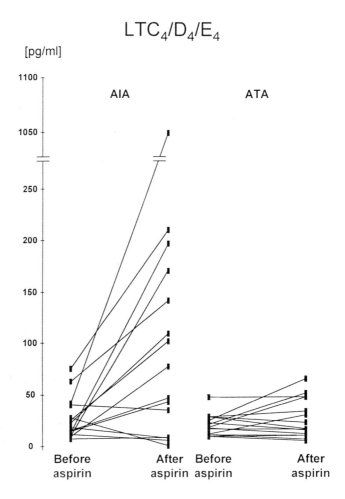

Figure 2 Release of cysteinyl-leukotrienes into bronchoalveolar lavage fluid 15 min after intrabronchial instillation of 10 mg lysine-aspirin. Individual data in 15 patients with AIA and 15 aspirin-tolerant asthmatics (ATA).

lease of leukotrienes by removing PGE_2 (67,68), a dominant COX product of airway (69). PGE_2 reduces LT synthesis in a number of inflammatory cells in vitro, including human eosinophils, neutrophils, and macrophages (70–72). In vivo, both aspirin-induced bronchoconstriction and the accompanying surge in urinary LTE_4 excretion can be completely abrogated by prior inhalation of PGE_2 (73,74). NSAID may, therefore, trigger adverse reactions by reducing PGE_2-dependent suppression of cys-LTs synthesis in the lung. However,

No aspirin   After aspirin

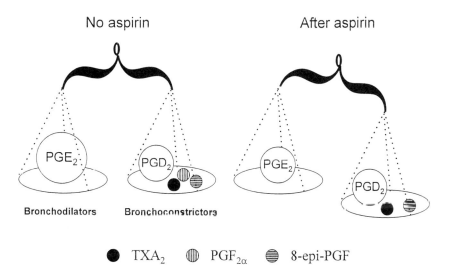

● TXA$_2$ ⦿ PGF$_{2\alpha}$ ⊜ 8-epi-PGF

Figure 3 In AIA aspirin causes specific prostanoid alteration in the lung (65). By removing bronchodilator PGE$_2$ and leaving unchecked bronchoconstrictor PGD$_2$ and PGF$_{2\alpha}$, aspirin might further tip the eicosanoid balance toward bronchial obstruction, the balance already disturbed by cysteinyl-leukotriene overproduction.

additional reasons are necessary to explain why NSAID do not trigger a similar rise in cys-LTs in aspirin-tolerant asthmatics. The finding of enhanced LTC$_4$ synthase expression in AIA (37) may resolve this paradox. NSAID may reduce PGE$_2$ synthesis equieffectively in all subjects, but more LTC$_4$-generation cells are then liberated from the suppression in AIA lung than in other subjects, leading to detectable cys-LTs release and bronchoconstriction only in AIA patients. Of additional importance might be profound inhibitory effects on inflammatory cells exerted by PGE$_2$ at concentrations known to occur in airway (69). Control of T-cell proliferation and cytokine production (75) might be particularly relevant (67). Finally, PGE$_2$ inhibits cholinergic transmission (69,76), which can be disregulated by chronic viral infection (77).

IX. Aspirin Desensitization

In most AIA patients, the state of aspirin tolerance can be introduced and maintained using desensitization. It is performed by giving incremental doses of aspirin in 2–3 days, until the well-tolerated dose of 600 mg is achieved. Aspirin is then administered regularly at a daily dose of 600–1200 mg (6,78).

The patients usually experience improvement in their underlying chronic respiratory symptoms, especially in the nose, during maintenance of the desensitized state for months or even years (79). The state of desensitization is possible because after each dose of aspirin there is a refractory period of 2–5 days' duration, during which aspirin and other COX inhibitors can be taken with impunity.

The mechanism of the desensitization remains elusive. Perhaps, during the period necessary for replacement of irreversibly inhibited COX, the functional balance in the bronchi is based on prostanoid-independent regulatory system, while hypersensitivity to aspirin reoccurs with the return of tissue capacity to generate prostaglandin after aspirin withdrawal (7). Desensitization could lead in AIA patients to reduction of airways responsiveness to LTE_4 due to cysteinyl receptor down-regulation (80). Depression of leukotriene production might be another possible explanation. Desensitization to aspirin results in decreased monocyte leukotriene B4 production (81). Patients maintained for months in the desensitized state still respond to oral aspirin challenge with rise in LTE_4 urinary excretion, though the response appears to be somewhat blunted (82).

X. Chronic Inflammation of Airways

Recent research concentrated on aspirin-precipitated bronchial respiratory reactions, because they are the hallmark of AIA and provide a unique model for study. It has to be remembered, however, that AIA is a chronic disease that runs a protracted course even if NSAID are totally avoided. Bronchial biopsy studies reveal a persistent inflammation of airways with marked eosinophilia, epithelial disruption, cytokine production, and up-regulation of adhesion molecules (7,36,37,83,84). Such pathological process could result from a non-IgE-mediated reaction to an endogenous or exogenous antigen. The HLA class II genes of the major histocompatibility complex are central to the immune processing of exogenous antigens, and finding of an HLA association with AIA might favor immunity as the underlying mechanism of the disease. In a relatively large sample of patients a strong positive association between the presence of HLA-DPB1*0301 and AIA has recently been reported (85). Interestingly, in another study (86) of a small group of AIA patients a possible increase in the frequency of DPB1*1041 was observed. Since the latter allele differs from DPB1*0301 by only a single amino acid in the first hypervariable region of the cell (β1) distal domain, it is possible that the two alleles may be functionally similar. The strength of the association suggests HLA DPB1*0301 may itself confer susceptibility to AIA. Therefore, AIA may be due in part to an inflammatory reaction to an antigen, possibly an autoantigen or a chronic viral infection (67). These possibilities are supported by the finding of elevated markers of autoimmunity (87,88) and enhanced IgG4 synthesis (89) in patients with AIA.

The course of AIA is reminiscent of persistent viral infection (67). Virus could either: (1) modify the genetic message for the COX molecule, making it prone to produce, in response to NSAID, unknown metabolites that stimulate LTs production (65), or (2) evoke an immunological response, perhaps dominated by specific cytotoxic lymphocytes and eosinophils, suppressed by PGE_2 (67). With the advent of molecular biology techniques it might be possible to probe the structure of COX genes and protein or look for the presence of a hypothetical virus in airway tissue of patients with AIA.

XI. Concluding Remarks

Clinical medicine has profited from the research in mechanisms operating in AIA. The important benefits include: development of safe and reliable diagnostic methods based on aspirin challenge, finding a rule for sorting NSAID into safe and contraindicated in AIA patients, and introduction of aspirin desensitization and antileukotriene drugs into therapy. There is now good evidence that aspirin-precipitated reactions result from inhibition of cyclooxygenase that is accompanied by release of cys-LTs. Eosinophils appear to be the best candidates for the cellular source of cys-LTs, while activation of mast cells is likely to affect the course of the reaction. The basis of the link between COX inhibition and LTs overproduction remains elusive, though interesting suggestions have recently been advanced. The least is known about the cause of the disease, which is acquired and runs a chronic course, even when NSAID are avoided. Search for the predisposing factors, especially of immunological origin, for aberrations in intracellular signal transduction, and for a virus as a possible principle initiating and driving the disease, seem to be promising avenues that might lead to solution of the enigma presented by this clinical syndrome.

References

1. Samter M, Beers RF. Intolerance to aspirin. Clinical studies and consideration of its pathogenesis. Ann Intern Med 1968; 68:975–983.
2. Szczeklik A, Gryglewski RJ, Czerniawska-Mysik G. Clinical patterns of hypersensitivity to nonsteroidal antiinflammatory drugs and their pathogenesis. J Allergy Clin Immunol 1977; 60:276–284.
3. Czerniawska-Mysik G, Szczeklik A. Idiosyncrasy to pyrazolone drugs. Allergy 1981; 36:381–384.

4. Hoigné RA, Szczeklik A. Allergic and pseudoallergic reactions associated with nonsteroidal anti-inflammatory drugs. In: Borda IT, Koff RS, eds. NSAIDs: A Profile of Adverse Effects. Philadelphia: Hanley & Belfus, 1992:157–184.
5. Quiralte J, Blanco C, Castillo R, Delgado J, Carillo T. Intolerance to nonsteroidal antiinflammatory drugs: results of controlled drug challenges in 98 patients. J Allergy Clin Immunol 1996; 98:678–685.
6. Stevenson DD. Diagnosis, prevention and treatment of adverse reactions to aspirin and nonsteroidal anti-inflammatory drugs. J Allergy Clin Immunol 1984; 74: 617–622.
7. Szczeklik A. Aspirin-induced asthma. In: Vane JR, Botting RM, eds. Aspirin and Other Salicylates. London: Chapman & Hall Medical, 1992:548–575.
8. Picado C, Castillo JA, Montserrat JM, Augusti-Vidal A. Aspirin-intolerance as a precipitating factor of life-threatening attacks of asthma requiring mechanical ventilation. Eur Respir J 1989; 2:127–129.
9. Marquette CH, Saulnier F, Leroy O, Wallaert B, Chopin C, Demarcq JM, Durocher A, Tonnel AB. Long-term prognosis for near-fatal asthma. A 6-year follow-up study of 145 asthmatic patients who underwent mechanical ventilation for near-fatal attack of asthma. Am Rev Respir Dis 1992; 146:76–81.
10. Settipane RA, Schrank PJ, Simon RA, Mathison DA, Christiansen SC, Stevenson DD. Prevalence of cross-sensitivity with acetaminophen in aspirin-sensitive asthmatic subjects. J Allergy Clin Immunol 1995; 96:480–485.
11. Simon RA. Adverse reactions to drug additives. J Allergy Clin Immunol 1984; 74: 623–630.
12. Weber RW, Hoffman M, Raine DA, Nelson HS. Incidence of bronchoconstriction due to aspirin, azo dyes, non-azo-dyes, and preservatives in a population of perennial asthmatics. J Allergy Clin Immunol 1979; 64:32–37.
13. Virchow C, Szczeklik A, Bianco S, Schmitz-Schumann M, Juhl E, Robuschi M, Damonte C, Menz G, Serwonska M. Intolerance to tartrazine in aspirin-induced asthma: results of a multicenter study. Respiration 1988; 53:20–23.
14. Bochenek G, Nizankowska E, Szczeklik A. Atopy trait in hypersensitivity to nonsteroidal anti-inflammatory drugs. Allergy 1996; 51:16–23.
15. Bianco S, Robuschi M, Petrigni G. Aspirin-induced tolerance in aspirin-induced asthma detected by a new challenge technique. IRCS J Med Sci 1977; 5:129–130.
16. Patriarca G, Ballioni P, Nucero E. Intranasal treatment with lysine-acetylsalicylate in patients with nasal polyposis. Ann Allergy 1991; 67:588–592.
17. Milewski M, Mastalerz L, Nizankowska E, Szczeklik A. Standardization of nasal provocation test with lysine-aspirin for diagnosis of aspirin intolerance in asthma. Allergy Clin Immunol News 1994; (Suppl 2):156.
18. Schlumberger HD. Drug-induced pseudo-allergic syndrome as exemplified by acetylsalicylic acid intolerance. In: Dukor P, Kallos P, Schlumberger HD, West GB, eds. Pseudo-allergic Reactions. Involvement of Drugs and Chemicals. Basel: Karger, 1980:125–203.
19. Dahlen B, Boreus LO, Anderson P, Anderson R, Zetterstrom O. Plasma acetylsalicylic acid and salicylic acid levels during aspirin provocation in aspirin-sensitive subjects. Allergy 1994; 49:43–49.

20. Capron A, Ameisen JC, Joseph M, Auriault C, Tonnel AB, Caen J. New function for platelets and their pathological implications. Int Arch Allergy Appl Immunol 1985; 77:107–114.
21. Pearson DJ, Suarez-Mendez VJ. Abnormal platelet hydrogen peroxide metabolism in aspirin hypersensitivity. Clin Exp Allergy 1990; 20:157–163.
22. Guez S, Gualde N, Bezian JH, Cabanieu G. In vitro study of platelets and circulating mononuclear cells of subjects presenting an intolerance to aspirin. Int Arch Allergy Immunol 1992; 97:233–236.
23. Bonne C, Moneret-Vautrin DA, Wayoff M, Descharmes A, Gazel P, Legrand A, Kalt C. Arachidonic acid metabolism and inhibition of cyclooxygenase in platelets from asthmatic subjects with aspirin intolerance. Ann Allergy 1985; 54:158–160.
24. Nizankowska E, Michalska Z, Wandzilak M, Radomski M, Marcinkiewicz F, Gryglewski RJ. An abnormality of arachidonic acid metabolism is not a generalized phenomenon in patients with aspirin-induced asthma. Eicosanoids 1988; 1:45–48.
25. Nizankowska E, Czerniawska-Mysik G, Szczeklik A. Lack of effect of i.v. prostacyclin on aspirin-induced asthma. Eur J Respir Dis 1986; 69:363–368.
26. Robuschi M, Gambaro G, Sestini P, Pieroni MG, Refini RM, Vaghi A, Bianco S. Attenuation of aspirin-induced bronchoconstriction by sodium cromoglycate and nedocromil sodium. Am J Respir Crit Care Med 1997; 155:1461–1464.
27. Szczeklik A. The cyclooxygenase theory of aspirin-induced asthma. Eur Respir J 1990; 3:588–593.
28. Vane JR. Inhibition of prostaglandin synthesis as a mechanism of action for aspirin-like drugs. Nature 1971; 231:232–234.
29. Szczeklik A, Gryglewski RJ, Czerniawska-Mysik G. Relationship of inhibition of prostaglandin biosynthesis by analgesics to asthma attacks in aspirin sensitive patients. Br Med J 1975; 1:67–69.
30. Stevenson DD, Lewis RA. Proposed mechanisms of aspirin sensitivity reactions. J Allergy Clin Immunol 1987; 80:788–790.
31. Lee TH. Mechanism of aspirin sensitivity. Am Rev Respir Dis 1992; 145:34–36.
32. Bazan N, Botting J, Vane JR. New Targets in Inflammation. Inhibitors of COX-2 or Adhesion Molecules. London: Kluwer Academic Publ. & William Harvey Press, 1996.
33. Mitchell JA, Belvisi MG, Akarasereenont PD, Robbins RA, Kwon OJ, Croxtall J, Barnes PJ, Vane JR. Induction of cyclooxygenase-2 by cytokines in human pulmonary epithelial cells: regulation by dexamethasone. Br J Pharmacol 1994; 113: 1008–1014.
34. Newton R, Kuitert LM, Slater DM, Adcock IM, Barnes PJ. Cytokine induction of cytosolic phospholipase A2 and cyclooxygenase-2 mRNA is suppressed by glucocorticoids in human epithelial cells. Life Sci 1997; 60:67–78.
35. Demoly P, Jaffuel D, Lequeux N, Weksler B, Creminon C, Michel F-B, Godard P, Bousquet J. Prostaglandin H synthase 1 and 2 immunoreactivities in the bronchial mucosa of asthmatics. Am J Respir Crit Care Med 1997; 155:670–675.
36. Nasser SMS, Pfister R, Christie PE, Sousa AR, Barker J, Schmitz-Schumann M, Lee TH. Inflammatory cell populations in bronchial biopsies from aspirin-sensitive asthmatic subjects. Am J Respir Crit Care Med 1996; 153:90–96.

37. Sampson AP, Cowburn AS, Sladek K, Adamek L, Nizankowska E, Szczeklik A, Lam BK, Penrose JF, Austen KF, Holgate ST. Profound overexpression of leukotriene C4 synthase in aspirin-intolerant asthmatic bronchial biopsies. Int Arch Allergy Immunol 1997; 113:355–357.
38. Bianco S, Robuschi M, Petrigni G, Scuri M, Pietroni MG, Refini RM, Vaghi A, Sestini PS. Efficacy and tolerability of nimesulide in asthmatic patients intolerant to aspirin. Drugs 1993; 46(suppl 1):115–120.
39. Busse WW. The role of leukotrienes in asthma and allergic rhinitis. Clin Exp Allergy 1996; 26:868–879.
40. Sampson AP. The leukotrienes: mediators of chronic inflammation in asthma. Clin Exp Allergy 1996; 26:995–1004.
41. Kumlin M. Measurements of leukotrienes in the urine: strategies and applications. Allergy 1997; 52:124–135.
42. Asano K, Lilly CM, O'Donnell WJ, Israel E, Fischer A, Ransil BJ, Drazen JM. Diurnal variation of urinary leukotriene E4 and histamine excretion rates in normal subjects and patients with mild-to-moderate asthma. J Allergy Clin Immunol 1995; 96:643–651.
43. Smith CM, Hawksworth RJ, Thien FC, Christie PE, Lee TH. Urinary leukotriene E4 in bronchial asthma. Eur Respir J 1992; 5:693–699.
44. Christie PE, Tagari P, Ford-Hutchinson AW, Charlesson S, Chee P, Arm JP, Lee TH. Urinary leukotriene E4 concentrations increase after aspirin challenge in aspirin-sensitive asthmatic subjects. Am Rev Respir Dis 1991; 143:1025–1029.
45. Kumlin M, Dahlen B, Bjorck T, Zetterstrom O, Granstrom E, Dahlen SE. Urinary excretion of leukotriene E4 and 11-dehydro-thromboxane B2 in response to provocations with allergen, aspirin, leukotriene D4 and histamine in asthmatics. Am Rev Respir Dis 1992; 146:96–103.
46. Sladek K, Szczeklik A. Cysteinyl leukotrienes overproduction and mast cell activation in aspirin-provoked bronchospasm in asthma. Eur Respir J 1993; 6:391–399.
47. Ortolani C, Mirone C, Fontana A, Folco GC, Miadonna A, Montalbetti N, Rinaldi M, Sala A, Tedeschi A, Valente D. Study of mediators of anaphylaxis in nasal wash fluids after aspirin and sodium metabisulfite nasal provocation in intolerant rhinitic patients. Ann Allergy 1987; 59:106–112.
48. Ferreri NR, Howland WC, Stevenson DD, Spiegelberg HL. Release of leukotrienes, prostaglandins and histamine into nasal secretions of aspirin-sensitive asthmatic during reaction to aspirin. Am Rev Respir Dis 1988; 137:847–854.
49. Picado C, Ramis I, Rosello J, Prat J, Bulbena O, Plaza V, Montserrat JM, Gelpi E. Release of peptido-leukotrienes into nasal secretions after local instillation of aspirin in aspirin-sensitive asthmatic patients. Am Rev Respir Dis 1992; 145:65–69.
50. Kowalski ML, Sliwinska-Kowalska M, Igarashi Y, White MV, Wojciechowska B, Brayton P, Kaulbach H, Rozniecki J, Kaliner MA. Nasal secretions in response to acetylsalicylic acid. J Allergy Clin Immunol 1993; 91:580–598.
51. Sladek K, Dworski R, Soja J, Sheller JR, Nizankowska E, Oates JA, Szczeklik A. Eicosanoids in bronchoalveolar lavage fluid of aspirin-intolerant patients with asthma after aspirin challenge. Am J Respir Crit Care Med 1994; 149:940–946.

52. Penrose JF, Spector J, Baldasaro M, Xu K, Arm JP, Austen KF, Lam BK. Molecular cloning for human LTC$_4$ synthase: organization, nucleotide sequence and chromosomal localization to 5q35. J Biol Chem 1996; 271:11356–11361.
53. Christie PE, Smith CM, Lee TH. The potent and selective sulfidopeptide leukotriene antagonist, SK&F 104353, inhibits aspirin-induced asthma. Am Rev Respir Dis 1991; 144:957–958.
54. Dahlen B, Margolskee DJ, Zetterstrom O, Dahlen S-E. Effect of the leukotriene receptor antagonist MK-0679 on baseline pulmonary function in aspirin sensitive asthmatic subjects. Thorax 1993; 48:1205–1210.
55. Fischer AR, Rosenberg MA, Lilly CM, Callery JC, Rubin P, Cohn J, White MV, Igarashi Y, Kaliner MA, Drazen JM, Israel E. Direct evidence for a role of the mast cell in the nasal response to aspirin in aspirin-sensitive asthma. J Allergy Clin Immunol 1994; 94:1046–1056.
56. Yamamoto H, Nagata M, Kuramitsu K, Tabe K, Kiuchi H, Sakamoto Y, Yamamoto K, Dohi Y. Inhibition of analgesic-induced asthma by leukotriene receptor antagonist ONO-1078. Am J Respir Crit Care Med 1994; 150:254–257.
57. Szczeklik A, Serwonska M. Inhibition of idiosyncratic reactions to aspirin in asthmatic patients by clemastine. Thorax 1979; 34:654–657.
58. Philips GD, Foord R, Holgate ST. Inhaled lysine-aspirin as a bronchoprovocation procedure in aspirin-sensitive asthma: its repeatability absence of a late-phase reaction and the role of histamine. J Allergy Clin Immunol 1989; 84:232–241.
59. Dahlen S-E, Nizankowska E, Dahlen B. Bochenek G, Kumlin M, Kastalerz L, Blomqvist H, Pinis G, Rasberg B, Swanson LJ, Larsson L, Dube L, Stensvad F, Zetterstrom O, Szczeklik A. The Swedish-Polish treatment study with the 5-lipoxygenase inhibitor Zileuton in aspirin-intolerant asthmatics. Am J Respir Crit Care Med 1995; 151:A376.
60. Kuna P, Malmstrom K, Dahlen S-E, Nizankowska E, Kowalski M, Stevenson DD, Bousquet J, Dahlen B, Picado C, Lumry W, Holgate ST, Pauwels R, Szczeklik A, Shahane A, Reiss TF. Montelukast (MK-0476), a cys-LT1 receptor antagonist, improves asthma control in aspirin-intolerant asthmatic patients. Am J Respir Crit Care Med 1997; 155:A975.
61. Sestini P, Ieroni MG, Refini RM, Robuschi M, Gambaro G, Spagnotto S, Vaghi A, Bianco S. Time-limited protective effect of inhaled frusemide against aspirin-induced bronchoconstriction in aspirin-sensitive asthmatics. Eur Respir J 1994; 7:1825–1829.
62. Bianco S, Pieroni MG, Refini RM, Robuschi M, Vaghi A, Sestini P. Inhaled loop diuretics as potential new anti-asthmatic drugs. Eur Respir J 1993; 6:130–134.
63. Kowalski ML, Grzegorczyk J, Wojciechowska B, Poniatowska M. Intranasal challenge with aspirin induces cell influx and activation of eosinophils and mast cells in nasal secretions of ASA-sensitive patients. Clin Exp Allergy 1996; 26:807–814.
64. Wong D-Y, Smitz J, Clement P. Prostaglandin D2 measurement in nasal secretions is not a reliable marker for mast cell activation in atopic patients. Clin Exp Allergy 1995; 25:1228–1234.
65. Szczeklik A, Sladek K, Dworski R, Nizankowska E, Soja J, Sheller J, Oates J. Bronchial aspirin challenge causes specific eicosanoid response in aspirin sensitive asthmatics. Am J Respir Crit Care Med 1996; 154:1608–1614.

66. Warren MS, Sloan SJ, Westcott JY, Hamilos D, Wenzel SE. LTE4 increases in bronchoalveolar lavage fluid (BALF) of aspirin-intolerant asthmatics (AIA) after instillation of indomethacin. J Allergy Clin Immunol 1995; 95:170.

67. Szczeklik A. Aspirin-induced asthma as a viral disease. Clin Allergy 1988; 18: 15–20.

68. Szczeklik A. Prostaglandin E and aspirin-induced asthma. Lancet 1995; 345:1056.

69. Pavord ID, Tattersfield AE. Bronchoprotective role for endogenous prostaglandin E_2. Lancet 1995; 345:436–438.

70. Kuehl FA, Dougherty WH, Ham EA. Interactions between prostaglandins and leukotrienes. Biochem Pharmacol 1984; 33:1–5.

71. Christman BW, Christman JW, Dworski R, Blair IA, Prakash C. Prostaglandin E_2 limits arachidonic acid availability and inhibits leukotriene B_4 synthesis in rat alveolar macrophages by a nonphospholipase A_2 mechanism. J Immunol 1993; 151: 2096–2104.

72. Tenor H, Hatzelmann A, Church MK, Schudt C, Shute JK. Effects of theophylline and rolipram on leukotriene C4 synthesis and chemotaxis of human eosinophils from normal and atopic subjects. Br J Pharmacol 1996; 118:1727–1735.

73. Szczeklik A, Mastalerz L, Nizankowska E, Cmiel A. Protective and bronchodilator effects of prostaglandin E and salbutamol in aspirin-induced asthma. Am J Respir Crit Care Med 1996; 153:567–571.

74. Sestini P, Armetti L, Gambaro G, Pieroni MG, Refini RM, Sala A, Vaghi A, Folco GC, Bianco S, Robuschi M. Inhaled PGE_2 prevents aspirin-induced bronchoconstriction and urinary LTE_4 excretion in aspirin-sensitive asthma. Am J Respir Crit Care Med 1996; 153:572–575.

75. Chan S, Henderson WR, Shi-Hua Li, Hanifin JM. Prostaglandin E_2 control of T-cell cytokine production is functionally related to the reduced lymphocyte proliferation in atopic dermatitis. J Allergy Clin Immunol 1996; 97:85–94.

76. Ellis JL, Conanan ND. Prejunctional inhibition of cholinergic responses by prostaglandin E_2 in human bronchi. Am J Respir Crit Care Med 1996; 154:244–246.

77. Kahn RM, Okanlami DA, Jacoby DB, Fryer AD. Viral infection induced dependence of neuronal M2 muscarinic receptors on cyclooxygenase in guinea pig lungs. J Clin Invest 1996; 98:299–307.

78. Kowalski ML, Grzelewska-Rzymowska I, Rozniecki J, Szmidt M. Aspirin tolerance induced in aspirin-sensitive asthmatics. Allergy 1984; 39:171–178.

79. Stevenson DD, Hankammer MA, Mathison DA, Christiansen SC, Simon RA. Aspirin desensitization treatment of aspirin-sensitive patients with rhinosinusitis asthma. Long-term outcomes. J Allergy Clin Immunol 1996; 98:751–758.

80. Arm JP, O'Hickey SP, Spur B, Lee TH. Airway responsiveness to histamine and leukotriene E_4 in subjects with aspirin-induced asthma. Am Rev Respir Dis 1989; 140:148–153.

81. Juergens UR, Christiansen SC, Stevenson DD, Zuraw BL. Inhibition of monocyte leukotriene B_4 production after aspirin desensitization. J Allergy Clin Immunol 1995; 96:148–156.

82. Nasser S, Patel M, Bell GS, Lee TH. The effect of aspirin desensitization on urinary leukotriene E_4 concentrations in aspirin-sensitive asthma. Am J Respir Crit Care Med 1995; 151:1326–1330.

83. Kawabori S, Denburg JA, Schwartz LB, Irani AA, Wong D, Jordana G, Evans S, Dolovich J. Histochemical and immunohistochemical characteristics of mast cell in nasal polyps. Am J Respir Cell Mol Biol 1992; 6:37–43.

84. Hamilos DL, Leung DYM, Wood R, Bean DK, Song YL, Schotman E, Hamid Q. Eosinophil infiltration in nonallergic chronic hyperplastic sinusitis with nasal polyposis (CHSINP) is associated with endothelial VCAM-1 upregulation and expression of TNF-α. Am J Respir Cell Mol Biol 1996; 15:443–450.

85. Dekker JW, Nizankowska E, Schmitz-Schumann M, Pile K, Bochenek G, Dyczek A, Cookson WOCM, Szczeklik A. Aspirin-induced asthma and HLA-DRB1 and HLA-DPB1 genotypes. Clin Exp Allergy 1997; 27:574–577.

86. Lympany PA, Welsh KI, Christie PE, Schmitz-Schumann M, Kemedy DM, Lee TH. An analysis with sequence-specific oligonucleotide probes of the association between aspirin-induced asthma and antigens of the HLA system. J Allergy Clin Immunol 1993; 92:114–123.

87. Lasalle P, Delneste Y, Gosset P, Grass-Masse H, Wallaert B, Tonnel AB. T and B cell immune response to a 55-kDa endothelial cell-derived antigen in severe asthma. Eur J Immunol 1993; 23:796–803.

88. Szczeklik A, Nizankowska E, Serafin A, Dyczek A, Duplaga M, Musial J. Autoimmune phenomena in bronchial asthma with special reference to aspirin intolerance. Am J Respir Crit Care Med 1995; 152:1753–1756.

89. Szczeklik A, Schmitz-Schumann M, Nizankowska E, Milewski M, Roehlig F, Virchow C. Altered distribution of IgG subclasses in aspirin-induced asthma: high IgG4, low IgG1. Clin Exp Allergy 1992; 22:283–287.

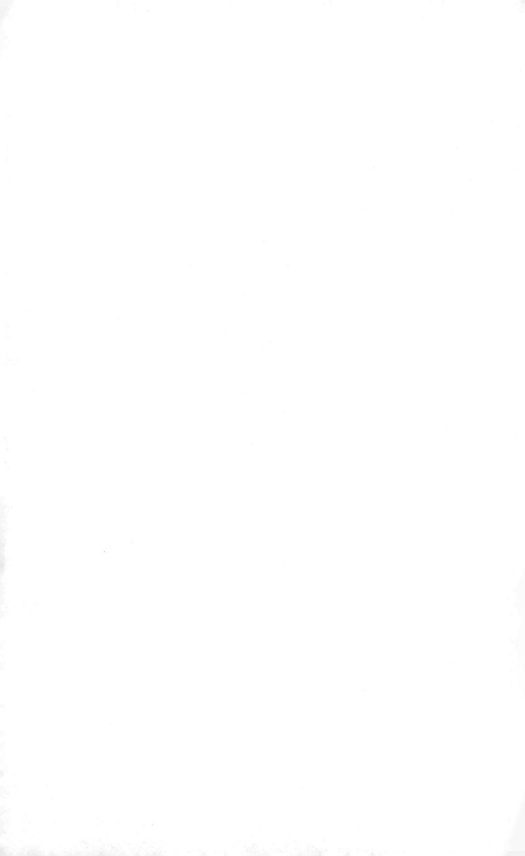

19

Leukotrienes in Aspirin-Sensitive Asthma

S. M. SHUAIB NASSER

Addenbrooke's Hospital
Cambridge, England

TAK H. LEE

Guy's Hospital
London, England

I. History of Aspirin-Induced Reactions

Aspirin was introduced into medicine in 1899 for the treatment of fever and inflammatory disorders (Table 1). In 1903 Franke, in Germany, described the first report of an aspirin-induced reaction when he gave himself 1 g aspirin and within 15 min developed angioedema of his face and larynx, tachycardia, and choking (1). The symptoms subsided after 2 hr. This was followed by a number of similar reports in patients who developed acute angioedema, generalized urticaria, or rhinoconjunctivitis after ingesting as little as 5 grains of aspirin (2–4). In 1905 Barnett published the first case reports of two patients who developed "difficulty in respiration" after ingesting 7.5 and 15 grains aspirin and this probably represents the first report of aspirin-induced bronchospastic reactions (5). Fifteen years later the first report of deaths from a therapeutic dose of aspirin was published (6). Francis reported the association between aspirin sensitivity and nasal polyps in 1919 and suggested that antipyrin and oxyquinothein could produce similar reactions and that phenacetin was safe in these patients (7). Three years later Widal et al. reported the association of aspirin sensitivity, asthma, and nasal polyps (8). In 1968 Samter and Beers

Table 1   History of Aspirin-Induced Reactions

1899	Aspirin introduced into medicine by Bayer in Germany
1903	Franke described first report of an aspirin-induced reaction in himself (1)
1905	Barnett describes first case report of aspirin-induced bronchospastic reactions (5)
1920	First report of deaths from a therapeutic dose of aspirin (6)
1919	Francis reports association between aspirin sensitivity and nasal polyps and suggests that phenacetin is safe (7)
1922	Widal reports the association of aspirin sensitivity, asthma, and nasal polyps (8)
1968	Samter and Beers rediscover syndrome and name it the "aspirin triad" (9)

rediscovered this association and named it the "aspirin triad" (9). Since then, much has been learned about the epidemiology, clinical features, and pathophysiology of aspirin intolerance and other nonsteroidal anti-inflammatory drugs (NSAIDs). In recent years the discovery of the involvement of mediators of both the cyclooxygenase and 5-lipoxygenase pathways in aspirin-sensitive asthma has provided new impetus to the quest for the underlying cause of this unique syndrome.

II. Clinical Presentation

Patients with sensitivity to aspirin are also sensitive to all drugs with anticyclooxygenase properties such as the NSAIDs. They form a distinct group of patients with bronchial asthma and frequent accompanying symptoms of rhinosinusitis including rhinorrhea, nasal congestion, anosmia, loss of taste, and recurrent severe nasal polyposis (9). These patients have aspirin-sensitive asthma (ASA) and their asthma can be severe and frequently requires maintenance therapy with oral corticosteroids and the almost invariable use of either inhaled or intermittent oral corticosteroids. Their nasal symptoms are often resistant to treatment and require topical corticosteroids together with oral courses for the treatment of exacerbations and they may give a history of repeated surgery to remove recurrent nasal polyps. However, despite the association between aspirin sensitivity and asthma the relationship is not causal, and indeed the patient may never have taken anticyclooxygenase drugs and therefore never elicited an intolerant reaction. Furthermore, avoidance of aspirin or NSAIDs appears to have little effect on the course of the chronic asthma or rhinosinusitis. Many patients do not appreciate that anticyclooxygenase drugs

Table 2   Clinical Symptoms Associated with Aspirin-Induced Reactions

Reproducible reaction occurs within 30–120 min
Systemic upset—facial flushing, perspiration, and intense lethargy
Nasal symptoms—rhinorrhea and nasal congestion
Conjunctivitis
Respiratory symptoms—cough and bronchospasm
Dermatological manifestations—urticaria and angioedema
Gastrointestinal symptoms—vomiting, diarrhea, and abdominal discomfort
Severe systemic reaction—respiratory arrest and shock

exacerbate their asthma, and because this relationship is not obvious, their physician is unable to advise on the use of appropriate therapy.

In ASA ingestion of any drug with anticyclooxygenase properties induces a reproducible reaction, which characteristically occurs within 30–120 min (Table 2). The form of the reaction is consistent within individual patients and any combination of symptoms may occur. These include systemic upset with facial flushing, perspiration, and intense lethargy, nasal symptoms with rhinorrhea and nasal congestion, conjunctivitis, and respiratory symptoms of cough and bronchospasm. Some patients experience dermatological manifestations of urticaria and angioedema, or may develop gastrointestinal symptoms of vomiting, diarrhea, and abdominal discomfort. In more sensitive individuals, or if a large dose has been taken, a severe reaction may ensue with the development of respiratory arrest and shock. Although any or all of these symptoms can occur in aspirin-sensitive individuals, in a prospective study of 1372 patients with asthma and rhinitis, the predominant symptom after aspirin ingestion in the asthmatic group was bronchospasm while that in the rhinitis-alone group was urticaria (10).

III. Epidemiology

Data on the epidemiology of aspirin intolerance are incomplete. However, it is clear that aspirin intolerance occurs more frequently in females (11) and most commonly presents in the third and fourth decades of life. In general, aspirin sensitivity occurs sporadically in the population and does not appear to have a genetic component. Familial clustering has been described but only in four families with asthma associated with aspirin intolerance either with or without nasal polyps (12–14). A relative risk of 4 for the HLA DQw2 locus has been reported in 26 subjects with aspirin sensitivity when compared to 22 normal controls (15).

The prevalence of aspirin-sensitive disease has proved difficult to assess and most studies have reported on information gathered either from hospitalized patients or from specialized respiratory and dermatology clinics. Initial reports based the prevalence of aspirin/NSAID sensitivity on patients attending allergy clinics supplying a history of intolerant reactions (11,16–19). The rates of 1.9% to 5.6% probably underestimated the prevalence as they excluded significant numbers of patients who had never taken aspirin/NSAIDS or had not associated drug ingestion with a subsequent bronchospastic reaction. More accurate prevalence data are provided by studies using aspirin challenge to identify sensitive patients. The lowest prevalence of 9% in 79 asthmatic subjects was reported by Stevenson et al., but this figure excluded those patients who gave a history of aspirin sensitivity (20). The true prevalence in their study population was 22% if all 93 consecutive asthmatic subjects were considered. The largest series reported a prevalence rate of 19% in 230 consecutive asthmatic subjects (21). Two large studies of adult asthmatic subjects reported a higher frequency of aspirin intolerance in asthmatic patients than in those with rhinitis alone (10,11).

Many authors on this topic have laid emphasis on the absence of atopy in aspirin-sensitive disease but this is not always the case. In a large study of asthmatic subjects 3.5% (18 of 518) of those with positive skin tests to common aeroallergens and 4.7% (10 of 213) of those with negative skin tests showed intolerance to aspirin (10). In an analysis of five selected studies with reasonably well-specified methods, sensitivity rates to aspirin were lowest (0.3–0.9%) in nonallergic patients. Furthermore, severe atopy was found to be a risk factor for aspirin sensitivity together with asthma and nasal polyposis (22).

IV. Relevance of Anticyclooxygenase Activity

Aspirin and all NSAIDs with anticyclooxygenase activity cross-react to cause intolerant reactions in aspirin-sensitive subjects. Furthermore, the potency of a drug to inhibit cyclooxygenase in vitro correlates well with its ability to induce intolerant reactions in these patients (23). After aspirin desensitization there is cross-desensitization with other inhibitors of cyclooxygenase. Since the first report of cross-reactivity between aspirin and indomethacin (24), a large number of NSAIDs have been marketed with similar effects, and patients with aspirin sensitivity should be warned to avoid them. Paracetamol is a weak inhibitor of cyclooxygenase and at doses of between 150 and 600 mg induces symptoms in approximately 6% (3/49) of aspirin-sensitive subjects (25). However, when the provoking dose of paracetamol is increased to 1000 mg there is a 28% (12/42) cross-reactivity to aspirin in ASA subjects (26).

From our current concepts on the pathogenesis of aspirin-sensitive disease, it is clear that the "affecter" mechanism is cyclooxygenase inhibition, but the interconnection with the downstream effects leading to aspirin-intolerant reactions have not yet been fully elucidated. In fact, experimental evidence has so far provided data that are difficult to interpret. Toogood (27) in an editorial in 1977 suggested that in ASA there is a relative deficiency of the bronchodilator prostaglandin PGE_2 in the respiratory tract compared to $PGF_{2\alpha}$, which increases bronchial smooth muscle tone. He postulated that in ASA, a dose of aspirin inhibits generation of PGE_2, which, in conjunction with its rapid clearance from the circulation due to a short half-life, could precipitate an acute insufficiency of PGE_2. The resultant unopposed action of $PGF_{2\alpha}$ would then lead to bronchoconstriction both by a direct action and by decreasing cAMP leading to enhanced release of other proinflammatory mediators. Support for this concept is provided by recent studies in which inhaled PGE_2 was shown to effectively inhibit the bronchoconstrictor effect of inhaled lysine-aspirin and this was accompanied by complete suppression of the rise in urinary LTE_4 suggesting that PGE_2 acts by an inhibitory activity on cysteinyl leukotriene generation (28,29). However, published studies do not support PGE_2 deficiency in the airways of patients with ASA, and by way of contrast, a study of 10 aspirin-sensitive and six non-aspirin-sensitive asthmatic subjects reported significantly higher baseline bronchoalveolar (BAL) fluid levels of PGE_2 and TXB_2 in the aspirin-sensitive group (30). Furthermore, pretreatment with inhaled salbutamol is as effective as PGE_2 in preventing the bronchoconstrictor effect of lysine-aspirin in ASA individuals, and this effect appears to be independent of its bronchodilator action (28).

V. Cysteinyl Leukotriene Release in ASA

The cysteinyl leukotrienes (LTC_4, LTD_4, and LTE_4) are products of arachidonic acid metabolism generated by the 5-lipoxygenase pathway and comprise the activity previously referred to as slow-reacting substance of anaphylaxis. They have a number of biological actions that can explain aspirin-induced reactions in sensitive individuals. The cysteinyl leukotrienes are potent bronchoconstrictors (31), stimulate bronchial mucus secretion (32), increase venopermeability (33), and increase bronchial hyperresponsiveness in asthmatic subjects (34). Recent evidence has also demonstrated their potent proinflammatory potential with inhaled LTE_4 recruiting both granulocytes and particularly eosinophils into the bronchial airways of asthmatic subjects (35). Leukotriene E_4 is the most stable of these compounds, and following intravenous infusion of either synthetic LTC_4 or LTE_4, 4–7% is excreted in urine as LTE_4 within 2 hr of the infusion. The proportion excreted is relatively constant

Table 3 Release of Leukotrienes in Aspirin-Sensitive Asthma

Biological fluid	Leukotriene release	Ref.
Urine	LTE$_4$ levels are 6-fold higher at baseline and increase a further 4-fold after aspirin challenge	Smith et al. (39) Christie et al. (40)
Nasal lavage	LTC$_4$ levels increase after aspirin challenge in 3/4 subjects who developed naso-ocular symptoms with bronchoconstriction	Ferreri et al. (43)
	Cysteinyl leukotrienes increase 3-fold in 10 subjects after nasal lysine-aspirin instillation	Picado et al. (44)
Bronchial lavage	Increased cysteinyl leukotriene levels after lysine-aspirin in 10 ASA subjects	Sladek et al. (30)

regardless of the infused dose (36,37). The excretion of urinary LTE$_4$ has also been found to correlate with the dose of both inhaled LTC$_4$ and LTE$_4$ (38), further supporting the use of urinary LTE$_4$ as a reliable measure of pulmonary cysteinyl leukotriene synthesis.

Patients with ASA have elevated release of cysteinyl leukotrienes compared to patients with non-ASA (Table 3). Resting mean urinary LTE$_4$ levels in ASA subjects are significantly higher than in normals or in non-aspirin-sensitive asthmatics. Smith and colleagues (39) reported that baseline urinary LTE$_4$ levels in 10 ASA subjects were 101 pg/mg creatinine compared to 43 pg/mg creatinine in 31 non-aspirin-sensitive asthmatic subjects and 34 pg/mg creatinine in 17 normals. However, there was substantial overlap between the groups and no correlation was found between urinary LTE$_4$ and histamine PD$_{20}$ or baseline forced expiratory volume in 1 sec (FEV$_1$). The authors therefore concluded that measurement of LTE$_4$ in a single sample of urine could not accurately predict the degree of resting airflow obstruction, the degree of bronchial hyperresponsiveness, or diagnose aspirin sensitivity despite the significantly higher mean cysteinyl leukotriene levels in the ASA population. Christie and colleagues reported sixfold higher baseline urinary LTE$_4$ levels in six aspirin-sensitive subjects compared to non-ASA controls. These patients were then challenged with a dose of oral aspirin, which led to a mean 21% decrease in FEV$_1$, and this resulted in a further fourfold elevation in urinary LTE$_4$ above baseline values. There was no change in lung function and no increase in urinary LTE$_4$ levels in the control asthmatic subjects following aspirin ingestion (40). Two subsequent studies have confirmed these findings. Sladek and Szczeklik reported a sevenfold increase in urinary LTE$_4$ levels within 6 hr of oral aspirin challenge in 10 aspirin-sensitive subjects (41), and Knapp and colleagues described a 3.6-fold increase in a similar study (42).

Mediator levels in nasal lavage samples have also been studied in patients with ASA and rhinosinusitis. After oral aspirin challenge, increased levels of both histamine and LTC_4 were detected in nasal lavage samples in three out of four ASA subjects who experienced both naso-ocular symptoms and a reduction in FEV_1. However, there was no increase in levels of these mediators after aspirin ingestion in normals, non-aspirin-sensitive asthmatics, desensitized aspirin-sensitive, or aspirin-sensitive subjects in whom aspirin did not provoke naso-ocular symptoms (43). Similarly, nasal instillation of aspirin in 10 ASA subjects, leading to both a nasal and bronchial reaction, resulted in a threefold increase in nasal lavage fluid cysteinyl leukotriene levels at 60 min (44). These studies have provided convincing evidence to support cysteinyl leukotrienes as mediators principally responsible for the symptoms experienced by aspirin-sensitive subjects in response to anticyclooxygenase action.

A number of studies have now documented hyperexcretion of cysteinyl leukotrienes following lysine-aspirin inhalation in ASA subjects, which further implicates the lung as the source for the increased release of these mediators. Christie and colleagues reported a threefold rise in urinary LTE_4 levels in six ASA subjects after lysine-aspirin inhalation challenge, which led to a mean 26% reduction in FEV_1 (45). Similar results were reported by Kumlin and colleagues in nine ASA subjects (46), and Sladek and colleagues demonstrated increased levels of BAL cysteinyl leukotrienes at 30 min after lysine-aspirin challenge in 10 ASA subjects (30).

VI. Antileukotriene Drugs

Although the cysteinyl leukotrienes have been shown to reproduce many of the symptoms and signs found in ASA and are found at higher levels in the biological fluids of these patients than in other forms of asthma, further proof of their critical role could only be provided by inhibiting their action during aspirin-induced reactions. With the arrival of antileukotriene drugs that were both safe for use in humans and had significant in vivo activity against the effect of inhaled LTD_4, there was a powerful tool to investigate the effect of cysteinyl leukotriene inhibition during aspirin challenge in subjects with ASA. The action of the cysteinyl leukotrienes may be suppressed either by antagonism at the human cysteinyl leukotriene receptor ($Cys\text{-}LT_1$) or by inhibition of their biosynthesis. Leukotriene generation is inhibited by interfering with the action of 5-lipoxygenase (5-LO) either by direct inhibition of the enzyme or by indirectly using compounds that bind with high affinity to 5-LO-activating protein

(FLAP) and therefore prevent arachidonic acid presentation to 5-LO. A number of antileukotrienes have been evaluated in ASA (Fig. 1).

A. Cysteinyl Leukotriene Antagonists

In a study of six aspirin-sensitive subjects, pretreatment with the weak Cys-LT$_1$ antagonist SK&F 104,353 administered by the inhaled route led to a partial inhibition of the bronchoconstrictor response to ingested aspirin by a mean 47% in 5/6 subjects (47). In a recent study of eight subjects with ASA, the more potent Cys-LT$_1$ antagonist MK-0679 significantly attenuated the airways obstruction produced by inhaled lysine-aspirin with a median 4.4-fold rightward shift in the dose-response curve compared to placebo. Indeed, after pretreatment with MK-0679, three of the eight subjects failed to achieve a decrease of 20% in FEV$_1$ despite receiving the maximum dose of lysine-aspirin (48). Bronchodilation has also been demonstrated with these agents. A single dose of 825 mg MK-0679 led to a mean peak increase in FEV$_1$ of 18% with a range of 5–34% in eight ASA subjects. The bronchodilation lasted for a minimum of 9 hr and strongly correlated with the baseline severity of asthma in individual patients (49). This has allowed us to conclude that the baseline up-regulation of cysteinyl leukotrienes found in ASA has an effect on intrinsic airway tone that can be reversed by antileukotriene treatment.

B. 5-Lipoxygenase Inhibitors

Inhibitors of cysteinyl leukotrienes biosynthesis are an alternative antileukotriene treatment that have been evaluated in ASA. The effect of aspirin ingestion was examined in a study of seven subjects with aspirin intolerance and hyperexcretion of urinary LTE$_4$. Premedication with a single dose of 350 mg of the 5-LO inhibitor ZD2138 in seven subjects with ASA resulted in substantial inhibition of both LTB$_4$ generation and urinary LTE$_4$ excretion. In response to oral aspirin challenge, the mean maximal fall in FEV$_1$ was 20.3% when patients were premedicated with placebo but only 4.9% after pretreatment with ZD2138, and this was associated with a reduction in systemic symptoms (Fig. 2). Consistent with the results obtained with the Cys-LT$_1$ antagonist MK-0679, administration of ZD2138 resulted in a 10% increase in FEV$_1$ compared to placebo at 3 hr after administration (50). In a separate study, predosing with zileuton reduced baseline urinary LTE$_4$ excretion by 70% and prevented the fall in FEV$_1$ in response to aspirin challenge. There was additional protection against the development of nasal, gastrointestinal, and dermal symptoms in response to aspirin ingestion (51). In a more recent placebo-controlled, crossover study, 40 ASA subjects received 6 weeks of treatment with the 5-LO inhibitor zileuton and placebo separated by a 4-week washout period. During zileuton treatment patients exhibited significant bronchodilation with an improve-

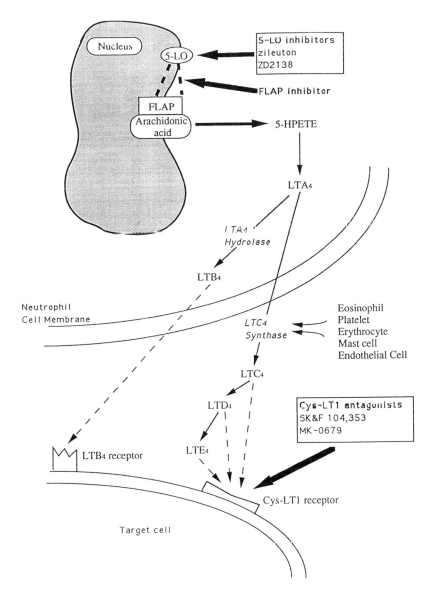

Figure 1 Sites of action of antileukotriene drugs.

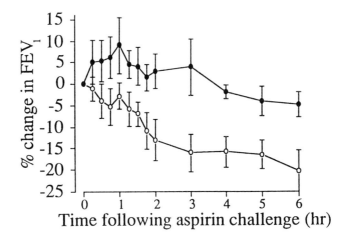

Figure 2 Percent change in FEV_1 for 6 hr following aspirin challenge. ZD2138 (closed circles) or placebo (open circles) was administered 4 hr prior to aspirin challenge. (From Ref. 50.)

ment in FEV_1 of 0.18 L, an improvement in nasal symptom scores, and a reduction in bronchial hyperreactivity with an increase in PD_{20} histamine of 0.5 log units (52).

VII. Aspirin Desensitization

In 1922 Widal desensitized an asthmatic individual who had previously experienced an asthmatic reaction to 100 mg aspirin. In 1976, Zeiss and Lockey (53) reported desensitization to both aspirin and indomethacin in ASA subjects using double-blind oral challenges. More recently, Stevenson (54) has advocated aspirin desensitization in aspirin-sensitive patients as a method of controlling symptoms of rhinosinusitis with the possibility of an improvement in asthma control. Desensitization is usually performed in aspirin-sensitive patients with intractable rhinosinusitis or in those who require regular aspirin or NSAID treatment for indications such as ischemic heart disease or arthritis. Typically, these patients are on large doses of intranasal and inhaled corticosteroids for rhinosinusitis and asthma and may also be taking oral corticosteroids. Aspirin desensitization is started with a dose of 10 mg or 30 mg aspirin, and increasing doses are given at two-hourly intervals in the order 30 mg, 60 mg, 100 mg, 300 mg, and finally 600 mg. If there is a 20% or greater reduction in FEV_1, desensitization is discontinued until the following day. The process usually takes between 2 and 4 days and the patient continues on a daily maintenance dose of 600–1200 mg. In a study of 107 aspirin-sensitive subjects from Stevenson's group (55), 42 were designated as controls and avoided aspirin. The remaining 65 patients were desensitized to aspirin, and of these, 30 discontinued aspirin within 12 months for reasons such as gastrointestinal intolerance, while a continuous group of 35 patients took up to 1200 mg aspirin daily and were followed for a mean of 46 months. Compared to the control group, those continuing on aspirin experienced significant improvements in rhinosinusitis symptom scores with a reduction in the appearance of nasal polyps and the number of surgical polypectomies. There was also a significant improvement in sense of smell in the treated group, and a reduction in the number of courses of oral corticosteroids required to treat exacerbations of rhinosinusitis as well as an average reduction of 5.5 mg in the maintenance dose of prednisone. Interestingly, improvements in chest symptoms were seen in both the treated and control groups.

The state of desensitization is made possible because after each dose of aspirin there is a refractory period during which a further equivalent dose produces no symptoms. The refractory period is individual to each patient and may last from less than 2 days to more than 7 days and is usually 2–4 days long. Furthermore, following aspirin desensitization there is cross-desensitization with other inhibitors of cyclooxygenase such as the NSAIDs. Recent studies have clarified the mechanism of acute aspirin desensitization, which may be explained by a reduction in airway receptor sensitivity to the biological effects of the cysteinyl leukotrienes. Arm et al. (56) demonstrated that inhaled LTE_4 was on average 145 times more potent than histamine in eliciting bronchoconstriction in aspirin-tolerant asthmatics and 1870-fold more potent than histamine in constricting the airways of aspirin-sensitive subjects. After aspirin desensitization there was a mean 20-fold decrease in the sensitivity of the airways to LTE_4 but not to histamine. In aspirin-sensitive subjects this selective hyperresponsiveness is exclusive to LTE_4 and not found with LTC_4 (57) suggesting an important role for LTE_4 in ASA.

An alternative or additional explanation for the efficacy of desensitization is that there is reduced leukotriene production in response to aspirin administration. Ferreri and colleagues reported that LTC_4 was released into nasal secretions of four subjects in whom aspirin sensitivity was associated with naso-ocular symptoms but not in those subjects who had been desensitized to aspirin (43). In a study of nine aspirin-sensitive subjects undertaken by our group (58), there was a mean sevenfold increase in urinary LTE_4 after administration of the threshold dose of aspirin producing a 15% decrease in FEV_1. Twenty-four hours after desensitization the nine subjects were rechallenged with 600 mg of aspirin and there was only a mean 3.3% decrease in FEV_1 with a twofold rise in urinary LTE_4. However, the absolute values of maximal urinary LTE_4 excretion on the two study days were similar, with 1714 pg/mg

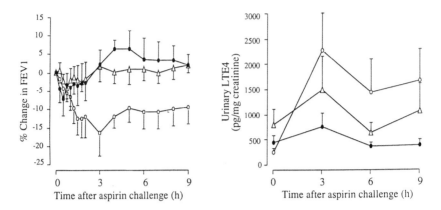

Figure 3   Percent change in FEV$_1$ (left) and urinary LTE$_4$ levels (right) in 5 subjects for 9 hr after challenge at the threshold dose of aspirin (open circles) and with 600 mg aspirin 24 hr (triangles) and at 9 (3.2) months following aspirin desensitization (closed circles). (From Ref. 58.)

creatinine on the threshold day and 1256 pg/mg creatinine following acute desensitization. Furthermore, after a period of chronic desensitization for a mean of 9 months with 600 mg aspirin daily in five subjects there was only an increase in urinary LTE$_4$ from a basal level of 432 pg/mg creatinine to 749 pg/mg creatinine 3 hr after 600 mg aspirin (Fig. 3). Therefore, although there is significantly less aspirin-induced LTE$_4$ excretion acutely after desensitization, substantial amounts of LTE$_4$ are still produced but without a significant change in lung function, thereby supporting a role for decreased airways responsiveness to LTE$_4$ during acute desensitization. However, with chronic aspirin therapy there is further down-regulation of urinary LTE$_4$ excretion in response to aspirin, suggesting that reduced airway release of leukotrienes becomes more important with chronic therapy.

VIII.   Cellular Source of Cysteinyl Leukotrienes

There is considerable indirect data to support both eosinophils and mast cells as the source for cysteinyl leukotrienes elease in the pathogenesis of ASA and rhinitis. However, because of the difficulty in obtaining appropriate tissue samples during aspirin-induced reactions, direct evidence has until recently proved difficult to obtain. Sladek and colleagues performed a study using BAL and found increased numbers of eosinophils and eosinophil cationic protein (ECP) in subjects with ASA compared to control individuals (30). The same authors also reported a significant fall in numbers of peripheral blood eosinophils and a rise in serum ECP and tryptase following oral aspirin ingestion in ASA subjects, thereby implicating both mast cells and eosinophils as the source of cysteinyl leukotriene generation (41). In a study of seven subjects with ASA, Yoshimi and colleagues reported a peripheral blood eosinophilia and increased numbers of activated eosinophils in their nasal polyps (59).

There is evidence supporting the mast cell as the origin for the mediators released in ASA reactions. Immunohistochemical examination of nasal polyps obtained from ASA patients demonstrated both abundant eosinophils and degranulated mast cells (60). Ferreri and colleagues reported increased levels of LTC$_4$ and histamine in nasal secretions following a reduction in FEV$_1$ in three out of four ASA patients who had nasal, ocular, and bronchospastic reactions to aspirin (43). Similarly, Bosso and colleagues demonstrated increased serum histamine and mast cell–derived tryptase levels after aspirin ingestion in ASA subjects, who manifested moderate to severe respiratory reactions associated with aspirin-induced reactions in other organs (61). These findings were confirmed by a further report of a significant rise in nasal lavage levels of mast cell–derived tryptase following aspirin ingestion in ASA subjects (62). A putative mast cell mediator, high-molecular-weight neutrophil chemotactic factor, has also been shown to be released into the serum of half of 22 subjects following aspirin-induced asthmatic reactions favoring the notion of mast cells as the source of increased cysteinyl leukotriene release in ASA (63).

A recent study supports the concept of both cell types playing an important role in ASA reactions. Intranasal lysine-aspirin instillation in six patients with ASA and rhinosinusitis resulted in a twofold increase in eosinophil recovery, a 15-fold increase in levels of eosinophil cationic protein, and an eightfold increase in mast cell tryptase levels in 5/6 subjects. There were no comparable changes in seven control aspirin-tolerant subjects (64). Our group has recently reported additional evidence supporting the involvement of both these cell types as sources for the cysteinyl leukotrienes released during aspirin-induced respiratory reactions. Using immunohistochemical techniques we have studied the inflammatory cell infiltrate and cellular expression of 5-LO in bronchial biopsies taken from asthmatic subjects with aspirin sensitivity both before (65) and after (66) endobronchial lysine-aspirin challenge (Fig. 4). Bronchial biopsies from subjects with ASA demonstrated significantly greater numbers of mast cells and eosinophils per square millimeter of tissue compared to similar biopsies from asthmatic subjects without aspirin sensitivity. Furthermore, 20 min after endobronchial challenge with lysine-aspirin solution in aspirin-sensitive individuals, there was a significant reduction in the numbers of mast cells staining for mast cell tryptase and an increase in the numbers of activated eosinophils, suggesting cellular activation and degranulation for both these cell types which are abundant sources for cysteinyl leukotrienes. Importantly,

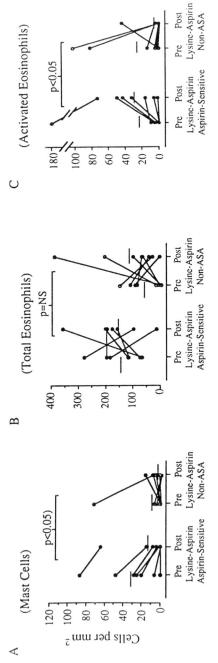

Figure 4 Results obtained from seven ASA and eight non-ASA subjects before and after endobronchial lysine-aspirin challenge. Total number of cells per mm^2 of bronchial biopsy tissue identified immunohistochemically as (A) mast cells; (B) total eosinophils; (C) degranulated eosinophils. (From Ref. 66.)

Table 4 Evidence for the Involvement of Cysteinyl Leukotrienes in Aspirin-Sensitive Asthma

1. Elevated cysteinyl leukotriene levels in ASA
2. Further elevation of cysteinyl leukotriene levels following aspirin ingestion
3. Biological actions of cysteinyl leukotriene consistent with symptoms experienced in ASA
4. Mast cells and eosinophils are important in ASA and are responsible for the generation of cysteinyl leukotrienes both in the chronic disease and following aspirin ingestion
5. Aspirin desensitization leads to down-regulation of cysteinyl leukotriene release
6. Antileukotriene drugs are effective bronchodilators and prevent aspirin-induced reactions in ASA

there was no change in numbers of cells expressing 5-LO after endobronchial lysine-aspirin challenge. These two studies therefore provide the first direct evidence that both mast cells and eosinophils may be responsible for the enhanced cysteinyl leukotrienes release both at baseline and following aspirin ingestion in aspirin-sensitive individuals.

IX. The Future

A number of theories on the pathogenesis of ASA have been proposed but so far none has been universally accepted either because of a lack of experimental evidence or because it does not answer the fundamental question of why inhibition of cyclooxygenase does not precipitate bronchoconstriction in the majority of asthmatics without the syndrome of aspirin sensitivity. Although, we still do not have an all-encompassing hypothesis to explain all the facets of this complex disease, significant strides have been made in understanding the underlying pathogenesis. We know that inhibition of cyclooxygenase is the precipitating event leading to acute bronchospastic and other reactions in ASA and that cysteinyl leukotrienes are the effector mediators for both the acute (following aspirin ingestion) and chronic pulmonary and rhinosinus symptoms experienced by these subjects (Table 4). Mast cells and eosinophils play a major role in the generation of cysteinyl leukotrienes both in the chronic disease and following aspirin ingestion. The symptoms experienced in ASA can be controlled either by aspirin desensitization, which affects the receptor sensitivity to LTE_4 and down-regulates cysteinyl leukotrienes generation, or with the use of the new generation of potent antileukotriene drugs. Further studies will aim to examine the effect of long-term antileukotriene treatment in the chronic phase of this disease and provide us with information on their steroid-sparing activity. Ultimately, we need to understand the fundamental basis of aspirin-intolerant disease to enable elucidation of the provoking event in previously naive patients.

References

1. Von Franke. Vergiftungserscheinungen nach Aspirin. Munch Med Wochenschr 1903; 1299–1300.
2. Von Otto. Aus der arztlichen praxis. Deutsche Med Wochenschr 1903; 123–124.
3. Von Mayer. Nebenwirkung nach dem gebrauch von Aspirin. Deutsche Med Wochenschr 1903; 124.
4. Lindsay J, Leckie AJB. A case of aspirin poisening. Br Med J 1913; 1:1108.
5. Barnett HN. Aspirin in rheumatism: a warning. Br Med J 1905; 2:21.
6. Van der Veer JJ. The asthma problem. N Y J Med 1920; 113:392.
7. Francis A. Aspirin idiosyncrasy. Br Med J 1919; 2:204.
8. Widal F, Abrami P, Lermoyez J. Anaphylaxie et idiosyncrasie. Paris: Presse Med, 1922:189–193.
9. Samter M, Beers RF. Intolerance to aspirin: clinical studies and consideration of its pathogenesis. Ann Intern Med 1968; 68:975–983.
10. Settipane GA, Chafee FH, Klein DE. Aspirin intolerance. II. A prospective study in an atopic and normal population. J Allergy Clin Immunol 1974; 53:200–204.
11. Chafee FH, Settipane GA. Aspirin intolerance. 1. Frequency in an allergic population. J Allergy Clin Immunol 1974; 53:193–199.
12. Miller FF. Aspirin-induced bronchial asthma in sisters. Ann Allergy 1971; 29: 263–265.
13. Lockey RF, Rucknagel DL, Vanselow NA. Familial occurrence of asthma, nasal polyps and aspirin intolerance. Ann Intern Med 1973; 78:57–63.
14. Von Maur K, Adkinson F Jr, Von Metre TE Jr, Marsh DG, Norman PS. Aspirin intolerance in a family. J Allergy Clin Immunol 1974; 54:380–395.
15. Mullarkey MF, Thomas PS, Hansen JA, Webb DR, Nisperos B. Association of aspirin-sensitive asthma with HLA-DQw2. Am Rev Respir Dis 1986; 133:261–263.
16. Prickman LE, Buchstein HF. Hypersensitivity to acetylsalicylic acid (aspirin). JAMA 1937; 108:445–448.
17. Walton CHA, Randle DL. Aspirin allergy. Can Med Assoc J 1957; 76:1016–1018.
18. Speer F. Aspirin allergy: a clinical study. South Med J 1975; 68:314–318.
19. Falliers CJ. Aspirin and subtypes of asthma: risk factor analysis. J Allergy Clin Immunol 1973; 52:141–147.
20. Stevenson DD, Mathison DA, Tan EM, Vaughan JH. Provoking factors in bronchial asthma. Arch Intern Med 1975; 135:777–783.
21. Spector SL, Wangaard CH, Farr RS. Aspirin and concomitant idiosyncrasies in adult asthmatic patients. J Allergy Clin Immunol 1979; 64:500–506.
22. Kwoh CK, Feinstein AR. Rates of sensitivity reactions to aspirin: problems in interpreting the data. Clin Pharmacol Ther 1986; 40:494–505.

23. Szczeklik A, Gryglewski RJ, Czerniawska-Mysik G. Relationship of inhibition of prostaglandin biosynthesis by analgesics to asthma attacks in aspirin-sensitive patients. Br Med J 1975; 1:67–69.
24. Vanselow NA, Smith JR. Bronchial asthma induced by indomethacin. Ann Intern Med 1967; 66:568–572.
25. Szczeklik A, Gryglewski RJ, Czerniawska-Mysik G. Clinical patterns of hypersensitivity to nonsteroidal anti-inflammatory drugs and their pathogenesis. J Allergy Clin Immunol 1977; 60:276–284.
26. Delaney JC. The diagnosis of aspirin idiosyncrasy by analgesic challenge. Clin Allergy 1976; 6:177–181.
27. Toogood JH. Aspirin intolerance, asthma, prostaglandins, and cromolyn sodium. Chest 1977; 72:135–137.
28. Szczeklik A, Mastalerz L, Nizankowska E, Cmiel A. Protective and bronchodilator effects of prostaglandin E and salbutamol in aspirin-induced asthma. Am J Respir Crit Care Med 1996; 153:567–571.
29. Sestini P, Armetti L, Gambaro G, Pieroni MG, Refini RM, Sala A, Folco GC, Bianco S, Robuschi M. Inhaled PGE_2 prevents aspirin-induced bronchoconstriction and urinary LTE_4 excretion in aspirin-sensitive asthma. Am J Respir Crit Care Med 1996; 153:572–575.
30. Sladek K, Dworski R, Soja J, Sheller JR, Nizankowska E, Oates JA. Eicosanoids in bronchoalveolar lavage fluid of aspirin-intolerant patients with asthma after aspirin challenge. Am J Respir Crit Care Med 1994; 149:940–946.
31. Drazen JM, Austen KF. Leukotrienes and airway responses. Am Rev Respir Dis 1987; 136:985–998.
32. Marom Z, Shelhamer JH, Bach MK, Morton DR, Kaliner M. Slow-reacting substances, leukotrienes C_4 and D_4, increase the release of mucus from human airways in vitro. Am Rev Respir Dis 1982; 126:449–451.
33. Dahlen SE, Bjork J, Hedqvist P, Arfors KE, Hammarstrom S, Lindgren JA, Samuelsson B. Leukotrienes promote plasma leakage and leukocyte adhesion in postcapillary venules: in vivo effects with relevance to the acute inflammatory response. Proc Natl Acad Sci USA 1981; 78:3887–3891.
34. Arm JP, Spur BW, Lee TH. The effects of inhaled leukotriene E_4 on the airway responsiveness to histamine in subjects with asthma and normal subjects. J Allergy Clin Immunol 1988; 82:654–660.
35. Laitinen LA, Laitinen A, Haahtela T, Vilkka V, Spur BW, Lee TH. Leukotriene E_4 and granulocytic infiltration into asthmatic airways. Lancet 1993; 341:989–990.
36. Sala A, Voelkel N, Maclouf J, Murphy RC. Leukotriene E_4 elimination and metabolism in normal human subjects. J Biol Chem 1990; 265:21771–21778.
37. Maltby NH, Taylor GW, Ritter JM, Moore K, Fuller RW, Dollery CT. Leukotriene C_4 elimination and metabolism in man. J Allergy Clin Immunol 1990; 85:3–9.
38. Christie PE, Tagari P, Ford-Hutchinson AW, Black C, Markendorf A, Lee TH. Increased urinary LTE_4 excretion following inhalation of LTC_4 and LTE_4 in asthmatic subjects. Eur Respir J 1994; 7:907–913.
39. Smith CM, Hawksworth RJ, Thien FC, Christie PE, Lee TH. Urinary leukotriene E_4 in bronchial asthma. Eur Respir J 1992; 5:693–699.

40. Christie PE, Tagari P, Ford-Hutchinson AW, Charlesson S, Chee P, Arm JP, Lee TH. Urinary leukotriene E₄ concentrations increase after aspirin challenge in aspirin-sensitive asthmatic subjects. Am Rev Respir Dis 1991; 143:1025–1029.

41. Sladek K, Szczeklik A. Cysteinyl leukotrienes overproduction and mast cell activation in aspirin-provoked bronchospasm in asthma. Eur Respir J 1993; 6:391–399.

42. Knapp HR, Sladek K, Fitzgerald GA. Increased excretion of leukotriene E₄ during aspirin-induced asthma. J Lab Clin Med 1992; 119:48–51.

43. Ferreri NR, Howland WC, Stevenson DD, Spiegelberg HL. Release of leukotrienes, prostaglandins, and histamine into nasal secretions of aspirin-sensitive asthmatics during reaction to aspirin. Am Rev Respir Dis 1988; 137:847–854.

44. Picado C, Ramis I, Rosellò J, Prat J, Bulbena O, Plaza V, Montserrat JM, Gelpí E. Release of peptide leukotriene into nasal secretions after local instillation of aspirin in aspirin-sensitive asthmatic patients. Am Rev Respir Dis 1992; 145: 65–69.

45. Christie PE, Tagari P, Ford-Hutchinson AW, Black C, Markendorf A, Lee TH. Urinary leukotriene E₄ after lysine-aspirin inhalation in asthmatic subjects. Am Rev Respir Dis 1992; 146:1531–1534.

46. Kumlin M, Dahlen B, Bjorck T, Zetterstrom O, Granstrom E, Dahlen SE. Urinary excretion of leukotriene E₄ and 11-dehydro-thromboxane B₂ in response to bronchial provocations with allergen, aspirin, leukotriene D₄, and histamine in asthmatics. Am Rev Respir Dis 1992; 146:96–103.

47. Christie PE, Smith CM, Lee TH. The potent and selective sulfidopeptide leukotriene antagonist, SK&F 104353, inhibits aspirin-induced asthma. Am Rev Respir Dis 1991; 144:957–958.

48. Dahlen B, Kumlin M, Margolskee DJ, Larsson C, Blomqvist H, Williams VC, Zetterstrom O, Dahlen SE. The leukotriene-receptor antagonist MK-0679 blocks airway obstruction induced by inhaled lysine-aspirin in aspirin-sensitive asthmatics. Eur Respir J 1993; 6:1018–1026.

49. Dahlen B, Margolskee DJ, Zetterstrom O, Dahlen SE. Effect of the leukotriene receptor antagonist MK-0679 on baseline pulmonary function in aspirin sensitive asthmatic subjects. Thorax 1993; 48:1205–1210.

50. Nasser SM, Bell GS, Foster S, Spruce KE, MacMillan R, Williams AJ, Arm JP. Effect of the 5-lipoxygenase inhibitor ZD2138 on aspirin-induced asthma. Thorax 1994; 49:749–756.

51. Israel E, Fischer AR, Rosenberg MA, Lilly CM, Callery JC, Shapiro J, Rubin P, Drazen JM. The pivotal role of 5-lipoxygenase products in the reaction of aspirin-sensitive asthmatics to aspirin. Am Rev Respir Dis 1993; 148:1447–1451.

52. Dahlén S-E, Nizankowska E, Dahlén B, Bochenek G, Kumlin M, Mastalerz L, Blomqvist H, Pinis G, Rasberg B, Swanson LJ, Larsson L, Dube L, Stensvad F, Zetterström O, Szczeklik A. The Swedish-Polish treatment study with the 5-lipoxygenase inhibitor zileuton in aspirin-intolerant asthmatics. Am J Respir Crit Care Med 1995; 151:A376.

53. Zeiss CR, Lockey RF. Refractory period to aspirin in a patient with aspirin-induced asthma. J Allergy Clin Immunol 1976; 57:440–448.

54. Stevenson DD. Desensitization of aspirin-sensitive asthmatics: a therapeutic alternative? J Asthma 1983; 20(Suppl 1):31–38.

55. Sweet JM, Stevenson DD, Simon RA, Mathison DA. Long-term effects of aspirin desensitization—treatment for aspirin-sensitive rhinosinusitis-asthma. J Allergy Clin Immunol 1990; 85:59–65.
56. Arm JP, O'Hickey SP, Spur BW, Lee TH. Airway responsiveness to histamine and leukotriene E_4 in subjects with aspirin-induced asthma. Am Rev Respir Dis 1989; 140:148–153.
57. Christie PE, Schmitz-Schumann M, Spur BW, Lee TH. Airway responsiveness to leukotriene C_4 (LTC_4), leukotriene E_4 (LTE_4) and histamine in aspirin-sensitive asthmatic subjects. Eur Respir J 1993; 6:1468–1473.
58. Nasser SM, Patel M, Bell GS, Lee TH. The effect of aspirin desensitization on urinary leukotriene E_4 concentrations in aspirin-sensitive asthma. Am J Respir Crit Care Med 1995; 151:1326–1330.
59. Yoshimi R, Takamura H, Takasaki K, Tsurumoto H, Kumagami H. Immunohistological study of eosinophilic infiltration of nasal polyps in aspirin-induced asthma. Nippon Jibiinkoka Gakkai Kaiho 1993; 96:1922–1925.
60. Yamashita T, Tsuji H, Maeda N, Tomoda K, Kumazawa T. Etiology of nasal polyps associated with aspirin-sensitive asthma. Rhinology 1989; 8(Suppl):15–24.
61. Bosso JV, Schwartz LB, Stevenson DD. Tryptase and histamine release during aspirin-induced respiratory reactions. J Allergy Clin Immunol 1991; 88:830–837.
62. Fischer AR, Rosenberg MA, Lilly CM, Callery JC, Rubin P, Cohn J, Israel E, Drazen JM. Direct evidence for a role of the mast cell in the nasal response to aspirin in aspirin-sensitive asthma. J Allergy Clin Immunol 1994; 94:1046–1056.
63. Szmidt M, Crzelewska-Rzymowska I, Roznecki J, Grzegorczyk J. Neutrophil chemotactic activity after administration of aspirin during aspirin tolerance in patients with asthma and aspirin hypersensitivity. Pneumonol Alergol Polska 1991; 59:16–21.
64. Kowalski ML, Grzegorczyk J, Wojciechowska B, Poniatowska M. Intranasal challenge with aspirin induces cell influx and activation of eosinophils and mast cells in nasal secretions of ASA-sensitive patients. Clin Exp Allergy 1996; 26:807–814.
65. Nasser SM, Pfister R, Christie PE, Sousa AR, Barker J, Schmitz-Schumann M, Lee TH. Inflammatory cell populations in bronchial biopsies from aspirin-sensitive asthmatic subjects. Am J Respir Crit Care Med 1996; 153:90–96.
66. Nasser SM, Christie PE, Pfister R, Sousa AR, Walls A, Schmitz-Schumann M, Lee TH. Effect of endobronchial aspirin challenge on inflammatory cells in bronchial biopsy samples from aspirin-sensitive asthmatic subjects. Thorax 1996; 51:64–70.

20

Mast Cell and Eosinophil Responses After Indomethacin in Asthmatics Tolerant and Intolerant to Aspirin

ESTHER L. LANGMACK and SALLY E. WENZEL

National Jewish Medical and Research Center
Denver, Colorado

I. Introduction

Over the last decade, a considerable body of evidence has accumulated in support of a central role for cysteinyl leukotrienes (cLTs) in the pathogenesis of aspirin-intolerant asthma. Aspirin-intolerant asthmatics (AIA) appear to release relatively large quantities of cLTs into nasal secretions, lung airways, and the systemic circulation after cyclooxygenase enzyme inhibition. Nasal and oral challenge with aspirin increased levels of LTC_4 in nasal secretions of AIA (1,2). Urinary LTE_4, a marker for systemic release of cLTs, was significantly elevated in AIA after oral (3) and inhaled (4,5) aspirin challenge. The ability of zileuton, a potent and selective 5-lipoxygenase (5-LO) inhibitor, to decrease nasal symptoms and leukotrienes (6) and prevent a decline in FEV_1 after oral aspirin (7) confirmed the critical role of cLTs in aspirin-tolerant asthma. Recent investigation in this area has focused on the release of eicosanoid mediators into bronchoalveolar lavage fluid (BALF). These studies showed that cLTs increased significantly in BALF of AIA after inhalation (8) and endobronchial instillation (9) of lysine-aspirin (L-ASA), a water-soluble form of aspirin.

Cysteinyl leukotrienes are potent bronchoconstrictors and vasodilators (10) and their release in AIA would plausibly explain many, if not all, of the nasoocular, pulmonary, and systemic features of the AIA response. However, the cellular and biochemical mechanisms that predispose AIA to produce this response are just beginning to be understood. Of particular interest is the identity of the cell, or cells, responsible for the rapid production and release of cLTs after cyclooxygenase inhibition. The eosinophil has emerged as an important potential source of cLTs in studies of endobronchial biopsy tissue and BAL cells from AIA. Human eosinophils have the capacity to rapidly produce significant quantities of cLTs (11); however, the modulation of eosinophil cLT production is poorly understood. The mast cell is another inflammatory cell of significant interest in AIA. Not only are mast cells capable of producing cLTs, but the modulation of the generation and release of other inflammatory mediators, such as histamine and PGD_2, may play a part in aspirin-induced bronchoconstriction.

II. The Eosinophil Response in AIA

AIA have greater numbers of eosinophils in bronchial mucosa than aspirin-tolerant asthmatics (ATA), and these eosinophils appear to be activated during cyclooxygenase inhibition. Nasser et al. compared baseline inflammatory cell populations in endobronchial biopsy tissue from 12 AIA and six ATA using cell-specific immunostaining techniques (12). They also evaluated the cell-type-specific location of 5-LO using a polyclonal antibody to the enzyme. They found more eosinophils in AIA tissue and a greater proportion of AIA cells double-immunostaining positive for the eosinophil marker BMK13 and 5-LO. Recently, this group examined endobronchial biopsies taken from AIA and ATA before and 20 min after application of L-ASA to carinae of subsegmental bronchi (13). Total eosinophils increased in both groups after L-ASA, as reflected by BMK13 immunostaining, but the increase was not statistically significant. However, there was a significant increase in activated, EG2-positive eosinophils in the AIA group. No significant changes in macrophage, neutrophil, or T-lymphocyte populations were observed. These biopsy data suggest that AIA not only have greater numbers of airway eosinophils, but that these eosinophils are uniquely equipped to release large quantities of cLTs, by virtue of their increased expression of 5-LO. The increase in EG2-positive cells after endobronchial L-ASA suggests that cyclooxygenase inhibition leads to overall activation of the eosinophil through unknown mechanisms.

Previous studies of inflammatory cell populations in BAL have demonstrated intriguing but inconsistent differences in eosinophils between AIA and ATA. Sladek et al. found more eosinophils and higher levels of eosinophil cationic protein (ECP), a marker for eosinophil degranulation, in BAL 30 min after placebo inhalation in AIA compared to ATA (8). After challenge with inhaled L-ASA, the number of eosinophils and ECP levels did not change significantly in AIA. ATA were not challenged with L-ASA; therefore, no control group was available for comparison. In a later study, this group examined BAL cells and BALF eicosanoid levels before and 15 min after endobronchial instillation of L-ASA (9). Using this technique, they found no differences in eosinophils at baseline between AIA and ATA. However, after endobronchial L-ASA, eosinophil numbers and cLT levels increased significantly in AIA compared to ATA. ECP levels did not change significantly. The inconsistencies in the eosinophil response to L-ASA are potentially related to differences in experimental technique. Airway L-ASA concentrations were likely lower after inhalational challenge than endobronchial challenge and may not have been sufficient to induce the eosinophil influx. In addition, the bronchoscopy was performed substantially later after inhalational challenge as compared to the endobronchial challenge model. Nonetheless, when the results of BAL and endobronchial biopsy studies utilizing endobronchial L-ASA are considered together, they provide evidence that pulmonary eosinophils are activated during cyclooxygenase inhibition and rapidly migrate into the airway lumen as part of this response.

Recent work in our laboratory confirms that eosinophils and cLTs increase in the airways of AIA following cyclooxygenase inhibition (14). Bronchoalveolar lavage cells and fluid were evaluated before and after endobronchial instillation of indomethacin in six AIA, seven ATA, and six normal subjects. Indomethacin, a cyclooxygenase inhibitor, was chosen because it elicits bronchospasm in AIA (15) and is available in an aqueous form (Indocin I.V., Merck and Co., West Point, PA). Lysine-aspirin is not currently available in the United States. Inclusion of a normal control group allowed us to demonstrate that the increase in cLTs may not be unique to AIA. In our studies, the magnitude of the increase in cLTs and the influx of eosinophils into the airways after cyclooxygenase inhibition are the factors that appear to distinguish AIA from ATA.

Subjects in our study ranged in age between 20 and 49 years. They had a baseline FEV_1 greater than 70% predicted and were otherwise healthy, without recent sinus or respiratory infections. To reduce the potentially confounding effects of medications, oral steroids, cromolyn, aspirin, and other nonsteroidal anti-inflammatory agents were not allowed for 1 month prior to or during the study. Antihistamines and theophylline were held 3 days prior to inhaled and endobronchial challenges. Beta$_2$-agonists were held 8 hr before all challenges. Inhaled steroids were stopped 7 days prior to endobronchial challenge.

Aspirin tolerance status was confirmed by oral aspirin challenge using a modified Scripps protocol (16) in all subjects, except for one AIA with a history of a life-threatening reaction to aspirin. At least 10 days later, an inhaled indomethacin challenge was performed to determine the endobronchial dose. Ten to 14 days after inhaled indomethacin challenge, subjects underwent bronchoscopy with BAL and endobronchial indomethacin challenge. Lavage fluid for "baseline" measurements was first collected from 150 ml of 37°C saline instilled into the lingula. A similar procedure was performed in the right middle lobe 15 min after endobronchial instillation of 4 ml of indomethacin solution. AIA received an average of one-third their PC_{20} FEV_1 for inhaled indomethacin (1.5 ± 0.6 mg/ml), while a twofold greater concentration (3 ± 0.8 mg/ml) was instilled in normals and ATA. Leukotriene levels in BALF were measured using a previously described enzyme immunoassay (EIA) (17). Differential counts of BAL cells were performed on cytospins using a modified Wright's stain (Diff Quik, American Scientific Products, MacGaw Park, IL).

cLT levels were elevated at baseline in both asthmatic groups compared with normals (overall $p = 0.016$). After indomethacin, cLTs increased markedly in AIA (approximately 30-fold over baseline) compared to normal controls ($p < 0.05$) (Fig. 1a). Interestingly, cLTs also increased in the ATA group after indomethacin, but to a lesser extent, such that no significant difference existed between the increases in the two asthmatic groups. Similar to the cLTs, LTB_4 also increased in both asthmatic groups, but the absolute change was much less than for cLTs. Although the increase in LTB_4 in AIA compared to controls was significant ($p < 0.05$, overall $p = 0.04$), as for cLTs, the difference between AIA and ATA was not significant. A significant correlation between the change in cLTs and change in LTB_4 was observed in all groups (Spearman's rho $= 0.70, p = 0.001$).

Baseline eosinophil concentrations in BALF were significantly higher in AIA compared to normals, but not ATA (overall $p = 0.03$). Fifteen minutes after indomethacin instillation, a rapid increase in eosinophils occurred in the AIA ($p = 0.06$), which was not observed in ATA or normals (Fig. 1b). Eosinophil concentrations nearly doubled in this relatively short period. Interestingly, the increase in eosinophils demonstrated a significant correlation with the increase in cLTs in the asthmatic groups (Spearman's rho $= 0.68, p = 0.01$). No significant changes were observed in lymphocyte, macrophage, monocyte, or neutrophil populations.

The increase in BALF cLT levels after indomethacin in AIA and, to a lesser extent, in ATA suggests that 5-LO activation occurs in all asthmatics, in varying degrees, after cyclooxygenase inhibition. In a separate study (18), we found further evidence of 5-LO activation in AIA and ATA, but not normal controls. BAL cells collected from AIA and ATA 15 min after endobronchial indomethacin were fractionated by ultracentrifugation. Western blotting with a 5-LO antibody identified a shift of 5-LO from the cytosolic to the membrane fraction after in vivo indomethacin in AIA and ATA but not normals.

a.

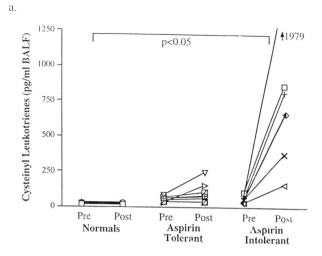

b.

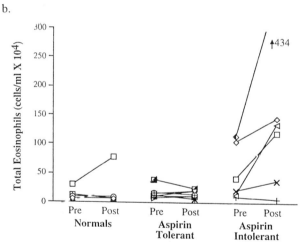

Figure 1 (a) Cysteinyl LT levels in BALF at baseline (Pre) and 15 min after indo-methacin (Post) in normals, aspirin-tolerant, and aspirin-intolerant asthmatics. Base-line cLT levels were different between the three groups, with ATA significantly higher than normals (overall $p = 0.016$). The change in AIA after indomethacin was statisti-cally different between the groups (overall $p = 0.0007$), with the increase in the AIA higher than normals ($p < 0.05$). (b) Total eosinophils (cells $\times 10^4$) in BALF at baseline (Pre) and 15 min after indomethacin (Post). The median number of total eosinophils in the AIA at baseline differed significantly among the three groups (overall $p = 0.03$). Following indomethacin the change in the total number of eosinophils approached significance among the groups ($p = 0.06$). AIA appeared to increase more than ATA and normals. The increase in eosinophils was significantly correlated with the increase in cLTs in AIA and ATA (Spearman's rho = 0.68, $p = 0.01$).

Translocation of 5-LO from the cytosol to the nuclear membrane, where it associates with 5-LO-activating protein (FLAP), is a necessary step in 5-LO activation (10). Because eosinophils are present as a much higher percentage of total cells than mast cells in postindomethacin BALF from AIA, it is likely that most of this shift is due to a response in eosinophils, or perhaps macrophages. In addition, a secondary 50-kDa band was found in all AIA and several ATA after indomethacin, which suggests the formation of an altered 5-LO enzyme or metabolite after activation that is not present in normal controls. Additional studies are needed to characterize this protein and determine its significance in the response of AIA.

The greater magnitude of cLT production in AIA may occur because there are more 5-LO-containing eosinophils and mast cells present in endobronchial tissue of AIA at baseline compared to ATA (12). Similarly, we found greater numbers of eosinophils in baseline BAL in AIA compared to controls, suggesting that more eosinophils are present in the peripheral airways of AIA. The rapid influx of eosinophils into BAL after cyclooxygenase inhibition that we and others (9) have observed could amplify the response of AIA by increasing the number of potential cLT-producing cells in the airway lumen. Finally, the positive correlation between the increase in eosinophils and the increase in cLTs that we observed strongly implicates the eosinophil as a major source of cLTs in AIA.

The mechanisms by which eosinophils move into the airway lumen after cyclooxygenase inhibition in AIA have not been studied. Serum eosinophils have been shown to decrease in AIA hours after aspirin ingestion (19), and it was hypothesized that this was due to recruitment of eosinophils to the lung. The technique of bronchoalveolar lavage has permitted direct verification that eosinophils move into the airway lumen. It seems unlikely that eosinophils increase in BALF as a result of a nonspecific increase in capillary permeability, because no similar increase was observed in other inflammatory cells. The influx of eosinophils into BALF may be related to increased production and release of a variety of eosinophil chemotaxins by mast cells, T lymphocytes, or, less likely, other inflammatory cells. Eosinophil chemoattractant cytokines include IL-4, IL-5 (20), IL-8 (21), RANTES (22), and eotaxin (23). IL-5 levels increased significantly in BALF from AIA but not ATA after endobronchial L-ASA (9). cLT themselves represent another potential chemoattractant for eosinophils in AIA. Eosinophils increased in bronchial mucosal biopsies from asthmatics 4 hr after LTE_4 inhalation (24). LTD_4 has been shown to be a potent chemoattractant for human eosinophils in vitro (25). Zileuton significantly decreased eosinophils in BAL fluid of nocturnal asthmatics (17), but studies of BAL or pulmonary biopsy from AIA in the presence of zileuton are not yet available.

To investigate the possible contribution of RANTES to the eosinophil influx in AIA, we measured levels of RANTES in BALF before and after endobronchial indomethacin in four AIA, four ATA, and six normal subjects using a specific immunoassay (R&D Systems, Minneapolis, MN) (26). Although differences between groups did not reach statistical significance, levels of RANTES were higher in AIA than controls at baseline (mean ± SEM for AIA 6.74 ± 2.14 pg/ml, ATA 4.85 ± 2.44 pg/ml, normals 2.72 ± 2.32 pg/ml), and a greater increase in RANTES was observed in AIA after indomethacin (AIA +7.32 ± 4.45 pg/ml, ATA +1.35 ± 1.42 pg/ml, normals +0.93 ± 0.99 pg/ml). Further studies with 5-LO inhibitors and cLT receptor antagonists in vivo, as well as neutralizing antibodies in vitro, are necessary before a definitive connection can be made between specific mediators and the eosinophil influx.

III. The Mast Cell Response in AIA

The contribution of mast cells to the pathogenesis of aspirin-intolerant asthma has been an area of controversy, largely because mast cell products, such as histamine and tryptase, have been inconsistently elevated in nasal secretions, blood, and BALF after cyclooxygenase inhibition. Levels of histamine (1,6) and tryptase (6) in nasal lavage fluid increased after oral aspirin challenge. Serum tryptase and histamine levels rose after oral ASA, particularly in patients with gastrointestinal manifestations of the reaction (6,27). Interestingly, treatment with zileuton blocked increases in both nasal tryptase and cLTs (6), raising the possibility that 5-LO inhibition attenuates mast cell degranulation. PGD_2 is the major cyclooxygenase product released from activated mast cells. $9\alpha,11\beta$-PGF_2, a urinary metabolite of PGD_2, increased in AIA after challenge with inhaled L-ASA (28), providing evidence of pulmonary mast cell activation. However, these findings are at odds with studies that showed PGD_2 levels in BALF either decreased (8) or were unchanged (9) after L-ASA, while $9\alpha,11\beta$-PGF_2 levels in BALF did not change (8,9). Although a nearly significant ($p = 0.06$) increase in histamine was observed in AIA after endobronchial L-ASA (9), tryptase failed to increase in BALF after inhaled (8) and endobronchial L-ASA (9). Therefore, conclusive evidence for mast cell activation specifically in AIA continues to be elusive.

In studies from our laboratory, histamine and tryptase increased in both AIA and ATA 15 min after endobronchial indomethacin, suggesting that cyclooxygenase inhibition produces a degree of mast cell activation in both asthmatic groups (14). Histamine was measured using a specific immunoassay (Immunotech, Marseilles, France). Tryptase was measured using the B12 ELISA (29). At baseline, histamine levels were higher in ATA compared with normals ($p < 0.05$, overall $p = 0.008$) but not AIA. Following indomethacin, histamine increased in the AIA to a greater, although not significant, degree than in the ATA. In AIA, the median histamine level increased 1327 pg/ml (169–4239 pg/ml) (median with interquartile range), while ATA histamine rose by 88 pg/ml (−234–888 pg/ml) (Fig. 2a). Normals did not change. Considerable variability in these responses in both AIA and ATA prevented significance ($p = 0.22$). Similarly, tryptase, a specific marker for mast cell degranulation, increased in both AIA and ATA after indomethacin (Fig. 2b). As individual groups, these changes did not reach statistical significance compared to normals ($p = 0.15$). However, when the two asthmatic groups were combined, a significant increase ($p = 0.05$) in tryptase occurred compared to normals. These data suggest that indomethacin causes some degree of mast cell degranulation in both ATA and AIA, but that the proportionately greater increase in 5-LO activation, as reflected by greater cLT release, is more specific for AIA. This dichotomy in response could be explained by differential control of degranulation as compared to phospholipase activation in mast cells (30), or, more likely, may reflect the contribution of a second cell, such as the eosinophil, to cLT production.

Studies of endobronchial biopsy tissue provide additional support for mast cell involvement in AIA, but here again, the results are subject to interpretation. Nasser et al. used an antibody against mast cell tryptase to localize mast cells in endobronchial tissue of AIA and ATA (12). At baseline, mast cells were present in greater numbers in AIA, and a greater proportion of mast cells stained positively for 5-LO compared to ATA. Like eosinophils, mast cells in AIA appear to have more 5-LO available for cLT production. Interestingly, after application of L-ASA to the bronchial mucosa, the number of tryptase-positive mast cells decreased significantly in AIA, as did the percentage of 5-LO-positive mast cells (13). This decrease in mast cell tryptase staining was interpreted as evidence of mast cell degranulation, although direct evidence for such dramatic degranulation is lacking. The decrease in 5-LO staining is less easily explained.

IV. The Role of Prostaglandins in AIA

It has been proposed that increased cLT production in AIA results from a decrease in the bronchoprotective prostanoid PGE_2, which may regulate 5-LO. We found PGE_2 levels to be lower in AIA at baseline compared to ATA ($p = 0.009$) (14). PGE_2 levels after indomethacin were highly variable in all groups, but the majority (5 of 6) AIA had increases in PGE_2 after indomethacin (Fig. 3a). PGE_2 was measured using standard EIA techniques (31) after derivatization with methoxamine (32). These results contradict those reported by Szczeklik et al., who found higher PGE_2 levels in AIA at baseline, and a

a.

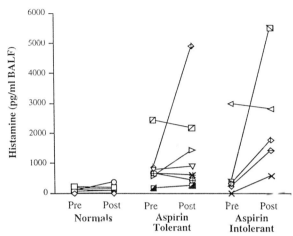

b.

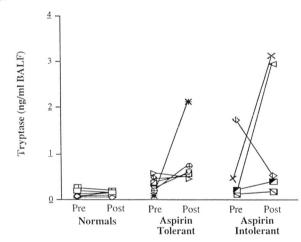

Figure 2 Histamine (a) and tryptase (b) levels in BALF at baseline (Pre) and 15 min after indomethacin (Post) in normals, ATA, and AIA. Baseline histamine levels were higher in both asthmatic groups compared to normals (overall $p = 0.008$). Histamine increases after indomethacin in both AIA and ATA were not significantly different. Tryptase levels in BALF at baseline followed the same pattern as histamine. Baseline tryptase levels and changes after indomethacin were not statistically different among the three groups. However, changes after indomethacin in the combined asthmatics were significantly increased compared to normal controls ($p = 0.05$).

a.

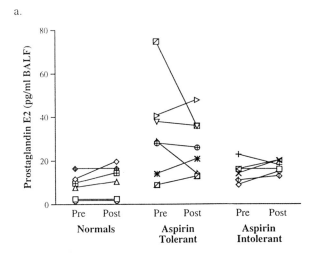

b.

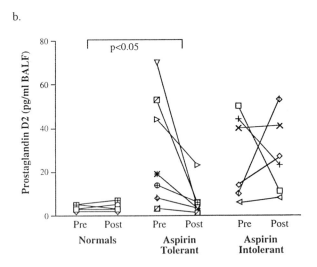

Figure 3 Prostaglandin E_2 (a) and prostaglandin D_2 (b) levels in BALF at baseline (Pre) and 15 min after indomethacin (Post) in the three groups. PGE_2 levels in BALF at baseline were significantly different among the three groups with the levels in AIA lower than ATA (overall $p = 0.009$). Changes in PGE_2 after indomethacin were not significant between the groups. PGD_2 levels at baseline were different between the groups (overall $p = 0.004$), with the AIA and ATA higher than normals ($p < 0.05$). PGD_2 levels decreased in the ATA significantly compared with the normals ($p < 0.05$).

significant reduction in PGE_2 in both AIA and ATA after endobronchial L-ASA (9). However, it is possible that diminished PGE_2 at baseline in AIA lowers the threshold for stimulation by cyclooxygenase inhibition. Two recent studies have shown that pretreatment with inhaled PGE_2 inhibits bronchospasm and the increase in urinary LTE_4 following inhaled L-ASA in AIA (33, 34). Although this may reflect the importance of PGE_2 in AIA, it should be noted that PGE_2 effects are rather nonspecific. PGE_2 has been shown to protect against other bronchoconstrictive stimuli such as exercise (35), allergen (36), and nebulized distilled water (37).

Prostaglandin D_2, a bronchoconstricting prostanoid, may contribute to aspirin-induced bronchospasm in AIA. PGD_2 levels were significantly higher in AIA and ATA compared to normals at baseline (overall $p = 0.004$). After indomethacin, PGD_2 levels fell significantly in ATA, as would be expected, but this consistent reduction was not seen in AIA (Fig. 3b). In fact, PGD_2 actually increased in four of six AIA after challenge. These results are in agreement with those of other investigators who have also been unable to demonstrate a consistent decrease in BALF and nasal lavage fluid PGD_2 (2,9). These results suggest that cyclooxygenase is incompletely suppressed following cyclooxygenase inhibition in AIA, possibly as a result of generalized activation of phospholipases and release of large quantities of arachidonic acid. Even if 90% of the cyclooxygenase were inhibited by indomethacin, 10% of the enzyme would still be available for PGD_2 production. If arachidonic acid levels were sufficiently high, enough substrate would be available to override the effects of cyclooxygenase inhibition and cause an increase in PGD_2 production.

V. Conclusions

Recent investigations into the pathogenesis of aspirin-intolerant asthma provide evidence that the eosinophil, in concert with the mast cell, plays a central role in determining the development of the clinical response to cyclooxygenase inhibition. Biopsy studies have shown more eosinophils and mast cells in endobronchial tissue of AIA compared to ATA. Considerable overlap exists in mast cell activation markers and changes in cLT levels among AIA and ATA after endobronchial indomethacin. This overlap in responses suggests that aspirin-intolerant asthma may, in fact, be more of an extreme manifestation of the cellular and eicosanoid inflammatory processes that characterize asthma, rather than a separate syndrome. The rapid influx of eosinophils into the airways of AIA after cyclooxygenase inhibition appears to be a distinctive feature of aspirin-intolerant asthma. The dramatic increase in cLTs that accompanies this eosinophil influx raises the possibility that eosinophils are a primary source of cLTs in this response, or, alternatively, that cLTs induce eosinophil migration. How this cellular influx and cLT production occur, and the role of cytokines, mast cell mediators, and prostaglandins in the modulation of this phenomenon, are areas for future research. In addition, the actual mechanism for the initiation of the response to cyclooxygenase inhibition in AIA deserves further investigation. Because overlap exists between the responses of AIA and ATA, studies of the cellular and biochemical processes in AIA may eventually provide insight into the role of leukotrienes in all asthmatics.

References

1. Ferreri NR, Howland WC, Stevenson DD, Spiegelberg HL. Release of leukotrienes, prostaglandins, and histamine into nasal secretions of aspirin-sensitive asthmatics during reaction to aspirin. Am Rev Respir Dis 1988; 137: 847–854.
2. Picado C, Ramis I, Rosello J, Prat J, Bulbena O, Plaza V, Montserrat JM, Gelpi E. Release of peptide leukotriene into nasal secretions after local instillation of aspirin in aspirin-sensitive asthmatic patients. Am Rev Respir Dis 1992; 145:65–69.
3. Christie PE, Tagari P, Ford-Hutchinson AW, Charlesson S, Chee P, Arm JP. Urinary leukotriene E_4 concentrations increase after aspirin challenge in aspirin-sensitive asthmatic subjects. Am Rev Respir Dis 1991; 143:1025–1029.
4. Christie PE, Tagari P, Ford-Hutchinson AW, Black C, Markendorf A, Schmitz-Schumann M, Lee TH. Urinary leukotriene E_4 after lysine-aspirin inhalation in asthmatic subjects. Am Rev Respir Dis 1992; 146:1531–1534.
5. Kumlin M, Dahlen B, Bjorck T, Zetterstrom O, Granstrom E, Dahlen SE. Urinary excretion of leukotriene E_4 and 11-dehydro-thromboxane B_2 in response to bronchial provocation with allergen, aspirin, leukotriene D_4, and histamine in asthmatics. Am Rev Respir Dis 1992; 146:96–103.
6. Fischer AR, Rosenberg MA, Lilly CM, Callery JC, Rubin P, Cohn J, White MV, Igarashi Y, Kaliner MA, Drazen JM, Israel E. Direct evidence for a role of the mast cell in the nasal response to aspirin in aspirin-sensitive asthma. J Allergy Clin Immunol 1994; 94:1046–1056.
7. Israel E, Fischer AR, Rosenberg AM, Lilly CM, Callery JC, Shapiro J, Cohn J, Rubin P, Drazen JM. The pivotal role of 5-lipoxygenase products in the reaction of aspirin-sensitive asthmatics to aspirin. Am Rev Respir Dis 1993; 148:1447–1451.
8. Sladek K, Dworski R, Soja J, Sheller JR, Nizankowska E, Oates JA, Szczeklik A. Eicosanoids in bronchoalveolar lavage fluid of aspirin-intolerant patients with asthma after aspirin challenge. Am J Respir Crit Care Med 1994; 149: 940–946.
9. Szczeklik A, Sladek K, Dworski R, Nizankowska E, Soja J, Sheller J, Oates J. Bronchial aspirin challenge causes specific eicosanoid response in aspirin-sensitive asthmatics. Am J Respir Crit Care Med 1996; 154:1608–1614.

10. Henderson WR. The role of leukotrienes in inflammation. Ann Intern Med 1994; 121:684–697.
11. Weller PF, Lee CW, Foster DW, Corey EJ, Austen KF, Lewis RA. Generation and metabolism of 5-lipoxygenase pathway leukotrienes by human eosinophils: predominant production of leukotriene C_4. Proc Natl Acad Sci USA 1983; 80: 7626–7632.
12. Nasser SMS, Pfister R, Christie PE, Sousa AR, Barker J, Schmitz-Schumann M, Lee TH. Inflammatory cell populations in bronchial biopsies from aspirin-sensitive asthmatic subjects. Am J Respir Crit Care Med 1996; 153:90–96.
13. Nasser S, Christie PE, Pfister R, Sousa AR, Walls A, Schmitz-Schumann M, Lee TH. Effect of endobronchial aspirin challenge on inflammatory cells in bronchial biopsy samples from aspirin-sensitive asthmatic subjects. Thorax 1996; 51:64–70.
14. Warren MS, Sloan SI, Westcott JY, Schwartz LB, Wenzel SE. Cell and mediator increases after endobronchial indomethacin challenge in aspirin-intolerant asthmatics: comparison with aspirin-tolerant asthmatics and normal controls. J Allergy Clin Immunol (submitted).
15. Martelli NA. Bronchial and intravenous provocation tests with indomethacin in aspirin-sensitive asthmatics. Am Rev Respir Dis 1979; 120:1073–9.
16. Stevenson DD. Oral challenges to detect aspirin and sulfite sensitivity in asthma. NER Allergy Proc 1998; 9:135–142.
17. Wenzel SE, Trudeau JB, Kaminsky DA, Cohn J, Martin RJ, Westcott JY. Effect of a 5-lipoxygenase inhibitor on bronchoconstriction and airway inflammation in nocturnal asthma. Am J Respir Crit Care Med 1995; 152:897–905.
18. Trudeau JB, Warren MS, Wenzel SE. Indomethacin challenge causes a cytosol-membrane shift of 5-lipoxygenase in aspirin intolerant asthmatics. Am J Respir Crit Care Med 1996; 153:A684 (abstract).
19. Sladek K, Szczeklik A. Leukotriene overproduction and mast cell activation during aspirin-provoked bronchoconstriction in aspirin-induced asthma. Am Rev Respir Dis 1992; 145:A17 (abstract).
20. Resnick MB, Weller PF. Mechanisms of eosinophil recruitment. Am J Respir Cell Mol Biol 1993; 8:349–55.
21. Erger RA, Casale TB. Interleukin-8 is a potent mediator of eosinophil chemotaxis through endothelium and epithelium. Am J Physiol 1995; 268:L117–22.
22. Rot A, Krieger M, Brunner T, Bischoff SC, Schall TJ, Dahinden CA. RANTES and macrophage inflammatory protein 1α induce the migration and activation of normal human eosinophil granulocytes. J Exp Med 1992; 176:1489–95.
23. Garcia-Zepeda EA, Rothenberg ME, Ownbey RT, Celestin J, Leder P, Luster AD. Human eotaxin is a specific chemoattractant for eosinophil cells and provides a new mechanism to explain tissue eosinophilia. Nature Med 1996; 2:449–456.
24. Laitinen LA, Laitinen A, Haahtela T, Vilkka V, Spur BW, Lee TL. Leukotriene E_4 and granulocytic infiltration into asthmatic airways. Lancet 1993; 341:989–90.
25. Spada CS, Nieves AL, Krauss AH-P, et al. Comparison of leukotriene B_4 and D_4 effects on human eosinophil and neutrophil motility in vitro. J Leukocyte Biol 1994; 55:183–91.
26. Warren MS, Sloan SI, Trudeau JB, Hoffman NE, Westcott JY, Wenzel SE. RANTES levels and eosinophils increase in bronchoalveolar lavage fluid (BALF) after

indomethacin in aspirin-intolerant asthmatics. J Allergy Clin Immunol 1996; 97: 318 (abstract).

27. Bosso JV, Schwartz LB, Stevenson DD. Tryptase and histamine release during aspirin-induced respiratory reactions. J Allergy Clin Immunol 1991; 88:830–837.

28. O'Sullivan S, Dahlen B, Dahlen SE, Kumlin M. Increased urinary excretion of the prostaglandin D_2, metabolite $9\alpha,11\beta$-prostaglandin F_2 after aspirin challenge supports mast cell activation in aspirin-induced airway obstruction. J Allergy Clin Immunol 1996; 98:421–432.

29. Schwartz LB, Bradford TR, Rouse C, Irani A-M, Rasp G, Van der Zwan JK, Van der Linden P-WG. Development of a more sensitive immunoassay for human tryptase: use in systemic anaphylaxis. J Clin Immunol 1994; 14:190–204.

30. Churcher Y, Allan D, Gomperts BD. Relationship between arachidonate generation and exocytosis in permeabilized mast cells. Biochem J 1990; 266:157–163.

31. Pradelles P, Grassi J, Maclauf J. Enzyme immunoassays of eicosanoids using acetylcholine esterase as label: an alternative to radioimmunoassay. Anal Chem 1985; 57:1170–1173.

32. Kelly RW, Deam S, Cameron MJ, Seamark RF. Measurement by radioimmunoassay of prostaglandins as their methyl oximes. Prostaglandins Leukotrienes Med 1986; 24:1–14.

33. Szczeklik A, Mastalerz L, Nizankowska E, Cmiel A. Protective and bronchodilator effects of prostaglandin E and salbutamol in aspirin-induced asthma. Am J Respir Crit Care Med 1996; 153:567–571.

34. Sestini P, Armetti L, Gambaro G, Pieroni MG, Refini RM, Sala A, Vaghi A, Folco GC, Bianco S, Robuschi M. Inhaled PGE_2 prevents aspirin-induced bronchoconstriction and urinary cLT excretion in aspirin-sensitive asthma. Am J Respir Crit Care Med 1996; 153:572–575.

35. Melillo E, Woolley KL, Manning PJ, Watson RM, O'Byrne PM. Effect of inhaled PGE_2 on exercise bronchoconstriction in asthmatic subjects. Am J Respir Crit Care Med 1994; 149:1138–1141.

36. Pavord ID, Wong CS, Williams J, Tattersfield AE. Effect of inhaled prostaglandin E_2 on allergen-induced asthma. Am Rev Respir Dis 1993; 148:87–90.

37. Pasargiklian M, Bianco S, Allegra L, Moavera NE, Petrigni G, Robuschi M, Grugni AA. Aspects of bronchial reactivity to prostaglandins and aspirin in asthmatic patients. Respiration 1977; 34:79–91.

21

Aspects of Mechanisms in Aspirin-Intolerant Asthma

BARBRO DAHLÉN

Karolinska Institute
Stockholm, Sweden

I. Introduction

It is well established that inhibition of the cyclooxygenase is central in the chain of events that in susceptible individuals brings about the intolerance reaction to aspirin and related nonsteroidal anti-inflammatory drugs (NSAIDs) (1). The reason why only certain asthmatics react in this way remains unknown, however, as do the exact mechanisms behind the intolerance reaction. Despite these areas of uncertainty, studies carried out during the last two decades have documented that leukotrienes are important mediators of NSAID-induced bronchoconstriction as well as the persistent airway obstruction in aspirin-intolerant asthmatics. This chapter will overview some of our findings relating to aspirin-intolerant asthma, with particular focus on the role of leukotrienes.

II. Bronchial Provocations for Diagnosis and Mechanistic Studies

While there are no in vitro tests available for routine clinical diagnosis, the introduction of lysine-aspirin bronchoprovocations by Bianco et al. (2) has been found useful in identifying aspirin-intolerant asthmatics. To study whether the bronchial challenge was as sensitive and predictive as an oral challenge, a prospective study was carried out (3). Since this is the only published comparison between the two methods, it appeared to be of interest to summarize the findings here.

On the basis of history and/or clinical findings (asthma, rhinorrhea, nasal polyposis) suggestive of aspirin intolerance, 22 consecutive patients were challenged by both routes in random order. The two challenges were separated by at least 2 weeks, to avoid false negative reactions due to the acute desensitization following a positive reaction (2–6). In addition, a group of aspirin-tolerant asthmatics were subjected to the bronchoprovocation challenge.

The diagnosis of aspirin-induced asthma was revealed in 10 subjects during either challenge. Both provocation methods caused significant decreases in FEV_1 ($>20\%$) in nine subjects. Thus, the sensitivity with respect to detection of airway obstruction was the same for the oral and the bronchial provocation (9/10). In contrast, the inhalation of lysine-aspirin caused insignificant changes of FEV_1 (mean ± SD: 99 ± 6% of baseline) in 19 aspirin-tolerant asthmatics whose FEV_1 percent of predicted was in the same range (43–109%, mean value 80%) as the 10 identified aspirin-intolerant asthmatics. These observations thus support the specificity of the bronchial provocation method.

The trial provided information also about the safety of bronchial provocation in comparison with the oral method. Thus, during the inhalation challenge the reactions were limited to the airways. This was despite the fact that some bronchial absorption of aspirin subsequently has been shown to occur during bronchial challenge (7). The airway obstruction also developed more promptly (20 min for the bronchial vs. 1 hr after the oral provocative dose). The reactions evoked by the oral provocations were more pronounced (mean ± SD fall in FEV_1 being 38 ± 16% vs. 29 ± 6% for the oral and the bronchial provocation, respectively), longer lasting, and often combined with generalized symptoms (6/10 subjects). These differences presumably explain why the oral tests required more extensive drug treatment for reversal, whereas the reactions following bronchial provocations always were reversed by inhalation of bronchodilators. As a practical result of the differences, the bronchial method gave considerably shorter test sessions (4 hr vs. 8 hr). The differences between the challenge methods are summarized in Table 1.

Almost 15 years of experience has since confirmed that the bronchial provocation method offers a diagnostic means for detection of aspirin-induced asthma that is easier to interpret and control than the oral method. The oral protocol has been replaced by the bronchial provocation in our outpatient clinic. This has been a great advantage in the acquisition of more knowledge about aspirin-induced asthma and in finding patients who are unaware of their sensitivity, which is not uncommon (3).

Table 1 Challenge with Aspirin by Different Routes in Aspirin-Sensitive Asthmatics

Summary of findings	Provocation method	
	Oral	Bronchial
Bronchoconstriction ($\geq$20% fall in FEV_1)	9/10	9/10
Maximal fall in FEV_1 (mean $\pm$ SD)	$-38 \pm 16\%$	$-29 \pm 6\%$
Drugs required for reversal	Bronchodilators and steroids systemically	Inhaled β-agonists
Duration of test session	>8 hr	<4 hr
Extrapulmonary reactions	6/10	0/10

Source: Ref. 3.

For pharmacological studies, the inhalation procedure has been further improved by the addition of a dosimeter allowing for determination of PD_{20} values. With this device and a protocol using approximately half-log increments in the cumulated dose of aspirin (Fig. 1), the repeatability of the challenge has been established to be very good (8). On the basis of the results of two challenges separated by 10–75 days, the 95% confidence interval for the PD_{20} value was between 0.6 and 1.8 times the observed value. For comparison, Phillips et al. (9), determining PC_{20} values using a range of increasing doubling concentrations of lysine-aspirin, had a larger variation in the PC_{20} (95% CI 0.3–2.9 of actual PC_{20} value). Concerning the occurrence of extrapulmonary reactions after bronchial challenges, this in part relates to the protocol used for the challenge. When higher doses of lysine-aspirin are inhaled, as may occur in subjects with a low degree of aspirin intolerance in the airways, some subjects also display local reactions in the upper airways.

Although oral administration is necessary for detection and investigation of reactions extraneous to the respiratory tract, the bronchial challenge has characteristics supporting it as the first choice both in routine clinical practice and in mechanistic investigations. For the latter purpose, safety aspects and the repeatability provide a considerable advantage over the oral challenge, in particular since a significant proportion of aspirin-intolerant asthmatics suffer from severe asthma.

III. Plasma Levels of ASA and SA During Intolerance Reactions

The plasma levels and metabolism of aspirin were studied to determine whether aspirin-intolerant subjects differed in this respect (7). Following oral aspirin

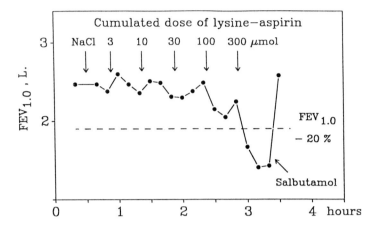

Figure 1   Recordings of pulmonary function (FEV₁) during lysine-aspirin broncho-provocations in an ASA-sensitive asthmatic, a 43-year-old woman, with the protocol used by the author.

provocations with up to 460 mg cumulated dose of acetylsalicylic acid (ASA), the plasma concentrations of ASA and its main metabolite salicylate (SA) were identical in nine aspirin-sensitive and nine aspirin-tolerant subjects. Therefore, it does not appear likely that differences in pharmacokinetics of ASA contribute to the disposition for being aspirin-intolerant.

For the aspirin-intolerant subjects, at the time of adverse reaction following oral provocations, the concentration range was 3–30 μM for ASA and 20–250 μM for SA. For ASA, these plasma concentrations are of the magnitude that has been established to inhibit cyclooxygenases in various test systems (10). These findings thus provided further support to the concept that cyclooxygenase inhibition is fundamental in the process leading to aspirin-elicited reactions.

Concerning SA, although the plasma levels at the time of the intolerance reactions were elevated compared to those of ASA, provocations with sodium salicylate yielding much higher concentrations failed to elicit intolerance reactions (7). This confirms previous indications that commonly used doses of SA (0.5–1.0 g) yielding plasma levels of SA below 0.5 mM can be tolerated by aspirin-sensitive individuals. In addition, the findings indicated that the metabolite SA is not responsible for the adverse reactions to aspirin. Interestingly, recently published in vitro studies in intact cells suggest that SA is about 150 times less potent than ASA as an inhibitor of COX-1, but only 3 times less potent as an inhibitor of COX-2 (11). The difference mainly relates to aspirin being almost 100-fold less potent as an inhibitor of COX-2, with an IC₅₀ value at 278 μM as compared with 1.67 for COX-1 (11). Therefore, the sensitivity to ASA but not SA in aspirin-intolerant subjects may suggest that inhibition of COX-1 rather than COX-2 is involved in the intolerance reaction.

The study of plasma levels also established that bronchial absorption of aspirin occurs after inhalation of lysine-aspirin (7). The obtained plasma levels were comparable in asthmatics and nonasthmatics, suggesting that the state of airway inflammation does not influence the absorption. However, the total systemic exposure to aspirin, reflected by the sum of ASA and SA concentrations in plasma, was much less during the inhalation challenge. A lower systemic load of aspirin would be consistent with the lack of symptoms extraneous to the airways during lysine-aspirin bronchoprovocations. Indeed, the plasma levels of ASA were about three times lower at the time of lysine-aspirin-induced bronchoconstriction, as compared with the levels measured in the same subjects during oral provocations (7). The findings of this pharmacokinetic study therefore support the view that the airway response during bronchial provocations mainly is triggered locally in the airways.

IV. Leukotrienes as Mediators of Aspirin-Induced Bronchoconstriction

Using the bronchial challenge method, we observed that lysine-aspirin-induced bronchoconstriction was associated with increased urinary excretion of LTE_4 (12). In contrast, the urinary levels of LTE_4 remained unchanged during the course of bronchoprovocation in five asthmatics who did not develop an airway obstruction to inhaled lysine-aspirin. This observation was in line with concurrent reports that oral aspirin challenge increased urinary LTE_4 (13,14), and strengthened our interest to evaluate the influence of a leukotriene antagonist on the airway response to aspirin.

The first pharmacological study intended to test whether leukotrienes mediated aspirin-induced bronchoconstriction involved oral challenge and pretreatment with the inhaled leukotriene antagonist SKF 104,353 (15). The study produced some support for leukotriene involvement, but the inhibition was incomplete and not observed among all the subjects. Using bronchial challenge with lysine-aspirin, we were able to find further supporting evidence for a major leukotriene component in aspirin-induced bronchoconstriction (8). In addition to the differences in challenge procedures, we used a more potent antagonist (MK-0679), which was given orally before the provocations.

One single dose of MK-0679 or placebo was given 1 hr before the start of lysine-aspirin bronchoprovocation. Pretreatment with MK-0679 caused a rightward shift in the dose-response relationship for all eight subjects (median shift in aspirin PD_{20} being 4.4-fold) when compared to placebo (Fig. 2). Thus,

higher cumulated doses of aspirin were required to elicit the stipulated 20%
fall in FEV_1. In the presence of MK-0679, three of the subjects even failed to
produce a 20% decrease in FEV_1 after inhalation of the highest available dose
of lysine-aspirin. Their PD_{20} values were set as equal to the highest cumulated
dose of aspirin given, and despite this underestimate of the influence of the
drug, the increase in the geometric mean aspirin PD_{20} was highly significant
($p < 0.001$). In addition, after treatment with MK-0679, the maximal fall in
FEV_1 (within 90 min after the last dose of aspirin) was significantly less than
after placebo ($29 \pm 6\%$ vs. $42 \pm 5\%$). MK-0679 did not, however, affect the
prechallenge FEV_1 values in the hour that passed between drug intake and the
start of the provocation. Bronchodilation was therefore not a probable reason
for the inhibition of response in this group of asthmatics (mean prestudy FEV_1
% predicted 84, range 60–99%). Thus, the investigation documented that leukotriene receptor blockade, by a specific competitive antagonist, could blunt
the response to lysine-aspirin. In addition, the study supported the excellent
repeatability of the bronchial challenge with lysine-aspirin (Fig. 2).

Another observation during this particular study deserves attention. While
the basal excretion of urinary LTE_4 was unaffected by MK-0679, the postchallenge urinary levels of LTE_4 were found to be much higher after MK-0679
(increase 626%) than after placebo (8). Thus, MK-0679 allowed an increase
in the dose of aspirin (stimulus) and caused increased excretion of LTE_4 (response), supporting a dose-dependent release of LTE_4 by aspirin in aspirin-

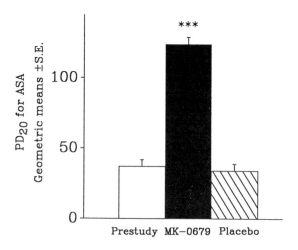

Figure 2   Group mean PD_{20} values for aspirin during screening, placebo session, and
active drug treatment session (MK-0679). (Modified from data in Ref. 8.)

sensitive asthmatics. In fact, the ratios between the dose of aspirin (expressed as either the aspirin PD_{20} value or the total dose of inhaled aspirin) and the urinary excretion of LTE_4 were found to be strikingly similar for each subject at the two challenge sessions ($r = 0.98$). The absolute magnitude of these ratios, however, showed quite large variations between subjects (range 0.3–100), which, assuming a similar urinary excretion fraction in each subject, would suggest a high degree of variation in the individual propensity to release leukotrienes. Therefore, although measurement of urinary LTE_4 in a group may establish that leukotrienes are released during a physiological or pathological reaction, it seems unlikely that measurement of urinary LTE_4 alone may predict the extent of leukotriene involvement in an asthmatic response in an individual subject. This conclusion is supported by the study of Smith et al. [16] where no correlations were found between urinary LTE_4 and baseline pulmonary function or bronchial responsiveness to histamine.

Israel and co-workers were able to show that pretreatment with the 5-lipoxygenase inhibitor Zileuton inhibited the bronchoconstriction induced by oral aspirin challenge [17]. Interestingly, they also reported that several of the extrapulmonary symptoms were blocked by Zileuton [17]. Nasser and co-workers confirmed that another 5-lipoxygenase inhibitor, ZD2138, was able to inhibit the bronchoconstriction induced by oral aspirin provocation [18]. Finally, using another leukotriene-antagonist (ONO-1078) and another NSAID (dipyrone), Yamamoto and co-workers have also provided evidence that the response to bronchial challenge has a major leukotriene component [19]. The published studies thus document that the leukotrienes fulfill two of the criteria required to prove a mediator function: (1) They are released in response to aspirin-elicited airway obstruction; (2) the airway reaction to aspirin can be blocked by a specific and potent leukotriene antagonist. Together with demonstrations that inhalation of leukotrienes induces airway obstruction in aspirin-sensitive asthmatics [20,21], it is possible to conclude that the cysteinyl-leukotrienes indeed fulfill all three criteria of being true mediators of aspirin-induced airway obstruction. Accordingly, treatment with antileukotriene drugs can prevent aspirin-induced bronchoconstriction.

V. Evidence for Mast Cell Activation During Aspirin-Induced Bronchoconstriction

One important step in the further understanding of the pathophysiology of aspirin-induced reactions is to define which cells are involved in the adverse reaction. From in vitro studies, no single cell type isolated from aspirin-intolerant subjects has consistently been shown to release mediators in direct response to cyclooxygenase inhibition alone. Hence a more complex cellular response in the intact tissue is expected. The demonstration that cysteinyl-leukotrienes are released in vivo during the reaction in fact allows for many different cells to be potential providers. Thus, mast cells, eosinophils, neutrophils, and macrophages are capable of generating cysteinyl-leukotrienes by themselves, whereas platelets, endothelial cells, lymphocytes, and epithelial cells may do so provided the precursor LTA_4 is supplied by cell-cell interaction (22–24).

The differences observed between oral and bronchial aspirin provocations may provide some clues as to where the reactions occur. Since inhalation challenges, despite a small amount of aspirin being absorbed (7), do not cause significant systemic symptoms, it seems unlikely that the reaction is triggered by circulating blood cells. In addition, Bianco et al. reported that it was possible to desensitize only the bronchial tree (inhalation via oral cavity) preserving the nasal reactivity or vice versa (nasal drops) (25). From the published studies on urinary LTE_4 excretion following aspirin challenge (8,12–14,26), it appears that the magnitude of the postchallenge increase is very similar after bronchial and oral provocations, which may support the pulmonary location of the cellular source for leukotrienes.

Mast cells located adjacent to the surface of the lumen would seem to be a likely primary source of mediators in the reaction following inhaled aspirin, just as they have been implicated in bronchoconstrictor responses following other trigger factors and in particular inhaled allergen. In addition to accommodating preformed mediators, human lung parenchymal mast cells generate significant amounts of both LTC_4 and PGD_2 (27–30). In the upper airways, it has indeed been possible during both local and systemic challenge with aspirin to document release of mast cell mediators (31–33). As a further indication that mast cells may be of central importance in the intolerance reactions, a marked overproduction of PGD_2, increased histamine excretion, and elevated serum tryptase levels have been found in a subset of patients with systemic mastocystosis who experienced respiratory and circulatory shock following ingestion of low doses of aspirin and aspirin-like drugs (34).

Nevertheless, it has been difficult to obtain evidence for mast cell activation during aspirin-induced bronchoconstriction. For example, measurements of histamine release into plasma and/or urine during oral provocations have yielded inconclusive data (35–38). Serum tryptase, a more specific marker of mast cell activation, was found to be elevated during airway and extrapulmonary reactions induced by oral aspirin (39,40), whereas the inhalation challenge did not change tryptase levels (40). One explanation could be that different mechanisms are involved in extrapulmonary and pulmonary symptoms. Another alternative is that the methods used for measuring mast cell markers distant from the affected tissue not have been sufficiently sensitive to detect reactions limited to the airways.

More recently, we have used the strategy to measure a PGD_2 metabolite in urine for assessment of the role of the mast cell in aspirin-induced broncho-constriction (41). The approach originated from several considerations. First, PGD_2 is the major cyclooxygenase product released upon activation of mast cells (27–29,34). Second, few, if any, of the other implicated cells have the capacity to synthesize this particular prostanoid in significant amounts (27,28). Third, a major caveat when measuring arachidonic acid metabolites in biological fluids such as plasma and lavage fluids is artifactual ex vivo formation of metabolites during sampling (42). Therefore, measurements of endogenously formed metabolites in urine are preferred as indicators of in vivo production of primary eicosanoids. Fourth, the easy and noninvasive access to urine obviously has advantages.

It was decided to measure (15S)-trihydroxy-prosta-(5Z,13E)-dien-1-oic acid ($9\alpha,11\beta$-PGF_2) because it constitutes one of the major urinary metabolites of PGD_2 (43). The NADPH-dependent enzyme 11-ketoreductase generates $9\alpha,11\beta$-PGF_2 from PGD_2 in the lung, and it is excreted intact into the urine. It was first documented that the basal levels of $9\alpha,11\beta$-PGF_2 were detectable, but low and without diurnal variation (41). Furthermore, allergen-induced bronchoconstriction was associated with increased urinary excretion of $9\alpha,11\beta$-PGF_2, whereas histamine-induced bronchoconstriction was not (41). These observations thus confirmed the hypothesis that release of PGD_2 occurred as a result of mast cell activation but not as a consequence of bronchocosntriction per se.

When bronchoconstriction was produced in a group of aspirin-intolerant asthmatics by inhalation of lysine-aspirin, there was a significant postchallenge increase in $9\alpha,11\beta$-PGF_2 (41). In fact, the time course of the increase in urinary $9\alpha,11\beta$-PGF_2 paralleled the concomitant increase in urinary LTE_4. Moreover, the postchallenge increase of $9\alpha,11\beta$-PGF_2 was dose-dependent, i.e., greater than the group was challenged with a higher dose of lysine-aspirin. The findings therefore support that mast cells are activated during aspirin-induced bronchoconstriction. This would argue for a common mechanism behind the intolerance reactions in the upper and lower airways. The parallel increase in urinary $9\alpha,11\beta$-PGF_2 and LTE_4 would also seem to indicate that mast cells are a major source for the cysteinyl-leukotrienes generated during the reaction. Since the findings were made in a group of subjects undergoing bronchial challenge and experiencing no extrapulmonary symptoms, it follows that the study also suggests that mast cells in the lungs primarily were involved. Recent morphological and biochemical studies in aspirin-intolerant asthmatics also lend support to the concept that mast cells are central effector cells in the intolerance reaction to aspirin and related NSAIDs (44,45).

The increased postchallenge level of $9\alpha,11\beta$-PGF_2 following aspirin-induced bronchoconstriction seems to introduce a conceptual paradox, namely that the cyclooxygenase inhibitor aspirin somehow should stimulate formation or release of the cyclooxygenase product PGD_2. Our findings measuring urinary excretion of a PGD_2 metabolite are, however, consistent with previous data on aspirin-induced release of PGD_2 in nasal fluid (31–33) and more recent observations following local segmental bronchial challenge with aspirin in aspirin-intolerant asthmatics (44,45). It has also been shown that certain patients with systemic mastocytosis exhibited increased formation of PGD_2 as well as histamine following ingestion of aspirin (34), supporting that cyclooxygenase inhibitor under certain circumstances may provoke mast cell activation, including the release of the cyclooxygenase product PGD_2. A biochemical explanation for these seemingly contradictory findings would be that there is a pool of preformed PGD_2 that is released despite inhibited de novo synthesis of prostaglandin endoperoxides. Alternatively, PGD_2 synthesis may be relatively less sensitive to diminished levels of prostaglandin endoperoxides.

Presumably, the solution of this seemingly inconsistent set of data may provide important clues in the search for the mechanisms involved in aspirin intolerance. Perhaps different cells in the airways, due to pharmacokinetic or pharmacodynamic differences, including differential expression of COX-1 and COX-2, exhibit differences with respect to the time course for inhibition of the cyclooxygenase. On a speculative note, the initial effect of cyclooxygenase inhibition would be to remove the production of an anti-inflammatory compound such as PGE_2 from a cell that is more sensitive to aspirin or exposed to higher doses. There is in fact some attraction to this hypothesis. It is established that PGE_2 has the capacity to inhibit mast cell mediator release in vivo (46). Therefore, removal of PGE_2 would be expected to alone, or in combination with some unknown additional trigger factor, favor mast cell activation and the release of preformed and newly formed substances, including the cyclooxygenase product PGD_2. In support of this possibility, inhalation of PGE_2 has been found to prevent both bronchoconstriction and urinary excretion of LTE_4 in response to aspirin-challenge (47,48). Moreover, many cells in the airways have the potential to generate PGE_2, including macrophages, bronchial smooth muscle, epithelial cells, endothelial cells, lymphocytes, eosinophils, and perhaps also mast cells themselves (49–51). However, since PGE_2 caused some bronchodilation and also prevents allergen and exercise-induced bronchoconstriction (52,53), the specificity of the effect of PGE_2 on aspirin-induced bronchoconstriction remains to be established.

VI. Leukotrienes as Mediators of Persistent Airway Obstruction in Aspirin-Intolerant Asthmatics

When we measured urinary LTE_4 in aspirin-intolerant asthmatics, it was observed that the baseline production of LTE_4 was significantly higher than in aspirin-tolerant asthmatics (12). Several investigations performed at this particular time (13,14,16) and subsequent studies have firmly confirmed that aspirin-intolerant asthmatics indeed have increased urinary excretion of cysteinyl-leukotrienes (41,54). In contrast, the basal excretion of urinary $9\alpha,11\beta$-PGF_2 in aspirin-intolerant asthmatics was not different from that of aspirin-tolerant asthmatics (41), suggesting that mast cell activation was not involved in the basal overproduction of cysteinyl-leukotrienes. On the basis of the well-established association between eosinophils and aspirin-intolerant asthma (55–57), and the indications that circulating eosinophils have enhanced capacity to generate leukotrienes (40), the findings would seem to fit with the hypothesis that the eosinophils are one major source of the baseline production of leukotrienes. This adds to the clinical indications that aspirin-induced brou choconstriction and the persistent airflow obstruction may be diffcient and mechanistically unrelated components in the syndrome.

In addition to the increased formation of cysteinyl-leukotrienes, there are reports that aspirin-intolerant asthmatics are particularly sensitive to inhalation of cysteinyl-leukotrienes (20), and in particular LTE_4 (21). Therefore, it may be that aspirin-intolerant asthmatics display both a basal overproduction of leukotrienes and an increased bronchial responsiveness to these compounds.

In support of such indications that even when not exposed to NSAIDs, airflow obstruction in aspirin-intolerant subjects has a leukotriene component, it was observed that one single dose of treatment with the leukotriene antagonist MK-0679 induced a prompt improvement in pulmonary function (58). The effect occurred within 30 min and was significantly different from placebo at all time points thereafter up to 5 hr, the mean increase varying between 11 and 15%. The mean maximal improvement in FEV_1 was 18% calculated from the peak effect in each individual. For comparison, inhalation of a nebulized solution of salbutamol (2500 μg) produced a 22.8% increase in FEV_1 in the same patients, which means that the response to this single dose of the leukotriene antagonist was about 80% of maximal reserve for bronchodilation. For the entire 12-hr observation period there was a significant increase in mean AUC (area under the FEV_1 curve vs. time) after MK-0679 compared with placebo (18.2 ± 6 units and –0.49 ± 7 units, $p < 0.05$). The change in AUC after active drug ($AUC_{MK-0679} - AUC_{placebo}$) was found to correlate strongly with the severity of asthma expressed as the sum of each subject's rank order score for FEV_1 percent of predicted and asthma medication. There was also a good correlation between the bronchodilator response to the drug and the individual's sensitivity to aspirin, expressed as prestudy PD_{20} for ASA.

Concerning the mechanism behind the bronchodilation produced by MK-0679, it is known that this drug, as well as other new leukotriene receptor antagonists, is very specific in mode of action and devoid of general smooth muscle relaxant properties (59–61). Initial studies with these leukotriene antagonists in healthy volunteers (62) or in subjects with mild asthma (63) failed to show evidence of bronchodilation. The finding of bronchodilation in a group of aspirin-sensitive asthmatics, differing with respect to asthma severity (for instance, range of FEV_1 % predicted was 58–99) and with best effect in the most severe subjects, adds support to the hypothesis that ongoing leukotriene formation in the airways is a prerequisite for a bronchodilator response to drugs that block the action or release of leukotrienes. Likewise, bronchodilator effects of antileukotrienes in asthmatics have been observed in studies of aspirin-tolerant subjects with compromised baseline pulmonary function (64–66).

Interestingly, the best effect of MK-0679 was seen in those patients who were kept on relatively high doses of inhaled corticosteroids. It is commonly believed that corticosteroids abrogate formation of all arachidonic acid metabolites. However, in vitro studies on isolated human neutrophils have shown that corticosteroids generally do not inhibit leukotriene production (67). In support of this observation, treatment with systemic or inhaled corticosteroids fails to alter urinary excretion of LTE_4 either at baseline (67,68) or after allergen bronchoprovocation in asthmatic patients (69). Therefore, one hypothesis that currently evolves is that leukotriene antagonists may add to the existing treatment strategies in asthma by blunting components of the airway inflammation that are unaffected by glucocorticosteroids.

Finally, a recently concluded treatment trial with the 5-lipoxygenase inhibitor Zileuton supports that leukotrienes indeed mediate persistent airway obstruction and other symptoms in aspirin-intolerant asthmatics (70). The study was conducted in collaboration between the group at our Institute and Professors Ewa Nizankowska and Andrew Szczeklik in Krakow, Poland. From each center, 20 aspirin-intolerant asthmatics were recruited. The aspirin intolerance had been diagnosed by an unequivocal history as well as a previously documented bronchoconstriction in response to challenge with inhaled or oral aspirin. Zileuton (600 mg q.i.d. orally) or placebo was administered during 6 weeks in a crossover, double-blind design with 4 weeks' washout period in between. The majority of subjects had suffered from asthma for 5 years or more, and all subjects had demonstrated reversibility of bronchoconstriction following inhalation of a beta-stimulant. This was an add-on study and all subjects were kept on their regular asthma therapy according to existing guidelines. It is noteworthy that 97.5% of the subjects in this study already were treated with glucocorticosteroids, and most often with high doses of inhaled preparations (>1200 μg budesonide or beclomethasone) or with prednisone orally. When the outcome of the treatment periods was evaluated, it was evident that Zileuton caused both acute and chronic improvement in pulmonary function, at the same time as there was a significant decrease in the use of beta-agonists. The bronchial hyperresponsiveness to histamine was evaluated before and at the end of each treatment period. There was a significant improvement also of this measure after treatment with Zileuton, possibly indicating a reduction in airway inflammation. In addition, consistent with previous preliminary findings, the treatment with Zileuton caused an improvement in nasal function and in particular return of the sensation of smell. Therefore, the study supported that inhibition of leukotrienes may provide a new therapeutic alternative in aspirin-intolerant asthma. The improvements observed were particularly encouraging because the 5-lipoxygenase inhibitor Zileuton at the employed dose level only caused partial inhibition of leukotriene biosynthesis, measured as urinary excretion of leukotriene E_4. Furthermore, the finding that addition of the 5-lipoxygenase inhibitor Zileuton caused improvement over and above that provided by treatment with glucocorticoids lends further support to the concept that antileukotrienes and glucocorticoids treat different parts of the airway inflammation. The effects of antileukotriene drugs in aspirin-intolerant asthma are summarized in Figure 3.

VII. Concluding Remarks

The last two decades have provided major advances in the understanding of the syndrome of aspirin-induced asthma. First, the establishment that inhibition of the cyclooxygenase is the common denominator of drugs that cause the intolerance reactions provided focus that has been instrumental for both clinical care and a mechanism-based research (1). Second, the discovery that leukotrienes mediate important components of both spontaneous and aspirin-induced airway obstruction has opened the path for a new treatment that appears likely to be beneficial for several manifestations of this syndrome (Fig. 3).

Effects of anti-leukotrienes

in Aspirin/NSAID-intolerant asthmatics:

*   Prevention of aspirin-induced bronchoconstriction

*   Reversal of baseline airway obstruction

*   Control of asthma

*   Reduction of extra-pulmonary symptoms,

   especially nasal manifestations

Figure 3   Summary of effects of antileukotrienes in aspirin-intolerant asthmatics.

Third, the creation of the AIANE network has resulted in a unique database that already has provided new findings on the clinical manifestations of aspirin-induced asthma. The AIANE network has the potential to be a fundamental resource in the further exploration of this truly intriguing syndrome, because, despite the achievements, there are yet many unanswered questions. Although the PGE_2 hypothesis currently best explains how the intolerance reactions may be triggered, it remains uncertain exactly how such a role is carried out, and in particular how the NSAID intolerance is acquired. Much more research on cellular and molecular mechanisms is needed. One poorly understood phenomenon relates to the desensitization following an adverse reaction, and the presumably associated consistent finding that intolerance to NSAIDs waxes and wanes over time. Neither are the reasons for the clinical association between NSAID intolerance and the two other manifestations of the aspirin triad, asthma and nasal polyposis, particularly well understood. It is possible that different mechanisms are involved and that the unifying hypothesis will remain elusive.

References

1. Szczeklik A, Gryglewski RJ, Czerniawska-Mysik G. Relationship of inhibition of prostaglandin biosynthesis by analgesics to asthma attacks in aspirin-sensitive patients. Br Med J 1975; 1:67–69.
2. Bianco S, Robuschi M, Petrini G. Aspirin-induced tolerance in aspirin-asthma detected by a new challenge test. IRCS J Med Sci 1977; 5:129.
3. Dahlén B, Zetterström O. Comparison of bronchial and per oral provocation with aspirin in aspirin-sensitive asthmatics. Eur Respir J 1990; 3:527–534.
4. Widal F, Abrami P, Lermoyez J. Anaphylaxie et idiosyncrasie. Presse Med 1922; 30:189–193.
5. Zeiss CR, Lockey RF. Refractory period to aspirin in a patient with aspirin-induced asthma. J Allergy Clin Immunol 1976; 57:440–48.
6. Pleskow WW, Stevenson DD, Mathison DA, Simon RA, Schatz M, Zeiger RS. Aspirin desensitization in aspirin-sensitive asthmatic patients: clinical manifestations and characterization of the refractory period. J Allergy Clin Immunol 1982; 69:11–19.
7. Dahlén B, Boréus LO, Anderson P, Andersson R, Zetterström O. Plasma acetylsalicylic acid and salicyclic acid levels during aspirin provocations in aspirin-sensitive subjects. Allergy 1994; 49:43–49.
8. Dahlén B, Kumlin M, Margolskee DJ, Larsson C, Blomqvist H, Williams VC, Zetterström O, Dahlén S-E. The leukotriene-receptor antagonist MK-0679 blocks airway obstruction induced by inhaled lysine-aspirin in aspirin-sensitive asthmatics. Eur Respir J 1993; 6:1018–1026.
9. Phillips GD, Foord R, Holgate ST. Inhaled lysine-aspirin as a bronchoprovocation procedure in aspirin-sensitive asthma: its repeatability, absence of late-phase reaction, and the role of histamine. J Allergy Clin Immunol 1989; 84:232–41.

10. Gryglewski RJ. Screening and assessment of the potency of anti-inflammatory drugs in vitro. In: Vane JR, Ferreira SH, eds. Anti-inflammatory Drugs. Handbook of Experimental Pharmacology. Berlin: Springer-Verlag, 1979:50/2:1–43.
11. Mitchell JA, Akarasereenont P, Thiemermann C, Flower RJ, Vane JR. Selectivity of nonsteroidal antiinflammatory drugs as inhibitors of constitutive and inducible cyclooxygenases. Proc Natl Acad Sci USA 1993; 90:11693–11697.
12. Kumlin M, Dahlén B, Björck T, Zetterström O, Granström E, Dahlén S-E. Urinary excretion of leukotriene E_4 and 11-dehydro-thromboxane B_2 in response to bronchial provocations with allergen, aspirin, leukotriene D_4, and histamine in asthmatics. Am Rev Respir Dis 1992; 146:96–103.
13. Christie PE, Tagari P, Ford-Hutchinson AW, Charlesson S, Chee P, Arm MP, Lee TH. Urinary leukotriene E_4 concentrations increase after ASA challenge in ASA-sensitive asthmatic subjects. Am Rev Respir Dis 1991; 143:1025–1029.
14. Knapp HR, Sladek K, FitzGerald GA. Increased excretion of leukotriene E_4 during aspirin-induced asthma. J Lab Clin Med 1992; 119.48-51.
15. Christie PE, Smith CM, Lee TH. The potent and selective sulfidopeptide leukotriene antagonist, SK&F 104353, inhibits aspirin-induced asthma. Am Rev Respir Dis 1991; 144:957–958.
16. Smith CH, Hawksworth RJ, Thien FCK, Christie PE, Lee TH. Urinary leukotriene E_4 in bronchial asthma. Eur Respir J 1992; 5:693–699.
17. Israel E, Fischer AR, Rosenberg MA, Lilly CM, Callery JC, Shapiro J, Cohn J, Rubin P, Drazen JM. The pivotal role of 5-lipoxygenase products in the reaction of aspirin-sensitive asthmatics to aspirin. Am Rev Respir Dis 1993; 148:1447–1451.
18. Nasser SM, Bell GS, Foster S, Spruce KE, MacMillan R, Williams AJ, Lee TH, Arm JP. Effect of the 5-lipoxygenase inhibitor ZD2138 on aspirin-induced asthma. Thorax 1994; 49:749–756.
19. Yamamoto H, Nagata M, Kuramitsu K, Tabe K, Kiuchi H, Sakamoto Y, Yamamoto K, Dohi Y. Inhibition of analgesic-induced asthma by leukotriene receptor antagonist ONO-1078. Am J Respir Crit Care Med 1994; 150:254–257.
20. Sakakibara H, Suetsugu S, Saga T, Handa M, Suzuki M, Doizoe T, Tsuda M, Horiguchi T, Konishi Y, Umeda H. Bronchial hyperresponsiveness in aspirin induced asthma. J Jpn Thorac Soc 1988; 26:612–619.
21. Arm JP, O'Hickey SP, Spur BW, Lee TH. Airway responsiveness to histamine and leukotriene E_4 in subjects with ASA-induced asthma. Am Rev Respir Dis 1989; 140:148–153.
22. Maclouf JA, Murphy RC. Transcellular metabolism of neutrophil-derived leukotriene A_4 by human platelets. A potential cellular source of leukotriene C_4. J Biol Chem 1988; 263:174–181.
23. Edenius C, Heidvall K, Lindgren JÅ. Novel transcellular interaction: conversion of granulocyte-derived leukotriene A_4 to cysteinyl-containing leukotrienes by human platelets. Eur J Biochem 1988; 178:81–86.
24. Claesson HE, Hæggström J. Human endothelial cells stimulate leukotriene synthesis and convert granulocyte released leukotriene A_4 into leukotrienes B_4, C_4, D_4, and E_4. Eur J Biochem 1988; 173:93–100.

25. Bianco S, Robuschi M, Damonte C, Simone P, Vaghi A, Pasargiklian M. Bronchial response to nonsteroidal anti-inflammatory drugs in asthmatic patients. Prog Biochem Pharmacol 1985; 20:132–142.
26. Christie PE, Tagari P, Ford-Hutchinson AW, Black C, Markendorf A, Lee TH. Urinary leukotriene E$_4$ after lysine-aspirin inhalation in asthmatic subjects. Am Rev Respir Dis 1992; 146:1531–1534.
27. Lewis RA, Soter N, Diamond P, Austen KF, Oates JA, Roberts LJI. Prostaglandin D$_2$ generation after activation of rat and human mast cells with anti-IgE. J Immunol 1982; 129:1627–1631.
28. MacGlashan DW, Schleimer RP, Peters SP, Schulman ES, Adams GK, Newball HH, Lichtenstein LM. Generation of leukotrienes by purified human lung mast cells. J Clin Invest 1982; 70:744–751.
29. Holgate ST, Burns GB, Robinson C, Church MK. Anaphylactic and calcium-dependent generation of prostaglandin D$_2$ (PGD$_2$), thromboxane B$_2$ and other cyclooxygenase products of arachidonic acid by dispersed lung cells an relationship to histamine release. J Immunol 1984; 133:2138–2144.
30. Sydbom A, Kumlin M, Dahlén SE. Stimulus-dependence and time-course of histamine and leukotriene release from chopped and dispersed human lung tissue. Agents Actions 1987; 20:198–201.
31. Ferreri NR, Howland WC, Stevenson DD, Spiegelberg HL. Release of leukotrienes, prostaglandins, and histamine into nasal secretions of aspirin-sensitive asthmatics during reaction to aspirin. Am Rev Respir Dis 1988; 137: 847–854.
32. Picado C, Ramis I, Roselló J, Prat J, Bulbena O, Plaza V, Montserrat JM, Gelpí E. Release of peptide leukotriene into nasal secretions after local instillation of aspirin in aspirin-sensitive asthmatic patients. Am Rev Respir Dis 1992; 145:65–69.
33. Fisher AR, Rosenberg MA, Lilly CM, Callery CP, Rubin P, Cohn J, White MA, Igarashi Y, Kaliner MA, Drazen JD, Israel E. Direct evidence for a role of the mast cell in the nasal response to aspirin in aspirin-sensitive asthma. J Allergy Clin Immunol 1994; 94:1046–1056.
34. Roberts LJ II, Sweetman BJ, Lewis RA, Austen KF, Oates JA. Increased production of prostaglandin D$_2$ in patients with systemic mastocytosis. N Engl J Med 1980; 303:1400–1404.
35. Stevenson DD, Arroyave CM, Bhat KN, Tan EM. Oral aspirin challenges in asthmatic patients: a study of plasma histamine. Clin Allergy 1976; 6:493–505.
36. Szmidt M, Grzelewska-Rzymowska I, Rozniecki I, Kowalski M, Rychlicka J. Histaminemia after aspirin challenge in aspirin-sensitive asthmatics. Agents Actions 1981; 11:105–107.
37. Wasserman SI, Sheffer AL, Soter NA, Austen KF, McFadden ER. Assessment of mast cell mediators and pulmonary function in aspirin (ASA) induced bronchospasm. J Allergy Clin Immunol 1978; 61:139 (abstract).
38. Simon RA, Pleskow W, Kaliner M, Wasserman S, Curd J, Stevenson D. Plasma mediator studies in aspirin-sensitive asthma: lack of a role for the mast cell. J Allergy Clin Immunol 1983; 71:146 (abstract).

39. Bosso JV, Schwartz LB, Stevenson DD. Tryptase and histamine release during aspirin-induced respiratory reactions. J Allergy Clin Immunol 1991; 88:830–837.

40. Sladek K, Szczeklik A. Cysteinyl-leukotriene overproduction and mast cell activation in aspirin-provoked bronchospasm in asthma. Eur Respir J 1993; 6:391–399.

41. O'Sullivan, Dahlén B, Dahlén S-E, Kumlin M. Increased urinary excretion of the prostaglandin D_2 metabolite $9\alpha,11\beta$-prostaglandin F_2 following aspirin challenge supports mast cell activation in aspirin-induced airway obstruction. J Allergy Clin Immunol 1996; 98:421–432.

42. Kumlin M. Analytical methods for measurement of leukotrienes and other eicosanoids in biological samples from asthmatic subjects. J Chromatogr 1996; 725: 29–40.

43. Liston TE, Roberts LJI. Metabolic fate of radiolabeled prostaglandin D_2 in a normal human male volunteer. J Biol Chem 1985; 260:13172.

44. Nasser SM, Christie PE, Pfister R, Sousa AR, Walls A, Schmitz-Schuman M, Lee TH. Effect of endobronchial aspirin challenge on inflammatory cells in bronchial biopsy samples from aspirin-sensitive asthmatic subjects. Thorax 1996; 51:64–70.

45. Szczeklik A, Sladek K, Dworski R, Nizankowska E, Soja J, Sheller J, Oates JA. Bronchial aspirin challenge causes specific eicosanoid response in aspirin-sensitive asthmatics. Am J Respir Crit Care Med 1996; 154:1608–1614.

46. Raud J, Dahlén SE, Sydbom A, Lindbom L, Hedqvist P. Enhancement of acute allergic inflammation by indomethacin is reversed by prostaglandin E_2: Apparent correlation with in vivo modulation of mediator release. Proc Natl Acad Sci USA 1988; 85:2315–19.

47. Szczeklik A, Mastalerz L, Nizankowska E, Cmiel A. Protective and bronchodilator effects of prostaglandin E_2 and salbutamol in aspirin-induced asthma. Am J Respir Crit Care Med 1996; 153:567–571.

48. Sestini P, Armett L, Gambaro G, Pieroni MG, Refini RM, Sala P, Vaghi A, Folco GC, Bianco S, Robuschi M. Inhaled prostaglandin E_2 prevents aspirin-induced bronchoconstriction and urinary LTE_4 excretion in aspirin-sensitive asthma. Am J Respir Crit Care Med 1996; 153:572–575.

49. MacDermot J, Kelsey CR, Waddel KA, Richmond R, Knight RK, Cole PJ, Dollery CT, Landon DN, Blair IA. Synthesis of LTB_4 and prostanoids by human alveolar macrophages: analysis by gas chromotography/mass spectrometry. Prostaglandins 1984; 27:163–179.

50. Haye-Legrand I, Cerrina J, Raffestin B, Labat C, Boullet C, Bayol A, Benveniste J, Brink C. Histamine contractions of isolated human smooth muscle preparations: role of prostaglandins. J Pharmacol Exp Ther 1986; 239:536–541.

51. Churchill L. Chilton FH, Resau JH, Bascom R, Hubbard WC, Proud D. Cyclooxygenase metabolism of endogenous arachidonic acid by cultured human tracheal epithelial cells. Am Rev Respir Dis 1989; 140:449–459.

52. Pavord ID, Wong CS, Williams J, Tattersfield AE. Effect of inhaled prostaglandin E_2 on allergen-induced asthma. Am Rev Respir Dis 1993; 148:87–90.

53. Melillo E, Woolley KL, Manning PJ, Watson RM, O'Byrne PM. Effect of inhaled PGE_2 on exercise-induced bronchoconstriction in asthmatic subjects. Am J Respir Crit Care Med 1994; 149:1138–1141.

54. Kumlin M, Stensvad F, Larsson L, Dahlén B, Dahlén S-E. Validation and application of a new simple strategy for measurements of leukotriene E_4 in human urine. Clin Exp Allergy 1995; 25:467–479.
55. Widal F, Abrami P, Lermoyez J. Anaphylaxie et idiosyncrasie. Presse Med 1922; 30:189–193.
56. Salén EB, Arner B. Some views on the aspirin-hypersensitive allergy group. Acta Allergol 1948; 1:47–84.
57. Samter M, Beers RF. Intolerance to aspirin. Clinical studies and considerations of its pathogenesis. Ann Intern Med 1968; 68:975–983.
58. Dahlén B, Margolskee DJ, Zetterström O, Dahlén S-E. Effect of the leukotriene-antagonist MK-0679 on baseline pulmonary function in aspirin-sensitive asthmatics. Thorax 1993; 48:1205–1210.
59. Jones TR, Zamboni R, Belley M, Champion E, Charette L, Ford-Hutchinson AW, Frenette R, Gauthier J-Y, Leger S, Masson P, McFarlane CS, Piechuta H, Rokach J, Williams H, Young RN, Dehaven RN. Pharmacology of L-660,711 (MK-571): a novel ptoent and selective leukotriene D_4 receptor antagonist. Can J Physiol Pharmacol 1989; 67:17–28.
60. Snyder DW, Giles RE, Keith RA, Yee YK, Krell RD. The in vitro pharmacology of ICI-198,615: a novel, potent selective peptide leukotriene antagonist. J Pharmacol Exp Ther 1987; 243:548–556.
61. Björck T, Dahlén S-E. Leukotrienes and histamine are the exclusive mediators of IgE-dependent contractions of human bronchi in vitro. Pulmon Pharmacol 1993; 6:87–96.
62. Kips JC, Joos GF, DeLepeleire I, Margolskee DJ, Buntix A, Pauwels R, Van Der Straeten ME. Mk-571: a potent antagonist of LTD_4-induced bronchoconstriction in the human. Am Rev Respir Dis 1991; 144:617–621.
63. Taylor IK, O'Shaoughnessy KM, Fuller RW, Dollery CT. Effect of cysteinyl-leukotriene receptor antagonist ICI 204,219 on allergen-induced bronchoconstriction and airway hyperreactivity in atopic subjects. Lancet 1991; 337:690–694.
64. Hui KP, Barnes NC. Lung function improvement in asthma with a cysteinyl-leukotriene receptor antagonist. Lancet 1991; 337:1062–1063.
65. Gaddy JN, Margolskee DJ, Bush RK, Williams VC, Busse WW. Bronchodilation with a potent and selective leukotriene D_4 (LTD_4) receptor antagonist (MK-571) in asthma patients. Am Rev Respir Dis 1992; 146:358–363.
66. Israel E, Rubin P, Kemp JP, Grossman J, Pierson W, Siegel SC, Tinkelman D, Murray JJ, Busse W, Segal AT, Fish J, Kaiser HB, Ledford D, Wenzel S, Rosenthal R, Cohn J, Lanni C, Pearlman H, Karahalios P, Drazen JM. The effect of inhibition of 5-lipoxygenase by Zileuton in mild-to-moderate asthma. Ann Intern Med 1993; 119:1059–1066.
67. Sebaldt RJ, Sheller JR, Oates JA, Roberts LJ II, FitzGerald GA. Inhibition of eicosanoid synthesis by glucocorticoids in humans. Proc Natl Acad Sci USA 1990; 87:6974–6978.
68. Manso G, Baker AJ, Taylor IK, Fuller RW. In vivo and in vitro effects of glucocorticosteroids on arachidonic acid metabolism and monocyte function in non asthmatic humans. Eur Respir J 1992; 5:712–716.

69. O'Shaughnessy KM, Wellings R, Gillies B, Fuller RW. Differential effects of fluticasone proprionate on allergen-evoked bronchoconstriction and increased urinary leukotriene E_4 excretion. Am Rev Respir Dis 1993; 147:1472–1476.

70. Dahlén S-E, Nizankowska E, Dahlén B, Bochenek G, Kumlin M, Mastalerz L, Blomqvist H, Pinis G, Råsberg B, Swanson LJ, Dubé L, Stensvad F, Zetterström O, Szczeklik A. The Swedish-Polish treatment study with the 5-lipoxygenase inhibitor Zileuton in aspirin-intolerant asthmatics. Am J Respir Crit Care Med 1995; 151:A376.

22

Aspirin-Intolerant Asthma

New Insights from Bronchial Mucosal Biopsies

ANTHONY P. SAMPSON

Southampton General Hospital
Southampton, England

I. Introduction

The central role of cysteinyl-leukotrienes (LTs) in causing bronchoconstriction, mucus hypersecretion, airway edema, bronchial hyperresponsiveness, and eosinophil infiltration in allergic asthma has been extensively reviewed (1–3). Cysteinyl-LTs may play a particularly prominent role in those asthmatics who experience adverse respiratory reactions to aspirin and other nonsteroidal anti-inflammatory drugs (NSAIDs) (4). Oral, inhaled, or endobronchial challenge with NSAIDs causes dramatic increments in cysteinyl-LT levels in bronchoalveolar lavage (BAL) fluid, plasma, and urine (5–9), and the resulting acute respiratory reactions are significantly blocked by cysteinyl-LT antagonists and leukotriene synthesis inhibitors (4,10–12).

Since acute reactions to NSAIDs are related to inhibition of prostanoid synthesis (13), and inhalation of prostaglandin (PG)E_2 blocks the rise in cysteinyl-LTs and restores normal lung function (14), the acute increment in cysteinyl-LT production may be due to removal of a putative PGE_2-dependent brake (15). However, this model does not explain why similar responses are not observed in aspirin-tolerant asthmatics (ATA) or normal subjects. A clue is provided by the persistent two- to sevenfold elevation in baseline production of cysteinyl-LTs in aspirin-intolerant asthmatics (AIA) compared to ATA, even in the absence of exposure to NSAIDs (5,10,16). This chronic cysteinyl-LT overproduction significantly impairs baseline lung function (17). There is therefore a persistent underlying anomaly in AIA that is not revealed, but only exacerbated, by NSAIDs. The anomaly may involve altered influx or survival of those inflammatory cells capable of generating cysteinyl-LTs or inhibitory prostanoids, or altered activity of leukotriene or prostanoid synthetic enzymes within a static population of resident cells, or a combination of both factors.

The advent of the flexible fiberoptic bronchoscope in the 1980s revolutionized immunopathological studies of allergic asthma, but relatively few workers have performed bronchoscopy studies in aspirin-intolerant patients. This chapter will use evidence from recent immunohistochemical studies on AIA bronchial biopsies (18–24) to address the following questions: Is there an unusual profile of inflammatory leukocytes in the lungs of AIA compared to other asthmatics, and what cytokine mechanisms bring this about? What are the cellular sources of acute and chronic cysteinyl-LT overproduction in the presence and absence of NSAIDs? What is the source of the endogenous PGE_2 brake and the site of action of NSAIDs? Finally, a new model for AIA will be proposed that describes how markedly enhanced expression of the terminal enzyme for cysteinyl-LT synthesis, LTC_4 synthase, within an enhanced population of eosinophils can explain both the acute and chronic features of AIA, without recourse to the hypothesis of a putative anomaly in prostanoid synthetic pathways.

II. Profile of Leukocytes in AIA Bronchial Biopsies

A. Leukocyte Sources of Cysteinyl-LTs In Vitro

The cellular sources of cysteinyl-LTs are thought to be mast cells, eosinophils, and macrophages, but as the evidence rests on cells isolated from lung, BAL fluid, or blood, their relative contributions within intact lung are poorly understood. Highly purified pulmonary mast cells are a strong source of LTC_4 after ionophore or IgE-dependent stimulation (25,26). Human lung fragments generate cysteinyl-LTs after IgE-dependent stimulation (27), and in atopic asthmatics, allergen inhalation leads to LTC_4 release into BAL fluid at the same time as the release of histamine, tryptase, and PGD_2 (28–31), suggestive of a mast cell source. Human blood eosinophils, but not neutrophils, secrete large amounts of LTC_4 in response to calcium ionophore and smaller amounts in response to receptor-dependent stimuli (32,33). Mature blood basophils also have a high capacity to generate LTC_4 (34). Monocyte-macrophages generate smaller amounts of cysteinyl-LTs (35), while human lymphocytes are not thought capable of generating cysteinyl-LTs.

B. Anomalies in Leukocyte Profile in AIA Biopsies

Early bronchoscopy studies in allergic asthma demonstrated inflammatory damage to bronchial epithelium and deposition of collagen beneath the basement membrane even in mild asthma (36,37). This was accompanied by histological and electron microscopic evidence of mast cell activation and of eosinophil and lymphocyte infiltration in the submucosa (38–41).

Bronchial biopsy studies in AIA have discovered marked differences in the profile of inflammatory leukocytes in comparison to ATA. Intriguingly, these differences are largely restricted to those few cell types capable of generating cysteinyl-LTs, namely eosinophils, mast cells, and macrophages. In one immunohistochemical study using frozen sections, a monoclonal antibody to mast cell tryptase (AA1) (42) demonstrated lower mast cell counts in unchallenged AIA biopsies than in ATA biopsies (21), suggestive of a loss of tryptase due to enhanced mast cell degranulation in the AIA group. In our collaborative studies with Prof. Andrzej Szczeklik (Krakow, Poland) and Drs. K. Frank Austen and John F. Penrose (Boston, USA) (19,22,23), thin sections (2 μm) were examined from acetone-fixed biopsies embedded in the water-permeable resin glycol methacrylate (GMA), a technique that is optimal for preservation both of high antigenicity and of good tissue morphology (43). No differences in AA1$^+$ mast cell counts were observed between AIA and ATA biopsies in either the absence or presence of NSAIDs (22,23). However, counts were lower in both asthmatic groups compared to normal biopsies, suggesting ongoing mast cell degranulation. The discrepancy between the studies may reflect the unusually high proportion of the AIA subjects who were atopic in the study by Shuaib Nasser et al. (21), as ongoing mast cell degranulation has been recognized by electron microscopy in the bronchial biopsies even of atopic subjects without asthma (44).

Both groups of workers have confirmed significant anomalies in eosinophil counts in steady-state AIA. Using the monoclonal antibody BMK13, total eosinophil counts were found to be 2.4-fold higher in unchallenged AIA biopsies compared to ATA biopsies (21). With the monoclonal antibody EG1, which recognizes eosinophil cationic protein (ECP) (45), total eosinophil counts are fourfold higher in AIA biopsies compared to ATA biopsies and 15-fold higher than in normal biopsies in both the presence and absence of NSAIDs (22,23). "Activated" eosinophils detected with the monoclonal antibody EG2 (46) are reported variously to be similar in AIA and ATA groups (21), or to be threefold and 10-fold higher in unchallenged AIA biopsies compared to ATA and normal biopsies, respectively (19,22,23). The assumption that EG2 directed against secretory ECP is a marker of activated eosinophils has recently been seriously questioned (46), and differences in methodology or in subject selection may also contribute to the discrepancy in EG2 results between the studies. However, taken together with the results for total eosinophil immunostaining, the overall picture is of profoundly exaggerated bronchial mucosal eosinophilia in AIA biopsies, even in the absence of exposure to NSAIDs, compared to those from ATA or normal subjects.

Macrophages immunostaining with the monoclonal antibody EBM11 directed against CD68 are reported to be slightly less numerous in AIA biopsies than in ATA biopsies (21); however, EBM11 also recognizes CD68 found on all myeloid cells and is therefore not a specific macrophage marker. Using the monoclonal PG-M1, which recognizes only the macrophage-restricted form of CD68 (47), we found in contrast a tendency for macrophage counts to be higher in unchallenged AIA biopsies than in ATA biopsies and to be significantly higher than in biopsies of normal subjects (23). However, these changes were modest in comparison to the profound eosinophilia observed in the same studies. Moreover, using an antibody against CD14 that is well expressed on monocytes and immature macrophages, no differences were observed between the subject groups (22). Overall, studies to date concur in finding no compelling evidence for a major anomaly in monocyte-macrophage counts in AIA bronchial biopsies.

No baseline differences have been reported between AIA and ATA biopsies in counts of NP57+ neutrophils (21) or CD3+, CD4+, or CD8+ T lymphocytes (21–23). The activation status of T cells has not been examined.

III. Expression of Cysteinyl-LT Synthetic Pathway Enzymes in AIA Bronchial Biopsies

A. Eicosanoid Pathway Enzymes

The biochemistry and molecular biology of the LT synthetic pathway enzymes have been elucidated within the last 10 years. During cell activation, arachidonic acid is released from membrane phospholipids by cytosolic phospholipase A_2 (cPLA$_2$) (48) and translocated to the integral membrane protein 5-lipoxygenase activating protein (FLAP) (49) (Fig. 1). Arachidonate is converted initially to 5-hydroperoxyeicosatetraenoic acid (5-HPETE) and then to leukotriene (LT) A_4 by cytosolic 5-lipoxygenase (5-LO) (50). LTA$_4$ is converted to the dihydroxy leukotriene, LTB$_4$, by cells expressing LTA$_4$ hydrolase (51), or to the cysteinyl-LT LTC$_4$ by cells expressing LTC$_4$ synthase, which conjugates LTA$_4$ to reduced glutathione (52). LTC$_4$ synthase is a 37-kDa dimeric integral membrane protein with a high degree of homology to FLAP (53). After carrier-mediated export, the sequential cleavage from LTC$_4$ of glutamate and glycine residues generates LTD$_4$ and LTE$_4$, respectively. In prostanoid biosynthesis, the released arachidonic acid is converted by constitutive cyclooxygenase-1 (COX-1) or by inducible COX-2 to the intermediate PGH$_2$, before conversion to biologically active prostanoids by synthases and isomerases (54).

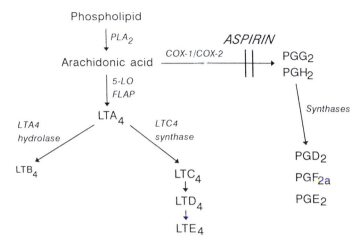

Figure 1 Enzymes of the leukotriene and prostanoid synthetic pathways: 5-lipoxy-genase (5-LO), 5-LO-activating protein (FLAP), LTA$_4$ hydrolase, LTC$_4$ synthase, cy-clooxygenase (COX)-1, and COX-2.

B. Expression of 5-LO, FLAP, and LTA$_4$ Hydrolase in AIA Biopsies

Surprisingly few studies have been performed to characterize the distribution of 5-LO pathway enzymes in normal or allergic asthmatic bronchial biopsies. In a preliminary report on paraffin-embedded bronchial biopsies from five normal subjects, 5-LO and FLAP have been colocalized to subepithelial mac-rophages, eosinophils, and mast cells (55). In two status asthmaticus biopsies, immunostaining for 5-LO was enhanced compared to normal biopsies com-mensurate with greater numbers of total leukocytes identified via leukocyte common antigen LCA (CD45) (55).

In aspirin-sensitive asthma, a study in frozen biopsy sections found no difference in the numbers of cells immunostaining for 5-LO between 12 AIA and eight ATA subjects in the absence of NSAID challenge (21). In our studies using GMA-embedded thin sections, we also found no differences in the counts of cells immunostaining for 5-LO in biopsies from 10 placebo-challenged AIA and 10 ATA patients, nor was either group different from nine nonatopic nor-mal subjects (22,23) (Fig. 2). There were also no differences between AIA, ATA, and normal groups in immunostaining for FLAP or for LTA$_4$ hydrolase (22,23). These results suggest that the capacity of steady-state AIA, ATA, and normal lung to initiate LT synthesis, or to generate LTB$_4$, is not different.

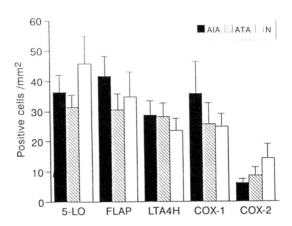

Figure 2   Counts of cells expressing enzymes of the leukotriene and prostanoid synthetic pathways in bronchial mucosal biopsies of aspirin-intolerant asthmatic (AIA), aspirin-tolerant asthmatic (ATA), and normal subjects. Mean ± SEM.

C. Profound Overexpression of LTC$_4$ Synthase in AIA Bronchial Biopsies

However, in the same subjects, we also identified cells immunostaining for LTC$_4$ synthase, the recently characterized terminal enzyme for cysteinyl-LT synthesis, using an affinity-purified rabbit polyclonal antibody to human lung LTC$_4$ synthase, which did not cross-react with FLAP (56). Cells expressing LTC$_4$ synthase were fivefold more numerous in AIA biopsies than in ATA biopsies ($p = 0.0006$), and 18-fold more numerous than in normal biopsies ($p = 0.0002$) (22,23) (Fig. 3). There was little overlap between the AIA and ATA subject groups. This is the first reported anomaly in the expression of any eicosanoid pathway enzyme in the AIA lung, and suggests a simple mechanism for the increased capacity to generate cysteinyl-LTs both basally and after aspirin challenge.

D. Cellular Localization of 5-LO Pathway Enzymes in AIA Biopsies

Colocalization of 5-LO pathway enzymes to cell markers has been performed using double immunostaining on frozen sections and by single immunostaining on serial adjacent GMA sections. Counts of cells immunostaining for 5-LO and FLAP correlate closely (23), and the majority of 5-LO$^+$ cells in AIA and ATA groups are macrophages and eosinophils, with a smaller proportion being mast cells (21,23). Most 5-LO$^+$ macrophages, however, coexpress LTA$_4$

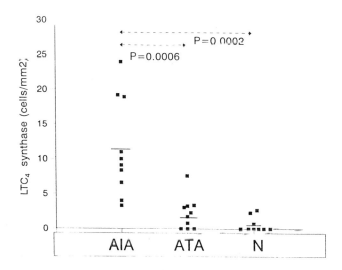

Figure 3 Counts of cells expressing LTC_4 synthase in bronchial mucosal biopsies of aspirin-intolerant asthmatic (AIA), aspirin-tolerant asthmatic (ATA), and normal subjects.

hydrolase but only rarely express LTC_4 synthase, and are thus adapted to generate LTB_4 not the cysteinyl-LTs.

Only cells expressing LTC_4 synthase can generate cysteinyl-LTs, and the predominance of these are eosinophils both in AIA biopsies (71%) and in ATA biopsies (45%), with a smaller porportion being mast cells (11% and 18%, respectively) and very few being macrophages (<5%) (23). In addition, the proportion of eosinophils expressing LTC_4 synthase is significantly higher in AIA biopsies (51%) than in ATA biopsies (21%), suggesting that LTC_4 synthase expression is enhanced by the lung microenvironment in AIA (23). The proportion of mast cells and macrophages expressing the enzyme is low (<15%) in all groups. Taken together, the significantly higher counts of eosinophils in AIA lung and the higher proportion of eosinophils that express LTC_4 synthase adequately account for the dramatically higher counts of LTC_4 synthase$^+$ cells in AIA biopsies.

IV. The Cellular Source of Cysteinyl-LT Overproduction in AIA

A. Chronic Cysteinyl-LT Overproduction in Steady-State AIA

The relative scarcity of LTC_4 synthase$^+$cells in all three subject groups compared to 5-LO and FLAP expression (Fig. 2) suggests that LTC_4 synthase expression is the rate-limiting factor in cysteinyl-LT synthesis. Indeed, the baseline levels of total cysteinyl-LTs were significantly higher in the broncho-alveolar (BAL) fluid of the AIA subjects compared to the ATA subjects, and overall, levels correlated significantly with the numbers of LTC_4 synthase$^+$ cells in the bronchial mucosa ($\rho = 0.86, p < 0.001$) (22,23). They did not correlate with the numbers of cells expressing any other eicosanoid pathway enzyme. Persistent cysteinyl-LT overproduction in AIA may therefore be due to profound and chronic overexpression of LTC_4 synthase within an increased population of bronchial eosinophils.

B. Acute Cysteinyl-LT Overproduction After Aspirin Challenge

Fifteen minutes after endobronchial challenge with lysine-aspirin, BAL fluid levels of cys-LTs rise significantly in AIA patients compared to prechallenge values, but there are no detectable changes in the ATA group (9,22,23). Although this difference is consistent with the much higher numbers of LTC_4 synthase$^+$ cells in the AIA bronchial mucosa compared to ATA biopsies, there was no direct linear correlation (22,23). This suggests that only a subgroup of the LTC_4 synthase$^+$ cell population is activated by aspirin. The identity of this subgroup remains unclear, as the rise in BAL fluid cysteinyl-LTs did not correlate with the counts of any individual cell type in the bronchial mucosa, but as the majority of LTC_4 synthase$^+$ are eosinophils it seems likely that they are a source. Moreover, the rise in cysteinyl-LTs was accompanied in the AIA subjects, but not the ATA subjects, by a rise in the percentage of eosinophils in the BAL fluid cell pellet (9,22,23), suggestive of a very rapid efflux of activated eosinophils into the airway lumen.

   Although, in parallel studies, the lysine-aspirin-induced rise in BAL fluid cysteinyl-LTs correlated with a rise in BAL fluid histamine levels, indicating mast cell or basophil activation, neither tryptase nor ECP levels changed (9). In our studies, local lysine-aspirin challenge did not change bronchial mucosal counts of any cell type, perhaps because the time interval after challenge (20 min) was too short (22,23), but a significant drop in mast cell counts after lysine-aspirin challenge has been reported in AIA with a similar protocol (20); this is argued to reflect loss of mast cell tryptase due to aspirin-induced mast cell degranulation, and was accompanied by marginal increases in eosinophil counts (20). Overall, however, evidence from studies to date for the cellular source of aspirin-induced cysteinyl-LT release remains ambiguous, although eosinophils and mast cells may both contribute.

   Endobronchial lysine-aspirin challenge does not affect the numbers of bronchial mucosal cells expressing 5-LO (20,22,23), or FLAP, LTA_4 hydrolase, or LTC_4 synthase (22,23) for 20 min after challenge. It is not yet known whether leukocyte counts or enzyme expression may alter several hours or days after aspirin challenge. Studies are also required to examine whether changes in leukocyte profile or enzyme expression are responsible for the reduced cysteinyl-LT responses to NSAIDs reported after aspirin desensitization therapy in AIA patients (57).

V. LTC$_4$ Synthase Expression Correlates Uniquely with Bronchial Responsiveness to Inhaled Lysine-Aspirin

Assays of BAL fluid mediators may not reflect mediator concentrations within the bronchial wall, but it is the action of the latter at their receptors on bronchial smooth muscle, mucus glands, and vascular endothelium within the bronchial submucosa that leads to aspirin-induced respiratory reactions. It is therefore important to relate anomalies in leukocyte profile or enzyme expression not only to BAL fluid mediator levels but also to the bronchoconstrictor response to challenge. We found a unique inverse relationship between the provocation dose of inhaled lysine-aspirin required to reduce the forced expiratory volume by 20% (lysine-aspirin PD$_{20}$ FEV$_1$), and the numbers of LTC$_4$ synthase$^+$ cells in the bronchial mucosa (22,23) (Fig. 4). The four- to fivefold higher counts of LTC$_4$ synthase$^+$ cells in the bronchial mucosa of AIA subjects equated to an approximately 200-fold greater bronchial sensitivity to

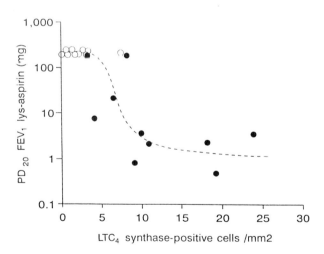

Figure 4 Relationship between bronchial mucosal counts of cells expressing LTC$_4$ synthase with bronchial responsiveness to inhaled lysine-aspirin challenge of aspirin-intolerant asthmatics (●) and aspirin-tolerant asthmatics (○). PD$_{20}$ FEV$_1$ is the provocation dose (mg) of inhaled lysine-aspirin required to reduce forced expiratory volume in 1 sec (FEV$_1$) by 20% of baseline.

inhaled lysine-aspirin. Importantly, the bronchial responsiveness to inhaled lysine-aspirin showed no relationship to immunostaining for any other eicosanoid pathway enzyme, or to individual cell counts, or to cytokine expression, or to any clinical characteristics of the AIA patient group. Overexpression of LTC_4 synthase in the bronchial wall, irrespective of cell type, may thus be the single most important determinant of adverse bronchial responses to aspirin.

VI. Suppression of Cysteinyl-LT Synthesis by Endogenous PGE_2

A. The Cellular Source of the Endogenous PGE_2 Brake

PGE_2 has been proposed as an important down-regulatory mediator in asthma (15) because NSAIDs enhance, and PGE_2 reduces, LT synthesis in a number of inflammatory cell types in vitro, including human eosinophils, neutrophils, and basophils, and rat macrophages (34,58–61). Even if eosinophils and/or mast cells are the source of acute cysteinyl-LT overproduction in AIA, they are not necessarily the source of the PGE_2 brake lifted by NSAIDs. Indeed, although mast cells generate a number of bronchoconstrictor prostanoids including PGD_2, they do not appear to generate PGE_2 (34). NSAIDs do not increase cysteinyl-LT release by stimulated human lung mast cells in vitro (26). In addition, although PGE_2 synthesis is clearly inhibited and cysteinyl-LT synthesis is strongly stimulated by lysine-aspirin challenge, levels of the mast cell–derived prostanoids PGD_2, $PGF_{2\alpha}$, and $9\alpha,11\beta$-PGF_2 in the nasal secretions, BAL fluid, and urine of aspirin-sensitive patients are not reduced (9,62,63), while NSAIDs reduce synthesis of all prostanoids in the BAL fluid of ATA patients (9). This relative refractoriness of the prostanoid synthetic pathway in the AIA mast cell to NSAIDs is paradoxical as the opposite might have been expected, and suggests the site of action of NSAIDs on PGE_2 synthesis is elsewhere. The refractoriness of the AIA mast cell may be due to enhanced expression of COX-2 (24), which is relatively resistant to aspirin. Combined with the fact that AIA patients tolerate the relatively selective COX-2 inhibitor nimesulide (64) and only respond adversely to COX-1-selective NSAIDs, this suggests that the PGE_2 brake is produced by constitutive COX-1 activity in a cell type other than the mast cell. This cell type may perhaps be the monocyte-macrophage, but as these are present in large numbers even in normal lung, it is unclear why aspirin does not enhance cysteinyl-LT release from normal human lung fragments (27). This supports the view that the cells that are the source of cysteinyl-LTs and/or the site of action of NSAIDs are not present in normal lung.

In contrast to the mast cell, normodense human blood eosinophils do produce nanomolar amounts of PGE_2 (58,65), probably via expression of small amounts of COX-1. Treatment of eosinophils with NSAIDs multiplies their synthesis of cysteinyl-LTs 10-fold, and this is restored to basal levels by nanomolar amounts of exogenous PGE_2 (58). We hypothesize that the eosinophil, which is virtually absent in normal bronchial biopsies, is present in modest numbers in ATA biopsies, and in very high numbers in AIA biopsies, is not only the major source of cysteinyl-LTs in AIA, but may also be the source of the PGE_2 brake. Aspirin sensitivity may thus form a continuum dependent on the degree of bronchial eosinophilia and on the degree of expression of LTC_4 synthase within those eosinophils.

B. Is There an Anomaly in the PGE$_2$ Brake in AIA?

A persistent failure in the PGE_2 braking mechanism causing hypersensitivity to inhibition by NSAIDs has been postulated to explain why AIA patients overproduce cysteinyl-LTs both chronically and after low doses of NSAIDs. However, baseline BAL fluid levels of PGE_2, PGD_2, $PGF_{2\alpha}$, thromboxane A_2, and other prostanoids are not different in AIA and ATA patients (9). There is no difference in the pharmacokinetics of aspirin in AIA and ATA patients (66). Inhaled lysine-aspirin can reduce BAL fluid and nasal PGE_2 levels in ATA patients to the same extent as in AIA patients (8,9,62), but only the AIA patients generate significant cysteinyl-LTs as a result. Our findings (22,23) resolve this apparent paradox, as the absence of significant LTC_4 synthase expression in ATA and normal biopsies prevents significant cysteinyl-LT production even if PGE_2 production is maximally inhibited by a large dose of NSAID. In AIA lung, in which LTC_4 synthase is profoundly overrepresented, any dose of NSAID sufficient to cause some degree of inhibition of PGE_2 synthesis would lead to a significant release of cysteinyl-LTs, possibly leading to an adverse respiratory reaction.

Corroborating this hypothesis, immunohistochemical studies on bronchial biopsies have found little evidence for a consistent or meaningful anomaly in the prostanoid synthetic pathway in AIA. Rabbit polyclonal and mouse monoclonal antibodies showed no differences in the expression of COX-1 in frozen or GMA-embedded biopsies from AIA, ATA, and normal subjects (18,22,23). Similarly, no differences have been observed in the numbers of COX-2$^+$ cells between AIA and ATA biopsies (18,22–24). Both AIA and ATA groups have been reported to express more COX-2 than normal subjects (18), although we and others found no difference (22,23,67); the discrepancy may be due to the use of polyclonal antibodies in the former study and monoclonal antibodies in the latter. Examination of the expression of enzymes upstream and downstream of COX-1/COX-2 is required, particularly of PGE_2 synthase, but the uniform expression of constitutive COX-1 and inducible COX-2 in

AIA and ATA subjects in all studies to date supports the view that the underlying anomaly in AIA does not lie in the PGE_2 synthetic pathway.

VII. Cytokine Regulation of Cysteinyl-LT Production

A.   Cytokine Expression in Allergic Asthmatic Bronchial Biopsies

We have seen that overexpression of LTC_4 synthase within an enhanced population of eosinophils is the principal determinant of bronchial hyperresponsiveness to NSAIDs. In the allergic asthmatic lung, correlations between submucosal eosinophil counts, activated T-cell counts, and nonspecific bronchial responsiveness suggested that allergic inflammation is driven by Th2-lymphocyte-derived cytokines (68–70). These include the eosinophilopoietic cytokines interleukin (IL)-3, IL-5, and granulocyte-macropahge colony-stimulating factor (GM-CSF), which promote eosinophil maturation, migration, activation, and survival, and IL-4, which is essential for IgE production by B lymphocytes. The capacity of human eosinophils and basophils to generate LTC_4 is enhanced by pretreatment with IL-3, IL-5, and GM-CSF (71), while in contrast, LTC_4 release from human lung mast cells is primed by stem cell factor (SCF; c-*kit* ligand) at low concentrations and directly triggered by SCF at high concentrations (72). Increases in expression of IL-4, IL-5, and GM-CSF have been reported in bronchial biopsies of atopic asthmatics 24 hr after inhaled allergen challenge (73), and symptomatic asthmatics have greater biopsy expression of IL-1, IL-2, IL-3, IL-5, GM-CSF, and tumor necrosis factor (TNFα) than asymptomatic asthmatics or normal controls (74). The cells expressing these cytokines are principally T cells with smaller numbers of mast cells and some eosinophils (74,75). Enhanced expression of IL-4 in lymphocytes in bronchial biopsies appears to distinguish atopic from nonatopic asthma (74).

B.   Enhanced IL-5 Expression in AIA Bronchial Biopsies

The reasons for the profound eosinophilia in AIA biopsies have been explored by immunohistochemical analysis of the expression of IL-3, IL-5, and GM-CSF in AIA and ATA bronchial biopsies (22,23). There are no differences in counts of cells expressing IL-3 or GM-CSF, but counts of cells expressing IL-5 are significantly (threefold) higher in AIA biopsies than in ATA biopsies. These IL-5[+] cells are predominantly mast cells, and the proportion of mast cells expressing IL-5 also tended to be higher in AIA than in ATA. This is consistent with the rapid and significant release of IL-5 into BAL fluid observed in AIA but not ATA subjects after endobronchial challenge with lysine-aspirin (9), as only mast cells store large quantities of IL-5. Counts of IL-5[+] cells correlated significantly with the numbers of eosinophils, suggesting that the intense eosinophilia in the AIA lung may be due at least in part to mast cell–derived IL-5.

The relative lack of intracellular storage of cytokines by T cells makes their immunohistochemical localization to T cells difficult. Expression of LTC_4 synthase is not observed in T cells, yet in AIA patients both the numbers of LTC_4 synthase$^+$ cells and the proportion of eosinophils expressing the enzyme correlated significantly with $CD4^+$ T-cell counts, but not with other cell types (22,23). Therefore $CD4^+$ T-cell products, perhaps IL-5, may also contribute to the up-regulation of eosinophil numbers and their expression of LTC_4 synthase in the AIA lung.

VIII. A New Model of Aspirin-Sensitive Asthma

The finding of profoundly enhanced LTC_4 synthase expression in AIA bronchial biopsies (22,23), against a background of no differences in expression of 5-LO, FLAP, LTA_4 hydrolase, COX-1, or COX-2, adds an entirely novel component to previous models, as it localizes the mechanism for enhanced cysteinyl-LT production in AIA within the cysteinyl-LT synthetic pathway itself. The enhanced LTC_4 synthase$^+$ cell counts, which correlated with basal levels of cysteinyl-LTs in BAL fluid and which were associated with enhanced release of cysteinyl-LTs in response to endobronchial lysine-aspirin challenge, link overexpression of the enzyme with overproduction of cysteinyl-LTs in both the presence and absence of exposure to NSAIDs. LTC_4 synthase$^+$ cell counts also correlated uniquely with bronchial responsiveness to inhaled lysine-aspirin challenge (23), linking overexpression of LTC_4 synthase directly to the exaggerated pathophysiological response to NSAIDs. A further attractive aspect of the model is that it has no requirement for any defect in the ability of NSAIDs to inhibit prostanoid synthesis in AIA lung. Instead, equieffective inhibition of COX in all asthmatic and normal subjects would lead to detectable synthesis of cysteinyl-LTs only in AIA patients, who have exaggerated expression of LTC_4 synthase, but not in ATA or normal subjects, in whom LTC_4 synthase expression is low or negligible.

The mechanisms causing overexpression of LTC_4 synthase and eosinophilia in the AIA lung remain undefined. Intriguingly, LTC_4 synthase is the only eicosanoid pathway enzyme whose gene localizes to human chromosome 5q (76), close to the loci of other candidate asthma genes including those of the IL-4 gene cluster (77). A polymorphism in the LTC_4 synthase gene leading to chronic overexpression of the enzyme in one or more leukocyte types would be an attractive hypothesis to explain several components of our model, as the products of LTC_4 synthase are not only bronchoconstrictor mediators but also potent and specific eosinophil chemoattractants (78,79). Alternatively, overexpression of LTC$_4$ synthase within eosinophils and/or mast cells could be secondary to a genetic anomaly in the activity of an eosinophilopoietic cytokine such as IL-5 and/or a mast cell growth factor such as stem cell factor.

Acknowledgments

APS is funded by the Frances and Augustus Newman Foundation and by the Royal College of Surgeons of England.

References

1. Arm JP, Lee TH. Sulphidopeptide leukotrienes in asthma. Clin Sci Colch 1993; 84:501–510.
2. Hay DWP, Torphy TJ, Undem BJ. Cysteinyl leukotrienes in asthma: old mediators up to new tricks. Trends Pharmacol Sci 1995; 16:304–309.
3. Sampson AP. The leukotrienes: mediators of chronic inflammation in asthma. Clin Exp Allergy 1996; 26:995–1004.
4. Israel E, Fischer AR, Rosenberg MA, Lilly CM, Callery JC, Shapiro J, Cohn J, Rubin P, Drazen JM. The pivotal role of 5-lipoxygenase products in the reaction of aspirin-sensitive asthmatics to aspirin. Am Rev Respir Dis 1993; 148:1447–1451.
5. Kumlin M, Dahlén B, Bjorck T, Zetterstrom O, Granstrom E, Dahlén SE. Urinary excretion of leukotriene E$_4$ and 11-dehydro-thromboxane B$_2$ in response to bronchial provocations with allergen, aspirin, leukotriene D$_4$, and histamine in asthmatics. Am Rev Respir Dis 1992; 146:96–103.
6. Christie PE, Tagari P, Ford-Hutchinson AW, Charlesson S, Chee P, Arm JP, Lee TH. Urinary leukotriene E$_4$ concentrations increase after aspirin challenge in aspirin-sensitive asthmatic subjects. Am Rev Respir Dis 1991; 143:1025–1029.
7. Sladek K, Szczeklik A. Cysteinyl leukotriene overproduction and mast cell activation in aspirin-provoked bronchospasm in asthma. Eur Respir J 1993; 6:391–399.
8. Sladek K, Dworski R, Soja J, Sheller JR, Nizankowska E, Oates JA, Szczeklik A. Eicosanoids in bronchoalveolar lavage fluid of aspirin-intolerant patients with asthma after aspirin challenge. Am J Respir Crit Care Med 1994; 149:940–946.
9. Szczeklik A, Sladek K, Dworski R, Nizankowska E, Soja J, Sheller JR, Oates J. Bronchial aspirin challenge causes specific eicosanoid response in aspirin sensitive asthmatics. Am J Respir Crit Care Med 1996; 154:1608–1614.
10. Christie PE, Smith CM, Lee TH. The potent and selective sulfidopeptide leukotriene antagonist SK&F 104353 inhibits aspirin-induced asthma. Am Rev Respir Dis 1991; 144:957–958.
11. Shuaib Nasser SM, Bell GS, Foster S, Spruce KE, MacMillan R, Williams AJ, Lee TH, Arm JP. Effect of the 5-lipoxygenase inhibitor ZD2138 on aspirin-induced asthma. Thorax 1994; 49:749–756.
12. Yamamoto H, Nagata M, Kuramitsu K, Tabe K, Kiuchi H, Sakamoto Y, Yamamoto K, Dohi Y. Inhibition of analgesic-induced asthma by leukotriene receptor antagonist ONO-1078. Am J Respir Crit Care Med 1994; 150:254–257.

13. Szczeklik A, Gryglewski RJ, Czerniawska-Mysik G. Relationship of inhibition of prostaglandin biosynthesis by analgesics to asthma attacks in aspirin-sensitive patients. Br Med J 1975; 1:67–69.
14. Sestini P, Armetti L, Gambaro G, Pieroni MG, Refini RM, Sala A, Vaghi A, Folco GC, Bianco S, Robuschi M. Inhaled PGE_2 prevents aspirin-induced bronchoconstriction and urinary LTE_4 excretion in aspirin-sensitive asthma. Am J Respir Crit Care Med 1996; 153:572–575.
15. Pavord ID, Tattersfield AE. Bronchoprotective role for endogenous prostaglandin E_2. Lancet 1995; 345:436–438.
16. Smith CM, Hawksworth RJ, Thien FC, Christie PE, Lee TH. Urinary leukotriene E_4 in bronchial asthma. Eur Respir J 1992; 5:693–699.
17. Dahlén B, Kumlin M, Margolskee DJ, Larsson C, Blomqvist H, Williams VC, Zetterstrom O, Dahlén SE. The leukotriene-receptor antagonist MK-0679 blocks airway obstruction induced by inhaled lysine-aspirin in aspirin-sensitive asthmatics. Eur Respir J 1993; 6:1018–1026.
18. Sousa AR, Pfister R, Lane SJ, Christie PE, Shuaib Nasser SM, Schmitz-Schumann M, Lee TH. Expression of COX-1 and COX-2 in aspirin-sensitive (ASA) and non-aspirin-sensitive (NASA) asthmatic and normal bronchial mucosa. J Allergy Clin Immunol 1996; 97(1):318 (abstract).
19. Cowburn A, Sladek K, Adamek L, Nizankowska E, Szczeklik A, Holgate S, Lam BK, Penrose JF, Austen KF, Sampson AP. Mast cell counts are lower and eosinophil counts are higher in bronchial biopsies of aspirin-sensitive asthmatics compared to aspirin-tolerant asthmatics. Am J Respir Crit Care Med 1996; 153:A683 (abstract).
20. Shuaib Nasser SM, Christie PE, Pfister R, Sousa AR, Walls A, Schmitz-Schumann M, Lee TH. Effect of endobronchial aspirin challenge on inflammatory cells in bronchial biopsies from aspirin-sensitive asthmatic subjects. Thorax 1996; 51: 64–70.
21. Shuaib Nasser SM, Pfister R, Christie PE, Sousa AR, Barker J, Schmitz-Schumann M, Lee TH. Inflammatory cell populations in bronchial biopsies from aspirin-sensitive asthmatic subjects. Am J Respir Crit Care Med 1996; 153:90–96.
22. Sampson AP, Cowburn AS, Sladek K, Adamek L, Nizankowska E, Szczeklik A, Penrose J, Austen KF, Holgate ST. Profound over-expression of leukotriene C_4 synthase in the bronchial biopsies of aspirin-intolerant asthmatics. Int Arch Allergy Immunol 1997; 113(1–3):355–357.
23. Cowburn AS, Sladek K, Soja J, Adamek L. Nizankowska E, Szczeklik A, Lam BK, Penrose J, Austen KF, Holgate ST, Sampson AP. Over-expression of leukotriene C_4 synthase in the bronchial biopsies of aspirin-intolerant asthmatics. J Clin Invest 1997 (submitted).
24. Sousa AR, Pfister R, Christie PE, Lane SJ, Nasser SSM, Schmitz-Schumann M, Lee TH. Enhanced expression of cyclooxygenase isoenzyme 2 (COX-2) in asthmatic airways and its cellular distribution in aspirin-sensitive asthma. J Allergy Clin Immunol 1997; 99:s376 (abstract).
25. Peters SP, Naclerio RM, Schleimer RP, MacGlashan DWJ, Pipkorn U, Lichtenstein LM. The pharmacologic control of mediator release from human basophils and mast cells. Respiration 1986; 50(Suppl 2):116–122.

26. Peters SP, MacGlashan DW, Schleimer RP, Hayes EC, Adkinson NF, Lichtenstein LM. The pharmacologic modulation of the release of arachidonic acid metabolites from purified human lung mast cells. Am Rev Respir Dis 1985; 132:367–373.

27. Salari H, Borgeat P, Fournier M, Hebert J, Pelletier G. Studies on the release of leukotrienes and histamine by human lung parenchymal and bronchial fragments upon immunologic and nonimmunologic stimulation: effects of nordihydroguaiaretic acid, aspirin, and sodium cromoglycate. J Exp Med 1985; 162:1904–1915.

28. Wenzel SE, Fowler AA, Schwartz LB. Activation of pulmonary mast cells by bronchoalveolar allergen challenge: in vivo release of histamine and tryptase in atopic subjects with and without asthma. Am Rev Respir Dis 1988; 137:1002–1008.

29. Wenzel SE, Westcott JY, Smith HR, Larsen GL. Spectrum of prostanoid release after bronchoalveolar allergen challenge in atopic asthmatics and in control groups: an alteration in the ratio of bronchoconstrictive to bronchoprotective mediators. Am Rev Respir Dis 1989; 139:450–457.

30. Wenzel SE, Larsen GL, Johnston K, Voelkel NF, Westcott JY. Elevated levels of LTC$_4$ in BAL fluid from atopic asthmatics after endobronchial allergen challenge. Am Rev Respir Dis 1990; 142:112–119.

31. Wenzel SE, Westcott JY, Larsen GL. Bronchoalveolar lavage fluid mediator levels 5 minutes after allergen challenge in atopic subjects with asthma: relationship to the development of late asthmatic responses. J Allergy Clin Immunol 1991; 87: 540–548.

32. Weller PF, Lee CW, Foster DW, Corey EJ, Austen KF, Lewis RA. Generation and metabolism of 5-lipoxygenase pathway leukotrienes by human eosinophils: predominant production of leukotriene C$_4$. Proc Natl Acad Sci USA 1983; 80: 7626–7630.

33. Bruynzeel PL, Kok PT, Hamelink ML, Kijne AM, Verhagen J. Exclusive LTC$_4$ synthesis by purified human eosinophils induced by opsonized zymosan. FEBS Lett 1985; 189:350–354.

34. Peters SP, Naclerio RM, Schleimer RP, MacGlashen DWJ, Pipkorn U, Lichtenstein LM. The pharmacologic control of mediator release from human basophils and mast cells. Respiration 1986; 50(Suppl 2):116–122.

35. Damon M, Chavis C, Godard P, Michel FB, Crastes-de-Paulet A. Purification and mass spectrometry identification of leukotriene D$_4$ synthesized by human alveolar macrophages. Biochem Biophys Res Commun 1983; 111:518–524.

36. Laitinen LA, Heino M, Laitinen A, Kava T, Haahtela T. Damage of the airway epithelium and bronchial reactivity in patients with asthma. Am Rev Respir Dis 1985; 131:599–606.

37. Ollerenshaw SL, Woolcock AJ. Characteristics of the inflammation in biopsies from large airways of subjects with asthma and subjects with chronic airflow limitation. Am Rev Respir Dis 1992; 145:922–927.

38. Beasley R, Roche WR, Roberts JA, Holgate ST. Cellular events in the bronchi in mild asthma and after bronchial provocation. Am Rev Respir Dis 1989; 139:806–817.

39. Bradley BL, Azzawi M, Jacobsen M, Assoufi B, Collins JV, Irani AM, Schwartz LB, Durham SR, Jeffery PK, Kay AB. Eosinophils, T-lymphocytes, mast cells, neutrophils and macrophages in bronchial biopsy specimens from atopic subjects

with asthma: comparison with biopsy specimens from atopic subjects without asthma and normal control subjects and relationship to bronchial responsiveness. J Allergy Clin Immunol 1991; 88:661–674.

40. Djukanović R, Wilson JW, Britten KM, Wilson SJ, Walls AF, Roche WR, Howarth PH, Holgate ST. Effect of an inhaled corticosteroid on airway inflammation and symptoms in asthma. Am Rev Respir Dis 1992; 145:669–674.

41. Laitinen LA, Laitinen A, Haahtela T. Airway mucosal inflammation even in patients with newly diagnosed asthma. Am Rev Respir Dis 1993; 147:697–704.

42. Walls AF, Bennett AR, McBride HM, Glennie MJ, Holgate ST, Church MK. Production and characterization of monoclonal antibodies specific for human mast cell tryptase. Clin Exp Allergy 1990; 20:581–589.

43. Britten KM, Howarth PH, Roche WR. Immunohistochemistry on resin sections: a comparison of resin embedding techniques for small bronchial biopsies. Biotech Histochem 1993; 68:271–280.

44. Djukanović R, Lai CK, Wilson JW, Britten KM, Wilson SJ, Roche WR, Howarth PH, Holgate ST. Bronchial mucosal manifestations of atopy: a comparison of markers of inflammation between atopic asthmatics, atopic nonasthmatics and healthy controls. Eur Respir J 1992; 5:538–544.

45. Tai PC, Spry CJF, Peterson C, Venge P, Olsson I. Monoclonal antibodies distinguish between storage and secretory forms of eosinophil cationic protein. Nature 1984; 309:182–185.

46. Jahnsen FL, Halstensen TS, Brandtzaeg P. Erroneous immunohistochemical application of monoclonal antibody EG2 to detect cellular activation. Lancet 1994; 344:1514–1515.

47. Falini B, Flenghi L, Pileri S, Gambacorta M, Bigerna B, Durkop H, Eitelbach F, Thiele J, Pacini R, Cavaliere A, Martelli M, Cardarelli N, Sabattini E, Poggi S, Stein H. PG-M1: a new monoclonal antibody directed against a fixative-resistant epitope on the macrophage-restricted form of the CD68 molecule. Am J Pathol 1993; 142(5):1359–1372.

48. Clark JD, Lin L-L, Kriz RW, Ramesha CS, Sultzman LS, Lin AY, Milona MN, Knopf JL. A novel arachidonic acid-selective cytosolic PLA_2 contains a Ca^{2+}-dependent translocation domain with homology to PKC and GAP. Cell 1991; 65:1043–1051.

49 Mancini JA, Abramowitz M, Cox ME, Wong E, Charleson S, Perrier H, Wang ZY, Prasit P, Vickers PJ. 5-lipoxygenase-activating protein is an arachidonate-binding protein. FEBS Lett 1993; 318:277–281.

50. Rouzer CA, Matsumoto T, Samuelsson B. Single protein from human leukocytes possesses 5-lipoxygenase and leukotriene A_4 synthase activities. Proc Natl Acad Sci USA 1986; 83:857–861.

51. Radmark O, Shimizu T, Jornvall H, Samuelsson B. Leukotriene A_4 hydrolase in human leukocytes: purification and properties. J Biol Chem 1984; 259:12339–12345.

52. Yoshimoto T, Soberman RJ, Spur B, Austen KF. Properties of highly purified leukotriene C_4 synthase of guinea pig lung. J Clin Invest 1988; 81:866–871.

53. Lam BK, Penrose JF, Freeman GJ, Austen KF. Expression cloning of a cDNA for human leukotriene C_4 synthase, an integral membrane protein conjugating reduced glutathione to leukotriene A_4. Proc Natl Acad Sci USA 1994; 91:7663–7667.

54. Vane JR. Towards a better aspirin. Nature 1994; 367:215–216.

55. Haley K, Sunday M, Reilly J, Sugerbaker D, Mentzer S, Evans J, Vickers P, Drazen J. Immunolocalization of 5-lipoxygenase activating protein and 5-lipoxygenase in normal and asthmatic lung. Am J Respir Crit Care Med 1995; 151(4):A677 (Abstract).

56. Penrose JF, Spector J, Lam BK, Friend DS, Xu K, Jack RM, Austen KF. Purification of human lung leukotriene C_4 synthase and preparation of a polyclonal antibody. Am J Respir Crit Care Med 1995; 152:283–289.

57. Shuaib Nasser SM, Patel M, Bell GS, Lee TH. The effect of aspirin desensitization on urinary LTE_4 concentrations in aspirin-sensitive asthma. Am J Respir Crit Care Med 1995; 151:1326–1330.

58. Tenor H, Hatzelmann A, Church MK, Schudt C, Shute JK. Effects of theophylline and rolipram on leukotriene C_4 synthesis and chemotaxis of human eosinophils from normal and atopic subjects. Br J Pharmacol 1996; 118:1727–1735.

59. Docherty JC, Wilson TW. Indomethacin increases the formation of lipoxygenase products in calcium ionophore stimulated human neutrophils. Biochem Biophys Res Commun 1987; 148:534–538.

60. Ham EA, Soderman DD, Zanetti ME, Dougherty HW, McCauley E, Kuehl FAJ. Inhibition by prostaglandins of LTB_4 release from activated neutrophils. Proc Natl Acad Sci USA 1983; 80:4349–4353.

61. Elliott GR, Lauwen APM, Bouta IL. Prostaglandin E_2 inhibits, and indomethacin and aspirin enhance, A23187-stimulated leukotriene B_4 synthesis by rat peritoneal macropahges. Br J Pharmacol 1989; 96:265–268.

62. Picado C, Ramis I, Rosello J, Prat J, Bulbena O, Plaza V, Montserrat JM, Gelpi E. Release of peptide leukotriene into nasal secretions after local instillation of aspirin in aspirin-sensitive asthmatic patients. Am Rev Respir Dis 1992; 145:65–69.

63. O'Sullivan S, Dahlén B, Dahlén SE, Kumlin M. Increased urinary excretion of the prostaglandin D_2 metabolite $9\alpha,11\beta$-prostaglandin F_2 after aspirin challenge supports mast cell activation in aspirin-induced airway obstruction. J Allergy Clin Immunol 1996; 98:421–432.

64. Bianco S, Robuschi M, Petrigni G, Scuri M, Refini RM, Vaghi A, Sestini PS. Efficacy and tolerability of nimesulide in asthmatic patients intolerant to aspirin. Drugs 1993; 46:115–120.

65. Kroegel C, Matthys H. Platelet-activating factor-induced human eosinophil activation: generation and release of cyclooxygenase metabolites in human blood eosinophils from asthmatics. Immunology 1993; 78:279–285.

66. Dahlén B, Boreus LO, Anderson P, Andersson R, Zetterstrom O. Plasma acetylsalicylic acid and salicyclic acid levels during aspirin provocation in aspirin-sensitive subjects. Allergy 1994; 49:43–49.

67. Demoly P, Jaffuel D, Lequeux N, Weksler B, Creminon C, Michel FB, Godard P, Bousquet J. Prostaglandin H synthase 1 and 2 immunoreactivities in the bronchial mucosa of asthmatics. Am J Respir Crit Care Med 1997; 155:670–675.

68. Bradley BL, Azzawi M, Jacobsen M, Assoufi B, Collins JV, Irani AM, Schwartz LB, Durham SR, Jeffery PK, Kay AB. Eosinophils, T-lymphocytes, mast cells, neutrophils and macrophages in bronchial biopsy specimens from atopic subjects with asthma: comparison with biopsy specimens from atopic subjects without asth-

ma and normal control subjects and relationship to bronchial responsiveness. J Allergy Clin Immunol 1991; 88:661–674.

69. Hamid Q. Barkans J, Robinson DS, Durham SR, Kay AB. Co-expression of CD25 and CD3 in atopic allergy and asthma. Immunology 1992; 75:659–663.

70. Ohashi Y, Motojima S, Fukuda T, Makino S. Airway hyperresponsiveness, increased intracellular spaces of bronchial epithelium, and increased infiltration of eosinophils and lymphocytes in bronchial mucosa in asthma. Am Rev Respir Dis 1992; 145:1469–1476.

71. Takafuji S, Bischoff SC, De Weck AL, Dahinden CA. IL-3 and IL-5 prime normal human eosinophils to produce LTC$_4$ in response to soluble agonists. J Immunol 1991; 147:3855–3861.

72. Bischoff SC, Dahinden CA. C-kit ligand: a unique potentiator of mediator release by human lung mast cells. J Exp Med 1992; 175:237–244.

73. Bentley AM, Meng Q, Robinson DS, Hamid Q, Kay AB, Durham SR. Increases in activated T lymphocytes, eosinophils, and cytokine mRNA for IL-5 and GM-CSF in bronchial biopsies after allergen inhalation challenge in atopic asthmatics. Am J Respir Cell Mol Biol 1993; 8:35–42.

74. Ackerman V, Marini M, Vittori E, Bellini A, Vassali G, Mattoli S. Detection of cytokines and their cell sources in bronchial biopsy specimens from asthmatic patients: relationship to atopic status, symptoms, and level of airway hyperresponsiveness. Chest 1994; 105:687–696.

75. Bradding P, Roberts JA, Britten KM, Montefort S, Djukanović R, Mueller R, Heusser CH, Howarth PH, Holgate ST. Interleukin-4, -5, and -6 and tumor necrosis factor-alpha in normal and asthmatic airways: evidence for the human mast cell as a source of these cytokines. Am J Respir Cell Mol Biol 1994; 10:471–480.

76. Penrose JF, Spector J, Baldasaro M, Xu K, Boyce J, Arm JP, Austen KF, Lam BK. Molecular cloning of the gene for human leukotriene C4 synthase: organization, nucleotide sequence, and chromosomal localization to 5q35. J Biol Chem 1996; 271:11356–11361.

77. Van Leeuwen BH, Martinson ME, Webb C, Young IG. Molecular organisation of the cytokine gene cluster involving the human IL-3, IL-4, IL-5, and GM-CSF genes on human chromosome 5. Blood 1989; 73:1142–1148.

78. Laitinen LA, Laitinen A, Haahtela T, Vilkka V, Spur BW, Lee TH. Leukotriene E$_4$ and granulocytic infiltration into asthmatic airways. Lancet 1993; 341:989–990.

79. Spada CS, Nieves AL, Krauss AH, Woodward DF. Comparison of leukotriene B$_4$ and D$_4$ effects on human eosinophil and neutrophil motility in vitro. J Leukoc Biol 1994; 55:183–191.

23

Pharmacological Intervention in Generation of Leukotrienes by Eosinophils

KLAUS F. RABE and GORDON DENT

Krankenhaus Grosshansdorf
Grosshansdorf, Germany

I. Introduction

Eosinophils are characteristic for acute and chronic inflammatory changes observed in bronchial asthma. They have also been implicated in many aspects of tissue damage occurring at sites of chronic inflammation. The proteins and lipids that these cells either contain or newly produce upon activation contribute profoundly to the pathophysiology of obstructive airways disease. This chapter concentrates on the physiological or pharmacological modulation of leukotriene generation by eosinophils.

II. Eosinophils as a Source of Leukotrienes

While a great deal of attention has been paid to the eosinophil's range of cytotoxic products, including cationic proteins and reactive oxygen species, eosinophils may also produce some of their physiological and pathological effects through the generation of lipid mediators, including leukotrienes. Here, we summarize the ability of eosinophils to generate lipoxygenase products of arachidonic acid.

A. Synthetic Enzymes

As described in Chapter 1, the generation of leukotrienes involves several stages, namely the liberation of arachidonic acid from membrane phospholipids, the 5-lipoxygenation of unesterified arachidonate to form 5-hydroperoxyeicosatetraenoic acid, the dehydration of 5-HPETE to form LTA_4 and then either hydrolysis of LTA_4 to produce LTB_4 or the conjugation of glutathione to LTA_4 to form LTC_4 and the further steps involved in transformation of LTC_4 to LTD_4, LTE_4, and, ultimately, the inert molecule LTF_4.

Phospholipase A_2, the arachidonate-liberating enzyme, is expressed in eosinophils developing from umbilical cord progenitor cells in culture under the influence of eosinopoietic cytokines at an early stage. 5-Lipoxygenase (5-LO) can also be found in these cells at about the same time. Approximately 4 days later the 5-LO-activating protein (FLAP) will also be expressed and after a further 3 days glutathione-transferring LTC_4 synthase appears, completing the apparatus for the generation of LTC_4 (1).

Eosinophils are distinct from other leukocytes in their expression of LTC_4 synthase. When HL-60 promyelocytes are cultured under conditions in which they differentiate into neutrophil-like or eosinophil-like cells, their expression of cytosolic phospholipase A_2 ($cPLA_2$) remains constant while FLAP and 5-LO protein synthesis increase. Expression of LTA_4 hydrolase—the synthetic enzyme for LTB_4—increases to approximately 100-fold higher levels in neutrophilic cells as compared to eosinophil-like cells, in which the expression of LTC_4 synthase mRNA and protein increases by approximately 75-fold (2), thus rendering eosinophils as predominantly LTC_4-producing cells and neutrophils as LTB_4 producers. Interestingly, during this differentiation process the cells also exhibit differential expression of cell surface leukotriene receptors, with HL-60 cells differentiating to a neutrophil-like or monocyte/macrophage-like phenotype producing receptors of the BLT class and those differentiating to an eosinophil-like phenotype producing CysLT receptors (3). Thus, the cells appear to selectively express receptors for their own predominant 5-LO products.

LTC_4 synthase has been purified from human lung tissue and identified as an approximately 18-kDa protein. An antibody raised against this protein has been used in immunoblotting experiments, allowing the expression of LTC_4 synthase in human eosinophils to be demonstrated directly (4). The enzyme is largely localized to the perinuclear region, placing it in close proximity to the activated 5-LO (5). Cloning of LTC_4 synthase from a KG-1 cDNA library permits the transfection of the gene to cell lines, where it can be shown to encode a 16.5-kDa cationic protein which, surprisingly, exhibits little homology with glutathione S-transferase but does share 31% of its sequence with FLAP and, in fact, LTC_4 synthase activity can be inhibited by MK 886, a FLAP inhibitor

(6). The LTC_4 synthase gene localizes to 5q35, near a cluster of genes that encode cytokines and receptors involved in allergic inflammation (7). Hybridization with a cDNA probe reveals the gene to be expressed in human eosinophils (6).

Species differences exist in the expression of leukotriene synthetic enzymes; notably, guinea pig peritoneal cavity eosinophils, frequently used to study eosinophil pharmacology, have been shown to lack the LTC_4 synthase completely (8,9).

Human eosinophils also differ from other leukocytes in expressing a Ca^{2+}/phosphatidylcholine-dependent 15-LO (10–13). 5-LO catalyzes the first two steps in the generation of leukotrienes from arachidonate, i.e., 5-lipoxygenation and 5,6-dehydration, while the latter activity—known as LTA_4 synthase—is also subserved by 15-LO in eosinophils (14). In addition, 15-LO under certain conditions synthesizes a range of products including 15-hydroxyeicosatetraenoic acid (15-HETE). In addition to exerting some actions on other cells, such as a slow contraction of airways smooth muscle (15), 15-HETE inhibits leukocyte 5-LO (16).

B. Range of Eicosanoids Produced

Human eosinophils stimulated with calcium ionophore A23187 (calcimycin) produce thromboxane A_2 (detected as its stable metabolite TxB_2) along with smaller quantities of other cyclooxygenase metabolites of arachidonic acid, including PGD_2, PGE_2, and prostacyclin (detected as 6-keto-$PGF_{1\alpha}$) (17,18). In addition, however, they produce a range of lipoxygenase metabolites. Granulocyte fractions from human blood produce 10–25 times more LTB_4 than LTC_4 in response to A23187 but the quantity of LTC_4 produced is directly proportional to the number of eosinophils (19), and when the fractions are enriched in eosinophils this balance shifts to favor the production of LTC_4 (20). This is due to the fact that, as a reflection of their synthetic enzyme complements, eosinophils produce 20–40 times more LTC_4 than neutrophils or mononuclear cells while neutrophils synthesize predominantly LTB_4 (19,21–26).

Apart from calcium ionophore, immune stimuli such as opsonized zymosan and IgG-coated Sepharose particles can induce LTC_4 generation by human eosinophils in vitro (27–30) or when allowed to attach to *Schistosoma mansoni* larvae (31). Immobilized IgG immune complexes also stimulate eosinophil LTC_4 generation but IgE is a weak stimulus (32). Unopsonized particles of zymosan also provoke LTC_4 production by eosinophils, apparently through a specific recognition mechanism for the glucan component of the polysaccharide (33,34). The magnitude of the leukotriene generation evoked by particulate stimuli is much smaller (approximately 100-fold) than the response to

A23187 (33). LTC_4 release can be measured in eosinophils incubated with fibronectin (35), and small responses can also be produced with soluble receptor agonists, such as the chemotactic tripeptide, fMet-Leu-Phe (fMLP) (36,37), or high concentrations of platelet-activating factor (PAF) (29,38,39). A high concentration of PAF has also been shown to enhance the LTC_4 generation induced by other stimuli, such as calcium ionophore, arachidonic acid, and opsonized zymosan (29,38,39).

The delivery of exogenous LTA_4 also causes eosinophils to produce LTC_4 (40). However, it is interesting that, as is the case when eosinophils are stimulated with calcium ionophore and arachidonic acid (33,34), the intracellular levels of LTC_4 continue to rise even though the extracellular level plateaus (40). This appears to reflect the existence of an energy-requiring export process that becomes saturated when LTC_4 synthase and LTA_4 uptake both continue to function within capacity (40).

In addition to LTC_4, human and monkey eosinophils produce smaller quantities of LTB_4 and 5-HETE when stimulated with calcium ionophore (9). Furthermore, as a consequence of their expression of 15-LO, human eosinophils also produce 15-HETE and small amounts of 5,15-diHETE and 8,15-diHETE under certain conditions, particularly in the presence of high concentrations of exogenous arachidonic acid (9,24,26,41–44). Curiously, under these conditions only the production of 5-LO metabolites is stimulated by PAF (44). In the presence of exogenous arachidonic acid or 15-HETE, other 15-LO products, including lipoxin-like derivatives and oxo-HETEs, have also been detected in human eosinophil supernatants (26,45).

Species differences in synthetic enzyme expression are reflected in the pattern of eicosanoid output from eosinophils. Murine eosinophils produce 12-HETE and 15-HETE, as well as smaller quantities of 5,15- and 5,12-diHETE and small quantities of LTA_4 hydrolysis products (46). Guinea pig peritoneal eosinophils, which do not contain LTC_4 synthase, produce predominantly LTB_4 when stimulated with calcium ionophore, fMLP, or unopsonized zymosan particles (8,25,47). Guinea pig eosinophils, like human cells, also produce TxA_2 on ionophore stimulation but, in addition, they produce a certain amount of 5-HETE (8,9,47). Bovine blood eosinophils have also been demonstrated to produce LTB_4 when stimulated (48) but equine eosinophils, like their human equivalent, produce predominantly LTC_4 (49).

C. Heterogeneity Among Eosinophils

Eosinophils can be separated by differential density centrifugation into fractions of different density ranges. It has been demonstrated often that asthmatic patients, as well as patients with other inflammatory conditions, have increased numbers of low-density cells in their circulation (50), although a fairly recent study failed to discern any difference in density profiles between nonasthmatic, allergic, and nonallergic asthmatic subjects (51). Where differences in density profiles can be demonstrated, several workers have sought to determine the influence of cell density of the capacity of eosinophils to generate leukotrienes.

Although it has been stated that low-density cells, which generally represent a greater proportion of the circulating eosinophils in asthmatic patients than in normals, produce greater quantities of LTC_4 (52), other workers have shown that low-density eosinophils actually produce less LTC_4 in response to calcium ionophore than do "normodense" cells (53–55). There is also disagreement over the relative LTC_4-producing capacity of normal and asthmatic eosinophils. Eosinophils from allergic or nonallergic asthmatic patients have been reported to produce up to three times more LTC_4 on ionophore stimulation than do eosinophils from normal donors (53,56). However, the capacity for producing LTC_4 does not correlate with disease severity; Laviolette et al. have pooled eosinophils from all density bands and shown that eosinophils from moderate asthmatics produce greater quantities of LTC_4 in response to ionophore than do those from either mild or severe asthmatics, as defined by the patients' requirements for treatment (57). Hodges and colleagues demonstrated that normal-density eosinophils from asthmatics and normal subjects produced similar quantities of LTC_4 whereas the low-density cells from asthmatics actually produced less than those from normals (58). Since, in their hands, the lower-density eosinophils produced greater quantities of LTC_4 than did the normal-density cells, the greater total leukotriene production from asthmatic eosinophils was presumed to reflect the shift in the cell profile to lower densities. There is some support for this position in the work of Roberge et al., who have demonstrated that the eosinophils at densities of 1.081–1.084 g/cm^3 are the most responsive and that the slight shift of the peak of the distribution to lower densities that characterizes asthma might account for the greater total LTC_4-producing capacity of eosinophils from asthmatic donors (55).

III. Physiological Significance of Leukotriene Production by Eosinophils

Eosinophils are a characteristic feature of inflammatory changes underlying bronchial asthma. Elevated numbers can be found in the serum, the sputum, in bronchial washes, bronchoalveolar lavage, airway mucosa, and peripheral lung tissue of asthmatic patients. Following specific challenge, i.e., with allergen, the numbers and the activation state of eosinophils are further increased in the airways, the lung, and the blood circulation.

Owing to the capacity of eosinophils to release a variety of preformed or newly synthesized mediators upon stimulation, these cells are capable of mediating a broad spectrum of responses, typical for clinical signs and symptoms seen in bronchial asthma. The physiology of eosinophils has been extensively reviewed elsewhere (59,60). The following section will briefly summarize the current knowledge of human eosinophil granule proteins and mediators generated de novo and their bioactivities.

Eosinophils contain a variety of preformed cationic proteins, some of which have been implicated in the pathophysiology of asthma. Major basic protein (MBP) has been shown to cause histamine release from basophils and rat mast cells, to cause bronchial constriction and hyperreactivity, to neutralize heparin, and to produce epithelial damage in guinea pig trachea and human bronchial rings. Eosinophil cationic protein (ECP) causes histamine release from rat mast cells and causes damage to guinea pig epithelium in vitro. Eosinophil-derived neurotoxin (EDN) acts as a mitogen and leads to fibroblast proliferation in culture. Eosinophil peroxidase (EPO) causes histamine release from rat mast cells and can, together with hydrogen peroxide (H_2O_2) lead to epithelial damage and may contribute to bronchial hyperreactivity.

Additionally, eosinophils generate toxic oxygen metabolites upon stimulation. Hydrogen peroxide may lead to smooth muscle contraction and singlet oxygen may damage pulmonary tissue.

Neuropeptides such as substance P and vasoactive intestinal polypeptide (VIP) have also been demonstrated to be released from eosinophils and this may result in smooth muscle contraction, edema formation, vasodilation, and degranulation of mast cells.

Among the range of cytokines known to be produced by eosinophils IL-3, IL-5, and GM-CSF promote priming and activation of inflammatory cells and granulocyte differentiation; they also enhance granulocyte survival. $TGF\beta_1$ has been found to regulate cell proliferation while $TGF\alpha$ promotes cell proliferation and angiogenesis and tumor necrosis factor-α ($TNF\alpha$) promotes fibroblast and lymphocyte proliferation. The C-C chemokine MIP1α acts as chemoattractant for B and T lymphocytes and eosinophils while the C-X-C chemokine IL-8 is a neutrophil chemoattractant and activator.

Eosinophils also synthesize a variety of lipid mediators and, of these, PAF activates mast cells, neutrophils, and eosinophils, causes platelet aggregation, mucus secretion, and edema, and can constrict bronchial and vascular smooth muscle. TxA_2 causes bronchial and vascular constriction and platelet aggregation, while PGD_2 is a bronchoconstrictor, causes pulmonary vasoconstriction, and increases vascular permeability and platelet aggregation. $PGF_{2\alpha}$ causes bronchoconstriction and platelet aggregation. Prostaglandin E_2 acts as a vasodilator, causes mucus secretion, and can inhibit inflammatory cell function.

Additionally, as stated above, eosinophils synthesize and release leukotrienes, mainly leukotriene C_4. Cysteinyl leukotrienes mediate a variety of responses in the human lung and, when applied exogenously, cause several symptoms resembling typical features of clinical asthma (5,61).

A. Bronchoconstriction

Leukotrienes are potent constrictors of human and animal airway smooth muscle. LTC_4 is approximately 1000 times more potent than histamine and equipotent to LTD_4 as a smooth muscle contractile agent (62). Cysteinyl leukotrienes cause bronchoconstriction in healthy individuals (63,64) and in patients with asthma (65,66), while the response in asthamtics is exaggerated compared to healthy individuals. In vivo, as under in vitro conditions, LTC_4 and LTD_4 have similar potency (66), although the effect of LTC_4 is somewhat delayed, taking 10–20 min to cause bronchoconstriction, compared to the immediate bronchoconstriction observed after LTD_4 and LTE_4 application (67,68).

Human airways, irrespective of airway hyperresponsiveness, possess inherent tone under resting conditions that is mainly due to cysteinyl leukotrienes (CysLT), since the application of the $CysLT_1$ receptor antagonist pobilukast or the 5-LO inhibitor zileuton relaxes inherent tone in isolated human airways in vitro (69,70). The source of the leukotrienes mediating this response has been shown not to be the epithelium and is believed to be resident inflammatory cells (70). The interaction of eosinophils with airway reactivity and smooth muscle tone has been addressed in a number of studies. Aizawa et al. (71) demonstrated that supernatants from ionophore-stimulated guinea pig peritoneal eosinophils induce histamine hyperresponsiveness in guinea pig tracheal smooth muscle and that this effect is abolished by pretreatment of eosinophils with AA 861, a 5-LO inhibitor. Subsequently, it was shown that fMLP-activated cultured eosinophils from human umbilical cord vein blood contract guinea pig trachealis in situ and increase cholinergic responsiveness (72); these effects were both inhibited by pretreatment with the 5-LO inhibitor, zileuton (Fig. 1). In human airways, Jongejan and colleagues demonstrated that human granulocytes activated with serum-opsonized zymosan contract human airways in vitro, and this effect was significantly reduced following pretreatment with the CysLT receptor antagonist FPL 55712 or the 5-LO inhibitor nordihydro-guaiaretic acid (NDGA). The magnitude of the effect was related to the number of eosinophils in the granulocyte preparation (73). Finally, it was shown that isolated human eosinophils activated with PAF contracted human airways in vitro, and that this contraction was mediated predominantly but not solely through products of 5-lipoxygenase (74), since the 5-LO inhibitor zileuton significantly inhibited eosinophil-induced airway contractions in a

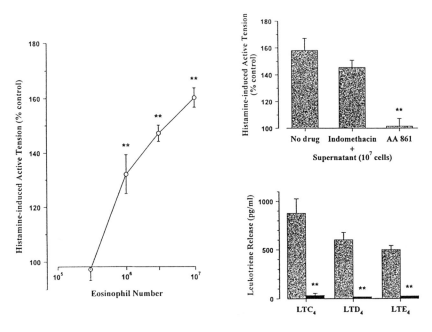

Figure 1 (Left) Effects of supernatants obtained from increasing numbers of iono-phore-stimulated eosinophils on the contractile response to histamine (3 μM). Results are reported as mean ± SEM of five guinea pigs. Significant differences from control values are indicated by **$p < 0.01$. (Top right) Effect of indomethacin (10 μM) and the 5-lipoxygenase inhibitor AA 861 (10 μM) on supernatant-induced increase in the contractile response to histamine (3 μM). Results are reported as mean ± SEM of five guinea pigs. Significant differences between conditions with and without treatment with the drugs are indicated by **$p < 0.01$. (Bottom right) Release of leukotrienes in the supernatant in the absence (dotted columns) and presence of pretreatment with AA 861, an inhibitor of 5-lipoxygenase (closed columns). Results are reported as mean ± SEM of supernatants (10^7 cells) obtained from three guinea pigs. Significant differences between results with and without AA 861 are indicated by *$p < 0.05$ and **$p < 0.01$. (Reproduced, with permission, from Ref. 71.)

concentration-dependent manner. Indomethacin had a small, but significant, effect on changes in luminal diameter under these conditions (Fig. 2).

B. Increased Vascular Permeability

Cysteinyl leukotrienes have been described to cause extravasation of a variety of markers such as Evans blue, radiolabeled albumin, or fluorescein-conjugated macromolecules in guinea pig and hamster cheek pouch and throughout the

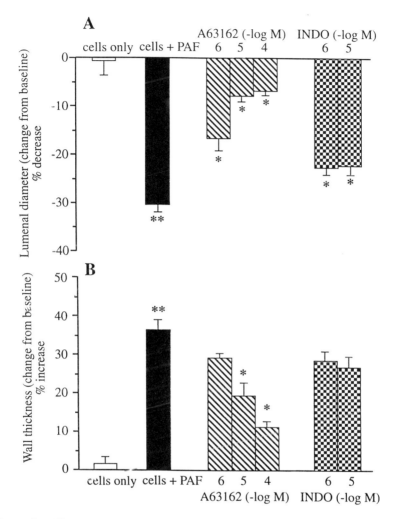

Figure 2 Effect of zileuton (A63162), a 5-lipoxygenase inhibitor, and indomethacin (INDO), a cyclooxygenase inhibitor, on airway narrowing and wall thickness. (A) Increasing concentrations of zileuton inhibited decrease in luminal diameter in a concentration-dependent manner. Indomethacin had a lesser, but statistically significant, effect in blocking luminal narrowing caused by activated eosinophils. $**p < 0.001$ versus untreated eosinophils (cells only). $*$Statistically significant differences ($p < 0.05$ to $p < 0.001$ versus cells + PAF). (B) PAF-activated cells caused substantial change in wall thickness versus nonactivated cells (cells only). This effect is attenuated by zileuton, but not indomethacin. Asterisks denote p values as above. (Reproduced, with permission, from Ref. 74.)

bronchial tree (75). In guinea pig preparations LTD_4 was 10 times less active than PAF but 1000 times more active than histamine in inducing bronchial plasma extravasation (76). In humans, intradermal cysteinyl leukotrienes cause a marked wheal-and-flare reaction (77,78).

C. Mucus Secretion

Cesteinyl leukotrienes are potent mucus secretagogues in human airways in vitro (79,80), and in dogs an enhancement of tracheal submucosal gland secretion has been observed after LTC_4 administration in vivo (81).

D. Cellular Infiltration

Cysteinyl leukotrienes are generally believed not to play a major role in chemotaxis (61), although in ovalbumin-sensitized guinea pigs it was demonstrated that treatment of the animals with the $CysLT_1$ receptor antagonist MK-571 (1 mg/kg p.o.) results in a significant inhibition of cysteinyl leukotriene-induced tissue eosinophilia (82), and, recently, Muñoz et al. have demonstrated that the BLT receptor antagonist LTB_4 dimethyl amide, the 5-LO inhibitor zileuton, and the $CysLT_1$ receptor antagonist zafirlukast all inhibited the fMLP-induced migration of human eosinophils into a guinea pig tracheal preparation (83). LTB_4 is a potent chemoattractant predominantly of neutrophils, and to a lesser extent of eosinophils (84,85).

IV. Modulation of Eosinophil Leukotriene Production

Since leukotrienes are involved in many physiological and pathological actions of eosinophils, the mechanisms mediating their generation may be considered as possible stages in the pathogenesis or pathology of inflammatory diseases and as potential targets for pharmacological intervention. Although numerous experiments have been described in which the influx of eosinophils to inflammatory sites is suppressed by drugs, it remains unclear whether the activation of the cells' functions can be inhibited, allowing a more immediate minimization of the risk of inflammatory amplification or tissue damage posed by eosinophils that are already at the appropriate site.

This section will describe both the factors that can promote eosinophil leukotriene generation through "priming" of cells and the influence that is exerted on eosinophil arachidonic acid metabolism by existing and potential anti-inflammatory drugs.

A. Priming

Conditioned media from resting or stimulated monocytes or U937 monocytic cell lines have been demonstrated to enhance the production of LTC_4 by eosinophils activated with calcium ionophore (86–88). Supernatants of cultured alveolar macrophages or epithelial cells obtained from asthmatic volunteers also prime eosinophils for increased production of LTC_4 in response to ionophore and phorbol ester (89,90); in both cases the priming activity was neutralized by an antibody against granulocyte-macrophage colony-stimulating factor (GM-CSF) and priming could be mimicked by recombinant human GM-CSF, indicating that the factor in the supernatants that accounts for the priming activity is GM-CSF. Supernatants of macrophages or epithelial cells from normal donors exhibited no priming activity in these experiments (89,90), and it is significant that GM-CSF concentrations in asthmatic epithelial cell culture supernatants were four times higher than those in cultures of normal subjects' epithelial cells (90).

Coculture of eosinophils with endothelial cells or culture with endothelial cell-conditioned medium prolongs eosinophil survival, reduces eosinophil density, and triples the A23187-induced production of LTC_4 (91). The property of priming eosinophils for increased LTC_4 generation is shared by recombinant GM-CSF and IL-3 (89,92–94), although culture of eosinophils with IL-3 and 3T3 fibroblasts has been reported to augment LTC_4 production only when the cells are stimulated with fMLP, and not with calcium ionophore or LTA_4 (95). GM-CSF also primes the eosinophil-differentiated HL-60 strain HL-60#7 to produce greater quantities of LTC_4 on ionophore stimulation; this property is not shared by IL-5 (96). In contrast, Laviolette et al. have shown that GM-CSF and IL-5 can prime eosinophils from both normal and asthmatic subjects to produce increased quantities of LTC_4 but that IL-3 exerts only a slight priming action on eosinophils from patients with moderate asthma and not at all on eosinophils from normal donors or from mild or severe asthmatics (57). Although two groups have reported that treatment of eosinophils with $TNF\alpha$ enhances LTC_4 generation, induced by either ionophore or soluble receptor stimuli such as fMLP (37,97,98), another reports shows that TNF promotes eosinophil cytotoxicity but not LTC_4 production (94).

Adherence to the extracellular matrix component fibronectin up-regulates eosinophil LTC_4 production in response to ionophore or to PAF (99,100). Fibronectin-ligated eosinophils, on stimulation with PAF, cause a greater narrowing of human bronchial rings in a microwell videomicrometry system than do eosinophils that have not attached to the matrix protein (Fig. 3); this up-regulation is prevented by blocking adherence with an antibody to $\alpha4\beta1$ integrin (VLA-4) (100).

Soluble, low-molecular-weight mediators can also increase the responsiveness of eosinophils. The mast cell–derived prostaglandin PGD_2 enhances

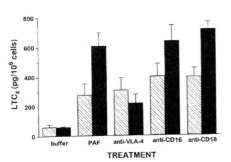 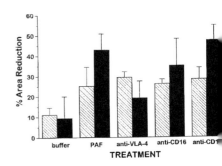

Figure 3 (Left) Effect of mAb blockade of adhesion ligands in PAF-induced eosinophil secretion of LTC$_4$. Eosinophils were preincubated for 15 min with either anti-VLA-4, anti-CD16, or anti-CD18 before 60 min exposure to protein-coated plates. Hatched bars, BSA coated; solid bars, FN coated; LTC$_4$ secretion was measured after 40 min treatment with PAF. (Right) Effect of mAb blockade of adhesion ligands on airway luminal narrowing. Augmented narrowing (% area reduction) was inhibited after pretreatment with anti-VLA-4 only in FN-exposed eosinophils. Hatched bars, BSA-coated plates; solid bars, FN-coated plates. In all groups studied, airway narrowing after pretreatment with nonbinding MAb remained unchanged. (Reproduced, with permission, from Ref. 100.)

ionophore-induced LTC$_4$ generation in eosinophils (101) and this activity is shared by PAF in asthmatic, but not normal, eosinophils (102). PAF, as well as LTB$_4$, also renders eosinophils capable of producing LTC$_4$ on attachment to IgE-coated schistosomula (31).

B. Pharmacological Modulation

Antileukotriene Drugs

Unsurprisingly, drugs that inhibit the biochemical pathways leading to leukotriene formation suppress the production of LTC$_4$ by eosinophils. Both mepacrine and the selective sPLA$_2$ inhibitor *p*-bromophenacylbromide abolish fMLP-induced LTC$_4$ generation by human eosinophils (103). Inhibition of FLAP with MK 886 or MK 571 or inhibition of 5-LO with E6080 abolishes ionophore-induced production of LTC$_4$ and B$_4$ by eosinophils without affecting production of 15-LO metabolites or PAF (104–106).

Cyclic AMP-Elevating Drugs

The β$_2$-adrenoceptor agonist salbutamol (albuterol) causes a concentration-dependent inhibition of fMLP-induced LTC$_4$ production in human eosinophils (107), up to a maximum of approximately 50% inhibition, that is reversed fully by the β-adrenoceptor antagonist propranolol (Fig. 4). This action is not

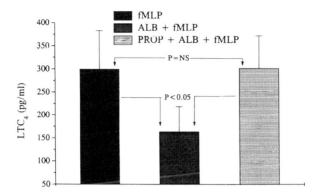

Figure 4 Effect of propranolol (PROP) on albuterol (ALB)-induced inhibition of LTC$_4$ secretion from eosinophils activated with 1 μM fMLP + 5 μg/ml of cytochalasin B (fMLP + B). Inhibition of LTC$_4$ secretion caused by 10 nM albuterol was attenuated completely by 10 nM PROP. $p < 0.05$ for PROP + ALB + fMLP + B versus ALB + fMLP + B; p = NS for PROP + ALB + fMLP + B versus fMLP + B alone. (Reproduced, with permission, from Ref. 107.)

exhibited by the long-acting β-agonist salmeterol, which produces no inhibition of LTC$_4$ release from activated cells (108,109). In fact, salmeterol actually antagonizes the inhibitory action of salbutamol (109), probably owing to its very low efficacy as a partial agonist at eosinophil β-receptors (110).

In contrast, nimesulide, which is thought to inhibit the PDE4 isoenzyme of cyclic nucleotide phosphodiesterase, the predominant PDE enzyme in the human eosinophil (111), and thereby elevate intracellular cyclic AMP in a similar way to β-agonists, does cause a concentration-dependent suppression of eosinophil LTC$_4$ production (108).

PAF is a weak stimulus of LTC$_4$ production in human eosinophils, and this appears to be accounted for in part by the stimulation of PGE$_2$ production, leading to receptor activation and an elevation of intracellular cyclic AMP that suppresses eosinophil functions. In the presence of a cyclooxygenase inhibitor, indomethacin, or an inhibitor of cyclic AMP-dependent protein kinase (PKA), PAF-induced LTC$_4$ production is greatly enhanced (112). In the presence of indomethacin the nonselective PDE inhibitor theophylline and the selective PDE4 inhibitor rolipram (Fig. 5), as well as a direct activator of PKA, (Sp)5,6-dichlor-1-β-D-ribofuranosylbenzimidazole (Fig. 6), cause profound inhibition of PAF or C5a-induced LTC$_4$ synthesis, indicating that elevation of cyclic AMP and activation of PKA is an effective way of suppressing LTC$_4$ production in eosinophils (112).

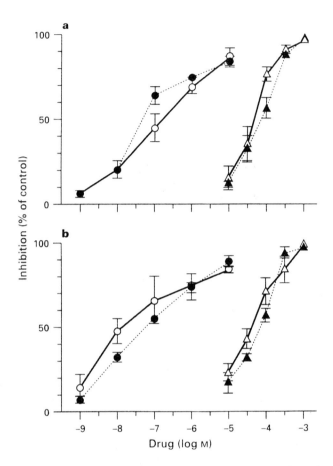

Figure 5 Effect of theophylline and rolipram on (a) PAF- and (b) C5a-stimulated human eosinophil LTC_4 generation. Human eosinophils (10^6 cells/200 μl) were obtained from normal (open symbols) and atopic (solid symbols) subjects and preincubated with theophylline (10 μM–1 mM; triangles) or rolipram (1 nM–10 μM; circles) in the presence of 10 μM indomethacin. Following incubation with either 100 nM PAF or 100 nM C5a for 15 min, LTC_4 was measured in ethanolic extracts. Results represent mean $\pm$ SEM from at least four experiments. (Reproduced, with permission, from Ref. 112.)

Protein Kinase C/Protein Tyrosine Kinase Inhibitors

Although it has been reported that activation of protein kinase C (PKC) with the phorbol ester phorbol 12-myristate,13-acetate (PMA) augments ionophore-induced LTC_4 production in eosinophils (39), an opposite action has been demonstrated by Ali et al., who showed an attenuation of A23187-

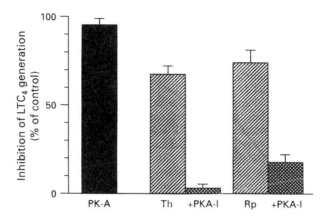

Figure 6 Effect of a protein kinase A activator on inhibition of eosinophil LTC_4 synthesis by theophylline or rolipram. Human eosinophils (10^6 cells/200 μl) were pre-incubated for 30 min with 1 mM Rp-8-Br-cyclic AMPS (protein kinase A-inhibitor; PKA-I) or vehicle and for 10 min with 100 μM 5.6DClcBIMPS (protein kinase A-activator; PK-A), 100 μM theophylline (Th), or 1 μM rolipram (Rp) and with 10 μM indomethacin. Eosinophils were stimulated with 100 nM PAF for 15 min and LTC_4 was measured by radioimmunoassay. Results are given as mean $\pm$ SEM from three experiments. (Reproduced, with permission, from Ref. 112.)

induced LTC_4 generation in HL-60#7 cells that was blocked by the PKC inhibitors staurosporine and bisindolylmaleimide I (113). Similarly, pretreatment of guinea pig eosinophils with PMA substantially suppresses subsequent responses to PAF and this suppression is also blocked by staurosporine (114).

It has been demonstrated in guinea pig eosinophils stimulated with LTB_4 and human eosinophils stimulated with PAF that the respiratory burst responses (generation of superoxide anion or H_2O_2) are suppressed much less potently by specific PKC inhibitors than are similarly sized responses induced by phorbol esters (Fig. 7), suggesting that respiratory burst is only partly mediated by PKC and that an alternative pathway for cell activation exists that may be sensitive to inhibition by activated PKC (115,116), particularly since the LTB_4-induced calcium signal in guinea pig eosinophils is greatly enhanced in the presence of a PKC inhibitor, Ro 31-8220 (115).

Since LTC_4 generation in human and guinea pig eosinophils is barely stimulated by PMA (116,117), it seems unlikely that this response is mediated by PKC. However, when PAF-stimulated LTC_4 release is measured in the presence of the PKC inhibitor bisindolylmaleimide I, the response is significantly enhanced (Fig. 8), suggesting that PKC activation occurring after PAF

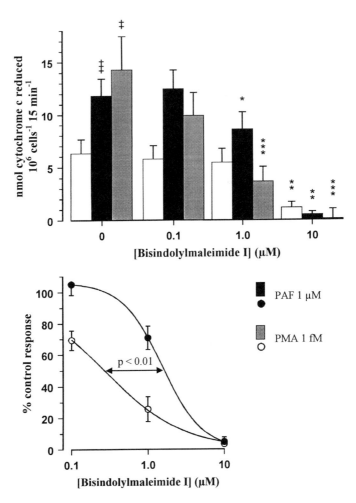

Figure 7 Effects of the PKC inhibitor bisindolylmaleimide I (Bis I) on respiratory burst responses of human eosinophils. Cells were preincubated at 37°C for 10 min in the absence or presence of Bis I at the indicated concentrations prior to addition of buffer (open bars), 1 μM PAF (solid bars and filled circles), or 1 fM PMA (shaded bars and open circles). Superoxide generation was measured as the SOD-inhibited reduction of ferricytochrome c per 10^6 cells in 15 min. (Top) Superoxide production: $^{++}p < 0.01$, $^{+++}p < 0.001$, compared to basal superoxide production; $^*p < 0.05$, $^{**}p < 0.01$, $^{***}p < 0.001$, compared to superoxide production in cells preincubated without Bis I. (Bottom) Data from upper panel expressed as percent of control response in cells preincubated without Bis I. Data are mean ± SEM from six experiments conducted in triplicate. (Reproduced from Ref. 116.)

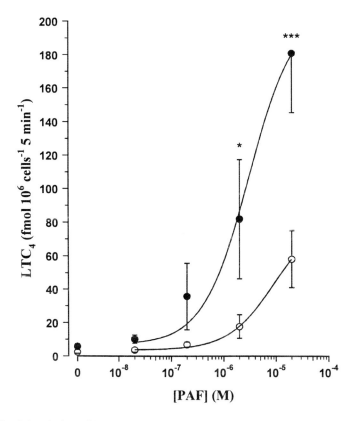

Figure 8 Stimulation of human eosinophil sulfidopeptide leukotriene generation and the effect of bisindolylmaleimide I (Bis I). Cells were preincubated at 37°C for 10 min in the absence (open circles) or presence of 1 μM Bis I (closed circles) prior to addition of PAF at the indicated concentrations. Leukotriene production is expressed as accumulation of LTC_4 in the cell supernatant per 10^6 cells in 5 min. Data are the mean ± SEM from six experiments conducted in duplicate. *$p < 0.05$, ***$p < 0.001$, compared to cells preincubated without Bis I. (Reproduced from Ref. 116.)

receptor stimulation is mediating a negative feedback pathway that minimizes the LTC_4 production (116).

In a preliminary report, PAF-induced LTC_4 production in human eosinophils has been described to be suppressed by genistein, a nonselective inhibitor of protein tyrosine kinases (PTK); however, a second inhibitor, tyrphostin A25, has no effect on PAF-induced LTC_4 release, so the response is probably mediated by an unknown PTK that is not sensitive to inhibition by the tyrophostin (118).

Glucocorticoids/Immunomodulators

Glucocorticosteroids inhibit the activity of both the cytosolic and secreted forms of phospholipase A_2 (cPLA$_2$ and sPLA$_2$) in cells in vitro (119) and this is associated with a decreased release of LTB$_4$ from monocytes and alveolar macrophages in vitro as well as a reduced release of TxA$_2$, PGF$_{2\alpha}$, and PGE$_2$ from monocytes and bronchoalveolar lavage (BAL) cells in vitro and ex vivo (119). Intravenous prednisone leads to a decrease in the ionophore-induced production of LTC$_4$ from peripheral blood eosinophils ex vivo (120) and a small ex vivo suppression can also be seen after 6 weeks' treatment with inhaled beclomethasone dipropionate 800 μg/day (121).

In contrast, treatment of atopic asthmatics with high doses of oral prednisone for 6–9 days had no significant effect on either BAL eicosanoid levels or urinary LTE$_4$ concentration despite the fact that a significant clinical improvement was observed and that, in these patients, the eicosanoid synthesis was reduced in BAL macrophages ex vivo (122).

In a further study in mild atopic asthmatics, a 2-week treatment with fluticasone propionate (1000 μg/day) significantly inhibited both early and late asthmatic responses to allergen and significantly reduced baseline bronchial reactivity without showing a significant effect on the increased urinary LTE$_4$ excretion following allergen challenge (123).

There appears, therefore, to exist a so far unexplained discrepancy between the demonstrated in vitro effects of glucocorticosteroids and the paucity of clinical effects of this class of drug on eicosanoid metabolism.

Other Antiallergy Drugs

At high concentrations, nedocromil sodium has been described to inhibit ionophore- and opsonized zymosan–induced LTC$_4$ release from human eosinophils (124,125), although this finding could not be reproduced with 10-min incubations of eosinophils with up to 100 μM nedocromil (34). This may simply reflect the fact that the inhibition is slight, amounting to a maximum of approximately 50% inhibition of A23187-induced leukotriene release at 10 μM nedocromil (126).

The piperazine antihistamine oxatomide and the phthalazinone antihistamine azelastine—both of which exert additional antiallergic actions mediated by uncharacterized mechanisms—suppress ionophore-induced LTC$_4$ release from human eosinophils at lower concentrations (15–35 μM) than those required of ketotifen to achieve the same effect (120 μM) (127), although ketotifen does cause some significant inhibition at lower concentrations (128,129).

Certain retinoids, which have anti-inflammatory actions when applied topically in psoriasis or acne, inhibit ionophore-induced LTC$_4$ production in equine eosinophils (130).

Antioxidants

LTC$_4$ is inactivated extracellularly by H$_2$O$_2$ and EPO, which oxidize LTC$_4$ to produce *trans*-isomers of LTB$_4$ and LTC$_4$ sulfoxides (21,36,131,132). L-Serine, which scavenges hydroxyl radicals, and catalase, which breaks down H$_2$O$_2$, increase the concentration of LTC$_4$ in the supernatant of stimulated eosinophils by preventing its breakdown (21,36).

V. Concluding Remarks

The generation of leukotrienes by eosinophils may account for several actions of these cells contributing to the pathogenesis and pathology of asthma. Few therapeutic agents in current use produce significant inhibition of eosinophil activation, and probably the most important action of drugs such as corticosteroids lies in the prophylactic prevention of eosinophil recruitment to inflammatory sites rather than in a direct inhibition of eosinophil function. The ability of cyclic AMP-elevating drugs to profoundly suppress eosinophil LTC$_4$ production may prove to have significance, i.e., in the development of selective PDE4 inhibitors. The relatively novel findings on the involvement of protein kinase C in the regulation of eicosanoid synthesis in human eosinophils may lead to novel therapeutic approaches in the future.

References

1. Boyce JA, Lam BK, Penrose JF, Friend DS, Parsons S, Owen WF, Austen KF. Expression of LTC$_4$ synthase during the development of eosinophils in vitro from cord blood progenitors. Blood 1996; 88:4338–4347.
2. Scoggan KA, Nicholson DW, Ford-Hutchinson AW. Regulation of leukotriene-biosynthetic enzymes during differentiation of myelocytic HL-60 cells to eosinophilic or neutrophilic cells. Eur J Biochem 1996; 239:572–578.
3. Patry C, Muller E, Laporte J, Rola-Pleszczynski M, Sirois P, de Brum-Fernandes AJ. Leukotriene receptors in HL-60 cells differentiated into eosinophils, monocytes and neutrophils. Prostaglandins Leukot Essent Fatty Acids 1996; 54: 361–370.
4. Penrose JF, Spector J, Lam BK, Friend DS, Xu K, Jack RM, Austen KF. Purification of human lung leukotriene C$_4$ synthase and preparation of a polyclonal antibody. Am J Respir Crit Care Med 1995; 152:283–289.
5. Drazen JM. Leukotrienes. In: Leff AR, ed. Pulmonary and Critical Care Pharmacology and Therapeutics. McGraw-Hill: New York, 1996:143–149.
6. Lam BK, Penrose JF, Freeman GJ, Austen KF. Expression cloning of a cDNA for human leukotriene C$_4$ synthase, an integral membrane protein conjugating reduced glutathione to leukotriene A$_4$. Proc Natl Acad Sci USA 1994; 91:7663–7667.

7. Penrose JF, Spector J, Baldasaro M, Xu K, Boyce J, Arm JP, Austen KF, Lam BK. Molecular cloning of the gene for human leukotriene C_4 synthase: organization, nucleotide sequence, and chromosomal localization to 5q35. J Biol Chem 1996; 271:11356–11361.

8. Sun FF, Czuk CI, Taylor BM. Arachidonic acid metabolism in guinea-pig eosinophils: synthesis of thromboxane B_2 and leukotriene B_4 in response to soluble or particulate activators. J Leukoc Biol 1989; 46:152–160.

9. Sun FF, Crittenden NJ, Czuk CI, Taylor BM, Stout BK, Johnson HG. Biochemical and functional differences between eosinophils from animal species and man. J Leukoc Biol 1991; 50:140–150.

10. Sigal E, Grunberger D, Cashman JR, Craik CS, Caughey GH, Nadel JA. Arachidonate 15-lipoxygenase from human eosinophil-enriched leukocytes: partial purification and properties. Biochem Biophys Res Commun 1988; 150:376–383.

11. Sigal E, Nadel JA. Arachidonic acid 15-lipoxygenase and airway epithelium: biologic effects and enzyme purification. Am Rev Respir Dis 1988; 138:S35–S40.

12. Nadel JA, Conrad DJ, Ueki IF, Schuster A, Sigal E. Immunocytochemical localization of arachidonate 15-lipoxygenase in erythrocytes, leukocytes, and airway cells. J Clin Invest 1991; 87:1139–1145.

13. Izumi T, Radmark O, Samuelsson B. Purification of 15-lipoxygenase from human leukocytes, evidence for the presence of isozymes. Adv Prostaglandin Thromboxane Leukot Res 1991; 21A:101–104.

14. MacMillan DK, Hill E, Sala A, Sigal E, Shuman T, Henson PM, Murphy RC. Eosinophil 15-lipoxygenase is a leukotriene A_4 synthase. J Biol Chem 1994; 269: 26663–26668.

15. Salari H, Schellenberg RR. Stimulation of human airway epithelial cells by platelet activating factor (PAF) and arachidonic acid produces 15-hydroxyeicosatetraenoic acid (15-HETE) capable of contracting bronchial smooth muscle. Pulm Pharmacol 1991; 4:1–7.

16. Cashman JR, Lambert C, Sigal E. Inhibition of human leukocyte 5-lipoxygenase by 15-HPETE and related eicosanoids. Biochem Biophys Res Commun 1988; 155:38–44.

17. Parsons WG III, Roberts LJ II. Transformation of prostaglandin D_2 to isomeric prostaglandin F_2 compounds by human eosinophils: a potential mast cell–eosinophil interaction. J Immunol 1988; 141:2413–2419.

18. Foegh ML, Maddox YT, Ramwell PW. Human peritoneal eosinophils and formation of arachidonate cyclooxygenase products. Scand J Immunol 1986; 23: 599–603.

19. Shaw RJ, Cromwell O, Kay AB. Preferential generation of leukotriene C_4 by human eosinophils. Clin Exp Immunol 1984; 56:716–722.

20. Borgeat P, Fruteau de Laclos B, Rabinovitch H, Picard S, Braquet P, Hebert J, Laviolette M. Eosinophil-rich human polymorphonuclear leukocyte preparations characteristically release leukotriene C_4 on ionophore A23187 challenge. J Allergy Clin Immunol 1984; 74:310–315.

21. Weller PF, Lee CW, Foster DW, Corey EJ, Austen KF, Lewis RA. Generation and metabolism of 5-lipoxygenase pathway leukotrienes by human eosinophils: predominant production of leukotriene C_4. Proc Natl Acad Sci USA 1983; 80: 7626–7630.

22. Tamura N, Agrawal DK, Townley RG. A specific radioreceptor assay for leuk-otriene C_4 and the measurement of calcium ionophore-induced leukotriene C_4 production from human leukocytes. J Pharmacol Methods 1987; 18:327–333.

23. Verhagen J, Bruynzeel PK, Koedam JA, Wassink GA, De Boer M, Terpstra GK, Kreukniet J, Veldink GA, Vliegenthart JF. Specific leukotriene formation by pu-rified human eosinophils and neutrophils. FEBS Lett 1984; 168:23–28.

24. Laviolette M, Picard S, Braquet P, Borgeat P. Comparison of 5- and 15-lipoxy-genase activities in blood and alveolar leukocyte preparations from normal sub-jects and patients with eosinophilia. Prostaglandins Leukot Med 1986; 23:191–199.

25. Sehmi R, Rossi AG, Kay AB, Cromwell O. Identification of receptors for leukotriene B_4 expressed on guinea-pig peritoneal eosinophils. Immunology 1992; 77:129–135.

26. Powell WS, Chung D, Gravel S. 5-Oxo-6,8,11,14-eicosatetraenoic acid is a potent stimulator of human eosinophil migration. J Immunol 1995; 154:4123–4132.

27. Bruynzeel PK, Kok PT, Hamelink ML, Kijne AM, Verhagen J. Exclusive leuk-otriene C_4 synthesis by purified human eosinophils induced by opsonized zymosan. FEBS Lett 1985; 189;350–354.

28. Shaw RJ, Walsh GM, Cromwell O, Moqbel R, Spry CJF, Kay AB. Activated human eosinophils generate SRS-A leukotrienes following IgG-dependent stimulation. Nature 1985; 316:150–152.

29. Bruijnzeel PL, de Monchy JG, Verhagen J, Kauffman HF. The eosinophilic granu-locyte: an active participant in the late phase asthmatic reaction? Bull Eur Physi-opathol Respir 1986; 22 Suppl 7:54–61.

30. Raible DG. Erythrocytes increase leukotriene C_4 release from human eosinophils: characterization and examination of possible mechanisms. J Leukoc Biol 1994; 56:65–73.

31. Moqbel R, MacDonald AJ, Cromwell O, Kay AB. Release of leukotriene C_4 (LTC_4) from human eosinophils following adherence to IgE- and IgG-coated schistosomula of *Schistomsoma mansoni*. Immunology 1990; 69:435–442.

32. Cromwell O, Moqbel R, Fitzharris P, Kurlak L, Harvey C, Walsh GM, Shaw RJ, Kay AB. Leukotriene C_4 generation from human eosinophils stimulated with IgG–*Aspergillus fumigatus* antigen immune complexes. J Allergy Clin Immunol 1988; 82:535–543.

33. Mahauthaman R, Howell CJ, Spur BW, Youlten LJ, Clark TJ, Lessof MH, Lee TH. The generation and cellular distribution of leukotriene C_4 in human eosino-phils stimulated by unopsonized zymosan and glucan particles. J Allergy Clin Im-munol 1988; 81:696–705.

34. Burke LA, Crea AE, Wilkinson JR, Arm JP, Spur BW, Lee TH. Comparison of the generation of platelet-activating factor and leukotriene C_4 in human eosino-phils stimulated by unopsonized zymosan and by the calcium ionophore A23187: the effects of nedocromil sodium. J Allergy Clin Immunol 1990; 85:26–35.

35. Yoshida K, Suko M, Matsuzaki G, Sugiyama H, Okudaira H, Ito K. Effect of fibronectin on the production of leukotriene C_4 by eosinophils. Int Arch Allergy Immunol 1995; 108:50–51.

36. Owen WF Jr, Soberman RJ, Yoshimoto T, Sheffer AL, Lewis RA, Austen KF. Synthesis and release of leukotriene C_4 by human eosinophils. J Immunol 1987; 138:532–538.

37. Takafuji S, Tadokoro K, Ito K, Dahinden CA. Effects of physiologic soluble agonists on leukotriene C_4 production and degranulation by human eosinophils. Int Arch Allergy Immunol 1995; 108 Suppl 1:36–38.

38. Bruijnzeel PLB, Kok PTM, Hamelink ML, Kijne AM, Verhagen J. Platelet-activating factor induces leukotriene C_4 synthesis by purified human eosinophils. Prostaglandins 1987; 34:205–214.

39. Tamura N, Agrawal DK, Townley RG. Leukotriene C_4 production from human eosinophils in vitro: role of eosinophil chemotactic factors on eosinophil activation. J Immunol 1988; 141:4291–4297.

40. Lam BK, Owen WF Jr, Austen KF, Soberman RJ. The identification of a distinct export step following the biosynthesis of leukotriene C_4 by human eosinophils. J Biol Chem 1989; 264:12885–12889.

41. Turk J, Maas RL, Brash AR, Roberts LJ II, Oates JA. Arachidonic acid 15-lipoxygenase products from human eosinophils. J Biol Chem 1982; 257:7068–7076.

42. Henderson WR, Harley JB, Fauci AS. Arachidonic acid metabolism in normal and hypereosinophilic syndrome human eosinophils: generation of leukotrienes B_4, C_4, D_4 and 15-lipoxygenase products. Immunology 1984; 51:679–686.

43. Kok PT, Hamelink ML, Kijne AM, Verhagen J, Koenderman L, Bruynzeel PL. Arachidonic acid can induce leukotriene C_4 formation by purified human eosinophils in the absence of other stimuli. Biochem Biophys Res Commun 1988; 153: 676–682.

44. Kok PT, Hamelink ML, Kijne GM, Verhagen J, Koenderman L, Veldink GA, Bruynzeel PL. Leukotriene C_4 formation by purified human eosinophils can be induced by arachidonic acid in the absence of calcium-ionophore A23187. Agents Actions 1989; 26:96–98.

45. Steinhilber D, Roth HJ. New series of lipoxins isolated from human eosinophils. FEBS Lett 1989; 255:143–148.

46. Turk J, Rand TH, Maas RL, Lawson JA, Brash AR, Roberts LJ II, Colley DG, Oates JA. Identification of lipoxygenase products from arachidonic acid metabolism in stimulated murine eosinophils. Biochim Biophys Acta 1983; 750:78–90.

47. Hirata K, Maghni K, Borgeat P, Sirois P. Guinea pig alveolar eosinophils and macrophages produce leukotriene B_4 but no peptido-leukotrienes. J Immunol 1990; 144:1880–1885.

48. Freiburghaus J, Jörg A. Isolation of bovine eosinophils and characterization of their leukotriene formation. Agents Actions 1990; 31:16–22.

49. Asmis R, Jörg A. Calcium-ionophore-induced formation of platelet-activating factor and leukotrienes by horse eosinophils: a comparative study. Eur J Biochem 1990; 187:475–480.

50. Spry CJF. Eosinophils: A Comprehensive Review and Guide to the Scientific and Medical Literature. Oxford: Oxford University Press, 1988.

51. Bruijnzeel PL, Virchow JC Jr, Rihs S, Walker C, Verhagen J. Lack of increased numbers of low-density eosinophils in the circulation of asthmatic individuals. Clin Exp Allergy 1993; 23:261–269.

52. Kajita T, Yui Y, Mita H, Taniguchi N, Saito H, Mishima T, Shida T. Release of leukotriene C_4 from human eosinophils and its relation to the cell density. Int Arch Allergy Appl Immunol 1985; 78:406–410.

53. Taniguchi N, Mita H, Saito H, Yui Y, Kajita T, Shida T. Increased generation of leukotriene C_4 from eosinophils in asthmatic patients. Allergy 1985; 40:571–573.
54. Kauffman HF, van der Belt B, de Monchy JG, Boelens H, Koeter GH, De Vries K. Leukotriene C_4 production by normal-density and low-density eosinophils of atopic individuals and other patients with eosinophilia. J Allergy Clin Immunol 1987; 79:611–619.
55. Roberge CJ, Laviolette M, Boulet LP, Poubelle PE. In vitro leukotriene (LT) C_4 synthesis by blood eosinophils from atopic asthmatics: predominance of eosinophil subpopulations with high potency for LTC_4 generation. Prostaglandins Leukot Essent Fatty Acids 1990; 41:243–249.
56. Sampson AP, Thomas RU, Costello JF, Piper PJ. Enhanced leukotriene synthesis in leukocytes of atopic and asthmatic subjects. Br J Clin Pharmacol 1992; 33: 423–430.
57. Laviolette M, Ferland C, Comtois JF, Champagne K, Bosse M, Boulet LP. Blood eosinophil leukotriene C_4 production in asthma of different severities. Eur Respir J 1995; 8:1465–1472.
58. Hodges MK, Weller PF, Gerard NP, Ackerman SJ, Drazen JM. Heterogeneity of leukotriene C_4 production by eosinophils from asthmatic and from normal subjects. Am Rev Respir Dis 1988; 138:799–804.
59. Hamann KJ. Inflammatory cells in airways. In: Leff AR, ed. Pulmonary and Critical Care Pharmacology and Therapeutics. McGraw-Hill: New York: 1996:355–369.
60. Kroegel C, Virchow J-C Jr, Luttmann W, Walker C, Warner JA. Pulmonary immune cells in health and disease: the eosinophil leukocyte. Eur Respir J 1994; 7: 519–543.
61. Chanarin N, Johnston SL. Leukotrienes as a target in asthma therapy. Drugs 1994; 47:12–24.
62. Dahlén S-E, Hedqvist P, Hammarström S, Samuelsson B. Leukotrienes are potent constrictors of human bronchi. Nature 1980; 228:484–486.
63. Holroyde MC, Altounyan REC, Cole M, Dixon M, Elliott EV. Bronchoconstriction produced in man by leukotrienes C and D. Lancet 1981; 2:17–18.
64. Barnes NC, Piper PJ, Costello JF. Comparative effects of inhaled leukotriene C_4, leukotriene D_4, and histamine in normal human subjects. Thorax 1984; 39:500–504.
65. Griffin M, Weiss JW, Leitch AG, McFadden ER Jr, Corey EJ, Austen KF, Drazen JM. Effects of leukotriene D_4 on the airways in asthma. N Engl J Med 1983; 308: 436–439.
66. Adelroth E, Morris MM, Hargreave FE, O'Byrne PM. Airway responsiveness to LTC_4 and D_4 and to methacholine in patients with asthma and normal controls. N Engl J Med 1986; 315:480–484.
67. Davidson AE, Lee TH, Scanlon PD, Solway J, McFadden ER Jr. Bronchoconstrictor effects of LTE_4 in normal and asthmatic subjects. Am Rev Respir Dis 1987; 135:333–337.
68. Drazen JM. Comparative contractile responses to sulfidopeptide leukotrienes in normal and asthmatic human subjects. Ann NY Acad Sci 1988; 524:289–297.
69. Ellis JL, Undem BJ. Role of cysteinyl-leukotrienes and histamine in mediating intrinsic tone in isolated human bronchi. Am J Respir Crit Care Med 1994; 149: 118–122.

70. Watson N, Magnussen H, Rabe KF. Inherent tone of human bronchus: role of eicosanoids and the epithelium. Br J Pharmacol 1997; 121:1099–1104.
71. Aizawa T, Sekizawa K, Aikawa T, Maruyama N, Itabashi S, Tamura G, Sasaki H, Takishima T. Eosinophil supernatant causes hyperresponsiveness of airway smooth muscle in guinea pig trachea. Am Rev Respir Dis 1990; 142:133–137.
72. Hamann KJ, Strek ME, Baranowski SL, Munoz NM, Williams FS, White SR, Vita A, Leff AR. Effects of activated eosinophils cultured from human umbilical cord blood on guinea pig trachealis. Am J Physiol 1993; 265:L301–L307.
73. Jongejan RC, De Jongste JC, Raatgeep RC, Bonta IL, Kerrebijn KF. Effects of zymosan-activated human granulocytes on isolated human airways. Am Rev Respir Dis 1991; 143:553–560.
74. Rabe KF, Muñoz NM, Vita AJ, Morton BE, Magnussen H, Leff AR. Contraction of human bronchial smooth muscle caused by activated human eosinophils. Am J Physiol 1994; 267:L326–L334.
75. Piacentini GL, Kaliner MA. The potential roles of leukotrienes in bronchial asthma. Am Rev Respir Dis 1991; 143:S96–S99.
76. Evans TW, Rogers DF, Aursudkij B, Chung KF, Barnes PJ. Regional and time-dependent effects of inflammatory mediators on airway microvascular permeability in the guinea pig. Clin Sci 1989; 76:479–485.
77. Camp RDR, Coutts AA, Greaves MW, Kay AB, Walfort MJ. Responses of human skin to intradermal injection of leukotrienes C_4, D_4, B_4. Br J Pharmacol 1983; 80:497–502.
78. Soter NA, Lewis RA, Corey EJ, Austen KF. Local effects of synthetic leukotrienes (LTC_4, LTD_4, LTE_4 and LTB_4) in human skin. J Invest Dermatol 1983; 80:115–119.
79. Coles ST, Neill KH, Reid LM, Austen KF, Nii Y. Effects of leukotrienes C_4 and D_4 on glycoproteins and lysozyme secretion by human bronchial mucosa. Prostaglandins 1983; 25:155–170.
80. Marom Z, Shelhamer JH, Bach MK, Morton DR, Kaliner MA. Slow reacting substances, leukotrienes C_4 and D_4 increase the release of mucus from human airways in vitro. Am Rev Respir Dis 1982; 126:449–451.
81. Johnson HG, Chinn RA, Chow AW, Bach MK, Nadel JA. Leukotriene C_4 enhances mucus production from submucosal glands in canine tracheas in vivo. Int J Immunopharmacol 1983; 5:391–396.
82. Foster A, Chan CC. Peptide leukotriene involvement in pulmonary eosinophil migration upon antigen challenge in actively sensitized guinea pig. Int Arch Allergy Appl Immunol 1991; 96:279–284.
83. Muñoz NM, Douglas I, Mayer D, Herrnreiter A, Zhu X, Leff AR. Eosinophil chemotaxis inhibited by 5-lypoxygenase blockade and leukotriene receptor antagonism. Am J Respir Crit Care Med 1997; 155:1398–1403.
84. Ford-Hutchinson AW, Bray WM, Doig MV, Shipley ME, Smith MJH. Leukotriene B_4, a potent chemokinetic and aggregating substance released from PMN leukocytes. Nature 1980; 286:264–268.
85. Nagy L, Lee TH, Goetzl EJ, Pickett WC, Kay AB. Complement receptor enhancement and chemotaxis of human neutrophils and eosinophils by leukotrienes and other lipoxygenase products. Clin Exp Immunol 1983; 71:394–398.

86. Dessein AJ, Lee TH, Elsas R, Ravalese J III, Silberstein D, David JR, Austen KF, Lewis RA. Enhancement by monokines of leukotriene generation by human eosinophils and neutrophils stimulated with calcium ionophore A23187. J Immunol 1986; 136:3829–3838.

87. Elsas P, Lee TH, Lenzi HL, Dessein AJ. Monocytes activate eosinophils for enhanced helminthotoxicity and increased generation of leukotriene C_4. Ann Inst Pasteur Immunol 1987; 138:97–116.

88. Elsas PX, Elsas MI, Dessein AJ. Eosinophil cytotoxicity enhancing factor: purification, characterization and immunocytochemical localization on the monocyte surface. Eur J Immunol 1990; 20:1143–1151.

89. Howell CJ, Pujol JL, Crea AE, Davidson R, Gearing AJ, Godard P, Lee TH. Identification of an alveolar macrophage-derived activity in bronchial asthma that enhances leukotriene C_4 generation by human eosinophils stimulated by ionophore A23187 as a granulocyte-macrophage colony-stimulating factor. Am Rev Respir Dis 1989; 140:1340–1347.

90. Soloperto M, Mattoso VL, Fasoli A, Mattoli S. A bronchial epithelial cell–derived factor in asthma that promotes eosinophil activation and survival as GM-CSF. Am J Physiol 1991; 260:L530–8.

91. Rothenberg ME, Owen WR Jr, Silberstein DS, Soberman RJ, Austen KF, Stevens RL. Eosinophils cocultured with endothelial cells have increased survival and functional properties. Science 1987; 237:645–647.

92. Rothenberg ME, Owen WF Jr, Silberstein DS, Woods J, Soberman RJ, Austen KF, Stevens RL. Human eosinophils have prolonged survival, enhanced functional properties, and become hypodense when exposed to human interleukin 3. J Clin Invest 1988; 81:1986–1992.

93. Fabian I, Kletter Y, Mor S, Geller-Bernstein C, Ben-Yaakov M, Volovitz B, Golde DW. Activation of human eosinophil and neutrophil functions by haematopoietic growth factors: comparisons of IL-1, IL-3, IL-5 and GM-CSF. Br J Haematol 1992; 80:137–143.

94. Silberstein DS, Owen WF, Gasson JC, Di Pierso JF, Golde DW, Bina JC, Soberman RJ, Austen KF, David JR. Enhancement of human eosinophil cytotoxicity and leukotriene synthesis by biosynthetic recombinant granulocyte-macrophage colony-stimulating factor. J Immunol 1986; 137:3290–3294.

95. Owen WF Jr, Petersen J, Austen KF. Eosinophils altered phenotypically and primed by culture with granulocyte/macrophage colony-stimulating factor and 3T3 fibroblasts generate leukotriene C_4 in response to FMLP. J Clin Invest 1991; 87: 1958–1963.

96. Scoggan KA, Ford-Hutchinson AW, Nicholson DW. Differential activation of leukotriene biosynthesis by granulocyte-macrophage colony-stimulating factor and interleukin-5 in an eosinophilic substrain of HL-60 cells. Blood 1995; 86: 3507–3516.

97. Roubin R, Elsas PP, Fiers W, Dessein AJ. Recombinant human tumour necrosis factor (rTNF) enhances leukotriene biosynthesis in neutrophils and eosinophils stimulated with the Ca^{2+} ionophore A23187. Clin Exp Immunol 1987; 70: 484–490.

98. Takafuji S, Bischoff SC, De Weck AL, Dahinden CA. IL-3 and IL-5 prime normal human eosinophils to produce leukotriene C_4 in response to soluble agonists. J Immunol 1991; 147:3855–3861.
99. Anwar AR, Walsh GM, Cromwell O, Kay AB, Wardlaw AJ. Adhesion to fibronectin primes eosinophils via $\alpha 4\beta 1$ (VLA-4). Immunology 1994; 82:222–228.
100. Muñoz NM, Rabe KF, Neeley SP, Herrnreiter A, Zhu X, McAllister K, Mayer D, Magnussen H, Galens S, Leff AR. Eosinophil VLA-4 binding to fibronectin augments bronchial narrowing through 5-lipoxygenase activation. Am J Physiol 1996; 270:L587–94.
101. Raible DG, Schulman ES, DiMuzio J, Cardillo R, Post TJ. Mast cell mediators prostaglandin-D_2 and histamine activate human eosinophils. J Immunol 1992; 148:3536–3542.
102. Shindo K, Koide K, Hirai Y, Sumitomo M, Fukumura M. Priming effect of platelet activating factor on leukotriene C_4 from stimulated eosinophils of asthmatic patients. Thorax 1996; 51:155–158.
103. White SR, Strek ME, Kulp GVP, Spaethe SM, Burch RA, Neeley SP, Leff AR. Regulation of human eosinophil degranulation and activation by endogenous phospholipase A_2. J Clin Invest 1993; 91:2118–2125.
104. Menard L, Pilote S, Maccache PH, Laviolette M, Borgeat P. Inhibitory effects of MK-886 on arachidonic acid metabolism in human phagocytes. Br J Pharmacol 1990; 100:15–20.
105. Menard L, Laviolette M, Borgeat P. Studies of the inhibitory activity of MK-0591 (3-[1-(4-chlorobenzyl)-3-(t-butylthio)-5-(quinolin-2-yl-methoxy)-indol-2-yl]-2,2 -dimethyl propanoic acid) on arachidonic acid metabolism in human phagocytes. Can J Physiol Pharmacol 1992; 70:808–813.
106. Fukuda T, Numao T, Akutsu I, Toda M, Motojima S, Makino S. Inhibition of leukotriene C_4 and B_4 release by human eosinophils with the new 5-lipoxygenase inhibitor 6-hydroxy-2(4-sulfamoylbenzylamino)-4,5,7-trimethylbenzothiazole hydrochloride. Arzneimittelforschung 1995; 45:1002–1004.
107. Muñoz NM, Vita AJ, Neeley SP, McAllister K, Spaethe SM, White SR, Leff AR. Beta adrenergic modulation of formyl-methionine-leucine-phenylalanine-stimulated secretion of eosinophil peroxidase and leukotriene C_4. J Pharmacol Exp Ther 1994; 268:139–143.
108. Tool AT, Mul FP, Knol EF, Verhoeven AJ, Roos D. The effect of salmeterol and nimesulide on chemotaxis and synthesis of PAF and LTC$_4$ by human eosinophils. Eur Respir J 1996; Suppl. 22:141s–145s.
109. Muñoz NM, Rabe KF, Vita AJ, McAllister K, Mayer D, Weiss M, Leff AR. Paradoxical blockade of beta adrenergically mediated inhibition of stimulated eosinophil secretion by salmeterol. J Pharmacol Exp Ther 1995; 273:850–854.
110. Rabe KF, Giembycz MA, Dent G, Perkins RS, Evans PM, Barnes PJ. Salmeterol is a comeptitive antagonist at β-adrenoceptors mediating inhibition of respiratory burst in guinea-pig eosinophils. Eur J Pharmacol 1993; 231:305–308.
111. Dent G, Giembycz MA, Evans PM, Rabe KF, Barnes PJ. Suppression of human eosinophil respiratory burst and cyclic AMP hydrolysis by inhibitors of type IV phosphodiesterase: interaction with the beta adrenoceptor agonist albuterol. J Pharmacol Exp Ther 1994; 271:1167–1174.

112. Tenor H, Hatzelmann A, Church MK, Schudt C, Shute JK. Effects of theophylline and rolipram on leukotriene C_4 (LTC_4) synthesis and chemotaxis of human eosinophils from normal and atopic subjects. Br J Pharmacol 1996; 118:1727–1735.

113. Ali A, Ford-Hutchinson AW, Nicholson DW. Activation of protein kinase C downregulates leukotriene C_4 synthase activity and attenuates cysteinyl leukotriene production in an eosinophil substrain of HL-60 cells. J Immunol 1994; 153: 776–788.

114. Kroegel C, Giembycz MA, Matthys H, Westwick J, Barnes PJ. Modulatory role of protein kinase C on the signal transduction pathway utilized by platelet-activating factor in eosinophil activation. Am J Respir Cell Mol Biol 1994; 11: 593–599.

115. Perkins RS, Lindsay MA, Barnes PJ, Giembycz MA. Early signalling events implicated in leukotriene B_4-induced activation of the NADPH oxidase in eosinophils: role of Ca^{2+}, protein kinase C and phospholipases C and D. Biochem J 1995; 310:795–806.

116. Dent G, Muñoz NM, Rühlmann E, Zhu X, Leff AR, Magnussen H, Rabe KF. Protein kinase C inhibition enhances platelet activating factor-induced eicosanoid production in human eosinophils. Am J Respir Cell Mol Biol (in press).

117. Giembycz MA, Kroegel C, Barnes PJ. Platelet activating factor stimulates cyclooxygenase activity in guinea pig eosinophils: concerted biosynthesis of thromboxane A_2 and E-series prostaglandins. J Immunol 1990; 144:3489–3497.

118. Dent G, Muñoz NM, Rühlmann E, Zhu X, Leff AR, Magnussen H, Rabe KF. Effects of protein tyrosine kinase inhibitors on platelet activating factor-induced respiratory burst and leukotriene production in human eosinophils. Am J Respir Crit Care Med 1997; 155:A59 (abstract).

119. Brattsand R, Selroos O. Current drugs for respiratory diseases: glucocorticosteroids. In: Page CP, Metzger WJ, eds. Drugs and the Lung. Raven Press: New York, 1994:101–220.

120. Shindo K, Hirai Y, Koide K, Sumitomo M, Fukumura M. In vivo effect of prednisolone on release of leukotriene C_4 in eosinophils obtained from asthmatic patients. Biochem Biophys Res Commun 1995; 214:869–8784.

121. Laviolette M, Ferland C, Trepanier L, Rocheleau H, Dakhama A, Boulet LP. Effects of inhaled steroids on blood eosinophils in moderate asthma. Ann NY Acad Sci 1994; 725:288–297.

122. Dworski R, Fitzgerald GA, Oates JA, Sheller JR. Effect of oral prednisone on airway inflammatory mediators in atopic asthma. Am J Respir Crit Care Med 1994; 149:953–959.

123. O'Shaughnessy KM, Wellings R, Gillies B, Fuller RW. Differential effects of fluticasone propionate on allergen-evoked bronchoconstriction and increased urinary LTE_4 excretion. Am Rev Respir Dis 1993; 147:1472–1476.

124. Bruijnzeel PL, Hamelink ML, Kok PT, Kreukniet J. Nedocromil sodium inhibits the A23187- and opsonized zymosan-induced leukotriene formation by human eosinophils but not by human neutrophils. Br J Pharmacol 1989; 96:631–636.

125. Bruijnzeel PL, Warringa RA, Kok PT, Hamelink ML, Kreukniet J. Inhibitory effects of nedocromil sodium on the in vitro induced migration and leukotriene formation of human granulocytes. Drugs 1989; 37:9–18.

126. Sedgwick JB, Bjornsdottir U, Geiger KM, Busse WW. Inhibition of eosinophil density change and leukotriene C_4 generation by nedrocromil sodium. J Allergy Clin Immunol 1992; 90:202–209.
127. Manabe H, Ohmori K, Tomioka H, Yoshida S. Oxatomide inhibits the release of chemical mediators from human lung tissues and from granulocytes. Int Arch Allergy Appl Immunol 1988; 87:91–97.
128. Nabe M, Miyagawa H, Agrawal DK, Sugiyama H, Townley RG. The effect of ketotifen on eosinophils as measured at LTC_4 release and by chemotaxis. Allergy Proc 1991; 12:267–271.
129. Chand N, Sofia RD. Azelastine—a novel in vivo inhibitor of leukotriene biosynthesis: a possible mechanism of action: a mini review. J Asthma 1995; 32:227–234.
130. Lehman PA, Henderson WRJ. Retinoid-induced inhibition of eosinophil LTC_4 production. Prostaglandins 1990; 39:569–577.
131. Lewis RA, Austen KF. Molecular determinants for functional responses to the sulfidopeptide leukotrienes: metabolism and receptor subclasses. J Allergy Clin Immunol 1984; 74:369–372.
132. Neill MA, Henderson WR, Klebanoff SJ. Oxidative degradation of leukotriene C_4 by human monocytes and monocyte-derived macrophages. J Exp Med 1985; 162:1634–1644.

24

Airway Ion Transport Mechanisms and Aspirin in Asthma

**SEBASTIANO BIANCO and
MARIA ROBUSCHI**

University of Milan
Milan, Italy

PIERSANTE SESTINI

University of Siena
Siena, Italy

ADRIANO VAGHI

Santa Corona Hospital
Garbagnate, Italy

I. Introduction

Despite the progress in our understanding of the actions of aspirin-like drugs (1) and of the mechanisms of aspirin-induced asthma, its pathogenesis remains largely undetermined (2,3). In the absence of animal or in vitro models of aspirin hypersensitivity, most of the recent knowledge of the mechanism of this type of asthma derives from studies involving measurement of arachidonic acid metabolites in urine or secretions and/or evaluation of the protective effect of different drugs against aspirin-induced reactions (2,4–7).

II. The Inhalation Challenge Test for Aspirin-Induced Asthma

The conventional provocation test consists of the oral administration of increasing doses of aspirin (ASA) under controlled conditions and the monitoring of the bronchial response for at least 1 hr after each dose with spirometric or plethysmographic parameters. Two main disadvantages of the conventional oral provocation test are the large amount of time required and the frequent occurrence of extrabronchial symptoms, which may at times be severe.

To make the ASA challenge less time-consuming and better tolerated, we developed in 1975 (8,9) an inhalation challenge test that involves nebulization of a freshly prepared solution of lysine-acetylsalicylate (LASA). For drug delivery, we originally used a method of continuous aerosol generation, in which the appropriate amounts of ASA progressively delivered to the mouth during tidal breathing were increased at 1-hr intervals through the appropriate combination of the concentration of the solution and the time of nebulization (8). More recently, we modified the procedure by using a MEFAR dosimeter and administering progressively doubling doses of LASA at 1-hr intervals.

The main advantages of inhalation over oral challenge, shown also by our previous studies (10–12), are that the response is more prompt, it is confined to the respiratory tract, and it is easily controlled with bronchodilators (13–15). These advantages are mostly due to the low dose of drug administered to the patient with this method; a dose between 1 and 10 mg of aspirin is sufficient to obtain a positive response in most aspirin-sensitive asthmatics (Fig. 1). We have the impression that the average provocative dose has tended to increase in recent years, as a result of the greater use of inhaled corticosteroids. This may also explain the sporadic occurrence of a negative bronchial

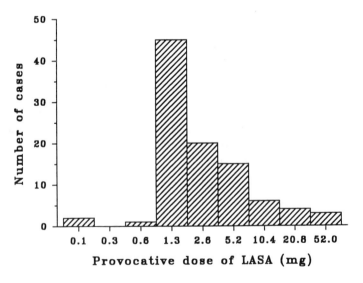

Figure 1 Distribution of the provocative dose of inhaled LASA (i.e., the dose that caused a decrease in FEV_1 of at least 20% of baseline) in 96 consecutive patients with aspirin-sensitive asthma.

challenge despite a positive oral test (16), since inhaled steroids are probably more effective against the effects of local rather than systemic administration of the drug.

The time course of the broncho-obstructive reaction that follows aspirin inhalation in aspirin-sensitive subjects is characteristically different from the responses induced by allergens and by most other bronchoconstrictor stimuli. The reaction usually begins 15–30 min after the challenge, peaks at 90–120 min, and lasts 4–5 hr. If the test is repeated on consecutive days, the bronchial response progressively fades and disappears after 3–4 days. This refractory state is then lost if ASA is withheld for a week, or if a substantially higher dose of ASA is administered. We have shown (8) that it is possible to desensitize aspirin-sensitive patients by progressively doubling the administered amount of ASA, initially by inhalation up to a dose of 64 mg, then by mouth, introducing the new dose only when the previous one has become ineffective. Within 15–20 days and without any trouble, we were able to make the patient tolerant to therapeutic doses of ASA or other cross-reacting nonsteroidal anti-inflammatory drugs (NSAIDs) (Fig. 2).

Other aspirin-like drugs vary in their asthmogenic potency in aspirin-sensitive asthmatics, largely depending on their cyclooxygenase inhibitory activity (17,18). For example, carprofen and nimesulide, two aspirin-like drugs with poor activity against constitutive cyclooxygenase (COX-1) but mostly active against inducible cyclooxygenase (COX-2) (1,19), are relatively well tolerated at commonly prescribed doses (20,21), although nimesulide may cause mild bronchoconstriction at higher doses (22). The time course of the asthmatic response to these drugs, however, is similar to the one observed with aspirin, with two exceptions. The first is that fenbufen can characteristically induce delayed reactions in some patients. These usually begin 3–4 hr after the administration of the drug and last for several hours. Interestingly, fenbufen (3-4 biphenylcarbonyl propionic acid) is a prodrug devoid of anti-COX activity, which is possessed instead by its principal active metabolite, biphenylacetic acid. Hence it is likely that the reaction starts only when there is a sufficient concentration of this active metabolite at the bronchial level.

III. Bronchial Obstructive Responses to Pyrazolone Derivatives

The second exception is in asthma induced by pyrazolones. Patients sensitive to pyrazolones may present two different patterns of reaction after specific challenge. A number of patients show the typical reaction to NSAIDs; it starts at 15–30 min, peaks 2–3 hr after challenge, and is inhibited by prior desensitization with ASA or pyrazolones. In some patients, however, the oral ingestion of pyrazolones is followed by an immediate bronchial reaction, with a pattern

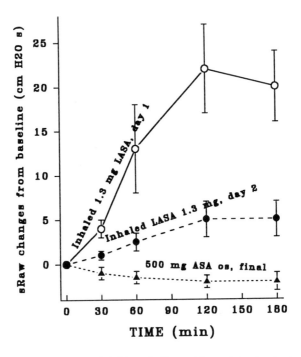

Figure 2 Bronchial response to LASA and effect of desensitization in six aspirin-sensitive asthmatics. The bronchial response to inhaled LASA was already attenuated at the second challenge. At the end of treatment, after less than 20 days, all the subjects tolerated an oral dose of 500 mg aspirin. (Modified from Ref. 8.)

similar to the early phase of the allergic asthmatic reaction (23). This reaction does not cross-react with other aspirin-like drugs, including pyrazolindirendiones, and is not inhibited by prior desensitization with ASA. Administration of repeated doses of pyrazolone may initially induce a partial desensitization, but escaping is frequent, hindering the induction and maintenance of desensitization.

Interestingly, some patients with aspirin-induced asthma may also present an immediate response to specific bronchial challenge. Whereas a recent report from Korea suggests that these patients are relatively common (24), our experience indicates that patients with this type of response are rather rare, representing less than 1% of the aspirin-sensitive asthmatics we tested. Furthermore, we recently observed (25) that one of these patients (Fig. 3) had a characteristic wheal-and-flare reaction upon skin testing with lysine-aspirin but not with sodium salicylate or lysine-ketoprofen; in contrast, the skinprick test with lysine-aspirin was negative in patients with a typical, late-onset aspi-

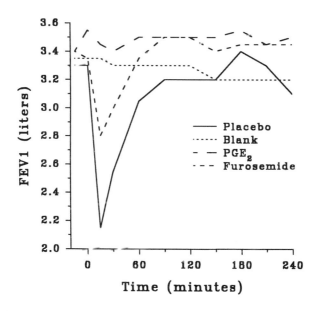

Figure 3 Atypical early response to inhaled LASA (8 mg) in a 25-year-old female patient with allergic asthma (predicted FEV₁ 3.33 L), presenting a wheal-and-flare reaction to skinprick test with LASA. The response was prevented by inhaled furosemide (dashed line) or PGE₂ (long dashed line).

rin-induced bronchoconstriction. These findings suggest that, unlike typical aspirin-induced asthma, the patient's reaction was due to a specific allergic response to acetylsalicylate.

IV. Bronchial Hypersensitivity to Hydrocortisone

It has been reported that hydrocortisone can induce asthmatic reactions in some ASA-sensitive patients (26,27). We have documented in one such patient that the two reactions develop through different mechanisms (28). In this subject, bronchial obstruction induced by inhaled hydrocortisone started and peaked earlier and was of shorter duration than that induced by LASA (Fig. 4). In addition, the patient could not be desensitized by repeated administration of hydrocortisone. Furthermore, after successful desensitization to ASA induced by repeated administration of increasing doses of LASA, the patient still responded to hydrocortisone. Thus, in its time course and characteristics, the response to hydrocortisone resembles that observed after oral challenge with pyrazolones rather than that after oral challenge with NSAIDs.

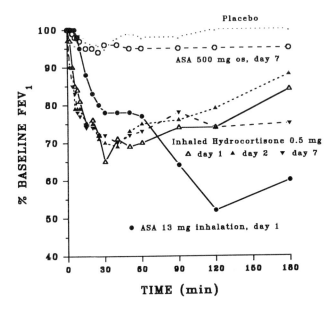

Figure 4 Bronchial obstructive response to inhaled LASA and to inhaled hydrocortisone in a sensitive subject. The response to hydrocortisone was not attenuated by repeated testing (day 2) and was unaffected after successful desensitization with ASA (day 7).

Therefore, when we challenge asthmatics with NSAIDs, three types of obstructive responses are possible: (1) the classic one, (2) a late reaction to fenbufen, and probably to other NSAID precursors, and (3) an immediate reaction to pyrazolones (Fig. 5). Classic and late reactions probably develop through the same mechanism, whereas the immediate reaction appears to have a completely different nature, possibly being mediated by an allergic mechanism.

V. Prevention of Aspirin-Induced Bronchoconstriction by Drugs Affecting Ion Transport Mechanisms

The specific bronchial challenge test offers the opportunity to evaluate the effect of pharmacological agents on aspirin-induced asthma, and several agents have been tested in this model. For example, a protective effect against aspirin-induced bronchoconstriction has been observed after treatment with beta$_2$-agonist (10,29), with PGE (9,29,30), with leukotriene-receptor antagonists (31,32), and with inhibitors of leukotriene synthesis (33). In the case of

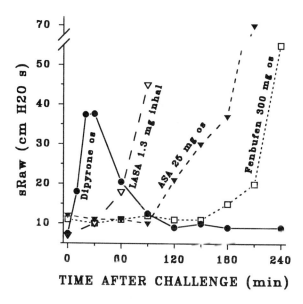

Figure 5 Early asthmatic response to oral dipyrone, compared to typical delayed responses to inhaled LASA, oral LASA, and oral fenbufen. The response to dipyrone is presented as the mean of six patients with a history of asthma caused by pyrazolone, while the other responses were all obtained in a single representative subject with aspirin-densitive asthma.

beta$_2$-agonist, the protective effect could be caused by a functional antagonism due to bronchodilator activity. However, the effect of inhaled PGE$_2$ is associated with inhibition of the urinary excretion of cysteinyl leukotrienes (30), suggesting that the effect is the result of the decreased release of these mediators. Thus, most of the agents that have proven effective in protection against aspirin-induced asthma appear to affect leukotriene activity, which confirms the importance of these mediators in the pathogenesis of aspirin-induced asthma (34–38).

Another interesting group of drugs that we have tested in this model includes those affecting ion transport mechanisms. It has been known for a long time that the ionic and osmotic characteristics of the bronchial lining fluid play a key role in the control of bronchomotor tone in asthmatics (reviewed in Ref. 39). More than 20 years ago, we developed a test of bronchial reactivity based on the inhalation of an ultrasonic mist of distilled water (ultrasonically nebulized water, UNW) (40). UNW-induced bronchoconstriction was dose-dependent and was more selective for asthma than other nonspecific stimuli, such as methacholine. However, inhalation of a similar volume of water in vapor had no effect, suggesting that bronchoconstriction was due to changes in the osmolarity of the bronchial lining in the sites of impact of the hypotonic droplets. This hypothesis has subsequently been confirmed through the use of different hypotonic solutions (41).

The mechanism of action of several other bronchoconstrictor stimuli, such as hypertonic solutions, dry-cold air, and exercise, probably involves a change in the osmolarity of the liquid bathing the bronchial mucosa. It has been suggested that alterations in osmolarity would cause bronchoconstriction on account of both an increased release of chemical mediators by superficial mast cells and the stimulation of cholinergic and noncholinergic nerve endings, resulting in the release of acetylcholine and neurokinins.

The osmolarity and ion composition of the bronchial lining fluid is regulated by complex cellular and intercellular mechanisms involving the integrity of tight junctions and the activity of ion channels asymmetrically distributed on the luminal and serosal sides of epithelial cells (reviewed in Refs. 42,43). These include the ouabain-sensitive, ATP-dependent Na/K pump and the loop diuretic-sensitive Na/Cl/K neutral cotransporter on the basolateral side of the cells, plus the Cl^- channels and amiloride-sensitive Na^+ channels on the apical side, along with other structures such as Na^+/H^+, Cl^-/HCO_3^- exchangers.

Given the sensitivity of bronchial tone to changes in osmolarity, it is not surprising that drugs affecting ion transport mechanisms also affect the response to osmotic bronchoconstrictor stimuli in asthma. Indeed, although ouabain (44) and strophanthus (45) failed to exhibit protective activity against histamine-induced bronchoconstriction in humans, and amiloride was ineffective against histamine-, metabisulfite-, or cold air–induced bronchoconstriction, inhalation of the loop diuretic furosemide has been found to effectively prevent bronchoconstriction induced by UNW (46), exercise (47), hypertonic solutions (48), and cold air. Perhaps more surprising is that furosemide also has protective activity against nonosmotic bronchoconstrictor stimuli, such as allergens (49), adenosine, metabisulfite, and neurokinins (39,50–52). These findings, along with the observation that furosemide equally affects both hypo- and hyperosmolar stimuli, suggest that the main site of action of the drug are probably not the structures responsible for ion and fluid secretion or reabsorption on the bronchial epithelial membrane, but rather the ion transport mechanisms of the cholinergic and noncholinergic nervous systems and inflammatory cells, which can modulate the release of chemical mediators triggered by these stimuli. This hypothesis is also supported by the fact that furosemide has little or no activity against bronchoconstrictor stimuli acting directly on the bronchial smooth muscle, such as methacholine, histamine, and prostaglandin F. Indeed, furosemide-sensitive ion transport mechanisms have been described

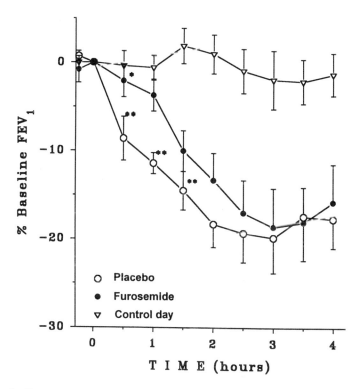

Figure 6 Protective effect of 40 mg inhaled furosemide on the bronchial response to a single provocative dose of LASA in eight sensitive asthmatics. *Not significant versus baseline. **$p < 0.05$ versus furosemide. (From Ref. 61.)

on several inflammatory cells (53), including mast cells (54), and this drug has been shown to inhibit both neural reflexes (55–57) and allergen-induced mediator release from lung tissue and isolated cells in vitro (58,59), as well as urinary excretion of cysteinyl leukotrienes after allergen challenge in vivo (60).

VI. Furosemide

We performed two studies to investigate the effect of furosemide on aspirin-induced bronchoconstriction. In both studies (one of which is illustrated in Fig. 6), we observed that inhaled furosemide affords good protection in the initial part of the obstructive response to aspirin, but this effect tends to fade away within 90–120 min after treatment (61). This is in contrast to the protective

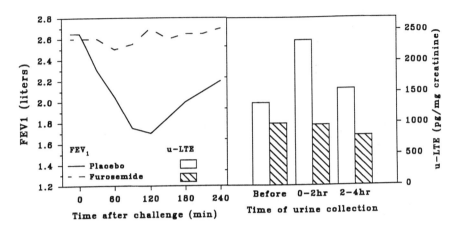

Figure 7   Effect of inhaled furosemide on the bronchial response (left) and on urine excretion of LTE$_4$ (right) in a single patient with aspirin-sensitive asthma. In this patient furosemide inhibited both bronchoconstriction and cysteinyl-leukotriene overproduction. LASA inhalation challenge (0.5 mg) was performed in an 18-year-old woman, with FEV$_1$ predicted 2.77.

activity against the late asthmatic response to allergen challenge, which occurs more than 4 hr after treatment (49). However, it is consistent with the duration of the protective effect of inhaled furosemide against UNW-induced bronchoconstriction, which has been found to last for less than 180 min. The most likely explanation for these apparently contrasting results is that, in the case of the allergic asthmatic reaction, the protection against the late response results from the inhibition of the release of mediators that occurs during the early phase of the response, resulting in blockage of any further development of the reaction even after the activity of furosemide is exhausted. By contrast, in aspirin-induced asthma, the prolonged duration of the response is probably the result of the permanence of the drug in the lung, causing continuous release of bronchoconstrictor mediators, notably cysteinyl-leukotrienes, which can be inhibited by furosemide only during its limited time of activity. Indeed, our preliminary results in one case (Fig. 7) indicate that the protective activity of inhaled furosemide against aspirin-induced bronchoconstriction is associated with decreased urinary excretion of cysteinyl-leukotrienes, although in this case furosemide afforded long-lasting protection. This observation supports the hypothesis that this treatment prevents local mediator release in the bronchi, which is considered to be the main cause of bronchoconstriction in aspirin-induced asthma (6,62,63).

VII. Chromones

Early in our studies of the effect of loop diuretics, we noted that the spectrum of the protective activities of inhaled furosemide against experimentally induced bronchoconstriction in asthma closely resembles that of sodium cromoglycate (49). Recent data indicate that the mechanism of action of chromones, such as disodium cromoglycate and nedocromil sodium, actually involves the modulation of ion transport mechanisms, namely Cl⁻ channel activity, in mast cells and possibly in other cell types (64–66). This suggests that they could act on cellular mechanisms in a manner similar to loop diuretics. Because the protective activity of chromones against aspirin-induced asthma had never been examined in controlled studies (9,67–71), we investigated the effect of nedocromil sodium and of cromoglycate on the inhalation challenge in aspirin-sensitive asthmatics (72). One of the reasons for comparing the effect of the two drugs was that in vitro nedocromil has been reported to be at least 500 times more potent than cromoglycate in inhibiting the aspirin-induced release of cytocidal oxygen mediators by platelets from aspirin-sensitive asthmatics (73), and nedocromil, but not cromoglycate, has been reported to be active on the same phenomenon after treatment in vivo (74). However, we found that both treatments significantly attenuated the response by about 60% with respect to placebo, without significant differences between the two drugs (Fig. 8). Thus, both furosemide and chromones exhibit protective activity against aspirin-induced asthma, although neither drug appears to be very efficacious: furosemide because of the short duration of action and chromones because of the modest overall (albeit longer) effect. It must be noted, however, that the degree of protection afforded by chromones appears to be similar to the one observed using antileukotriene drugs in the same model (31–33). In comparison, when investigated with a similar protocol, inhaled PGE_2 afforded almost complete protection in all patients, with a mean protection greater than 80% (30). In addition, the lack of difference between the activity of nedocromil and cromoglycate in this model suggests that their mechanism of action against aspirin-induced bronchoconstriction is independent of their activity on the platelets of these patients.

Although these data, taken together, suggest that the antiasthmatic activities of loop diuretics and chromones are mediated by a common final mechanism, probably involving ion transport and mediator release in inflammatory cells, a few differences in the activities of these compounds have been reported, suggesting that at least the initial steps of their mechanism of action may be different. First, although no correspondence has been found between the protective activity of different loop diuretics against bronchoconstrictor stimuli and their inhibitory potency on the Na/K/Cl transporter (50,51,75), there is currently no evidence that the latter activity is not necessary to their

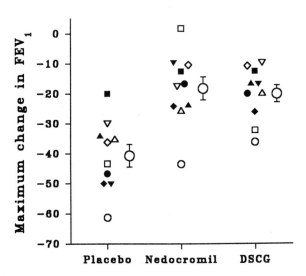

Figure 8 Effect of 4 mg nedocromil and of 10 mg cromoglycate on the maximum decrease in FEV1 after bronchial challenge with LASA in 10 sensitive subjects. Each symbol identifies a single patient. Symbols with bars represent the mean and SE for each treatment.

antiasthmatic effect, and even their inhibitory effect on Cl⁻ channel opening in mast cells could be mediated by this phenomenon (54). By contrast, chromones have no effect on the Na/K/Cl transporter, and their effect on Cl⁻ transport appears to be mediated by an effect on intracellular nucleosides (76). A second difference is in the shape of the dose-response curve of the activity of the two groups of compounds in vitro. While the effects of loop diuretics always increase with the dose, chromones typically exhibit a bell-shaped dose-response curve; i.e., they reach a maximum activity, which then fades at increasing doses (77). A third difference has been observed in the effect of these drugs on nerve transmission. While loop diuretics have been reported to inhibit both inhibitory and excitatory nonadrenergic noncholinergic neurotransmission in the guinea pig, nedocromil appears to inhibit only the excitatory neurotransmission in the same model (78).

VIII. Protective Activity of Furosemide and Aspirin-like Drugs

Interestingly, a further difference between the antiasthmatic effects of furosemide and cromoglycate involves their interaction with aspirin-like drugs, although this phenomenon is not limited to aspirin-sensitive asthmatics. In fact, we observed that inhalation of LASA attenuates the obstructive response to several bronchoconstrictor stimuli (79,80). Furthermore, the protective activity of furosemide against UNW-induced bronchoconstriction is strongly potentiated by inhalation of LASA, indicating a positive interaction between the mechanisms of action of these two treatments (81). By contrast, the protective activity of disodium cromoglycate against the same stimulus is unaffected by LASA or by furosemide, resulting in a simple additive effect (82,83). Since inhibition of COX is considered to be the main pharmacological effect of aspirin-like drugs (1), these data suggest that the protective activity of furosemide is normally reduced by the release of endogenous prostaglandins, while the mechanism of action of cromoglycate is insensitive to local prostaglandins.

The latter results are somewhat surprising, since the diuretic and vasodilator effects caused by systemic administration of furosemide are known to be partially mediated by the release of prostaglandin E and are attenuated by the simultaneous administration of aspirin-like drugs. Furthermore, inhalation of PGE affords protection against several bronchoconstrictor stimuli (9) and would therefore appear to be a likely mediator of the protective activity of furosemide. If this were the case, an inhibition, rather than potentiation, of the effect of furosemide would be expected after inhalation of an inhibitor of prostaglandin synthesis such as LASA. However, although inhibition of prostaglandin synthesis by systemic treatment with indomethacin resulted in attenuation of the protective activity of inhaled furosemide against exercise-induced bronchoconstriction in one study (84), in other studies the same treatment failed to affect the activity of furosemide against bronchoconstriction induced by exercise (85), metabisulfite (86), UNW (unpublished), and hypertonic saline (87). In addition, although UNW is the only stimulus for which a potentiating protective effect of inhaled LASA and furosemide has been reported, an additive effect of the two treatments has been observed against allergen- (88) and exercise-induced (89) bronchoconstriction. This indicates that, even at the relatively high local concentration of the drug obtained by inhalation, LASA has no inhibitory effect on the antibronchoconstrictor activity of furosemide.

On the basis of these experimental studies, we also performed clinical trials to investigate whether the combination of inhaled LASA and furosemide could be of benefit in patients with steroid-dependent asthma. In these studies, a remarkable steroid-sparing effect of more than 80% was observed both in patients with severe asthma requiring oral steroids (one of whom, incidentally, had aspirin-induced asthma) (90) and in patients receiving high doses of inhaled beclomethasone (91). Although we were not able to differentiate the effects of LASA and furosemide in these studies, it seems unlikely that such brilliant results would have been achieved if one of the drugs had a detrimental effect on the other. Taken together, these data indicate that the antibroncho-constrictor activity of furosemide in humans is not inhibited by prostaglandin inhibitors and that it is probably not mediated by the release of PGE. This conclusion is further supported by the observation that furosemide fails to induce PGE production by human epithelial cells in vitro (92,93).

IX. Conclusion

In conclusion, study of the effects on aspirin-induced asthma of drugs affecting ion transport mechanisms has demonstrated that such mechanisms play an important role in control of the bronchoconstrictor response to this stimulus. It has also been confirmed that they act on some basic mechanism controlling the bronchial response to several stimuli. Further knowledge of these mechanisms could help to explain the pathogenesis of asthma and possibly to develop new effective treatments for it, including the aspirin-induced form.

References

1. Vane JR, Botting RM. New insights into the mode of action of anti-inflammatory drugs. Inflamm Res 1995; 44:1–10.
2. Szczeklik A. Aspirin-induced asthma: an update and novel findings. Adv Prostaglandin Thromboxane Leukot Res 1994; 22:185–198.
3. Szczeklik A, Nizankowska E, Serafin A, Dyczec A, Duplaga M, Musial J. Autoimmune phenomena in bronchial asthma with special reference to aspirin intolerance. Am J Respir Crit Care Med 1995; 152(6 Pt 1):1753–1756.
4. Ortolani C, Mirone C, Fontana A, Folco GC, Miadonna A, Montalbetti N, Rinaldi M, Sala A, Tedeschi A, Valente D. Study of mediators of anaphylaxis in nasal wash fluids after aspirin and sodium metabisulfite nasal provocation in intolerant rhinitic patients. Ann Allergy 1987; 59:106–112.
5. Lee TH. Mechanism of bronchospasm in aspirin-sensitive asthma. Am Rev Respir Dis 1993; 148:1442–1443.
6. Sladek K, Dworski R, Soja J, Sheller JR, Nizankowska E, Oates JA, Szczeklik A. Eicosanoids in bronchoalveolar lavage fluid of aspirin-intolerant patients with asthma after aspirin challenge. Am J Respir Crit Care Med 1994; 149:940–946.
7. Szczeklik A. Mediator assays in aspirin-induced asthma. Allergy Proc 1994; 15: 135–138.
8. Bianco S, Robuschi M, Petrigni G. Aspirin induced tolerance in aspirin asthma detected by a new challenge test. IRCS J Med Sci 1977; 5:129.
9. Pasargiklian M, Bianco S, Allegra L, Moavero NE, Petrigni G, Robuschi M, Grugni AA. Aspects of bronchial reactivity to prostaglandins and aspirin in asthmatic patients. Respiration 1977; 34:79–91.

10. Bianco S, Robuschi M, Petrigni G. Aspirin sensitivity in asthmatics. Br Med J 1981; 282:116 (letter).
11. Bianco S, Robuschi M, Damonte MC, et al. Bronchial response to nonsteroidal anti-inflammatory drugs in asthmatic patients. Prog Biochem Pharmacol 1985; 20:132.
12. Bianco S. Asthme et médicaments antiinflammatoires non stéroidiens. In: Charpin S, ed. Allergology, 2nd ed. Paris: Flammarion, 1986:683–693.
13. Schmitz-Schuman M, Schaub E, Virchow C. Inhalative provocation mit Lysin-Azetylsalicylsaeure bei Analgetika-Asthma-Syndrom. Praxis Klin Pneumol 1982; 36:17.
14. Dahlén B, Zetterström O. Comparison of bronchial and per oral challenge with ASA in ASA-sensitive asthmatics. Eur Respir J 1990; 3:527–534.
15. Melillo G, Padovano A, Masi C, Melillo E, Cocco G. Aspirin-induced asthma and bronchial hyperresponsiveness. Allergia Immunologia 1991; 23:423–426.
16. Bestynska A, Cmiel A, Dworski R, Nizankowska E, Szczeklik A. Oral or inhaled aspirin challenge for diagnosis of aspirin induced asthma? International symposium, Eicosanoids, Aspirin and Asthma, Krakow, 1996, Abstract p. 190.
17. Szczeklik A, Griglewsky RJ, Czerniawska-Mysik G. Relationship of inhibition of prostaglandin biosynthesis by analgesics to asthma attacks in aspirin-sensitive patients. Br Med J 1975; 1:67–69.
18. Szczeklik A. The cyclooxygenase theory of aspirin-induced asthma. Eur Respir J 1990; 3:588–593.
19. Tavares IA, Bishai PM, Bennett A. Activity of nimesulide on constitutive and inducible cyclooxygenase. Arznheim-Forsch/Drug Res 1995; 45(2):1093–1095.
20. Bianco S, Robuschi M, Simone P, Vaghi A, Pasarkiklian M. Tolerance of carprofen in patients with asthma caused by nonsteroidal anti-inflammatory drugs. J Int Med Res 1985; 13:294–299.
21. Bianco S, Robuschi M, Petrigni G, Vaghi A, Refini RM, Pieroni MG, Sestini P. Efficacy and tolerability of nimesulide in asthmatic patients intolerant to aspirin. Drugs 1993; 46(Suppl 1):115–120.
22. Robuschi M, Gambaro G, Spagnotto S, Refini RM, Pieroni MG, Sestini P, Bianco S, Vagliasindi M. Tolerance of high dose nimesulide by patients with aspirin-induced asthma. Am J Respir Crit Care Med 1994; 149:A947.
23. Robuschi M, Spagnotto S, Gambaro G, Petrigni G, Vaghi A, Pieroni M, Sestini P, Bianco S. Characterization of the bronchial obstructive reactions to pyrazolones. Am J Respir Crit Care Med 1994; 149:A197.
24. Park HS. Early and late onset asthmatic response following lysine-aspirin inhalation in aspirin-sensitive asthmatic patients. Clin Exp Allergy 1995; 25:38–40.
25. Sestini P, Refini M, Pieroni MG, Vaghi A, Sala A, Armetti L, Robuschi M. An aspirin-sensitive patient with an early asthmatic response and a wheal and flare skin reaction to lysine aspirin. Am J Respir Crit Care Med 1996; 153:A684.
26. Partridge MR, Gibson GJ. Adverse bronchial reactions to intravenous hydrocortisone in two aspirin-sensitive asthmatic patients. Br Med J 1978; 1:1521.
27. Szczeklik A, Nizankowska E, Czerniawska-Mysik G, Sek S. Hydrocortisone and airflow impairment in aspirin-induced asthma. J Allergy Clin Immunol 1986; 76:530–536.

28. Vaghi A, Robuschi M, Petrigni G, et al. Characterization of the bronchial response to aspirin and hydrocortisone by inhalation challenge test and desensitization procedures in a sensitive patient. Am Rev Respir Dis 1993; 147:A556.
29. Szczeklik A, Mastalerz L, Nizankowska E, Cmiel A. Protective and bronchodilator effects of prostaglandin E and salbutamol in aspirin-induced asthma. Am J Respir Crit Care Med 1996; 153:567–571.
30. Sestini P, Armetti L, Gambaro G, Pieroni MG, Refini RM, Sala A, Vaghi A, Folco GC, Bianco S, Robuschi M. Inhaled PGE2 prevents aspirin-induced bronchoconstriction and urinary LTE4 excretion in aspirin-sensitive asthma. Am J Respir Crit Care Med 1996; 153:572–575.
31. Christie PE, Smith CM, Lee TH. The potent and selective sulfidopeptide leukotriene antagonist, SK&F 104353 inhibits aspirin-induced asthma. Am Rev Respir Dis 1991; 144:957–958.
32. Dahlén B, Kumlin M, Margolskee DJ, Larsson C, Blomqvist H, Williams VC, Zetterström O, Dahlén S. The leukotriene-receptor antagonist MK-0679 blocks airway obstruction induced by inhaled lysine-aspirin in aspirin-sensitive asthmatics. Eur Respir J 1993; 6:1018–1026.
33. Nasser SMS, Bell GS, Foster S, Spruce KE, MacMillan A, Williams AJ, Lee TH, Arm JP. Effect of the 5-lipoxygenase inhibitor ZD21138 on aspirin-induced asthma. Thorax 1994; 49:749–756.
34. Szczeklik A. Asthme, aspirine et leukotriènes. Bull Eur Physiopathol Respir 1983; 19:531–538.
35. Szczeklik A. The cyclooxygenase theory of aspirin-induced asthma. Eur Respir J 1990; 3:588–593.
36. Sladek K, Szczeklik A. Cysteinyl leukotrienes overproduction and mast cell activation in aspirin-provoked bronchospasm in asthma. Eur Respir J 1993; 6:391–399.
37. Lee TH, Christie PE. Leukotrienes and aspirin induced asthma. Thorax 1993; 48: 1189–1190.
38. Dahlén B, Margolskee DJ, Zetterström O. Dahlén S-E. Effect of the leukotriene receptor antagonist MK-0679 on baseline pulmonary function in aspirin sensitive asthmatic subjects. Thorax 1993; 488:1205–1210.
39. Bianco S, Robuschi M, Sestini P, Vaghi A, Refini M, Pieroni M, Gambaro G, Spagnotto S, Rossoni G, Berti F, Pasargiklian M. Osmolarity, bronchial reactivity, and the protective effect of loop diuretics. In: Melillo G, Norman PS, Marone G, eds. Respiratory Allergy. Clinical Immunology, Vol 2. Toronto: BC Decker, 1990: 119–130.
40. Allegra L, Bianco S. Non-specific broncho-reactivity obtained with an aerosol of distilled water. Respiration 1980; 61(Suppl):41–49.
41. Eschenbacher WL, Boushey HA, Sheppard D. Alteration in osmolarity of inhaled aerosols cause bronchoconstriction, but absence of a permanent anion causes cough alone. Am Rev Respir Dis 1984; 129:211–215.
42. Welsh M. Electrolyte transport by airway epithelia. Physiol Rev 1987; 67:1143–1183.
43. Boucher RC. State of the art: human airway ion transport. Am J Respir Crit Care Med 1994; 150:271–281, 581–593.

44. Knox AJ, Tattersfield AE, Britton JR. The effect of inhaled ouabain on bronchial reactivity to histamine in man. Br J Clin Pharmacol 1988; 24:758–760.
45. Vaghi A, Robuschi M, Pieroni MG, Refini RM, Sestini P, Bianco S. Effect of inhaled strophanthus on histamine-induced bronchoconstriction. Eur Respir J 1993; 6(Suppl 17):200s.
46. Robuschi M, Gambaro G, Spagnotto S, Vaghi A, Bianco S. Inhaled furosemide is highly effective in preventing ultrasonically nebulized distilled water bronchoconstriction. Pulm Pharmacol 1989; 1:187–191.
47. Bianco S, Vaghi A, Gambaro G, Pasargiklian M. Prevention of exercise-induced bronchoconstriction by inhaled furosemide. Lancet 1988; 2:252–255.
48. Robuschi M, Vaghi A, Gambaro G, Spagnotto S, Bianco S. Inhaled furosemide is effective in preventing ultrasonically nebulized 5.8% NaCl bronchoconstriction. Eur Respir J 1988; 1:194s.
49. Bianco S, Pieroni M, Refini R, Rottoli L, Sestini P. Protective effect of inhaled furosemide on allergen-induced early and late asthmatic reactions. N Engl J Med 1989; 321:1069–1073.
50. Bianco S, Pieroni MG, Refini RM, Robuschi M, Vaghi A, Sestini P. Inhaled loop diuretics as potential new anti-asthmatic drugs. Eur Respir J 1993; 6:130–134.
51. Barnes PJ. Diuretics and asthma. Thorax 1993; 48:195–196.
52. Bianco S, Pieroni MG, Refini RM, Sestini P, Robuschi M, Vaghi A. Protective effect of inhaled loop diuretics on experimentally induced bronchoconstriction. In: Spector SL, ed. Provocation Testing in Clinical Practice. New York: Marcel Dekker, 1994:411–423.
53. Gallin E. Ion channels in leukocytes. Physiol Rev 1991; 71:775–810.
54. Meyer G, Doppierio S, Vallin P, Daffonchio L. Effect of furosemide on Cl⁻ channel in rat peritoneal mast cells. Eur Respir J 1996; 9:2461–2467.
55. Elwood W, Lotvall JO, Barnes P, Chung KF. Loop diuretics inhibit cholinergic and noncholinergic nerves in guinea-pig. Am Rev Respir Dis 1991; 143:1345–1349.
56. Molimard M, Advenier C. Effect of furosemide on bradykinin- and capsaicin-induced contraction of the guinea-pig trachea. Eur Respir J 1993; 6:434–439.
57. Verleden GM, Pype JL, Deneffe G, Demetz MG. Effect of loop diuretics on cholinergic neurotransmission in human airways in vitro. Thorax 1994; 49:657–663.
58. Anderson SD, Wey H, Temple DM. Inhibition by furosemide of inflammatory mediators from lung fragments. N Engl J Med 1991; 234:131.
59. Berti F, Rossoni G, Buschi A, Zuccari G, Villa LM. Protective activity of inhaled furosemide against immunological respiratory changes and mediator release in guinea-pigs. Pulm Pharmacol 1992; 5:115–120.
60. Sala A, Arnetti L, Sestini P, Bianco S, Folco GC. Effect of furosemide on urinary LTE4 in asthmatic patients. Eur Respir J 1993; 6(Suppl 17):493s.
61. Sestini P, Pieroni MG, Refini RM, Robuschi M, Gambaro G, Spagnotto S, Vaghi A, Bianco S. Time-limited protective effect of inhaled furosemide against aspirin-induced bronchoconstriction in aspirin sensitive asthmatics. Eur Respir J 1994; 7:1825–1829.
62. Fischer AR, Rosenberg MA, Lilly CM, Callery JC, Rubin P, Cohn J, White MV, Igarashi Y, Kaliner MA, Drazen JM, Israel E. Direct evidence for a role of the

mast cell in the nasal response to aspirin-sensitive asthma. J Allergy Clin Immunol 1994; 94:1046–1056.

63. O'Sullivan S, Dahlen B, Dahlén SE, Kumlin M. Increased urinary excretion of the prostaglandin D_2 metabolite $9\alpha,11\beta$-prostaglandin F_2 after aspirin challenge supports mast cell activation in aspirin-induced airway obstruction. J Allergy Clin Immunol 1996; 98:421–432.

64. Reinsprecht M, Pecht I, Schinder H. Potent block of Cl^- channels by antiallergic drugs. Biochem Biophys Res Commun 1992; 188:957–963.

65. Paulmichl M, Norris AA, Rainey DK. Role of chloride channel modulation in the mechanism of action of nedocromil sodium. Int Arch Allergy Immunol 1995; 107:416.

66. Alton EWFW, Kingsleigh-Smith DJ, Munkonge F, Smith SN, Lindsay ARG, Gruenert DC, Jeffery PK, Norrs A, Geddes D, Williams AJ. Asthma prophylaxis agents alter the function of an airway epithelial chloride channel. Am J Respir Cell Mol Biol 1996; 14:380–397.

67. Basomba A, Romar A, Pelaez A, Villalmanzo IG, Campos A. The effect of sodium cromoglycate in preventing aspirin induced bronchospasm. Clin Allergy 1976; 6: 269–275.

68. Delaney JC. The effect of sodium cromoglycate on analgesic-induced asthmatic reactions. Clin Allergy 1976; 13:365–368.

69. Martelli NA, Usandivaras G. Inhibition of aspirin-induced bronchoconstriction by sodium cromoglycate inhalation. Thorax 1977; 32:684–690.

70. Wuthric B. Protective effect of ketotifen and disodium cromoglycate against bronchoconstriction induced by aspirin, benzoic acid or tartrazine in intolerant asthmatics. Respiration 1980; 37:224–231.

71. Dahl R. Oral and inhaled disodium cromoglycate in challenge test with food allergens or acetylsalicyclic acid. Allergy 1981; 36:161–165.

72. Robuschi M, Gambaro G, Sestini P, Pieroni MG, Refini RM, Vaghi A, Bianco S. Attenuation of aspirin-induced bronchoconstriction by sodium cromoglycate and nedocromil sodium. Am J Respir Crit Care Med 1997; 155 (in press).

73. Joseph M, Thorel T, Tsicopulos A, Tonnel AB, Capron A. Nedocromil sodium inhibition of IgE-mediated activation of human mononuclear phagocytes and platelets from asthmatics. Drugs 1989; 37(Suppl 1):32–36.

74. Marquette CH, Joseph M, Tonnel AB, Vorng H, Lassalle P, Tsicopulos A, Capron A. The abnormal in vitro response to aspirin of platelets from aspirin-sensitive asthamtics is inhibited after inhalation of nedocromil sodium but not of sodium cromoglycate. Br J Clin Pharmacol 1990; 29:525–531.

75. Bianco S, Robuschi M, Vaghi A, Pieroni MG, Sestini P. Protective effect of inhaled piretanide on the bronchial obstructive response to ultrasonically nebulized H_2O. A dose-response study. Chest 1993; 104:185–188.

76. Mackay GA, Pearce FL. Extracellular guanosine 3′,5′-cyclic monophosphate and disodium cromoglycate share a similar spectrum of activity in the inhibition of histamine release from isolated mast cells and basophils. Int Arch Allergy Immunol 1995; 109:258–265.

77. Napier FE, Shearer MA, Temple DM. Nedocromil sodium inhibits antigen-induced contraction of human lung parenchymal and bronchial strips, and the re-

lease of sulphidopeptide-leukotrienes and histamine from human lung fragments. Br J Pharmacol 1990; 100:247–250.

78. Verleden GM, Pypc JL, Demedts NJ. Furosemide and bumetanide but not nedocromil sodium modulate nonadrenergic relaxation in guinea-pig trachea in vitro. Am J Respir Crit Care Med 1994; 149:138–144.

79. Bianco S, Vaghi A, Pieroni MG, Robuschi M, Refini RM, Sestini P. Protective activity of inhaled nonsteroidal antiinflammatory drugs on bronchial responsiveness to ultrasonically nebulized water. J Allergy Clin Immunol 1992; 90: 833–839.

80. Bianco S, Pieroni MG, Refini RM, Robuschi M, Vaghi A, Sestini P. Could NSAIDs have a role as antiasthmatic agents? Drugs 1994; 48:9–15.

81. Bianco S, Vaghi A, Pieroni MG, Robuschi M, Refini RM, Berni F, Sestini P. Potentiation of the antireactive, antiasthmatic effect of inhaled furosemide by inhaled lysine acetylsalicylate. Allergy 1993; 48:570–575.

82. Sestini P, Robuschi M, Vaghi A, Refini RM, Pieroni MG, Bianco S. Effect of inhaled lysine acetylsalicylate on the protective activity of cromolyn sodium against the bronchial obstructive response to ultrasonically nebulized water. Am Rev Respir Dis 1993; 147:836A.

83. Sestini P, Refini RM, Pieroni GM, Ferretti B, Bianco S, Vagliasindi M. Effect of inhaled furosemide on the protective activity of cromolyn sodium against the bronchial obstructive response to ultrasonically nebulized water. Eur Respir J 1993; 6(Suppl 17):199s.

84. Pavord ID, Wisniewski A, Tattersfield AE. Inhaled furosemide and exercise-induced asthma: evidence of a role for inhibiting prostanoids. Thorax 1992; 47: 797–800.

85. Vaghi A, Berni F, Robuschi M, Sestini P, Bianco S. Indomethacin (I) does not influence the protective effect of furosemide (F) against exercise-induced bronchoconstriction (EIB). Eur Respir J 1989; 2(Suppl 8):790s.

86. O'Connor BJ, Barnes PJ, Chung KF. The role of cyclooxygenase products in the inhibition of sodium metabisulphite-induced broncho-constriction by furosemide in asthma. Thorax 1994; 54:307–311.

87. Rodwell LT, Anderson SD, Spring J, Mohamed S, Seale JP. Effect of inhaled furosemide and oral indomethacin on the airway response to hypertonic saline challenge in asthmatic subjects. Thorax 1997; 52:59–66.

88. Bianco S, Refini RM, Pieroni MG, Ferretti B, Sestini P, Vagliasindi M. Potentiation of the protective effect of inhaled furosemide on allergen-induced bronchoconstriction by inhaled lysine acetylsalicylate. Eur Respir J 1991; 4:235s.

89. Robuschi M, Scuri M, Vaghi A, Spagnotto S, Gambaro G, Fai V, Sestini P, Bianco S. Inhaled acetylsalicylic acid enhances the protective activity of furosemide against exercise-induced bronchoconstriction. Am Rev Respir Dis 1992; 145:729.

90. Bianco S, Vaghi A, Robuschi M, Pieroni MG, Refini RM, Sestini P. Steroid-Sparing Effect of Inhaled Lysine-Aspirin and Furosemide in Steroid-Dependent Asthma. In: Melillo G, O'Byrne PH, Marone G, eds. Respiratory Allergy—Advances in Clinical Immunology and Pulmonary Medicine. Amsterdam: Elsevier, 1993: 261–269.

91. Bianco S, Vaghi A, Robuschi M, Refini RM, Pieroni MG, Sestini P. Steroid-sparing effect of inhaled lysine acetylsalicylate and furosemide in high-dose bechlomethasone-dependent asthma. J Allergy Clin Immunol 1995; 95:937–943.

92. Mullol J, Ramis I, Prat J, Rosselló-Cafatau J, Xaubet A, Piera C, Gelpi E, Picado C. Failure of furosemide to increase production of prostaglandin E_2 in human nasal mucosa in vitro. Thorax 1993; 48:260–263.

93. Levasseur-Acker GM, Molimard M, Regnard J, Naline E, Freche C, Lockart A. Effect of furosemide on prostaglandin synthesis by human nasal and bronchial epithelial cells in culture. Am J Respir Cell Mol Biol 1994; 10:378–383.

25

Role of Autoantibodies Against Endothelial Cells in Severe Asthma

PHILIPPE LASSALLE, MICHEL JOSEPH, and ANDRE-BERNARD TONNEL

Institut Pasteur
INSERM U416
Lille, France

I. Introduction

Among patients suffering from bronchial asthma, a few subjects require continuous treatment with oral steroids to control the airflow obstruction. They report a longer history of asthma, with more nocturnal wheezing, more dipping of morning PEF values, and also more severe bronchial hyperresponsiveness to methacholine. These symptoms constitute severe asthma, and, in the absence of recognized allergen sensitivity in skin tests and in the triggering of asthma attacks, they are generally referred to as nonallergic or *intrinsic* asthma. Between 10 and 20% of adults with severe asthma experience asthma attacks after ingestion of aspirin and nonsteroidal anti-inflammatory drugs (NSAID). In most cases, allergic mechanisms based on classic specific antigen-antibody reactions have been excluded. Among other arguments, the most compelling is the diversity of chemical agents, such as NSAID with totally different structures, which, besides aspirin, precipitate asthma attacks in sensitive patients. The symptoms associate aspirin sensitivity, asthma, and nasal polyps, an observation first reported by Widal and co-workers in

1922 (1) and named "the aspirin (or Widal) triad." For years the etiology of aspirin-induced asthma (AIA) has been a matter of successive hypotheses and sustained controversy.

Several concepts, reviewed a few years ago (2,3), were put forward to explain the pathogenesis of AIA. Most hypotheses were based on the inhibition of cyclooxygenase, a common property of the various drugs precipitating the rhinorrhea and the acute bronchospasm observed in these patients (4). However cyclooxygenase metabolites—i.e., prostanoids—do not seem to be involved directly, or at least solely, in the onset of asthma attacks. Among other compounds pointed out in conjunction with prostanoids, leukotrienes have been involved through the diversion of the arachidonic acid pathway induced by the inhibition of cyclooxygenase (5), with the possibility of an abnormal reactivity of AIA patients to leukotrienes or an impaired reciprocal control of lipoxygenase metabolites and of prostanoids on the functions of target cells and tissues (6).

In the perspective of a cyclooxygenase-dependent mechanism, the implication of chronic viral infections as triggering agents in aspirin-sensitive asthmatics has also been suggested (7). In this hypothesis, anticyclooxygenase compounds would inhibit the alveolar macrophage-mediated generation of PGE_2, which modulates the antiviral effects of cytotoxic lymphocytes toward lung cells chronically infected with virus. Chronically stimulated cytotoxic lymphocytes would therefore provoke deleterious effects in the respiratory tract with subsequent direct impact on smooth muscles.

In 1985, we proposed the participation of blood platelets in AIA, through an abnormal behavior of these cells in vitro in the presence of aspirin and NSAID (8). The metabolic parameter used to detect platelet sensitivity was the generation of cytotoxic mediators toward bystander *Schistosoma* larvae. In these conditions, platelets not only generated cytotoxic properties against schistosomules but were the only blood cell population to express such properties in vitro in the presence of aspirin and NSAID. However, we failed to detect other secreted metabolites that could be potentially and specifically involved in the bronchospastic response of patients. Furthermore, with the accumulation of experiments, although we never observed false negative tests (with aspirin-sensitive asthmatics exhibiting aspirin-insensitive platelets), about 10% patients with severe asthma gave false positive results in vitro (with aspirin-reactive platelets from patients tolerating aspirin perfectly well). We suggest that such a discrepancy might reflect a potential (and forthcoming?) evolution of severe asthmatics from the status of aspirin-tolerant to aspirin-sensitive patients. Nevertheless, a practical and relevant metabolic parameter in blood platelets from aspirin-dependent asthmatics is still lacking to validate our hypothesis (9).

II. Autoimmune Features in Severe Asthma and More Particularly AIA

More recently, autoimmunity was postulated as a background status characterizing the immune system of aspirin-dependent asthmatics, and more generally patients with severe asthma. There are few reports on clinical symptoms of autoimmunity in patients with severe asthma in spite of a high proportion of aspirin intolerance in asthmatics with autoantibodies (10). Therefore, the concept of autoimmune parameters associated with aspirin intolerance seems more or less a paradox. Immunosuppressive treatments, based on methotrexate, cyclosporin, or azathioprine, were evaluated in severe asthma with a certain degree of success (11–14). However, these tests were based uniquely on the clinical criterion of the severity. The lack of efficient markers allowing identification of autoimmunity in asthma has limited such clinical investigations.

In 1995, Szczeklik and co-workers published two papers closely linked to this subject. In the first (10) the authors have identified, in a large number of patients with asthma, the presence of antinuclear antibodies (ANA). ANA were found in 55% of AIA, the highest proportion among the 185 patients with asthma in this study, since ANA were present in 41% of aspirin-tolerant intrinsic asthmatics, 39% of atopic asthmatics, and only 11% of healthy subjects. These antibodies were directed against single-stranded DNA. No antinative double-stranded DNA nor antineutrophil cytoplasmic antibodies (ANCA) could be detected. ANA were frequently associated with various physiopathological manifestations such as signs of complement activation, circulating immune complexes, presence of rheumatoid factor, and clinical signs of autoimmunity (rheumatic symptoms—myalgias, arthralgias, morning stiffness, or transient arthritis—cold sensitivity, and Raynaud's phenomenon). Such a coincidence does not prove a causative link between the clinical symptoms of autoimmunity and asthma, but it provides a first interesting piece of information.

A second association of AIA with autoimmunity was reported (15) when it was observed that peripheral vasculitis, expressed on distal parts of the body by limited scleroderma in one patient or perniosis in another, together with ANA and circulating immune complexes, preceded by 5 years the onset of AIA. In these patients, autoimmune symptoms were precipitated by aspirin. The authors stressed the vascular abnormalities frequently observed in the lungs of patients with cold-sensitive peripheral vasculitis. They also underlined a suggestion by McFadden (16) to consider asthma as a vascular illness. The authors concluded that it was tempting to make a link between increased leukotriene generation in AIA, bronchial reactions, and increased vascular disorders.

At this point of the overview, our attention is focused on a new factor in the physiopathology of asthma (of the atopic or of the intrinsic form), namely the endothelial cell. Besides their role as filters for circulating inflammatory leukocytes between the blood flow and inflamed tissues, endothelial cells have to be considered as accessory cells of the immune response, especially as cytokine producers, with particular emphasis on eosinophil maturation and survival.

III. Involvement of Antiendothelial Antibodies

We have identified antiendothelial cell antibodies in cyclic angioedema with eosinophilia, in allergic granulomatosis and angiitis (against a 120-kDa antigen), in bronchial asthma (against a major antigen of 55 kDa present in endothelial cell and platelet lysates) (17). The anti-55-kDa antibodies were of various isotypes and found in the serum of 49% of patients with corticodependent severe asthma and 70% of patients with AIA, whereas they were present in the serum of 37% of intrinsic asthmatics and only 31% of allergic asthmatics. These sera induced platelet cytotoxicity against helminth larvae in a test similar to that described above for aspirin-sensitive platelets. T lymphocytes reactive to the same 55-kDa antigen were also found in patients with severe asthma (18). The T-cell proliferation was inversely correlated with pulmonary functions, returning to control level after treatment and normalization of FEV values in patients admitted in the emergency unit for acute asthma attacks. In another case report (19), a patient suffering from severe asthma and exhibiting circulating anti-55-kDa antibodies was given plasma exchanges. Unexpectedly, asthma symptoms progressively decreased, leading to a complete remission within 4 weeks of treatment. To our knowledge, only a few authors have reported some beneficial effects of plasma removal in severe asthma. Gartmann et al. (20) have reported clinical improvement following plasma exchange in a 54-year-old woman with severe and corticosteroid-dependent asthma. Bambauer et al. (21) have also reported clinical improvement following plasma exchange in two patients with severe asthma, one of whom had aspirin-sensitive asthma. These authors have also suggested that plasma exchange could rapidly remove antigen-antibody complexes as well as vasoactive or anaphylactic substances from plasma, which might be involved in the pathogenesis of asthma.

The mechanism of induction of autoantibodies in bronchial asthma is unknown. Are autoantibodies a cause or a consequence of the pathology? As observed by Szczeklik et al. (10), if they were a consequence of damaged cells and tissues, they should also be present for example in chronic bronchitis or emphysema, which is not the case in spite of smooth muscle or lung parenchyma destruction. One hypothesis could be that, in asthmatics, ineffective antigen elimination or exposure of autoantigens in the inflammatory process may cause chronic immune stimulation and autoantibody production. In severe asthma, circulating factor(s) involved in the severity of the disease do exist. One can speculate that anti-55-kDa autoantibodies might represent at least one of these, thus supporting the concept of autoimmunity in a subgroup of patients with severe and nonallergic asthma. To examine in more detail the effects of plasma exchanges in patients suffering from severe asthma, we have performed a clinical trial, the results of which are summarized below.

A. Effects of Plasma Exchanges on the Clinical Symptoms of Severe Asthmatics

Twelve patients fulfilling the criteria of asthma as defined by the American Lung Association were included in the clinical trial. The inclusion criteria were based on the degree of severity of asthma (FEV_1 < 70% after β_2 mimetic inhalation, duration of asthma up to 5 years, and continuous oral steroid therapy up to 10 mg/day for more than 4 years), and on the ability to tolerate plasma exchanges. The proposed treatment consisted of a series of two plasma exchanges per week for 3 weeks and one plasma exchange per week for the following 3 weeks. The plasma exchanges were replaced by methotrexate 7.5 mg per week, beginning at week 4, in association with one plasma exchange per week. Methotrexate was increased to 15 mg/week from the seventh week, when plasma exchanges were stopped. During the period of plasma exchanges, the accompanying oral and inhaled regimen was strictly unchanged. The follow-up was every 3 weeks for the first 6 months and every 6 weeks for the next 6 months. The progressive decrease of daily oral steroid therapy was proposed from the 10th week. The decrease and discontinuation of methotrexate was 1 year after inclusion.

Table 1 summarizes the clinical and biological characteristics of each patient. At the end of the 3 weeks of plasma exchanges the patients and their physicians gave their respective opinion on the efficacy of the treatment. The scale was 1 = very efficient; 2 = efficient; 3 = slightly efficient; 4 = no effect; 5 = side effects. Neither patients nor physicians quoted 5. The responsive patients included scores 1 and 2 (six patients, R group). The nonresponsive patients included scores 3 and 4 (six patients, NR group). The mean clinical and biological characteristics of the R and NR groups are shown in Table 2. The two groups of patients were very similar in most of the chosen criteria except that in the R group the sex ratio was three men–three women, whereas the other group was exclusively male. A second difference was that in the R group asthma symptoms presented no detectable allergic component, in contrast to the NR group which included three out of six severe asthmatics with an allergic component (positive skin tests toward at least two allergens).

Table 1 Clinical and Biological Characteristics of the Patients Included in the Clinical Trial

	Patient no.											
	1	2	3	4	5	6	7	8	9	10	11	12
Age, years	52	50	45	46	27	41	40	41	51	53	58	51
Sex	M	M	F	M	F	F	M	M	M	M	M	M
Atopy	0	0	0	0	0	0	+	0	0	0	+	+
ASA	0	0	0	0	+	+	+	0	0	0	0	0
Duration, years	17	3	4	2	4	8	5	2	6	3	3	11
Total IgE, RIU/L	140	1080	98	69	135	46	955	15	51	85	413	158
Rheumatoid factor	0	0	0	0	0	0	0	0	0	0	0	0
Antinuclear antibody	0	0	0	0	0	0	0	0	0	1:5	0	1:64
CIC, mg/L	0	0	3.1	0	0	2.5	0	0	0	0	0	0
Anti-55-kDa antibody	0	+	0	+	+	+	+	0	0	0	0	0

ASA, documented aspirin-sensitive asthma; antinuclear antibodies determined by indirect immunofluores cence and expressed in the highest positive dilution. CIC, circulating immune complexes; anti-55-kDa, posi tive (+) or negative (0) as determined by a 55-kDa band in Western blot with human umbilical vein endo thelial cell extracts.

In the R group, the plasma exchanges induced significant reduction of the dyspnea (scaled from 1 to 10 by the patient), of the number of daily inhaled β_2 puffs (Table 3). There was also a significant increase of the morning peak flow values (Table 3). Although the mean FEV_1 change was not significant, there was a strong increase of FEV_1 values in some patients (Table 3).

The presence of the circulating anti-55-kDa autoantibodies was found in five of 12 patients (Table 1). Four of them were in the R group and one in the NR group. In addition to the isolated case reported above (19), in five of seven patients plasma exchanges have been efficient against the severity of asthma. The patient with anti-55-kDa antibodies in the NR group exhibited an allergic component to both house dust mite and *Candida albicans*, which may account in part for his unresponsiveness.

These results suggest an association between the presence of the anti-55-kDa autoantibodies and the efficiency of the plasma exchanges. Thus, one can speculate that these autoantibodies may reveal a particular pathological pathway involving circulating factor(s) in the severity of asthma.

Table 2 Mean Clinical Characteristics of the Responsive and the Nonresponsive Groups Before Plasma Exchanges

	Responsive group	Nonresponsive group
Age, years	45 ± 9.2	50.5 ± 8.40
Sex (F/M)	3/3	0/6
Atopy	0/6	3/6
Aspirin-sensitive asthma	2/6	1/6
Duration of asthma, years	7.2 ± 6.0	12.5 ± 7.60
Duration of oral steroid therapy, years	4.8 ± 2.6	5.3 ± 3.2
Oral steroid therapy, mg/24 hr	21.7 ± 11.3	25 ± 9.5
Total IgE, kIU/L	261 ± 203	280 ± 260
CIC, mg/L	0.83 ± 1.35	0
Dyspnea, scale 1–10	4.3 ± 3.1	4.8 ± 1.7
$FEV_1\%$	69.7 ± 20.7	62.5 ± 14.8
No. of β_2 puffs per 24 hr	15.3 ± 5.60	11.7 ± 3.01
Nocturnal asthma, scale 0–4	1.41 ± 1.27	1.27 ± 1.20
Diurnal asthma, scale 0–4	1.51 ± 1.13	1.80 ± 1.24
Morning peak flow value, L/min	295 ± 131	275 ± 112

The data represent the mean ± SD of individual values.

Table 3 Mean Clinical Characteristics of the Responsive and Nonresponsive Groups After a 3-Week Treatment by Plasma Exchanges

	J 0	J 21	p (Student's t-test)
R group			
Dyspnea, scale 1–10	4.3 ± 3.1	2.2 ± 2.6	0.015
$FEV_1\%$	62.7 ± 20.7	84.1 ± 25.7	ns
No. of β_2 puffs per 24 hr	15.3 ± 5.60	5.3 ± 5.6	0.022
Nocturnal asthma, scale 0–4	1.41 ± 1.27	0.76 ± 1.17	ns
Diurnal asthma, scale 0–4	1.51 ± 1.13	0.54 ± 1.21	ns
Morning peak flow value, L/min	295 ± 131	343 ± 135	0.019
NR group			
Dyspnea, scale 1–10	4.8 ± 1.7	4.8 ± 2.1	ns
$FEV_1\%$	62.5 ± 14.8	59.7 ± 14.3	ns
No. of β_2 puffs per 24 hr	11.7 ± 3.01	10.8 ± 2.23	ns
Nocturnal asthma, scale 0–4	1.27 ± 1.20	1.03 ± 1.03	ns
Diurnal asthma, scale 0–4	1.80 ± 1.24	1.69 ± 1.33	ns
Morning peak flow value, L/min	275 ± 112	284 ± 079	ns

The data are the mean ± SD. The statistical analysis was performed with the paired Student's t-test.

B. Long-Term Evolution of the Disease After Plasma Exchange

The patients in the NR group followed the clinical trial for 6 months. Based on the absence of efficacy, the trial was stopped. Patients were followed monthly for 6 months with their initial treatment. Among the patients in the R group, two of them (one with, the other without autoantibodies) were followed up to 2 years with an apparent complete remission. In these two cases, the oral steroid therapy and the methotrexate were progressively stopped without reappearance of asthma symptoms. In the other four responsive patients, a relapse of asthma was observed, occurring upon the arrest of methotrexate for side effects (two cases), or reduction of daily oral steroid therapy (two cases). These patients were excluded from the clinical trial and followed up every 3 weeks for 6 months to 2 years.

As a whole, our clinical trial has induced transient remission in six of 12 patients suffering from severe asthma, and apparent stable remission in two of 12 patients. From these results it may be concluded that if anti-55-kDa autoantibodies represent a good marker of the short-term efficacy of plasma exchange therapy, their presence on long-term efficacy of this treatment appears questionable.

C. Dynamic Aspects of Asthma Noted During Follow-Up

During the course of the follow-up, the patients were asked to quote daily their clinical scores, the mean peak flow values, and the treatment received. The FEV_1 values and the biological data were recorded every 3 weeks. Unexpectedly, we have found, in three patients, that blood eosinophilia reappeared 2–4 weeks before asthma relapse. The 8-month follow-up of one of these three patients is shown in Figure 1. This patient, like the other two, belongs to the R group. The graphic follow-up shows that under plasma exchanges the peak flow values increased and the blood eosinophil counts decreased concomitantly. As indicated before, after the series of plasma exchanges a clinical state of remission was observed based on the clinical scores, peak flow values, FEV_1, and blood eosinophil counts. During the remission phase, the initial change observed was an increase of the blood eosinophil count, which was still observed 3 weeks later. Starting at this time, an increase of the peak flow instability was observed, which was associated with a progressive decrease of the mean peak flow. The asthma relapse occurred progressively to reach the level observed before the inclusion of this patient in the clinical trial. In this case, it was surprising that the relapse occurred progressively out of any infectious context. A second point is that the blood eosinophil count can represent a predictive marker, its increase preceding relapse from 2–4 weeks (4 weeks in this case). It is now clear from our own and several other studies that the level

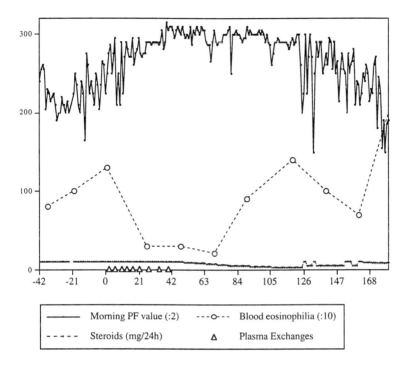

	Morning PF value (:2)	---o---	Blood eosinophilia (:10)
- - - - -	Steroids (mg/24h)	Δ	Plasma Exchanges

Figure 1   Evolution of the clinical and biological parameters during treatment with plasma exchanges in one patient. The time in the *X*-axis is recorded in days. Day 1 is the beginning of the treatment. The *Y*-axis is an arbitrary linear scale corresponding to (1:2) × (L/min) for the daily recorded morning peak flow values; to (1:10) × (blood eosinophil number per mm^3) for blood eosinophilia; and to mg/24 hr for oral steroid therapy.

of blood eosinophilia and the severity of asthma were strictly correlated (22–24). Here we have observed not only the same correlation, but that blood eosinophilia may be a predictive parameter, preceding the bronchial tissue infiltration and asthma. This particular feature was observed in three patients suffering from severe nonallergic asthma. Hypereosinophilia is the result of activated T-cell-derived cytokines, like IL-5. Such a T-cell activation can be detected through the dosage of soluble CD25 in plasma recovered at the same periods. We have found that sCD25 paralleled, but did not precede, the blood eosinophil increase. However, from these data, one can raise the hypothesis that, in a subgroup of nonallergic severe asthmatics, the chronic inflammatory bronchial disease may be the consequence of a chronic infiltration of eosinophils mediated by autoreactive or dysregulated T cells.

D. Comments

Plasma exchanges were effective in a subgroup of nonallergic and severe asthmatics. The effects of plasma exchanges were clinically detectable beginning at the fourth plasma exchange, after the second week of treatment. However, the remission state was transient, between 2 and 4 months. The relapse seemed to depend on several factors, including discontinuation of the immunosuppressive treatment and a too rapid decrease of oral steroids.

The pathogenesis of severe nonallergic asthma is thought to be due to T-cell-mediated hyperreactivity, including hypereosinophilia in both the bloodstream and bronchial tissues. Soluble IL-2 receptor (sCD23) is one marker of T-cell activation. Soluble CD25 in the plasma of severe asthmatics has been found elevated (24). It was associated with blood eosinophilia, and inversely correlated with the level of oral steroid therapy and lung function (as measured by FEV_1). Based on these data, one can suggest that in severe asthma there is a dynamic equilibrium between the cells and factors involved in the pathogenesis and the level of anti-inflammatory steroid therapy. The detailed follow-up of the patients undergoing a relapse of their disease clearly indicates that plasma sCD25 and blood eosinophilia preceded the relapse by a few weeks. The T-cell hyperreactivity that controls eosinopoiesis and hypereosinophilia in the bloodstream is the first step of the disease. The second step might include colonization of the bronchial tissues by eosinophils and the onset of asthma symptoms. Plasma exchanges were initiated at a stable state of the disease. With no change in the inhaled and oral therapy of patients, plasma exchanges have induced in the responsive group a decrease of blood eosinophilia. It is not known whether bronchial tissues underwent a similar decrease, but if they did, one can speculate that mediators involved in this process do exist in the bloodstream and can be removed by plasma exchange.

The factors responsible for such an abnormal T-cell reactivity are unknown. One can suggest that the anti-55-kDa autoantibodies might be one of these. The presence of such antibodies is associated with the responsive group of asthmatics. However, no real decrease of these antibodies was found during the plasma exchanges (evaluated by Western blot). Since the 55-kDa antigen can be released by blood platelets, we cannot exclude a possible decrease of the 55-kDa antigen concentration as a consequence of plasma exchanges immediately counterbalanced by platelets. The antigen has not been cloned yet. Much work has to be done to examine this speculative hypothesis. Hundreds of other plasmatic factors are removed by plasmapheresis, and it is unwise, at this stage, to attribute to the above biological parameters the origin of pathological symptoms. Nevertheless, the common characteristics of the above reports are the onset of vascular inflammation or disorders together with autoantibodies, some of which seem to be specific for endothelial cells and platelets.

IV. Conclusion

If autoimmune phenomena are so frequently present in severe asthmatics and in patients with aspirin-intolerant asthma, why are they so underestimated or ignored by clinicians? Szczeklik et al. made a relevant observation (10): only occasionally do autoimmune symptoms prompt patients to seek medical attention, either because they are of weak intensity or because their presence is overshadowed by major problems related to asthma. One explanation of such a low symptomatology is that severe asthmatics are under strong corticotherapy, which may keep autoimmune symptoms below detectable levels. Still unknown is the actual link between autoimmune manifestations and intrinsic severe asthma, with particular emphasis on AIA. Are autoimmune processes, fortuitously, simultaneous with other abnormal metabolic pathways involved in asthma, without any causative link? Or are modifications of endothelial functions, induced by autoantibodies, the cause of a precise but unclear disturbance of eicosanoid metabolism? Rather than providing definitive conclusions about the problem, the purpose of this short review was to stimulate speculation and new possibilities in the search for evidence on a connection between autoimmune phenomena and severe asthma.

References

1. Widal MF, Abramin P, Lermoyez J. Anaphylaxie et idiosyncrasie. Presse Med 1922; 30:198–192.
2. Szczeklik A, Virchow C, Schmitz-Schumann M. Pathophysiology and pharmacology of aspirin-induced asthma. In: Page CP, Barnes PJ, eds. Pharmacology of Asthma. Heidelberg: Springer Verlag, 1991:291–314.
3. Szczeklik A. Aspirin-induced asthma: pathogenesis and clinical presentation. Allergy Proc 1992; 13:163–173.
4. Szczeklik A, Gryglewski RJ, Czerniawska-Mysik G. Relationship of inhibition of prostaglandin biosynthesis by analgesics to asthma attacks in aspirin-sensitive patients. Br Med J 1975; 1:67–69.
5. Lee TH, Christie PE. Leukotrienes and aspirin induced asthma. Thorax 1993; 48: 1189–1190.
6. Christie PE, Tagari P, Ford-Hutchinson AW, Charlesson S, Chee P, Arm JP, Lee TH. Urinary leukotriene E4 concentrations increase after aspirin challenge in aspirin-sensitive subjects. Am Rev Respir Dis 1991; 143:1025–1029.
7. Szczeklik A. Aspirin-induced asthma as a viral disease. Clin Allergy 1988; 18:15–20.
8. Ameisen JC, Capron A, Joseph M, Maclouf J, Vorng H, Pancré V, Fournier E, Wallaert B, Tonnel AB. Aspirin-sensitive asthma: abnormal platelet response to drugs inducing asthmatic attacks. Diagnostic and physiopathological implications. Int Arch Allergy Appl Immun 1985; 78:438–448.

9. Ameisen JC, Capron A, Joseph M, Tonnel AB. Platelets and aspirin-induced asthma. In: Kay AB, ed. Asthma: Clinical Pharmacology and Therapeutic Progress. Oxford: Blackwell Scientific Publications, 1986:226–236.

10. Szczeklik A, Nizankowska E, Serafin A, Dyczek A, Duplaga M, Musial J. Autoimmune phenomena in bronchial asthma with special reference to aspirin intolerance. Am J Respir Crit Care Med 1995; 152:1753–1756.

11. Mullarkey MF, Blumenstein BA, Andrade WP, Olason I, Wetzel CE. Methotrexate in the treatment of corticosteroid-dependent asthma. A double-blind crossover study. N Engl J Med 1988; 318:603–607.

12. Alexander AG, Barnes NC, Kay AB. Trial of cyclosporin in corticosteroid-dependent chronic severe asthma. Lancet 1992; 339:324–328.

13. Nizankowska E, Soja J, Pinis G, Bochenek G, Sladek K, Domagala B, Pajak A, Szczeklik A. Treatment of steroid dependent bronchial asthma with cyclosporin. Eur Respir J 1995; 8:1091–1099.

14. Irwin RS, Curley FJ, French CL. Difficult-to-control asthma. Contributing factors and outcome of a systematic management protocol. Chest 1993; 103:1662–1669.

15. Szczeklik A, Musial J, Dyczek A, Bartosik A, Milewski M. Autoimmune vasculitis preceding aspirin-induced asthma. Int Arch Allergy Immunol 1995; 106:92–94.

16. McFadden ERJ. Microvasculature and airway responses. Am Rev Respir Dis 1992; 145:S42–S43.

17. Lassalle P, Gosset P, Gruart V, Prin L, Capron M, Lagrue G, Kusnierz JP, Tonnel AB, Capron A. Presence of antibodies against endothelial cells in the sera of patients with episodic angioedema and hypereosinophilia. Clin Exp Immunol 1990; 82:38–43.

18. Lassalle P, Delneste Y, Gosset P, Gras Masse H, Wallaert B, Tonnel AB. T and B cell immune response to a 55-kDa endothelial cell-derived antigen in severe asthma. Eur J Immunol 1993; 23:796–803.

19. Lassalle P, Joseph M, Ramon P, Dracon M, Tonnel AB, Capron A. Plasmapheresis in a patient with severe asthma associated with auto-antibodies to platelets. Clin Exp Allergy 1990; 20:707–712.

20. Gartmann J, Grob P, Frey M. Plasmapheresis in severe asthma. Lancet 1978; 1:40.

21. Bambauer R, Jutzler GA, Micka K, Austgen M, Schlimmer P, Trendelenburg F. Drug-resistant bronchial asthma successfully treated with plasma exchange. J Clin Apheresis 1984; 2:200–205.

22. Horn BR, Robin ED, Theodore J, van Kesel A. Total eosinophil counts in the management of bronchial asthma. N Engl J Med 1975; 292:1152–1155.

23. Bousquet J, Chanez P, Lacoste JY. Eosinophilic infiltration in asthma. N Engl J Med 1990; 323:1033–1039.

24. Lassalle P, Sergant M, Delneste Y, Gosset P, Wallaert B, Zandecki M, Capron A, Joseph M, Tonnel AB. Levels of soluble IL-2 receptor in plasma from asthmatics. Correlations with blood eosinophilia, lung function, and corticosteroid therapy. Clin Exp Immunol 1992; 87:266–271.

26

Clinical Course of Aspirin-Induced Asthma
Results of AIANE*

EWA NIŻANKOWSKA, MARIUSZ DUPLAGA, GRAŻYNA BOCHENEK, and ANDRZEJ SZCZEKLIK

Jagiellonian University School of Medicine
Krakow, Poland

I. The AIANE Project

Since its rediscovery in the late 1960s by Samter (1), aspirin-induced asthma (AIA) has been inspiring a lot of interest among basic and clinical researchers. In 1993 21 university departments from 14 European countries jointly set up the European Network on Aspirin-Induced Asthma (AIANE). The Department of Medicine in Krakow has been the coordinating center, and the whole project was financially aided by the Commission of the European Communities. One of the chief aims of the AIANE has been to provide a good insight into the clinical course of AIA. For this purpose a relational database has been developed.

---

*On behalf of the AIANE Project. AIANE participating centers: Barcelona (C. Picado), Berlin (G. Kunkel, J. Niechus), Jena (L. Jäger, A. Machnik), Lille (M. Joseph), London (T. Lee), Łódź (J. Rożniecki, P. Kuna, M. L. Kowalski), Marseille (D. Vervloet), Milan (S. Bianco), Montpellier (J. Bousquet, P. Godard), Porto (M. Vaz Azavedo, J. Rodrigues), Rome (G. Patriarca, C. D'Ambrosio), Sophia (T. A. Popov).

II. Software Tool Development

The database of the AIANE network was developed with the use of MS access 1.1 package. The choice of the database software was dictated by such criteria as cost-effectiveness, user friendliness of the interface, and the possibility of quick modification of the software. Work on the database was initiated in the University Department of Medicine, Krakow in 1993, before the final acceptance of the AIANE project by European Community.

The prototype version of the AIANE database was distributed to the chosen centers of the AIANE project, and was subsequently amended, following intensive discussions during the workshops held in 1994 and 1995.

The final version of the software was issued in October 1995. Simultaneously, all AIANE centers involved in data collection on AIA obtained software tools enabling them to transfer the data gathered in previous versions of the AIANE database to the final one. The present structure of the database covers most of research areas on AIA in Europe.

III. The AIANE Database Structure

The structure of the database is patient-oriented. The main form consists of three sections. The first section enables the selection of conditions that are used to create the list of patients that will be available during further use of the database. The second section is devoted to data entry. The data are entered in four clusters: personal and demographic data, medical history, results of laboratory and diagnostic tests, and follow-up of the patient. The third section of the main form enables quick presentation of charts showing basic statistical data.

Data on 365 aspirin-intolerant asthmatics from 14 university departments in eight countries have been collected in the main database (Figs. 1, 2).

A. Sex

Among 365 patients, there were 254 women and 111 men. This proportion was observed not only in the whole population of the AIANE patients, but also in nearly all groups of patients from the countries participating in the project.

The predominance of women in AIA had already been noticed by Widal et al. (2) and then repeatedly confirmed by many clinicians. The group of 45 patients with AIA reported by Friedlaender and Feinberg included 28 women and 17 men (3). Samter and Beers reported that the proportion of women to men in their group of patients was three to two (1), while of 37 AIA patients of Settipane et al. (4), women constituted 76%. The analysis of questionnaires obtained from 457 patients with bronchial asthma carried out by Enomoto et al. also confirmed that female patients more frequently reported symptoms of

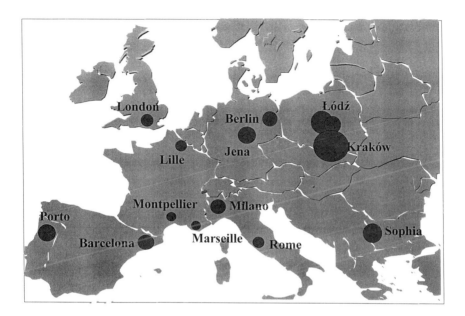

Figure 1 Centers participating in the data collection. The diameter of the circles varies depending on the number of patients entered in the database.

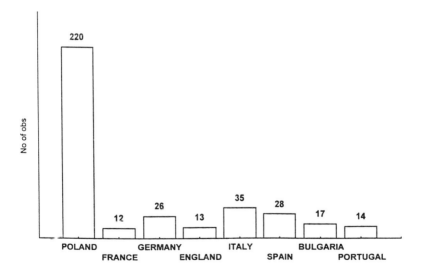

Figure 2 Numbers of patients from different European countries.

aspirin intolerance (5). The same is true for the pediatric patients: Giraldo et al. described seven patients with AIA under 20 years of age, all of them female (6). On the basis of studies in a large group of asthmatic children, Falliers concluded that females were more prone to develop asthma and aspirin intolerance even though in this age group the males prevailed among the asthmatic patients (7).

B. Age

The mean age of patients was 46.0 ± 12.4 years. There were no significant differences between the mean age of males and females (45.9 vs. 46.1 years, respectively). The age distribution in the whole population of AIANE patients is shown in Figure 3; the majority of patients were in their thirties to sixties.

C. Age of Appearance of Symptoms

Figures 4 and 5 present the age of appearance of the first symptoms of bronchial asthma and aspirin intolerance.

The mean age of the appearance of bronchial asthma was 32.1 ± 13.6 years. It was preceded by symptoms of rhinosinusitis (30.1 ± 12.8 years). The diagnosis of nasal polyps and appearance of aspirin intolerance was delayed by about 3 years in relation to bronchial asthma (35.4 ± 12.1 and 35.5 ± 12.4 years, respectively; Fig. 6).

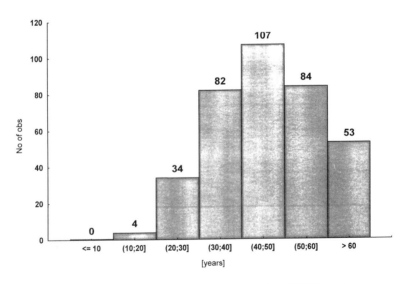

Figure 3   Ages of the patients registered in the AIANE database.

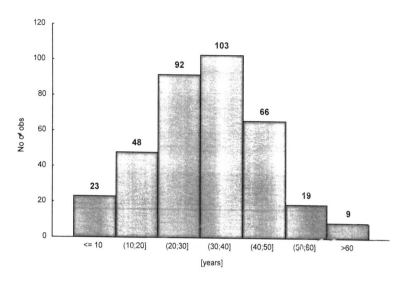

Figure 4 Age at appearance of bronchial asthma symptoms.

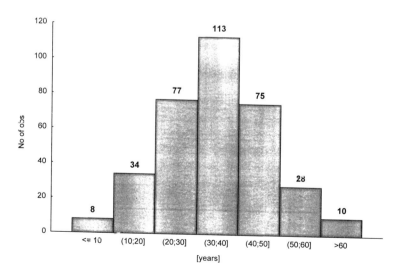

Figure 5 Age at appearance of first symptoms of aspirin intolerance.

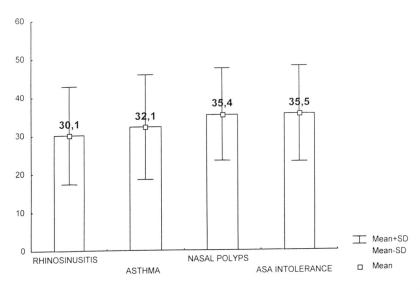

Figure 6 Age at appearance of rhinosinusitis, bronchial asthma, nasal polyps, and aspirin intolerance.

The same mean age of bronchial asthma appearance (32.1 years of life) was reported by Ogino et al. in a group of 18 patients with symptoms of asthma and/or rhinorrhea provoked by ingestion of nonsteroidal anti-inflammatory drugs, while rhinosinusitis occurred earlier than in AIANE patients (25.4 years) (8).

In the majority of AIANE patients the first symptoms of aspirin intolerance appeared during the third, fourth, or fifth decade of life. In some cases, symptoms developed before puberty—as early as at the age of 6. In other cases they occurred after 60 years of age. In most cases the appearance of aspirin intolerance took the patients by surprise. Many of them used to take aspirin without adverse reactions in the past. The occurrence of aspirin intolerance in the wide interval from 1 to 60 years of life was underlined by Speer et al. (9). These authors emphasized also that women of "childbearing age" were particularly at risk of developing aspirin intolerance (9).

In the group of 21 patients described by Pina et al. that revealed various reactions after ingestion of aspirin, women also prevailed (81%) (10). The onset of bronchial asthma with aspirin intolerance in children was analyzed by Falliers (7). She found that AIA appeared decidedly later than asthma without aspirin intolerance (medians; 11 vs. 2 years). Grzelewska-Rzymowska et al. observed that in 52 aspirin-intolerant asthmatics only 11.5% revealed symptoms of aspirin intolerance before the development of bronchial asthma (11).

D. Overall Incidence of ASA Intolerance in Asthma

The issue of incidence of aspirin intolerance in patients with bronchial asthma has not been the subject of our study. The values reported by various authors differed between 2% and 20%, and it seems that overall incidence of aspirin intolerance depends on the method used for setting diagnosis (history of adverse reaction vs. challenge test with aspirin) (5–7,12–17). The data on the incidence of aspirin intolerance among patients with bronchial asthma according to the literature are included in Table 1. The lowest incidence of aspirin intolerance was generally reported in children with bronchial asthma (7). On the other hand, aspirin intolerance appears to be more frequent in patients with severe asthma (15,17,18). Confusion could stem from the fact that some authors included urticarial reactions in their reports. It seems that most of these reactions have other etiopathogenesis (19,20).

E. Frequency and Symptoms of Intolerance to NSAIDs

Most patients (86.6%) indicated aspirin as the drug precipitating first symptoms of intolerance; derivatives of pyrazolones (aminophenazone, noramidopirine) were second. Patients who had first symptoms following pyrazolones administration usually experienced one or several episodes following ingestion of aspirin.

Table 1 Incidence of Aspirin Intolerance Among Patients with Bronchial Asthma According to the Data from Literature

Author	Year of publication	Method	Frequency of aspirin intolerance (%)
Van Leeuwen (12)	1928	Oral challenge	16.0
Giraldo et al. (6)	1969	History	5.8
			3.0
McDonald et al. (14)	1972	Oral challenge	8.0
Chafee and Settipane (13)	1973	History	4.3
Falliers (7)	1973	History	1.9
Settipane et al. (4)	1973	History	3.8
Harnett et al. (15)	1976	Oral challenge	11.6/54.0[a]
Kosturkov et al. (16)	1980	History	8.7
Scherrer et al. (17)	1984	History	4.5
Picado et al. (18)	1989	History	8
Enomoto et al. (5)	1995	History	12.0/29.0[a]

[a]The second value refers to those patients from the entire study group who had particularly severe bronchial asthma.

F. Symptoms of Aspirin Intolerance

After ingestion of aspirin most patients experienced an acute asthma attack. In nearly half of them, it was accompanied by nasal symptoms (nasal blockage, rhinorrhea).

A considerable number of patients gave a history of skin symptoms: rash or a distinct redness of head and neck, urticaria, or seldom angioedema. In 15 patients (4.1%) aspirin ingestion led to anaphylactic(oid) shock (Fig. 7). The data concerning the frequency of anaphylactic(oid) shock are not easy to interpret. In some cases very severe, dramatic dyspnea caused by acute bronchospasm might have led to acute asphyxia with subsequent loss of consciousness. These reactions could have been erroneously classified as anaphylactic shock. The anaphylactic shock caused by aspirin may occur after a prolonged latent period (21).

The symptoms related to bronchospasm were reported as the most frequent manifestation of aspirin intolerance by Chafee and Settipane (13). Its frequency in 89 aspirin-intolerant patients was 66% whereas urticaria or angioedema occurred in 33% of patients and rhinosinusitis in 10%. In the prospective study of Speer et al. (9) the most frequent manifestation of aspirin intolerance was urticaria or angioedema, the second most common being asthma. However, the group of patients revealing symptoms of aspirin intolerance were not necessarily asthmatic patients. Other authors confirmed a high frequency

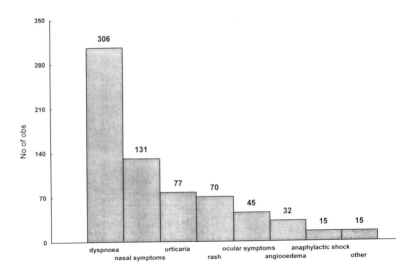

Figure 7 Frequency of symptoms of aspirin intolerance.

of bronchospastic reactions after ingestion of NSAIDs (10,16). Pina et al. reported that of 21 patients with aspirin intolerance 11 showed symptoms of bronchial asthma and in two patients aspirin provoked anaphylactic shock.

G. Symptoms of Intolerance to Pyrazolones and Other NSAID

Among symptoms caused by pyrazolones acute dyspnea prevailed, followed by nasal symptoms and skin reactions (Fig. 8). This frequency of symptoms is somewhat different from that manifested by subjects, usually nonasthmatics, who are exclusively sensitive to pyrazolones, but tolerate aspirin well (19). Their main manifestation consists of angioedema, urticaria, and anaphylactic shock. The etiopathogenesis of this type of reaction to pyrazolones seems to be quite different from that in patients sensitive to aspirin and pyrazolones (20).

Hypersensitivity to other NSAIDs (arylaliphatic acids, diclofenac; acetic acids, indomethacin; enolic acids, piroxicam) was reported by about 20% of all patients in the database.

H. History of Hypersensitivity to Other Than NSAID Drugs

Nearly 20% of patients reported sensitivity to antibiotics; however, we did not have any objective confirmation of this hypersensitivity. Sensitivity to

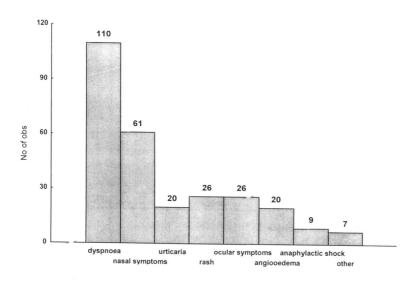

Figure 8 Frequency of symptoms of pyrazolones intolerance.

sulfonamides was reported by 6.6% of patients, and to local anesthetics and vitamins by 3.3% of patients.

A few authors dealt with the frequency of hypersensitivity to drugs other than NSAIDs in patients with aspirin sensitivity. Multiple drug allergy was reported in 18% of 89 patients with aspirin intolerance by Chafee and Settipane (13). Among the patients described by Speer et al. (9) in 43% of patients the sensitivity to other drugs was found.

I. Family History of NSAIDs Intolerance

Only 19 of 365 (5.2%) patients in the AIANE database reported a positive family history of NSAIDs intolerance. This was mainly rhinitis, but in some cases also bronchoconstriction with wheezing, sporadically urticaria. The occurrence of NSAIDs intolerance in the family of the patients was addressed in some previous studies. None of 45 aspirin-intolerant asthmatics described by Friedlaender and Feinberg (3) had a positive family history of NSAIDs intolerance. Among 25 children suffering from bronchial asthma and aspirin intolerance, only in one was intolerance to NSAIDs present in the family (7). The incidence of NSAIDs intolerance in the family of a group of 52 aspirin-intolerant asthmatics studied by Grzelewska-Rzymowska et al. (11) (5.8%) was nearly equal to that found in the AIANE patients. A few reports on clustering of aspirin intolerance in families were published (22–25); the concept of aspirin intolerance as an autosomal recessive trait remains unproved.

J. Main Asthmatic Complaints and Factors Associated with Their Appearance

The chief complaint was dyspnea (93.4%) followed by cough (77.3%), wheezing (51.8%), and increased sputum production (40.3%).

Patients were asked to determine, if possible, factors coinciding with their first asthmatic symptoms. Nearly half of the patients indicated infection of the respiratory tract (Fig. 9). Interestingly, 14.4% of patients reported ingestion of NSAIDs as the cause of the first asthmatic attack. AIA often begins as an upper respiratory tract illness, resembling a viral infection. However, unlike most viral infections of the upper respiratory tract, inflammation in nasal and sinus membranes persists and evolves into a chronic eosinophilic rhinosinusitis with or without nasal polyps and secondary purulent infection in the paranasal sinuses (26–29).

K. Triggering Factors of Bronchial Asthma

Among the factors that may exacerbate the course of asthma or provoke the appearance of symptoms, the AIANE patients most frequently enumerated psychological stress and physical exercise (both in nearly two-thirds of patients; Fig. 10). Some of the patients linked the exacerbation of their symptoms with

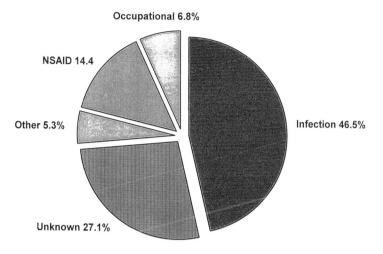

Figure 9 Factors associated with appearance of the first asthma symptoms.

clear-cut exposure to inhaled allergens; they had positive skin prick tests with some inhaled allergens (Table 2).

L. Total IgE (AIANE Patients from Krakow)

The differences in methods of total IgE measurement, number, and interpretation of skin tests in participating European centers made the comparison of

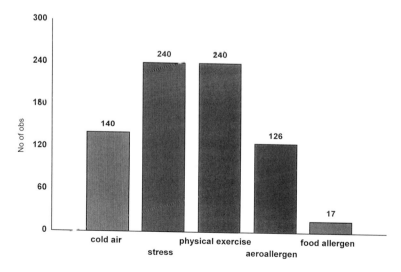

Figure 10 Potential triggering factors in relation to asthma symptoms.

Table 2 Contribution of Inhaled Allergens to
Asthma Symptom Exacerbations in History of the
AIANE Patients

Allergen	% of patients ($n = 126$)
Mites	65
Grasses	48
Trees	21
Weeds	12
Animal dander	41
Moulds	23

these data unreliable. The results presented below were obtained in a group
of AIANE patients from Krakow. In this group total IgE was determined by
particle-enhanced nephelometry with the Na-Latex IgE test (Behring, Germany). Most patients had values below 100 IU/ml, which is frequently considered the upper limit of the normal range. However, the upper limits of normal
IgE values are also a matter of controversy, because serum levels of IgE vary
according to sex, age, race, smoking habits, and concomitant disease (30,31).
The geometric mean in this group of patients was 80.6 IU/ml. In 38.2% of
patients this value exceeded 100 IU/ml. As reported earlier, the total IgE

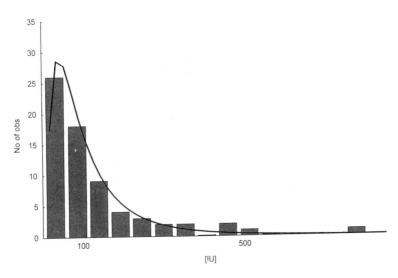

Figure 11 Distribution of total IgE values in patients from Krakow.

values had log-normal distribution (Fig. 11); this distribution pattern was not different from that observed in the general population.

M. Pulmonary Function Tests and Atopy (AIANE, Krakow)

FEV_1 measurements in the AIANE patients from Krakow are shown in Figure 12. In about 6% of examined patients symptoms were difficult to control despite the therapy, as evidenced by FEV_1 below 50% of the predicted value. Half of the patients had mild or moderate bronchial obstruction at the time of the data entry.

Skin prick tests were positive in 19% of patients examined ($n = 63$). They were considered positive if at least one allergen produced a wheal of at least 3 mm. The most common inhaled allergens were house dust, mixed grasses, mixed trees, *Dermatophagoides pteronyssinus*, animal dander and *Alternaria*.

The features of atopy in patients with AIA were analyzed by Van Leeuwen (12), who found relative paucity of positive skin tests; cutaneous and intracutaneous tests with food were always negative. Twenty years later, Friedlaender and Feinberg (3) reported that 16 of 42 patients with AIA had positive skin tests with at least one common inhalant or food allergen. In the group of patients with aspirin intolerance described by Samter and Beers, only 3.0% also had a personal history of atopy, and surprisingly, 50% of them had a positive family history of atopy (1). In a later publication of Samter, family history of atopy was positive in 22.5% of 284 aspirin-intolerant patients (32). In the same group skin reactions to seasonal and environmental inhalant allergens

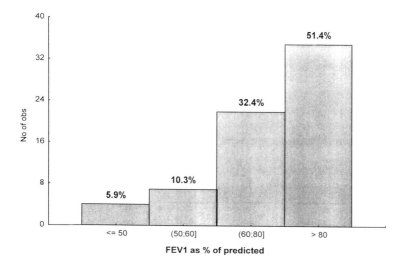

Figure 12 Distribution of FEV_1 values in the AIANE patients from Krakow.

were positive in 11.3% of subjects. In the group of 89 subjects with aspirin intolerance studied by Giraldo et al. (6) family history of atopy was positive in 65.6%, and skin tests in 50%. Walton and Randle reported a 65% frequency of positive family history of atopy in their patients with aspirin intolerance (33). Among 89 aspirin-intolerant patients analyzed by Chafee and Settipane (13) family history of asthma or rhinitis was positive in 51% of patients and positive skin tests occurred in 65%. Falliers (7) reported a 28% frequency of positive history of asthma, eczema, or rhinitis among 25 children with AIA. In the analysis of 52 aspirin-intolerant asthmatics, Grzelewska-Rzymowska et al. found that 70% of patients exhibited at least two features of atopy (positive history and positive skin tests) (11). Skin tests were also positive in seven of nine patients with AIA in the study reported by Ogino et al. (8). In another group of patients from Krakow, studied by Bochenek et al. (34), the geometric mean of total IgE was 62.2 IU/ml in aspirin-intolerant asthmatics. In the same group at least one positive skin test with common allergens was noted in 43.6% of patients (34 of 78 patients). Family history was positive in 34.6% and personal history of atopy in 21.8% of these patients. In this study, no difference in frequency of positive personal or family history or positive skin tests was found between aspirin-intolerant asthmatics and patients with exclusive hypersensitivity to pyrazolones.

N. Corticosteroid Therapy

The use of inhaled steroids was high: 79.2% of study patients were treated with them in the course of their illness (beclomethasone or budesonide). The dose of inhaled steroids used before registration in the AIANE database was also recorded. The differences between mean doses used in seven countries were not considerable (range: 902–1384 μg; Table 3).

Oral corticosteroids were used in the years before registration in the AIANE database by more than half of all patients (51.2%). A dose of oral corticosteroids ingested by the patients for the longest interval during 12 months preceding registration of the patient in the AIANE database was 8.7 $\pm$ 5.9 mg of prednisone equivalent (Table 4).

Nearly 20% (71 of 365) of the patients were treated with intravenous corticosteroids in the year preceding registration in the database. This number is consistent with the frequency of emergency interventions in this population of patients.

Depot preparations of corticosteroids administered during the preceding year were given to 18 patients, mainly in the group from Poland (9 of 220 patients) and Spain (9 of 28 patients).

All patients registered in the AIANE database who were treated with oral corticosteroids were questioned about the occurrence of side effects. The data are presented in Table 5.

Table 3 Mean Doses of Inhaled Corticosteroids in Patients During 12 Months Before Registration in the AIANE Database, According to the Country[a]

Country	Number of patients	Mean dose ± SD
Bulgaria	10	945 ± 492
France	12	1316 ± 522
Germany	17	1384 ± 1907
Italy	11	1064 ± 753
Poland	173	1167 ± 471
Portugal	12	1054 ± 564
Spain	27	902 ± 475
All patients	270	1137 ± 669

[a]Values expressed in μg.

O. Admissions to Hospital and Emergency Interventions due to Exacerbations of Asthma in the Preceding 12 Months

Of 365 patients registered in the AIANE database, 35 subjects were hospitalized at least once because of exacerbation of bronchial asthma during the year preceding the AIANE registration.

Most of them were hospitalized once or twice, but a few were admitted 3–7 times (Fig. 13). Among the patients admitted to hospital more than 3 times in the preceding 12 months were three patients from Poland and four from

Table 4 Mean Maintenance Doses of Oral Corticosteroids Used by Patients for the Longest Interval During 12 Months Before Registration in the AIANE Database, According to the Country[a]

Country	Number of patients (% of total population)	Mean dose ± SD
Bulgaria	12 (70.6)	14.6 ± 5.0
France	3 (25)	13.7 ± 11.0
Germany	4 (15.4)	5.5 ± 1.4
Italy	4 (11.4)	8.0 ± 4.0
Poland	102 (46.4)	8.2 ± 5.6
Portugal	5 (35.7)	10.8 ± 9.4
Spain	9 (32.1)	5.4 ± 1.6
All patients	139	8.7 ± 5.9

[a]Values expressed as dose of prednisone in mg.

Table 5 Frequency of Side Effects of Oral Corticosteroid
Therapy

Side effect	% of patients
Obesity	26.5
Osteoporosis	25.9
Arterial hypertension	17.3
Gastrointestinal ulcers	15.1
Myopathy	8.1
Modification of behavior	7.6
Acne	5.4
Hypertrichosis	4.9
Impairment of glucose tolerance	4.3
Cataract	2.7

Bulgaria. They suffered from severe corticodependent asthma and they usually
were hospitalized in internal medicine wards of local hospitals. All of them
received at least 10–20 mg of prednisolone for prolonged periods. The remaining 330 patients had no history of hospital admission in the preceding year or
the data on this event were not included.

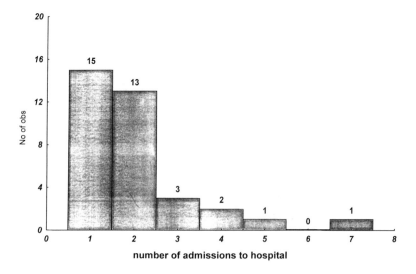

Figure 13 Frequency of admissions to hospital in the 12 months before registration
of the patient in the AIANE database ($n = 35$).

P. Emergency Care

The number of AIANE patients who needed emergency intervention due to an attack of asthma during the 12 months preceding history taking was nearly twice as high as the number of patients admitted to hospital ($n = 61$). The number of emergency interventions ranged from one to even 12 in one patient.

The need for emergency intervention as well as the necessity of hospital admission due to exacerbations of bronchial asthma indicates a severe course of asthma in a fairly large group of the AIANE patients. It goes along with the suggestions made in the twenties (12) and forties (3) about aspirin sensitivity as an indicator of the severity of asthma. This "unusual severity and chronicity" of asthmatic symptoms in patients with aspirin intolerance was repeatedly described by many authors during the last decades. Moreover, Picado et al. (18) found that 8% of patients admitted to the intensive care unit because of asthmatic attack were patients with aspirin intolerance. The severe course of AIA was also emphasized in the report of Enomoto et al. (5), who described more frequent use of ambulance, treatment in emergency rooms, and hospitalizations in aspirin-intolerant than aspirin-tolerant asthmatics.

Q. Use of Drugs Other Than Corticosteroids for Treatment of Asthma

The majority of patients with AIA used inhaled β-mimetics, similarly to the general population of asthmatics. Relatively large groups of patients were also treated with methyloxanthines and cromoglycates (Fig. 14).

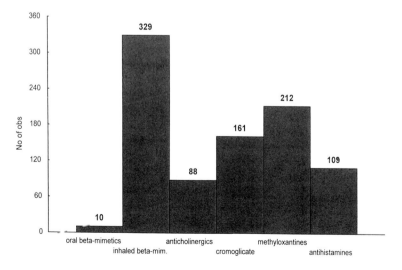

Figure 14 Use of drugs other than corticosteroids for treatment of asthma.

There are no controlled studies on the effects of prolonged treatment with methyloxanthines or cromoglycates on the clinical course of AIA. However, in many experimental challenges both drugs seemed to attenuate or prevent adverse effects provoked by aspirin challenge. Pasargiklian et al. commented on the favorable influence of aminophylline in protecting against aspirin-induced bronchospasm (35). The effect of cromolyn sodium on aspirin-induced reactions were studied in the seventies and eighties (36–38). These authors usually found only mild or moderate attenuation of aspirin-provoked reactions. Similarly, antihistamines, such as clemastine and ketotifen, were found to have only a moderate protective effect on aspirin-induced bronchospasm, but they significantly diminished extrabronchial symptoms of untoward aspirin reactions like rash, sneezing, and rhinorrhea (39–41). The results of the above-mentioned clinical experimental studies could explain the widespread usage of these drugs by physicians participating in the AIANE project.

R. Incidence and Symptoms of Rhinosinusitis

The majority of AIANE patients (77.5%) suffered from the symptoms of rhinosinusitis and complained of nasal blockage accompanied by rhinorrhea. Loss of smell occurred in 67.5% of these patients. Numerous patients also indicated sneezing as a symptom of rhinosinusitis.

In 71% of 34 AIANE patients from Krakow we found significant abnormalities in almost all paranasal sinuses. Minor abnormalities were found in another 14% of patients examined. A normal computed-tomography (CT) image was seldom observed.

In a group of patients described by Ogino et al. (8), the sinusitis was confirmed in 81.8% of X-rays. Any combination of air fluid levels, mucosal thickening, or opacification of one or more paranasal sinuses was present in over 90% of ASA-sensitive patients in other studies (27,42). These lesions can usually be demonstrated with routine roentgenograms or more clearly and in greater detail with CT (43,44).

S. Factors Coinciding with Appearance of First Symptoms of Rhinosinusitis

Only about 40% of patients with rhinosinusitis were able to determine clearly factors coinciding with the beginning of symptoms. Respiratory infection was most frequently indicated. Aspirin or other NSAID were reported rarely as a precipitating factor (4.8% of all patients with rhinosinusitis).

T. Nasal Polyps

Nasal polyps were diagnosed in 58.1% of the AIANE patients (212 of all 365 patients registered in the database). Friedlaender and Feinberg found

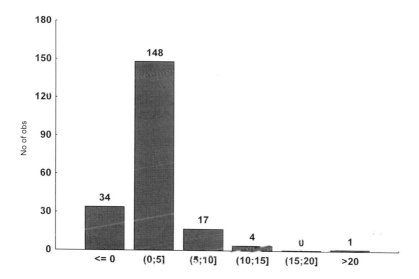

Figure 15 Number of polypectomies in patients with nasal symptoms.

rhinosinusitis with polyposis in 21 of 45 patients with AIA (3). In the study of Chafee and Settipane (13), 36% of aspirin-intolerant patients had nasal polyps. The incidence of nasal polyps in patients with AIA reported by Grzelewska-Rzymowska et al. (11) and by Ogino et al. (8) was even higher (77.0% and 72.2%, respectively). The latter authors pointed out that polyps had a tendency to recur, and seven of 13 patients had to have repeated polypectomies.

Multiple polypectomies were common among AIANE patients. On average they did not exceed five but in sporadic patients they were as high as 10–15 (Fig. 15).

The evident tendency of nasal polyps to recur observed in patients with AIA was emphasized earlier (45).

U. Nasal Corticosteroid Therapy for Rhinosinusitis

A total of 65.7% of patients suffering from rhinosinusitis were treated with nasal corticosteroids. The positive effects of corticosteroids on diminishing the recurrences in most patients with polyposis were described earlier (46,47). Many authors confirm that sinusitis associated with AIA is often difficult to treat. Antibiotics, decongestants, and a prolonged use of systemic corticosteroids, followed by topical corticosteroid therapy for maintenance, seems to produce the best pharmacological results. Reformation of polypoid tissue may occur even with corticoid treatment. However, repeated polypectomies at a later date are required in a substantial number of aspirin-sensitive patients (48).

References

1. Samter M, Beers RF. Intolerance to aspirin: clinical studies and consideration to its pathogenesis. Ann Intern Med 1968; 68:975–983.
2. Widal F, Abramin P, Lermoyez J. Anaphylaxis et idiosyncrasie. Presse Med 1922; 30:189–193.
3. Friedlaender S, Feinberg SM. Aspirin allergy: its relationship to chronic intractable asthma. Ann Intern Med 1947; 26:734–740.
4. Settipane GA, Chafee FH, Klein DE. Aspirin intolerance. II. A prospective study in an atopic and normal population. J Allergy Clin Immunol 1974; 4:200–204.
5. Enomoto T, Okada T, Ichihashi K, Horikoshi S, Matsuura T, Imai T, Mita S, Adachi M, Miura Y. Examination on aspirin-induced asthma and hypersensitivity to steroids—a questionnaire to 850 asthmatics on hypersensitivity to non-steroidal anti-inflammatory drugs and hypersensitivity to steroids. Arerugi 1995; 44:534–539.
6. Giraldo B, Blumenthal MN, Spink WW. Aspirin intolerance and asthma. A clinical and immunological study. Ann Intern Med 1969; 68:975–496.
7. Falliers CJ. Aspirin and subtypes of asthma: risk factor analysis. J Allergy Clin Immunol 1973; 3:141–147.
8. Ogino S, Harada T, Okawachi I, Irifune M, Matsunaga T, Nagano T. Aspirin-induced asthma and nasal polyps. Acta Otolaryngol Suppl Stockh 1986; 430:21–27.
9. Speer F, Denison TR, Baptist JE. Aspirin allergy. Ann Allergy 1981; 3:123–126.
10. Pina J, Barbado A, Marques D, Leitao MC, Duarte C, Gomes MJ, Amaral-Marques R. Our experience with acetylsalicyclic acid hypersensitivity. Allergol Immunopathol Madr 1984; 3:217–223.
11. Grzelewska-Rzymowska I, Rożniecki J, Szmidt M, Kowalski ML. Asthma with aspirin intolerance. Clinical entity or coincidence of nonspecific bronchial hyperreactivity and aspirin intolerance. Allergol Immunopathol Madr 1981; 9:533–538.
12. Van Leeuwen WS. Pathognomonishe Bedeutung der Ueberempfindlichkeit gegen Aspirin bei Asthmatikern. Munch Med Wochenschr 1928; 75:1588–1592.
13. Chafee FH, Settipane GA. Aspirin intolerance. I. Frequency in an allergic population. J Allergy Clin Immunol 1974; 53:193–199.
14. McDonald JR, Mathison DA, Stevenson DD. Aspirin intolerance in asthma, detection by oral challenge. J Allergy Clin Immunol 1972; 50:198–207.
15. Harnett JC, Spector SL, Farr RS. Aspirin idiosyncrasy. Asthma and urticaria. In: Middleton E Jr, Reed CE, Ellis EF, eds. Allergy. Principles and Practice. St. Louis: CV Mosby, 1978:1002–1022.
16. Kosturkov G, Staneva-Stoianova M, Mileva Z. Hypersensitivity to acetysal in bronchial asthma. Vutr Boles 1980; 19:50–53.
17. Scherrer M, Zeller C, Berger M. Bronchial asthma, nasal polyposis and analgesic intolerance (the ASA triad). A successful computer based analysis of free texts. Schweiz Med Wochenschr 1984; 114:337–342.

18. Picado C, Castillo JA, Montserrat JM, Augusti-Vidal A. Aspirin-intolerance as a precipitating factor of life-threatening attacks of asthma requiring mechanical ventillation. Eur Respir J 1989; 2:127–129.
19. Szczeklik A, Gryglewski RJ, Czerniawska-Mysik G. Clinical patterns of hypersensitivity to nonsteroidal anti-inflammatory drugs and their pathogenesis. J Allergy Clin Immunol 1977; 60:276–284.
20. Czerniawska-Mysik G, Szczeklik A. Idiosyncrasy to pyrazolone drugs. Allergy 1981; 36:381–384.
21. Flarup M, Udholm S. Tardive anaphylactic shock caused by intolerance to aspirin. Ugesk Laeger 1989; 151:2211–2212.
22. Delaney JC. Asthma, nasal polyposis, and aspirin sensitivity. Ann Intern Med 1973; 8:239–246.
23. Lockey R, Rucknagel DL, Vanselow NA. Familial occurrence of asthma, nasal polyps and aspirin intolerance. Ann Intern Med 1973; 54:380–389.
24. Kvon M, Adkinson NF Jr, van Metre TE, Marsh DG, Norman PS. Aspirin intolerance in a family. J Allergy Clin Immunol 1974; 54:380–389.
25. Settipane GA, Paddupakkam RK Aspirin intolerance. III. Subtypes, familial occurrence, and cross-reactivity with tartrazine. J Allergy Clin Immunol 1975; 56: 215–221.
26. Stevenson DD. Diagnosis, prevention and treatment of adverse reactions to aspirin and nonsteroidal anti-inflammatory drugs. J Allergy Clin Immunol 1984; 74:617–622.
27. Spector SL, Wangaard CH, Farr RS. Aspirin and concomitant idiosyncrasies in adult asthmatic patients. J Allergy Clin Immunol 1979; 64:500–508.
28. Lumry WR, Curd JG, Stevenson DD. Aspirin-sensitive asthma and rhinosinusitis: current concepts and recent advances. Ear Nose Throat J 1984; 63:66, 68–70, 72–74 passim.
29. Lumry WR, Curd JG, Zeiger RS, Pleskow WW, Stevenson DD. Aspirin sensitive rhinosinusitis: the clinical syndrome and effects of aspirin administration. J Allergy Clin Immunol 1983; 71:580–587.
30. Peltonen L, Havu VK, Mattila L. Serum IgE in non-atopic adults and in dermatitis patients. Allergy 1988; 43:152–158.
31. Zetterström O, Johansson SGO. IgE concentrations measured by PRIST in serum of healthy adults and in patients with respiratory allergy. Allergy 1981; 36:537–547.
32. Samter M. Intolerance to aspirin. Hosp Pract 1973; 8:85–90.
33. Walton CH, Randle DL. Aspirin allergy. Can Med Assoc J 1957; 76:1016–1018.
34. Bochenek G, Niżankowska E, Szczeklik A. The atopy trait in hypersensitivity to nonsteroidal anti-inflammatory drugs. Allergy 1996; 51:16–23.
35. Pasargiklian M, Bianco S, Allegra L, Moavero NE, Petrigni G, Robuschi M, Grugni A. Aspects of bronchial reactivity to prostaglandins and aspirin in asthmatic patients. Respiration 1977; 34:79–91.
36. Basomba A, Romar A, Pelaez Z, Villamanzo IG, Campos A. The effect of sodium cromoglycate in preventing aspirin-induced bronchospasm. Clin Allergy 1976; 6: 269–275.
37. Martelli NA, Usandivaras G. Inhibition of aspirin-induced bronchoconstriction by sodium cromoglycate inhalation. Thorax 1977; 32:684–690.

38. Dahl R. Oral and inhaled sodium cromoglycate in challenge test with food allergens or acetylosalicyclic acid. Allergy 1981; 36:161–165.
39. Szczeklik A, Czerniawska-Mysik G, Serwońska M, Kukliński P. Inhibition by ketotifen of idiosyncratic reactions to aspirin. Allergy 1980; 35:421–424.
40. Szczeklik A, Serwońska M. Inhibition of idiosyncratic reactions to aspirin in asthmatic patients by clemastine. Thorax 1979; 34:654–657.
41. Delany JC. The effect of ketotifen on aspirin-induced asthmatic reactions. Clin Allergy 1983; 13:247–251.
42. Stevenson DD, Simon RA. Sensitivity to aspirin and nonsteroidal antiinflammatory drugs. In: Middleton E Jr, Reed CE, Ellis EF, Adkinson NF Jr, Younginger JW, Busse WW, eds. Allergy. Principles and Practice. St. Louis: CV Mosby, 1993: 1747–1766.
43. Bilaniuk LT, Zimmerman RA. Computed tomography in the evaluation of the paranasal sinuses. Radiol Clin North Am 1982; 20:51–66.
44. Kuhn JP. Imaging of the paranasal sinuses: current status. J Allergy Clin Immunol 1986; 77:6–8.
45. Jantti Alanko S, Holopainen E, Malmberg H. Recurrence of nasal polyps after surgical treatment. Rhinol Suppl 1989; 8:59–64.
46. Schapowal AG, Simon HU, Schmitz-Schumann M. Phenomenology, pathogenesis and treatment of aspirin-sensitive rhinosinusitis. Acta Otorhinolaryngol Belg 1995; 49:235–250.
47. Mastalerz L, Milewski M, Duplaga M, Niżankowska E, Szczeklik A. Intranasal fluticasone propionate for chronic eosinophilic rhinitis in patients with aspirin-induced asthma. Allergy 1997; 52:895–900.
48. Lawson W. The intranasal ethmoidectomy: an experience with 1077 procedures. Laryngoscope 1991; 101:367–371.

27

Nasal Polyposis

NIELS MYGIND and RONALD DAHL

Aarhus University Hospital
Aarhus, Denmark

TORBEN LILDHOLDT

Vejle Hospital
Vejle, Denmark

PER L. LARSEN

Hillerød Hospital
Hillerød, Denmark

CLAUS BACHERT

University Hospital
Ghent, Belgium

I. Introduction

Hippocrates, in 400 B.C., described nasal polyps, named them "polypous" (poly = many; pous = footed or feet), and developed a surgical method for their removal. Nasal polyps are protrusions of an edematous mucous membrane, originating in the upper part of the nose around the openings to the ethmoidal sinuses (see later). The polyps protrude into the nasal cavity from the middle (and superior) meatus, resulting in nasal blockage and abolished airflow to the olfactory region. Nasal polyposis, consisting of recurrent, multiple polyps, is part of an inflammatory reaction involving the mucous membrane of the nose, paranasal sinuses, and often the lower airways. The polyps are easily accessible for immunological and histological studies, and an increasing number of publications have appeared in recent years, including two monographs (1,2). As polyps frequently occur in patients with intolerance to nonsteroidal anti-inflammatory drugs, it is relevant to describe nasal polyposis in a volume on aspirin intolerance.

In this chapter we will describe the pathogenesis of nasal polyposis in detail as polyps are ideal models for the study of eosinophil-dominated immune inflammation in the airway mucous membrane. Finally, we will give a short description of the clinical presentation and treatment of nasal polyposis.

II. Occurrence and Prevalence

The exact prevalence rate of nasal polyposis in the general population is not known, because there are few epidemiological studies and their results depend on the diagnostic methods used (history, rhinoscopy, endoscopy, CT-scan examination). The overall prevalence rate is probably about 2% (3,4), and it increases with age of the study population. Nasal polyposis occurs with a high frequency in groups of patients having specific airway diseases (Table 1).

Although nasal polyposis is rare in the general population, much higher figures of the occurrence of isolated nasal polyps have been obtained in autopsy studies. A thorough endoscopic examination of removed nasoethmoidal blocks and endoscopic examination of unselected autopsy specimens have shown polyps in as many as 26–42% of the specimens (6,7).

III. Etiology

A. Eosinophil-Dominated Inflammation and Allergy

As most polyps are characterized by tissue eosinophilia, it has been the belief for decades that allergy is a significant cause of nasal polyposis. However, this

Table 1 Prevalence of Nasal Polyposis in Different Population Subgroups

Aspirin intolerance	36–72%
Adult asthma	7%
IgE-mediated	5%
Non-IgE-mediated	13%
Chronic sinusitis in adults	2%
IgE-mediated	1%
Non-IgE-mediated	5%
Childhood asthma/sinusitis	0.1%
Cystic fibrosis	
Children	10%
Adults	50%
Allergic fungal sinusitis	66–100%
Primary ciliary dyskinesia[a]	40%

[a]According to Pedersen and Mygind (5).
Source: Adapted from Ref. 1.

view has been challenged because most studies have failed to show a higher occurrence of positive skin tests to inhaled allergens in patients with polyps than in the general population (3,8–10). In addition, conditions associated with a high prevalence of polyposis (Table 1) are not based on IgE-mediated allergy. For example, the prevalence of nasal polyps is higher in nonallergic rhinitis and asthma than in their allergic counterparts (3,8–10). It is striking that children with perennial allergic rhinitis, who can have markedly swollen nasal mucous membranes, almost never develop polyps (Table 1).

Even the pathogenetic contribution of allergic reactions in patients with simultaneous occurrence of the two conditions can be questioned. Keith and co-workers (11) were unable to show any deterioration of nasal symptoms or eosinophilia during the pollen season in polyp patients having a positive skin test to pollen (Fig. 1). Thus, in our opinion, allergy to inhaled allergens is not a well-documented cause of eosinophil-dominated polyps, and the etiology is unknown, as is the case for nonallergic rhinitis and asthma.

B. Neutrophil-Dominated Inflammation and Infection

There is an association between polyps and bacterial infection, as both disease manifestations frequently occur in patients with cystic fibrosis and primary ciliary dyskinesia (Kartagener's syndrome). The polyps associated with these diseases are not characterized by tissue eosinophilia but by lymphocytes in the tissue and neutrophil leukocytes in the secretions (12).

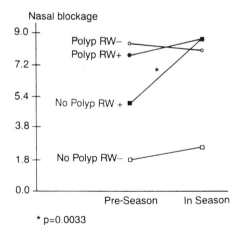

Figure 1 Symptoms preseason and in pollen season in four groups of subjects [with or without nasal polyps, and with or without allergy to ragweed (RW)]. Symptoms increased only in allergic patients without polyps. (From Ref. 11.)

IV. Anatomy and Histology

A. Site of Polyp Formation

Nasal endoscopy of a large number of patients with nasal polyposis (13) and a detailed anatomic examination of autopsy specimens (6,7) have shown that nasal polyps are mainly situated in the middle meatus and they originate from the mucous membrane of the outlets (ostia, clefts, recesses) from the paranasal sinuses. This area, so critical for sinus pathology, is also referred to as "the ostiomeatal complex."

It is remarkable that polyps exclusively develop from a few square centimeters of an airway mucous membrane that often is universally inflamed. The reason for this is unknown and one can only speculate about the nature of a "localization factor." In the upper part of the nose, including the middle meatus, the airway lumen is a narrow slit with only a few millimeters between opposing mucous membranes. Stammberger (14) has observed that polyp formation predominantly occurs in contact areas between two opposing mucous membranes. It is known that stimulation of epithelial cells induces the generation and release of a series of proinflammatory cytokines (see later), and one can therefore hypothesize that mechanical stimulation of the surface epithelium in contact areas contributes, or even initiates, the inflammatory reaction in the polyps.

Other "localization factors" may be related to the anatomy of nerve endings, blood vessels, and mucociliary flow in the thin mucous membrane near the borderline between the nose and paranasal sinuses.

B. Gross Anatomy

A polyp is a pedunculating process with a slim or broad stalk or base, protruding into the nasal cavity. The polyp stroma is highly edematous with a varying density of inflammatory cells. There are few glands and few blood vessels.

C. Surface Epithelium

The entire polyp is covered by a surface epithelium. The major part of the surface is covered by a typically ciliated pseudostratified epithelium of various heights, but transitional and squamous epithelium is also found, especially in anterior polyps, influenced by the inhaled air currents (15).

Epithelial Defects

There is experimental evidence that cytotoxic proteins from eosinophil leukocytes can damage the respiratory epithelium and induce bronchial hyperreactivity in asthma (16). Epithelial defects have apparently also been described in nasal polyps (17), but when polyps are removed carefully and gentle methods are used for fixation, dehydration, and cutting, the polyp epithelium appears well preserved without defects in the scanning electron microscope (18). Although gross epithelial defects do not seem to appear in carefully prepared polyp specimens, the function of the epithelium may be impaired and epithelial cell kinetics altered (19).

Biology of the Surface Epithelium

Perturbation of the epithelium, as occurs on exposure to chemical, physical, and immunological stimuli, can contribute to inflammation by release and activity of metabolites of arachidonic acid and cytokines, which influence the growth, differentiation, migration, and activation of inflammatory cells (20, 21). Recent studies have suggested that the airway epithelium may play a more important role and influence the pathogenesis of inflammatory airway diseases. Possibly, contact between epithelial surfaces in the narrow middle meatus is part of the explanation why polyps are formed specifically in this location, as discussed above.

Electrolyte and Water Transport

The basic elements of Na^+ and Cl^- movement in the respiratory surface epithelium may be relevant for the understanding of nasal polyp formation. In the normal nasal mucosa, there is a net absorption of Na^+ and very little Cl^- secretion (22,23). In cystic fibrosis, a disease often associated with polyp formation, there is both an absence of the cyclic AMP–controlled Cl^- channel and abnormal regulation of the Na^+ channel (22,23). An increased Na^+ and a decreased Cl^- secretion in cystic fibrosis result in dehydration of mucus because of the net movement of water into the interstitial space. Possibly, this may also contribute to the formation of tissue edema.

Increased Na^+ absorption may also be secondary to chronic inflammation, which is the hallmark of nasal polyposis. Recent findings on the effect of chronic inflammation in different types of polyps indicate that there is an altered Na^+ absorption not only in CF polyps but also in non-CF polyps (22,23). These results suggest that factors leading to the development of nasal polyposis include pathophysiological changes in the electrolyte and water transport in the surface epithelium.

D. Innervation

The sensory nerves, and the autonomic vasomotor and secretory nerves, invariably found in normal and abnormal nasal mucosa, cannot be identified within the stroma of polyps, either in the vicinity of the epithelial basement membrane or within the walls of blood vessels or glands. A few nerve fibers can be seen in the stalk of some polyps (24).

It is assumed, therefore, that denervation of nasal polyps causes a decrease in secretory activity of the glands and induces an abnormal vascular permeability, leading to an irreversible tissue edema. Nasal polyps develop in areas where the lining of the nasal cavity joins that of the sinuses, and these marginal zones contain thin nerve fascicles (24), which may be more sensitive to damage, from, e.g., eosinophil-derived proteins (25).

While the exact cause and mechanism of the denervation of the nasal polyps are unknown, there is little doubt that the complete loss of autonomic innervation is an important pathogenetic factor in the formation of polyps.

E. Goblet Cells

The histopathological picture shows great variations, not only in type of epithelium, but also in goblet cell density in different locations on the single polyp. The density is lower in anterior than in posterior polyps, and much lower than in the normal nasal mucosa (15).

F. Submucosal Glands

The glands of nasal polyps differ markedly from normal nasal glands (26). While normal glands are small, branched tubuloalveolar glands, those in the polyps are long, tubular, and of varying shape, size, and type. The normal glands are evenly distributed over the mucous membrane, while the glands in the polyps are very unevenly distributed. Their density is more than 10 times less than in the nasal mucosa (26).

All glands in the polyps are pathological showing signs of cystic degeneration with stagnation of mucus within the distended tubules (12,26), and without the normal production of secretory component (27). Apparently, all glands are newly formed during the growth of the polyps, which is consistent with their lack of innervation.

G. Blood Vessels and Exudation of Plasma

The vascularity of polyps is minimal compared to normal nasal mucosa (24), and neither venous sinusoids nor arteriovenous anastomoses are present. The venules of the polyps show unusual organization with respect to their endothelial cell junctions and the basement membrane. Many cell junctions have the appearance of a web of villous processes and are incompletely sealed, while others are wide open (24). As mentioned above, the blood vessels of polyps are devoid of nerves.

The release of histamine and other inflammatory mediators (see below) may be an important factor in causing microvascular plasma exudation, which is highly characteristic of nasal polyps. The vascular exudation of plasma suggests that the lamina propria, the basement membrane, the airway epithelium, and the mucosal surface are furnished by potent plasma-derived peptides and proteins, and that the mucosal macromolecular milieu in nasal polyposis therefore is dramatically different from that of the normal nasal mucosa (19). It is of particular interest that the process of microvascular exudation of plasma may participate in the chronic generation of edema fluid in nasal polyposis.

V. Pathogenesis: Immune Inflammation

Nasal polyposis is the ultimate form of inflammation of the upper airways, which, for unknown reasons, preferably develops in subtypes of inflammatory diseases. As mentioned above, the factors determining the localization of the disease to a few square centimeters of the airways are still poorly understood. Although IgE-mediated allergy does not seem to be an important etiological factor for the development of polyps, recent data indicate that IgE, mast cells, and histamine are involved in the immune inflammation and in the pathogenesis of polyps.

As shown in Table 1, nasal polyposis is very frequent in patients with intolerance to acetylsalicyclic acid and in patients with allergic fungal sinusitis. These two etiologically different diseases have an eosinophil-dominated inflammation as a common feature, and apparently the degree of tissue eosinophilia is an important denominator of the recurrence rate of nasal polyps (3,4). In non-eosinophil-dominated inflammation (cystic fibrosis, primary ciliary dyskinesia) other pathophysiological mechanisms may be of importance.

A. IgE, Mast Cells, and Histamine

There is a large number of epithelial mast cells in nasal polyps (28) (Fig. 2). Electron microscopic studies have shown marked and widespread mast cell degranulation in all polyps studied, and the degree of degranulation is more marked than in allergic rhinitis (29,30) (Fig. 3). There is some evidence that the changes may extend into the nasal mucosa of the inferior turbinate in some patients, indicating the existence of a more widespread inflammation of the airway mucosa (31). Total histamine of polyps is far above other tissues, and large quantities of free histamine can be measured in the edema fluid (32), which concurs with the ultrastructural findings. Arachidonic acid–generated mediators are also found in polyp fluid (33). Measurable levels of IgE decapeptide in polyp fluid (34) (Fig. 4) support the idea that a membrane event induces the degranulation of mast cells. However, as described above, an inhaled or ingested antigen cannot be identified in the large majority of patients. Probably other immune mechanisms are at work, for example, the interaction between autoantibodies and membrane-bound IgE or IgE receptor.

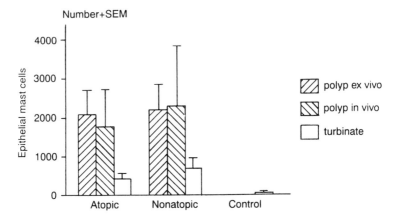

Figure 2   Epithelial mast cells on scrapings from polyps and turbinates of atopic and nonatopic polyp subjects as well as turbinate tissue from normal controls. (Based on data from Ref. 28.)

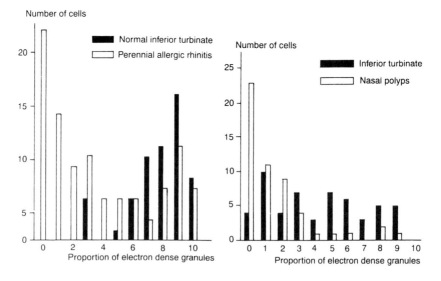

Figure 3   Degree of degranulation of mast cells in inferior turbinates from normal controls and from perennial allergic rhinitis (left), and from inferior turbinates and nasal polyps from patients with polyposis (right). A score of 0 indicates complete degranulation. (From Ref. 31.)

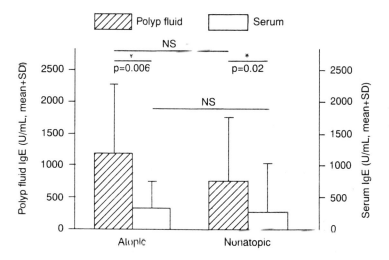

Figure 4 Polyp fluid and serum IgE concentrations in 29 polyp patients. While the IgE level was the same in atopic and nonatopic patients, it was significantly higher in polyp fluid than in serum. (From Ref. 32.)

B. Adhesion Molecules, Cytokines, and Inflammatory Cells

Today the pathogenesis of inflammatory airway diseases cannot be discussed without a description of adhesion molecules, cytokines, and chemokines, which are instrumental in orchestrating the cell infiltration of immune inflammation. Representing a chronic, eosinophil-dominated inflammation, nasal polyposis is well suited for study of cellular and molecular mechanisms involved in rhinitis and asthma.

Extravasation of leukocytes is a coordinated multistep event with several molecular choices at each step. This process therefore provides great combinatorial signal diversity, which can display remarkable specificity in relation to the inflammatory stimulus, the stage of the inflammatory response, and the tissue site or organ involved. A good example of such selectivity is the preferential recruitment of eosinophils in nasal polyps (35).

Convincing immunohistochemical data strongly suggest that VLA-4/VCAM-1 interactions play an important role for extravasation of eosinophils into polyps. Two independent studies have found considerable upregulation of VCAM-1 (36,37), which supports adhesion and transmigration of eosinophils without having any effect on neutrophils. Both IL-3 and IL-4 as well as IL-1 and TNFα can induce VCAM-1 expression in microvascular endothelium from the polyps. All these cytokines are expressed in the polyps, and in various combinations they may have synergistic effects on VCAM-1 expression (35). Another adhesion molecule, P-selectin, probably plays a role in the initial adhesion of eosinophils to the polyp endothelium. Interestingly, it has recently been reported that prolonged endothelial surface expression of P-selectin is induced by IL-3 and TNFα. Both these cytokines are expressed in polyp tissue indicating that P-selectin may be persistently expressed in this chronic inflammatory disorder (35).

Finally, chemokines most likely are involved as eosinophil attractants. Although limited information exists with regard to their possible role in vivo, reports on RANTES and eotaxin expression in nasal polyps indicate a role for these chemoattractants in accumulation of eosinophils (37).

Several hematopoietic and proinflammatory cytokines (GM-CSF, IL-6, IL-8, SCF), capable of recruiting and activating mast cells and eosinophils in particular, are up-regulated in various tissue compartments (epithelium, stroma) of nasal polyps (38–40). The inflammatory cells themselves, eosinophils especially, are rich sources of many cytokines, including those capable of inducing their own differentiation and activation in an autocrine fashion. Thus, nasal polyps can be looked upon as a type of self-perpetuating inflammatory process (41).

C. Comparison Between Polyps Tissue, Diseased Sinus Mucosa, and Normal Nasal Mucosa

We have learned to differentiate nasal and sinus diseases on the basis of histological features and clinical symptoms. Today, sinus diseases may also be differentiated on the basis of cytokine patterns creating a specific inflammatory milieu that may be linked to morphology (39).

In acute infectious sinusitis, the proinflammatory cytokines IL-1, IL-6, and IL-8 orchestrate the ongoing inflammatory reaction and cause a strong tissue neutrophilia. The levels of proinflammatory cytokines are low in chronic recurrent sinusitis, but IL-3 seems to unfold a multicell stimulating activity (Fig. 5). Although presenting clinically as a polyp, the antrochoanal polyp resembles an acute or chronic sinusitis rather than a polyp disease judged from the cytokine pattern.

The finding of high amounts of IL-5 protein in the majority of nasal polyp specimens, but in none of the normal control or sinusitis samples, indicates that IL-5 plays a key role in the pathophysiology of eosinophil-dominated polyps (39). This contrasts to other cytokines, which demonstrate only marginal quantitative differences between polyps and other sinus diseases. IL-5 levels are significantly higher in polyps of asthmatic subjects compared to those of nonasthmatics, relating this cytokine to clinical data on associations of asthma

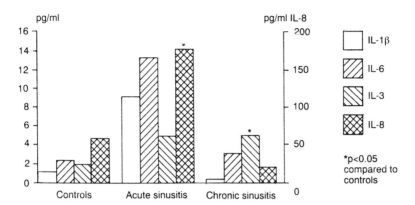

Figure 5 Cytokine profiles in acute and chronic recurrent sinusitis compared to control turbinate mucosa. Proinflammatory cytokines IL-1β, IL-6, and IL-8 were elevated in the acute sinusitis mucosa, whereas IL-3 was dominant in chronic sinusitis. (From Ref. 39.)

and polyposis (Fig. 6). In the study by Bachert (39), there was a tendency of higher IL-5 concentrations in aspirin-sensitive patients than in nonsensitive patients. The three highest IL-5 concentrations in polyp tissue were found in patients with asthma and aspirin sensitivity, linking this cytokine to pseudoallergic mechanisms as well. Immunohistochemistry reveals that IL-5 may be

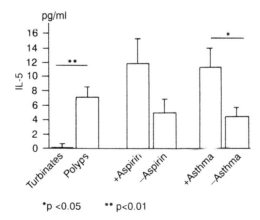

Figure 6 High IL-5 levels were detected in polyp samples compared to turbinate specimens (mean + SEM). IL-5 concentrations were higher in polyps from aspirin-sensitive patients than from nonsensitive patients and from asthmatics compared to nonasthmatics. (From Ref. 39.)

predominantly produced by eosinophils, which creates a possible autocrine loop in nasal polyps tissue, as mentioned earlier. The investigation of cytokines may give new insights into the underlying pathomechanisms, may help to differentiate subgroups of sinus diseases, and possibly open new approaches for therapy. Increasing evidence suggests that eosinophils can cause tissue damage by release of their cytotoxic granule proteins. Enhanced knowledge about the molecules that take part in the recruitment of these cells might create the basis for a future rational therapeutic intervention based on blocking one or more crucial steps in eosinophil extravasation, thereby controlling the development of several important airway diseases. IL-5 represents a main target for therapy, and nasal polyposis may serve as a good model for other eosinophil-related diseases, such as asthma.

VI. Clinical Presentation

A. Rhinitis

Nasal polyps, as a rule, develop in a patient who has suffered from perennial nonallergic rhinitis (vasomotor rhinitis) with profuse watery rhinorrhea for some years. A sensation of "secretion," which cannot be expelled, is often the first symptom of polyp formation. Nasal blockage gradually develops and can be complete. Impairment or loss of the sense of smell, and with that "taste," due to obstruction of the upper part of the nasal airway, is characteristic. This symptom is very annoying as it mars the pleasure of eating and drinking.

The disease can vary in severity from a single episode of nasal blockage to constant daily symptoms, requiring continuous therapy. Nasal polyposis can be the most severe manifestation of eosinophil inflammation in the upper airways.

B. Sinusitis

As nasal blockage progresses, secretions become more viscous and difficult to expell. Involvement of the paranasal sinuses, the mucosa of which has many goblet cells, but few seromucous glands (42), contributes to the viscosity of the discharge.

There is hyperplasia of the maxillary mucous membrane, and the ethmoidal cells are filled with polypous transformed mucous membrane. This increases the tendency to bacterial infection in the nose and paranasal sinuses, especially following a common cold.

C. Asthma

Severe cases, with an increased blood eosinophil count, are usually associated with asthma. The classic ASA triad, consisting of asthma, sinusitis/polyposis, and aspirin intolerance, is described elsewhere in this volume. Questioning about adverse reactions to acetylsalicylic acid is obligatory in patients with nasal polyps.

VII. Diagnosis

The diagnosis is easily made by rhinoscopy, preferably using an endoscope. The use of a vasoconstrictor spray may be necessary. Nasal polyps are typically multiple and bilateral. Unilateral masses should alert the physician to other conditions, such as malignant tumors, invert papillomata, and meningoceles, all of which may masquerade as simple polyps. For that reason, microscopy is always necessary when polyps occur for the first time. A CT scan of the nose and paranasal sinuses gives an excellent presentation of abnormal anatomical conditions and is indicated when there is a suspicion of malignancy or meningocele, and also in all cases before endoscopic surgery.

VIII. Treatment

Nasal polyps represent a clinical manifestation resulting from a number of possible pathophysiological processes. No one medical or surgical therapy guarantees cure, and most clinicians treat patients on an individual basis, modulating medical and surgical therapy as appropriate (Table 2).

A. Medical Treatment

Corticosteroids are the only type of drug having a proven effect on symptoms and signs of nasal polyposis. Corticosteroids probably relieve symptoms by down-regulating the expression and production of cytokines, such as IL-5,

Table 2 Characteristics of the Ideal Treatment

Elimination or considerable reduction in polyp size
Reestablishment of open nasal airways and nasal breathing
Freedom from rhinitis symptoms
Normalization of sense of smell
Prevention of recurrence of polyps
High patient compliance
Minimal risk of side effects
Preservation of normal nasal anatomy and physiology

which effectively reduce the number of eosinophils. The effects of corticosteroids on these processes may be enhanced by effects on hematopoietic
mechanisms arising in the bone marrow (43).

Topically applied steroids are the type of therapy that has been best
studied in controlled clinical trials (44,45). They reduce rhinitis symptoms,
improve nasal breathing, reduce the size of polyps, and prevent, in part, their
recurrence, but they have no or little effect on the sense of smell. Topical
steroids can, as basic long-term therapy, be used alone in mild cases, and together with systemic steroids and/or surgery in severe cases.

Systemic steroids, less well studied, have an effect on all types of symptoms and pathology, including the sense of smell (46). This type of treatment,
which can serve as "medical polypectomy," is only used for short periods owing
to the risk of adverse effects.

B. Surgical Treatment

In common with many surgical problems, the literature is lacking in prospective, double-blinded, randomized trials. Even relatively simple comparative
studies of medical and surgical therapies (46) have not proved popular, and
we find a miscellany of studies, most of which rely on subjective patient improvement, gross polyp recurrence, or, more rarely, macroscopic normalization of sinonasal mucosa.

The choice of surgical approach will depend greatly on the individual
surgeon's experience and philosophy. The precise evaluation of extent of disease by CT scanning and endoscopy holds much intellectual appeal, and this
is supported by imperfect historical comparisons that suggest that endoscopic
polypectomy/sinus surgery offers better results than the conventional intranasal ethmoidectomy of the past or even simple polypectomy, with no evidence
that this is associated with any greater morbidity in terms of surgical complications. Whether a more conservative or more radical approach offers better
long-term results remains to be determined, but in either case, even the most
enthusiastic surgeon would accept that this must be combined with long-term
topical medication (47).

C. Combined Treatment

Therapy is in most cases a combination of (a) long-term local corticosteroid
therapy, (b) short-term systemic corticosteroid treatment, and (c) simple polypectomy (45). Endonasal ethmoidectomy is indicated in cases resistant to this
treatment schedule. Treatment plans have been summarized as algorithms by
Naclerio and Mackay (48) (Fig. 7).

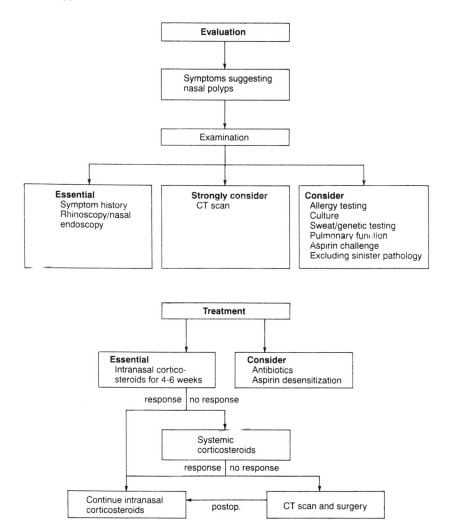

Figure 7 Management plan for diagnosis and treatment of nasal polyposis. (From Ref. 48.)

IX. Conclusions

Nasal polyposis, occurring in about 2% of the general population, is the ultimate form of inflammation of the upper airways. For unknown reasons, polyps preferably develop in subtypes of inflammatory diseases, and they are associated with nonallergic rhinitis and asthma, aspirin intolerance (eosinophildominated inflammation), or cystic fibrosis and primary ciliary dyskinesia (neutrophil-dominated inflammation). In contrast to common belief, IgE-mediated allergy does not seem to be an important etiological factor. The majority of polyps originate from the mucosa around the ostiomeatal complex of the nasal cavity. The factors determining the localization of the disease to a few square centimeters of the airways are poorly understood. Polyps are edematous sacks covered by a normal airway epithelium and containing very few blood vessels and cystic degenerated glands. They contain a high number of degranulated mast cells and activated eosinophils, which accumulate due to up-regulation of vascular VCAM-1 and a high local level of IL-5 (in eosinophil-dominated polyps). As eosinophils can generate IL-5, this creates a possible autocrine loop in nasal polyps, which can be considered as a type of self-perpetuating inflammatory process. Treatment consists of corticosteroids and in severe cases surgery.

References

1. Settipane GA, Lund VJ, Bernstein JM, Tos M, eds. Nasal Polyps: Epidemiology, Pathogenesis and Treatment. Providence, RI: The New England and Regional Allergy Proceedings, 1997.
2. Mygind N, Likdholdt T, eds. Nasal Polyposis: An Inflammatory Disease and Its Treatment. Copenhagen: Munksgaard, 1997.
3. Settipane GA. Nasal polyps: pathology, immunology and treatment. Am J Rhinol 1987; 1:119–126.
4. van der Baan B. Epidemiology and natural history. In: Mygind N, Lildholdt T, eds. Nasal Polyposis: An Inflammatory Disease and Its Treatment. Copenhagen: Munksgaard, 1997:13–16.
5. Pedersen M, Mygind N. Rhinitis, sinusitis and otitis media in Kartagener's syndrome. Clin Otolaryngol 1982; 7:373–380.
6. Larsen PL, Tos M. Site of origin of nasal polyps. Transcranially removed naso-ethmoidal blocks as a screening method for nasal polyps in autopsy material. Rhinology 1995; 33:185–188.
7. Larsen PL, Tos M. Anatomic site of origin of nasal polyps. Am J Rhinol 1996; 10: 211–216.
8. Caplin I, Haynes TJ, Spahn J. Are nasal polyps an allergic phenomenon? Ann Allergy 1971; 29:631–634.
9. Drake-Lee AB, Lowe D, Swanston A, Grace A. Clinical profile and recurrence of nasal polyps. J Laryngol Otol 1984; 98:783–793.
10. Braun JJ, Haas F, Conraux C. Polyposis of the nasal sinuses. Epidemiology and clinical aspects of 350 cases. Treatment and results with a follow-up over 5 years on 93 cases. Ann Otolaryngol Chir Cervicofac 1992; 109:189–199.
11. Keith PK, Conway M, Evans S, Wong S, Jordana G, Pengelly D, Dolovich J. Nasal polyps: effects of seasonal allergen exposure. J Allergy Clin Immunol 1994; 93: 567–574.

12. Sørensen H, Mygind N, Tygstrup I, Flensborg EW. Histology of nasal polyps of different etiology. Rhinology 1977; 15:121–128.
13. Stammberger H. Functional Endoscopic Sinus Surgery. The Messerklinger Technique. Toronto: BC Dekker, 1991.
14. Stammberger H. Examination and endoscopy of the nose and paranasal sinuses. In: Mygind N, Lildholdt T, eds. Nasal Polyposis: An Inflammatory Disease and Its Treatment. Copenhagen: Munksgaard, 1997:120–136.
15. Larsen PL, Tos M. Nasal polyps. Epithelium and goblet cell density. Laryngoscope 1990; 99:1274–1280.
16. Garrison HA, Leonard CA, et al. Injurious effect of the eosinophil peroxide-hydrogen peroxide-halide system and major basic protein on human nasal epithelium in vitro. Am Rev Respir Dis 1989; 140:125–131.
17. Wladislavosky-Wasserman P, Kern EB, Holley KE, Eisenbrey AB, Gleich GJ. Epithelial damage in nasal polyps. Clin Allergy 1984; 14:241–247.
18. Larsen PL, Qvortrup K, Rostgaard J, Rasmussen N. Ultrastructural analyses of human nasal polyps employing an improved method for immersion fixation 1997 (in preparation).
19. Greiff L, Erjefält JS, Andersson M, Svensson C, Persson CGA. Microvascular exudation of plasma and epithelial shedding-restitution processes as causative events in inflammatory airway diseases. In: Mygind N, Lildholdt T, eds. Nasal Polyposis: An Inflammatory Disease and Its Treatment. Copenhagen: Munksgaard, 1997: 50–60.
20. Devalia JL, Davies RJ. Airway epithelial cells and mediators of inflammation. Respir Med 1993; 87:405–408.
21. Devalia JL, Campbell AM, Sapsford RJ, et al. Effect of nitrogen dioxide on synthesis of inflammatory cytokines expressed by human bronchial epithelial cells in vitro. Am Rev Respir Cell Mol Biol 1993; 9:271–278.
22. Bernstein JM, Yankaskas JR. Increased ion transport in cultured nasal epithelial cells. Arch Otolaryngol Head Neck Surg 1994; 120:993–996.
23. Bernstein JM, Yankaskas JR. Electrolyte and water transport and biophysical properties of nasal polyps. In: Mygind N, Lildholdt T, eds. Nasal Polyposis: An Inflammatory Disease and Its Treatment. Copenhagen: Munksgaard, 1997: 44–49.
24. Cauna N, Hinderer KH, Manzetti GW, Swanson EW. Fine structure of nasal polyps. Ann Otol Rhinol Laryngol 1972; 81:41–48.
25. Mygind N. Nasal polyposis. J Allergy Clin Immunol 1982; 86:827–829 (editorial).
26. Tos M, Mogensen C. Mucous glands in nasal polyps. Arch Otolaryngol 1977; 103: 407–413.
27. Nakashima T, Hamashima Y. Loss of secretory activity in the glands of nasal polyps. Ann Otol Rhinol Laryngol 1979; 88:210–216.
28. Ruhno J, Howie K, Anderson M, Andersson B, Vanzieleghem M, Hitch D, Lapp P, Denburg J, Dolovich J. The increased number of epithelial mast cells in nasal polyps and adjacent turbinates is not allergy-dependent. Allergy 1990; 45:370–374.
29. Drake-Lee A, Price J. Ultrastructure of mast cells in normal subjects and patients with perennial allergic rhinitis. J Laryngol Otol 1991; 105:1006–1013.

30. Drake-Lee A, Price J. Mast cell ultrastructure in the inferior turbinate and stroma of nasal polyps. J Laryngol Otol 1996 (in press).

31. Drake-Lee A. Mast cells, histamine and other mediators. In: Mygind N, Lildholdt T, eds. Nasal Polyposis: An Inflammatory Disease and Its Treatment. Copenhagen: Munksgaard, 1997:61–67.

32. Drake-Lee AB, McLauhlan P. Clinical symptoms, free histamine and IgE in nasal polyps. Int Arch Allergy Appl Immunol 1982; 69:268–271.

33. Salari H, Borgeat P, Steffenrud S, Richard J, Bedard P, Hebert J, Pelletier G. Immunological and non-immunological release of leukotrienes and histamine from nasal polyps. Clin Exp Immunol 1986; 63:711–717.

34. Drake-Lee AB, Jones V, Lewis I, Nayyar S, Wells A, Stanworth D. Levels of substance p and IgE decapeptide in nasal polyp fluid and matching sera: a preliminary study. J Laryngol Otol 1996; 110:225–227.

35. Jahnsen FL, Haraldsen G, Haye R, Brandtzaeg P. Adhesion molecules and recruitment of eosinophils. In: Mygind N, Lildholdt T, eds. Nasal Polyposis: An Inflammatory Disease and Its Treatment. Copenhagen: Munksgaard, 1997:88–97.

36. Jahnsen FL, Haraldsen G, Aanesen JP, Haye R, Brandtzaeg P. Eisonphil infiltration is related to increased expression of vascular cell adhesion molecule-1 in nasal polyps. Am J Respir Cell Mol Biol 1995; 12:624–632.

37. Beck L, Stellato C, Beall D, et al. Detection of chemochine RANTES and endothelial adhesion molecules in nasal polyps. J Allergy Clin Immunol 1996; 98: 766–780.

38. Jordana M, Dolovich J, Ohno I, Finotto S, Denburg J. Nasal polyposis: a model for chronic inflammation. In: Busse WW, Holgate ST, eds. Asthma and Rhinitis. Boston: Blackwell Scientific Publications, 1995:156–164.

39. Bachert C. Comparison between polyp tissue, diseased sinus mucosa and normal nasal tissue. In: Mygind N, Lildholdt T, eds. Nasal Polyposis: An Inflammatory Disease and Its Treatment. Copenhagen: Munksgaard, 1997:98–104.

40. Bachert C, Wagenman M, Hauser U, Rudack C. IL-5 synthesis is upregulated in human nasal polyp tissue. J Allergy Clin Immunol 1997 (in press).

41. Denburg J. Nasal polyposis: cytokines and inflammatory cells. In: Mygind N, Lildholdt T, eds. Nasal Polyposis: An Inflammatory Disease and Its Treatment. Copenhagen: Munksgaard, 1997:78–87.

42. Tos M. Distribution of mucus producing elements in the respiratory tract. Differences between upper and lower airways. Eur J Respir Dis 1982; 64(Suppl 128): 269–279.

43. Kanai N, Denburg J, Jordana M, Dolovich J. Nasal polyp inflammation. Effect of topical nasal steroid. Am J Respir Crit Care 1994; 150:1094–1100.

44. Mygind N, Lund V. Topical corticosteroid therapy of rhinitis. Clin Immunother 1996; 5:122–136.

45. Lildholdt T, Mygind N. Effect of corticosteroids on nasal polyps. In: Mygind N, Lildholdt T, eds. Nasal Polyposis: An Inflammatory Disease and Its Treatment. Copenhagen: Munksgaard, 1997:160–169.

46. Lindholdt T, Fogstrup J, Gammelgaard N, Kortholm B, Ulsøe C. Surgical versus medical treatment of nasal polyps. Acta Otolaryngol (Stockh) 1988; 105: 140–143.

47. Lund V. Surgical treatment. In: Mygind N, Lildholdt T, eds. Nasal Polyposis: An Inflammatory Disease and Its Treatment. Copenhagen: Munksgaard, 1997: 170–176.
48. Naclerio RM, Mackay IS. Guidelines for the management of nasal polyposis. In: Mygind N, Lildholdt T, eds. Nasal Polyposis: An Inflammatory Disease and Its Treatment. Copenhagen: Munksgaard, 1997:177–180.

28

The Nose in Aspirin-Sensitive Asthma

CÉSAR PICADO and JOAQUIM MULLOL

Hospital Clinic
Barcelona, Spain

I. Introduction

The association of nasal polyps, chronic rhinosinusitis, asthma, and aspirin intolerance constitutes an intriguing syndrome often referred to as the "asthma triad." The relationship between these different processes is an unresolved enigma. This chapter confines itself to analysis of the similarities between the diseases affecting the nose and the bronchial tree in patients with aspirin intolerance. A great deal of evidence suggests that the same disease affects both the nose and the bronchi and that the two processes share common pathogenic mechanisms. We also present data showing that the nose may be used both in the diagnosis of aspirin sensitivity and in the study of the mechanisms responsible for an adverse response to anti-inflammatory drugs.

II. Nasal Polyps, Chronic Rhinosinusitis, and Aspirin-Sensitive Asthma

Most patients with aspirin-induced asthma develop a characteristic pattern of chronic tissue inflammation associated with marked sinus mucosal thickening and nasal polyposis. Using the modern techniques of exploration of the nose and sinuses, such as endoscopy and computerized-tomography (CT) scan, the presence of a sinus disease is detected in almost all patients with aspirin-induced asthma. In several recent series on patients with chronic sinusitis undergoing functional endoscopic surgery, the prevalence of aspirin sensitivity was 11–20% (1).

A. Pathogenesis

Although many theories on the pathogenesis of polyposis have been presented, at present the origin of polyps is unknown. The most common disease associated with nasal polyps is asthma with aspirin intolerance. Other diseases, such as cystic fibrosis, primary ciliary dyskinesia, and Young's syndrome, also have a high frequency of nasal polyps.

Inflammation, obstruction of sinus drainage, and infection are the factors that may contribute to the development of chronic rhinosinusitis. However, histopathological studies reveal similar inflammatory changes in both the sinus tissues and the nasal polyps. This finding suggests that inflammation appears to be the most important contributing factor to chronic rhinosinusitis.

B. Anatomy

Macroscopically, nasal polyps of aspirin-sensitive asthma (ASA) patients are similar to other types of polyposis. They are usually bilateral and multiple evaginations of the nasal mucosa attached by a pedicle and arising from the ethmoid sinus, the middle turbinate, and the maxillary sinus. Nasal polyps have a characteristic appearance. They are smooth, soft, light gray, semitranslucent, movable structures. Nasal polyps in aspirin-sensitive asthma subjects most commonly follow an aggressive course filling the nasal cavity and often protruding from the anterior nares and/or projecting posteriorly into the nasopharynx. Facial deformation is not uncommon and it is due to midfacial expansion, which occurs as a consequence of the increased pressure on bones caused by nasal polyps and inflamed sinus.

C. Histopathology

The general histological appearance of nasal polyps and chronic rhinosinusitis associated with aspirin intolerance bears many similarities to that of bronchial asthma. As in the bronchi of asthmatic patients, epithelial damage (desquamation) is frequently found in nasal polyps (2). Small areas of epithelial metaplasia without atypia can also be seen. As in the typical findings in bronchial asthma, a thickened basement membrane is a prominent characteristic of nasal polyps. Nasal polyps contain myofibroblast-like cells (2), which have also been described in asthma (3). The stroma of polyps and sinus mucosa is very edematous and contains a mixed inflammatory reaction with neutrophils, activated lymphocytes, mast cells, and eosinophils (2). Eosinophils are the most abundant inflammatory cell type and the majority of them are EG2 positive, indicating that they are activated (2).

There are no clear histological differences between polyps and sinusitis in ASA-sensitive patients with respect to nonsensitive subjects. However, eosinophilic infiltration in nasal polyps and sinus mucosa from patients with ASA sensitivity is in general more prominent than in allergic and nonallergic rhinitis without aspirin sensitivity.

As in asthma, the presence of epithelial cell desquamation in polyps has been related to the presence of cytotoxic eosinophil-derived products. A strong positive correlation has also been found between the number of polypectomies and the peripheral blood eosinophil count (4).

A recent comparison study of the inflammatory cell infiltrate in bronchial biopsies revealed, as in polyps, significantly more eosinophils in ASA (37%) than in aspirin-tolerant patients (11%) (5).

The similarities in the profile of inflammatory cells in polyps/sinus and the airway suggest that they are responding to similar inflammatory signals from these tissues. However, recent studies have shown some differences in the type of T lymphocytes and the cellular sources and nature of the cytokines promoting eosinophilia in nonallergic asthma and nonallergic chronic sinusitis with polyposis and aspirin intolerance (6).

In contrast to polyps from asthmatic patients with aspirin sensitivity, polyps from patients with cystic fibrosis, primary ciliary dyskinesia, and Young's syndrome usually lack an eosinophil component and have neutrophils as a predominant cell.

D. Cytokines

Recent studies indicate that inflammatory and structural cells within nasal polyps are an important source of cytokines (6–11). Activated eosinophils produce a variety of cytokines including IL-3, IL-5, and GM-CSF. Eosinophils have been shown to express mRNA for GM-CSF in nasal polyps (7). The demonstration that eosinophils can both produce and respond to GM-CSF suggests that activated eosinophils may autostimulate themselves to produce this and other cytokines. Furthermore, IL-3, IL-5, and GM-CSF enhance the production of leukotrienes, which have the capacity to promote tissue inflammation and bronchoconstriction.

Nasal fibroblast and nasal epithelial cells derived from nasal polyps release GM-CSF, TNFα, IL-8, and RANTES (2,7,9–11). Epithelial cells from nasal mucosa and polyps enhance eosinophil survival, suggesting that this can be a mechanism for eosinophil accumulation in the nose (7,9–11). Epithelial cells obtained from nasal polyps are more active in inducing eosinophil survival than those obtained from nasal mucosa (9). Recent studies have shown that GM-CSF, and to a lesser extent IL-8 and TNFα, are the main contributors to increased eosinophil survival induced by supernatants obtained from cultured epithelial cells (11). It has also been reported that the spontaneous production of GM-CSF is higher in cultures from nasal polyps compared with those from normal mucosa (7). All these findings suggest that polyp epithelial cells represent a very active inflamed tissue (7,9,11).

Lymphocytes are also present in nasal polyps and sinusitis. Recent studies have shown that TH2-type T lymphocytes in sites of allergic inflammation produce GM-CSF, IL-3, IL-5, and IL-4 (12). All these cytokines contribute to eosinophil accumulation. Hamilos et al. (8) have recently reported evidence that in patients with atopy and nasal polyposis eosinophil recruitment is associated with T-lymphocyte infiltration and the production of GM-CSF, IL-3, IL-5, and IL-4. In contrast, however, Hamilos et al. (8) did not find any evidence of T-lymphocyte infiltration or production of IL-4 and IL-5 in nonatopic nasal polyposis. These patients had a significantly higher tissue expression of GM-CSF, IL-3, and IFNγ. Interestingly, a clinical history of aspirin sensitivity was strongly correlated with the nonallergic profile of cytokines. This suggests that eosinophil infiltration in nasal polyps in nonallergic, aspirin-sensitive patients is not regulated by T lymphocytes and IL-5. Hamilos et al. (8) postulate that other mechanisms exist at the level of the sinus mucosa to account for the eosinophil infiltration in nonallergic chronic rhinosinusitis and polyposis. Such mechanisms might include the production of cytokines and/or different mediators (leukotrienes, PAF) by epithelial cells, fibroblasts, or mast cells.

Unfortunately, the characteristics of the cellular infiltrate present in the nasal polyps of aspirin-sensitive patients cannot be compared with bronchial mucosa obtained from the same patients, because there are no studies investigating the characteristics and cytokine profile of lymphocytes in the bronchial mucosa of these patients.

III. Arachidonic Acid Metabolites in Nasal and Bronchial Secretions in Aspirin-Sensitive Patients

In the majority of aspirin-sensitive patients, aspirin ingestion precipitates both an asthmatic reaction and a nasal reaction. This finding provides additional evidence for a common pathogenic mechanism in chronic sinusitis/nasal polyps and bronchial asthma in these patients.

Aspirin-induced attacks of asthma and rhinitis appear to be precipitated by inhibition of cyclooxygenase (COX) in the airways and nose. There is evidence that these reactions are directly related to the generation of cysteinyl leukotrienes (13–19).

A. Production of Eicosanoids in the Nose and Airways in Aspirin-Sensitive Patients

At baseline no differences in the production of eicosanoids have been detected in either nasal lavages or bronchoalveolar lavages between aspirin-intolerant and aspirin-tolerant subjects (18,19). The nasal and bronchial levels of PGE_2, $PGF_{2\alpha}$, PGD_2, and TXB_2 are similar in patients with and without aspirin intolerance (18,19).

Several studies have documented with aspirin-intolerant asthmatic subjects an increased excretion of urinary LTE_4 compared with other asthmatic subjects (16,17). This finding suggests that aspirin-intolerant asthmatic patients have an overproduction of cysteinyl-leukotrienes. This is in contrast with the demonstration of a similar production of cysteinyl-leukotrienes in the nose (18) and airways (19) in asthma patients with and without aspirin sensitivity. The reasons for this difference are unclear. It is possible that the area studied by BAL and nasal lavages is too small to allow for the detection of differences in the release of mediators. The participation of other cells, isolated or in combination, such as activated blood eosinophils and platelets, in the overproduction of cysteinyl-leukotrienes detected in urine is possible but not proved.

B. Effect of Aspirin on COX and Lipoxygenase Metabolites in the Nose and Airways in Aspirin-Sensitive Patients

Oral and inhaled aspirin provocation is associated with increased excretion of cysteinyl-leukotrienes in nasal lavages (15), bronchoalveolar lavages (13), and urine in ASA (16,17). Direct challenge of the nose (18) and the bronchial mucosa (19) also induces an increase in cysteinyl-leukotrienes release in these patients. No significant changes have been detected after aspirin challenge in the release of other lipoxygenase metabolites such as LTB_4 and 15-HETE, either in the nose (18) or in the airways (13).

The metabolic response to local instillation of aspirin in the nose and airways is similar. After aspirin deposition on the nose or on the bronchi, PGE_2, $PGF_{2\alpha}$, and PGD_2 became significantly depressed in aspirin-tolerant asthmatics, whereas cysteinyl-leukotriene remained unchanged (18,19). In contrast, in the intolerant group, PGE_2 levels were reduced, but mean PGD_2 and $PGF_{2\alpha}$ showed no changes (18,19). In the intolerant group, aspirin also caused a three-fold rise in cysteinyl-leukotriene release in both nasal washings and bronchoalveolar lavage (18,19). These impressive similarities in the response to aspirin challenge provide clear evidence that the nose and airways share common abnormalities of similar significance in the arachidonic acid pathway.

The different susceptibility of PGD_2 and $PGF_{2\alpha}$ to aspirin between aspirin-tolerant and -intolerant patients detected in nasal and bronchial challenges has no clear explanation. Interestingly, aspirin-sensitive patients are also less reactive to $PGF_{2\alpha}$ than aspirin-tolerant patients (20). It has been suggested that the disparate effect of aspirin on PGE_2 and $PGF_{2\alpha}$ in aspirin-sensitive patients might potentiate the eicosanoid balance toward bronchial obstruction by removing the bronchodilator effect of PGE_2 and leaving the bronchoconstrictor effect of $PGF_{2\alpha}$ unchecked (19).

The relative resistance of $PGF_{2\alpha}$ to inhibition by aspirin, and its poor bronchoconstrictor effect on ASA compared to tolerant patients, is an intriguing phenomenon, the origin of which remains to be clarified. Whether the phenomenon of aspirin sensitivity is somehow related to the resistance of $PGF_{2\alpha}$ to inhibition by aspirin is unknown.

IV. Effects of Aspirin on the Release of Mast Cells and Eosinophil Products in the Nose and Airways

The eosinophil has been implicated in the pathogenesis of nasal and bronchial aspirin-induced reactions. Recently it has been shown that nasal (21) and bronchial (19) aspirin challenges caused an early influx of eosinophils into nasal and bronchial secretions. The eosinophil cationic protein (ECP), considered a marker of eosinophil activation, increased significantly in nasal secretions 30 min after the challenge, reached the highest value at 60 min, and remained significantly elevated at 120 min (21). ECP values also increased after bronchial challenge (from 3.9 ± 6.5 to 10 ± 15 ng/ml) but they did not reach statistical significance, probably because bronchoalveolar lavages were carried out only once, 15 min after aspirin challenge (19). The time course of eosinophil activation obtained in the nose suggests that a period of 30 min or more between challenge and lavage is necessary to detect significant changes in eosinophil influx (21).

The possible role of mast cells during aspirin-induced respiratory reactions has been a matter of debate, with studies both denying and supporting their participation. Fischer et al. (15) found that tryptase, a marker of mast cell activation, increased in nasal lavages several hours after challenge. Kowalski et al. (21) also found a significant increase in the tryptase level in nasal secretions 60 min after aspirin challenge. In contrast, Sladek et al. (13) and Szczeklik et al. (19) did not find significant changes in tryptase levels in bronchoalveolar lavages, possibly because BAL was carried out at 30 (13) and 15 (19) min post aspirin challenge, and according to nasal studies (21), the release of mast cell products usually peaks at 60 min post challenge.

Recently, Nasser et al. (22) have reported increased percentages of 5-lipoxygenase immunostaining cells, identified as mast cells and eosinophils, in bronchial biopsies from aspirin-intolerant patients compared with those from aspirin-tolerant patients. After aspirin instillation, a decrease in the number of mast cells and activation of eosinophils was detected. These findings suggest that the degranulation of mast cells and the activation of eosinophils are involved in ASA.

No similar studies have been carried out so far in the nose.

V. Clinical Manifestations

The typical patient with aspirin-induced asthma starts to experience intense vasomotor rhinitis characterized by a profuse rhinorrhea, eventually followed by chronic nasal congestion and loss of smelling capacity (hyposmia or anasmia) (23). The patient often seeks medical attention at this point and physical examination frequently reveals nasal polyps. CT scans help to identify extended sinusitis mostly located in the maxillar and ethmoidal sinus. Bronchial asthma and aspirin intolerance develop during subsequent stages of the illness. This course of events may progress over a few months or last for years.

There are cases where the first asthma attack is precipitated by aspirin or related drugs. In these patients asthma and aspirin sensitivity are detected at the same time.

Asthma never develops in some patients and aspirin only precipitates nasal symptoms. In contrast, in some unusual patients with aspirin-induced asthma, nasal symptoms never develop, or they begin several months or years after the appearance of bronchial symptoms.

A typical aspirin-induced reaction occurs within 30 min to 2 hr of intake of an aspirin or other nonsteroidal anti-inflammatory drug (NSAID). Symptoms include bronchospasm, profuse rhinorrhea, and nasal congestion. In addition to the symptoms from the airways and nose, the patients often experience ocular injection, nausea, vomiting, diarrhea, and abdominal cramps.

However, many patients with an identical clinical picture (rhinosinusitis, polyps, and asthma) never develop aspirin intolerance. More intriguing is the group of patients with nasal polyps and chronic rhinosinusitis whose asthma and rhinitis are relieved by aspirin (24,25).

VI. Diagnosis of Aspirin Sensitivity

An asthmatic with chronic rhinitis, loss of smelling capacity, and nasal polyps should always be considered a candidate for the development of aspirin intolerance. In some patients with these characteristics, and repetitive attacks of bronchospasm and rhinitis precipitated by NSAID, the diagnosis of aspirin-induced asthma and rhinitis is easily established. However, in patients only suspected of aspirin intolerance, the diagnosis can be established with certainty only by aspirin challenge.

There are three types of provocation tests, oral, inhaled, and nasal, depending on the route of aspirin administration. Oral provocation with aspirin has been used for many years to diagnose aspirin-induced asthma (26,27). The procedure has a high risk of provoking severe bronchial and/or systemic reaction and is not suitable for routine clinical practice. Inhalation challenge is safer than the oral challenge but cannot be used on patients with a moderate-severe bronchial obstruction (a baseline FEV_1 higher than 65–70% predicted is usually required) (28). Nasal challenge with aspirin is a safe, easily performed test, but its diagnostic value is limited by its moderate sensitivity (29,30).

VII. Treatment of Rhinosinusitis and Nasal Polyposis in Aspirin-Sensitive Patients

Treatment for patients with the asthma triad involves avoidance of NSAID, glucocorticoid therapy (systemic and topical), aspirin desensitization, and surgical therapy.

A. Avoidance of NSAID

Patients with nasal polyps, chronic rhinosinusitis, and aspirin sensitivity should avoid all products that inhibit COX. Most patients will tolerate paracetamol at a dose not exceeding 1000 mg daily. They can safely take codeine, dextro-poxyphene, opiates, and their derivatives (tramadol, pentazocin). However, the avoidance of NSAID is not a specific therapy because even a strict control of NSAID intake does not alter the course of bronchial and nasal disease.

As anti-inflammatory drugs, glucocorticoids are recommended if anti-inflammation therapy is required for a short period. If prolonged anti-inflammatory therapy is necessary, the majority of patients will tolerate choline magnesium trisalicylate, nimesulide, and sodium salicylate. Because some aspirin-sensitive patients do not tolerate some of these products, it is important to perform a controlled challenge test with the proposed anti-inflammatory drug.

B. Glucocorticoids

Systemic steroids are effective when given in a dose of 30–50 mg daily for 2 or more weeks. In some patients, a poor response to high doses of systemic doses can be detected. The mechanisms responsible for this relative steroid resistance are unclear. Hydrocortisone, and in particular succinate salts, have been reported to precipitate adverse reaction in some ASA (31), an old observation that has been questioned in a recent study (32).

Topical glucocorticoids are the drugs of choice for nasal polyposis and chronic sinusitis. These patients need regular therapy with topical glucocorticoids. Topical steroids should be given in a dose higher than that usually recommended. Six hundred micrograms or more of budesonide is necessary to obtain relatively good results. Several studies have shown that topical glucocorticoids both reduce the size of polyps and prevent or delay recurrence of nasal polyps after surgery and therefore repolypectomies (33–36). Unfortunately, the smelling capacity is only occasionally recovered with topical steroid therapy.

C. Desensitization

Aspirin desensitization was discovered following the observation of a refractory period to aspirin after repeated aspirin-induced bronchoconstriction (37). The duration of refractoriness varies individually from a few hours to 7 days. The mechanisms for desensitization are unknown. A permanent state of tolerance to aspirin can be achieved by giving aspirin regularly. Hypersensitivity to aspirin recurs within 2–7 days of discontinuing aspirin administration.

Aspirin desensitization in ASA should be performed only by experienced physicians in a specialized clinic. Desensitization can be carried out using a rapid or slow procedure. In the rapid method desensitization can be achieved in a few days by giving increasing doses of aspirin (38–40). With this procedure the initial dose(s) precipitate bronchospastic reaction until the well-tolerated dose of 500 mg is reached. Aspirin is then administered regularly at a daily dose of 500–1000 mg.

In the slow procedure a dose of 30 mg of aspirin is initially given and the dose is doubled every 1 or 2 days, up to the maintenance dose of 500–1000 mg. Gastrointestinal side effects occur in 15–20% of the patients. Sweet et al. (40) found that aspirin desensitization is effective in the treatment of rhinosinusitis and that a high proportion of patients recovered partially or totally from their anosmia.

Aspirin desensitization by local instillation of aspirin is not effective and patients only occasionally respond clinically to this therapy. Conversely, some patients may even show a progressive deterioration of their nasal symptoms.

D. Surgical Therapy

When nasal respiration is severely compromised by polyps and chronic rhinosinusitis not responding to medical therapy, surgery should be considered (41). The goal for surgical management of nasal polyps should be to restore nasal function. Unfortunately, nasal polyps recur very early and more often in aspirin-sensitive patients than in aspirin-tolerant subjects. Early introduction of corticosteroid therapy immediately after surgery is mandatory to prevent or at least delay polyp recurrence.

There are different techniques for the surgical management of nasal polyps. If the nose is blocked by a few large polyps, they can be removed by a simple polypectomy. Functional endoscopy sinus surgery is a second-step therapy in patients with nasal polyps. When patients with nasal polyps require polypectomy several times or suffer from severe chronic rhinosinusitis, ethmoidectomy can be performed. In general, this procedure resulted in long-term reduction of recurrent sinusitis and nasal airway patency improvement (41). Unfortunately, recurrence of nasal polyps is still frequent after this extensive surgery, especially in those patients not adequately managed with post-surgery medical therapy.

Surgical therapy does not aggravate asthma. On the contrary, the amelioration of nasal function can even improve the course of asthma with a substantial reduction in the dosage of systemic glucocorticoids.

E. Prospects for Future Therapy

Since aspirin-sensitive subjects characteristically show an overproduction of cysteinyl-leukotrienes, it is conceivable that this subgroup of asthmatic subjects should respond better to antileukotriene drugs than aspirin-tolerant patients. Recent studies have shown that regular therapy of aspirin-intolerant asthmatics with a 5-lipoxygenase inhibitor (Zileuton) leads to improvement in both bronchial and nasal symptoms (42). Zileuton treatment blocked the increase in nasal symptoms after aspirin challenge. It also blocked the rise in nasal tyrptase and nasal leukotrienes (15).

VIII. Summary

Nasal polyps and chronic rhinosinusitis are present in the majority of ASA. In these patients, aspirin ingestion or instillation into the nose or airways induces both a nasal and bronchial reaction. These reactions are accompanied by a concomitant increase in cysteinyl-leukotriene release. The parallel release of tryptase and the presence of high numbers of eosinophils and increased levels of ECP suggest that mast cells and eosinophils are involved in the adverse reaction. The similarities in the reaction between the nose and airways in aspirin-sensitive subjects provide compelling evidence for common pathogenic mechanisms for both nasal polyps/chronic rhinosinusitis and bronchial asthma. Direct challenge of nasal mucosa with aspirin is a very safe test that can be used in the diagnosis of aspirin intolerance, and in the study of the mechanisms responsible for this intriguing phenomenon.

References

1. Terries MH, Davidson TM. Review of published results for endoscopic sinus surgery. Ear Nose Throat J 1994; 73:574–580.
2. Jordana M, Dolovich J, Ohno I, Finotto S, Denburg J. Nasal polyposis: a model for chronic inflammation. In: Holgate ST, Busse W, eds. Asthma and Rhinitis. Boston: Blackwell, 1995:156–163.
3. Brewster CEP, Howarth PH, Djucanovic R, Wilson J, Holgate ST, Roche WR. Myofibroblasts and subepithelial fibrosis in bronchial asthma. Am J Respir Cell Mol Biol 1990; 3:507–511.
4. Wong GG, Jordana M, Denburg J, Dolovich J. Blood eosinophilia and nasal polyps. Am J Rhinol 1992; 6;195–198.
5. Nasser SMS, Pfister R, Christie PE, Sousa AR, Barker J. Schmitz-Schumann M, Lee TH, Inflammatory cell populations in bronchial biopsies from aspirin-sensitive asthmatic subjects. Am J Respir Crit Care Med 1996; 153:90–96.
6. Hamilos D, Leung DYM, Wood R, Cunningham L, Bean DK, Yasruel Z, Schotman E, Hamid Q. Evidence for distinct cytokine expression in allergic versus nonallergic chronic sinusitis. J Allergy Clin Immunol 1995; 96:537–544.
7. Ohno I, Lea R, Finotto S, Marshall J, Denburg J, Dolovich J, Gauldie J, Jordana M. Granulocyte/macrophage colony-stimulating factor (GM-CSF) gene expression by eosinophils in nasal polyposis. Am J Respir Cell Mol Biol 1991; 5:505–510.
8. Hamilos DL, Leung DYM, Wood R, Schotman E, Hamid Q. Chronic hyperplastic sinusitis: association of tissue eosinophilia with mRNA expression of granulocyte-macrophage colony-stimulating factor and interleukin-3. J Allergy Clin Immunol 1993; 92:39–48.
9. Xaubet A, Mullol J, Lopez F, Roca-Ferrer J, Rozman M, Carrion T, Fabra JM, Picado C. Comparison of the role of nasal polyp and normal nasal mucosa epithelial cells on in vitro eosinophil survival. Mediation by GM-CSF and inhibition by dexamethasone. Clin Exp Allergy 1994; 24:307–317.
10. Mullol J, Xaubet A, Lopez E, Roca-Ferrer J, Picado C. Comparative study of the effects of different glucocorticoids on eosinophil survival primed by cultured epithelial cell supernatant obtained from nasal mucosa and nasal polyps. Thorax 1995; 50:270–274.
11. Mullol J, Xaubet A, Gaya A, Roca-Ferrer J, Lopez E, Fernandez JC, Fernandez MD, Picado C. Cytokine gene expression and release from epithelial cells. A comparison study between healthy nasal mucosa and nasal polyps. Clin Exp Allergy 1995; 25:607–615.
12. Durham SR, Ying S, Varney VA, Jacobson MR, Sudderick RM, Mackay IS, Kay AB, Hamid QA. Cytokine messenger RNA expression for IL-3, IL-4, IL-5 and granulocyte/macrophage-colony-stimulating factor in the nasal mucosa after local allergen provocation: relationship to tissue eosinophilia. J Immunol 1992; 148: 2390–2394.
13. Sladek K, Dworski J, Soja J, Sheller E, Nizankowska E, Oates JA, Szczeklik A. Eicosanoids in bronchoalveolar lavage fluid of aspirin-intolerant patients with asthma after aspirin challenge. Am J Respir Crit Care Med 1994; 149:940–946.

14. Ferreri NR, Howland WC, Stevenson DD, Spiegelberg HL. Release of leuko-trienes, prostaglandins and histamine into nasal secretion of aspirin-sensitive asthmatics during reaction to aspirin. Am Rev Respir Dis 1988; 137:847–854.

15. Fischer AR, Rosenberg MA, Lilly CM, Callery JC, Rubin P, Cohn J, White MV, Igarashi Y, Kaliner MA, Drazen JM, Israel E. Direct evidence for a role of mast cell in the nasal response to aspirin in aspirin-sensitive patients. J Allergy Clin Immunol 1994; 94:1046–1056.

16. Christie PE, Tagari P, Ford-Hutchinson AW, Charlesson S, Chee J, Arm JP, Lee TH. Urinary leukotriene E$_4$ concentrations increase after ASA challenge in ASA-sensitive subjects. Am Rev Respir Dis 1991; 143:1025–1029.

17. Kumlin M, Dahlén B, Björck T, Zetterström O, Granström E, Dahlén SE. Urinary excretion of leukotriene E$_4$ and 11-dihydro-thromboxane B$_2$ in response to bronchial provocations with allergen, aspirin, leukotriene D$_4$ and histamine in asthmatics. Am Rev Respir Dis 1992; 146:96–103.

18. Picado C, Ramis I, Rosellò J, Prat J, Bulbena O, Plaza V, Montserrat JM, Gelpí E. Release of peptide leukotriene into nasal secretions after local instillation of aspirin in aspirin-sensitive asthmatic patients. Am Rev Respir Dis 1992; 145:65–69.

19. Szczeklik A, Sladek K, Dworski R, Nizankowska E, Soja J, Sheller J, Oates J. Bronchial aspirin challenge causes specific eocisanoid response in aspirin-sensitive asthmatics. Am J Respir Crit Care Med 1996; 154:1608–1614.

20. Pasargiklian M, Bianco S, Allegra L, Moavero NE, Petrigine G, Robuschi M, Grugni A. Aspects of bronchial reactivity to prostaglandins and aspirin in asthmatic patients. Respiration 1977; 34:79–91.

21. Kowalski ML, Grzegorczyk J, Wojciechowska B, Poniatowska M. Intransal challenge with aspirin induces cell influx and activation of eosinophils and mast cells in nasal secretions of ASA-sensitive patients. Clin Exp Allergy 1996; 26: 807–814.

22. Nasser SMS, Christie PE, Pfister R, Sousa AR, Barker J, Schmitz-Schumann M, Lee TH. Effects of endobronchial challenge of inflammatory cells in bronchial biopsy samples from aspirin-sensitive asthmatic subjects. Thorax 1996; 51:64–70.

23. Szczeklik A. Aspirin-induced asthma. Pathogenesis and clinical presentation. Allergy Proc 1992; 13:32–37.

24. Kodansky D, Adkinson F, Norman PS, Rosenthal RR. Asthma improved by nonsteroidal anti-inflammatory drugs. Ann Intern Med 1978; 88:508–511.

25. Szczeklik A, Nizankowska E. Asthma improved by aspirin-like drugs. Br J Dis Chest 1983; 77:153–158.

26. Stevenson DD. Diagnosis, prevention and treatment of adverse reactions to aspirin and nonsteroidal anti-inflammatory drugs. J Allergy Clin Immunol 1984; 74:617–622.

27. Castillo JA, Picado C. Prevalence of aspirin-intolerance in a hospital population. Respiration 1986; 50:153–157.

28. Dahlén B, Zetterström O. Comparison of bronchial and per oral provocation with aspirin in aspirin-sensitive asthmatics. Eur Respir J 1990; 3:527–534.

29. Patriarca G, Nucera E, DiRienzo V, Schiavino D, Pellegrino S, Fais G. Nasal provocation test with lysine acetylsalicylate in aspirin-sensitive patients. Ann Allergy 1991; 67:60–62.

30. Casadevall J, Mullol J, Picado C. Intranasal challenge with aspirin in the diagnosis of aspirin sensitive asthma. Evaluation of nasal response by acoustic rhinometry. Eur Respir J (in press).
31. Dajani BM, Sliman NA, Shubair KS, Hamzeh YS. Bronchospasm caused by intravenous hydrocortisone sodium succinate (Solu-Cortef) in aspirin-sensitive asthmatics. J Allergy Clin Immunol 1981; 68:201–204.
32. Feigembaum BA, Stevenson DD, Simon RA. Hydrocortisone sodium succinate does not cross-react with aspirin in aspirin-sensitive patients with asthma. J Allergy Clin Immunol 1995; 96:545–548.
33. Mygind N, Pedersen CB, Prytz S, Sörensen H. Treatment of nasal polyps with intranasal beclomethasone nasal aerosol. Clin Allergy 1975; 5:159–164.
34. Deutschl H, Drettner B. Nasal polyps treated by beclomethasone nasal aerosol. Rhinology 1977; 15:159–164.
35. Lidholt T, Rundcratz H, Lindqvist N. Efficacy of topical corticosteroid power for nasal polyps: a double-blind, placebo-controlled study of budesonide. Clin Otolaryngol 1995; 20:26–30.
36. Hartwig S, Linden M, Laurent C, Vargö AK, Lindqvist N. Budesonide nasal spray as prophylactic treatment after polypectomy. J Laryngol Otol 1988; 102:148–151.
37. Zeiss CR, Lockey RF. Refractory period to aspirin in a patient with aspirin-induced asthma. J Allergy Clin Immunol 1976; 57:440–448.
38. Stevenson DD, Simon RA, Mathinson DA. Aspirin-sensitive asthma: tolerance to aspirin after positive oral aspirin challenges. J Allergy Clin Immunol 1980; 66:82–88.
39. Lumry WR, Lurd JG, Zeiger RS, Pleskow WW, Stevenson DD. Aspirin-sensitive rhinosinusitis: the clinical syndrome and effects of aspirin administration. J Allergy Clin Immunol 1983; 71:580–587.
40. Sweet JM, Stevenson DD, Simon RA, Mathinson DA. Long-term effects of aspirin desensitization. Treatment for aspirin-sensitive rhinosinusitis-asthma. J Allergy Clin Immunol 1990; 85:59–65.
41. Holmberg K, Karlsson W. Nasal polyps: medical or surgical management? Clin Exp Allergy 1996; 26(Suppl 3):23–30.
42. Dahlen SE, Nizankowska E, Dahlen B, Bochenek G, Kumlin M, Mastlerz L, Blomqvist H, Pinis G, Rasberg B, Swanson LJ, Larsson L, Dube L, Stensvad F, Zetterström O, Szczeklik A. The Swedish-Polish treatment study with the 5-lipoxygenase inhibitor Zileuton in aspirin-intolerant asthmatics. Am J Respir Crit Care Med 1995; 151:A376 (abstract).

29

The Role of Glucocorticoids in the Modulation of Eicosanoid Metabolism in Asthma

ISABELLE VACHIER, PASCAL CHANEZ, CLAUDE CHAVIS, JEAN BOUSQUET, and PHILIPPE GODARD

Hôpital Arnaud de Villeneuve
INSERM U454
Montpellier, France

I. Introduction

Bronchial asthma is now clearly defined as an inflammatory disorder of the bronchi. Glucocorticoids, which are actually the most potent anti-inflammatory agents, are very effective in controlling inflammation and are the treatment of choice for long-term management. The therapeutic development has mainly been governed by results in clinical improvement but the mechanistic explanations of the effects of glucocorticoids are still unclear, despite recent advances in the understanding of the molecular mechanisms of their action.

Patients with asthma have increased numbers of various types of inflammatory cells, such as eosinophils and neutrophils, within their airways (1). These cells are activated and produce a variety of inflammatory mediators including histamine, reactive oxygen species, cytokines, prostaglandins, and leukotrienes, for example (2,3). There is increasing evidence that leukotrienes play an important role in the pathophysiology of asthma (4–9).

Since glucocorticoids have been shown to inhibit the release of some arachidonic acid metabolites (10), the purpose of this review is to summarize and analyze current concepts of asthma therapy with glucocorticoids, especially in their effects on inflammatory cells regulating eicosanoid production.

II. Mechanisms of Glucocorticoid Action

A. Functional Study of the Glucocorticoid Receptor (GR)

Glucocorticoids control a wide range of processes in a variety of cells. GR is expressed in most cell types and tissues, but GR levels vary among different tissue types (11). The amino acid sequence for human GR consists of 777 residues with greater than 90% homology with GR sequences from other species (12).

The carboxy-terminus of GR is the hormone-binding domain (about 300 amino acids). This hormone-binding domain contains nuclear localization signals (13). This domain is also implicated in the binding with heat shock protein 90 (hsp 90), and these hsp 90-GR complexes are destabilized by ligand binding (14). The hormone-binding domain contains also one of the two dimerization contact regions.

GR regulates the transcription of target genes by its binding to glucocorticoid responsive element (GRE). The domain responsible for this binding is the central DNA-binding domain, which contains a "zinc finger" structure (15). Two monomers of the DNA-binding domain bind symmetrically to the surface of the DNA, at the consensus GRE (16).

The transcriptional activation domain in the amino-terminal region of the protein is a region that increases the RNA polymerase-initiated transcription (17). This region requires ligand binding to induce transcriptional activity. The dimerization is also necessary for this region to be functional.

B. Molecular Mechanism of Anti-inflammatory Action of Glucocorticoids

Glucocorticoid hormones are effective in controlling inflammation, but the mechanisms that confer this action are largely unknown. In asthmatic airways, the biological action of glucocorticoids' effect on responsive cells is mediated by intracellular GR that binds to homologous ligand function as DNA-binding protein, directly or indirectly enhanced or suppressed basal transcription of target cells (18,19). Glucocorticoids act through an inactive GR (94 kDa). This inactivated GR is bound to a protein complex, two subunits of the hsp 90 (20) and a 59-kDa immunophilin protein (21). Hsp 90 significantly facilitates GR function, since its association with the receptor is essential for obtaining the high-affinity steroid-binding conformation (22). With glucocorticoid binding, the DNA-binding site of GR is revealed and the complex migrates to the nucleus. GR forms a homodimer that binds to a consensus *cis*-acting DNA sequence, GRE, in the upstream regulatory region of genes that either inhibits or stimulates transcription of target gene (18,19). GR may also form complexes with activating transcription factors in the nucleus to inhibit their effects. Proinflammatory transcription factors, such as activator protein-1 (AP-1) (23) and nuclear factor kappa B (NF-κB), can form a complex with GR to modulate the transcription of various genes including GR itself (Fig. 1).

Recent studies have shown that both positive and negative regulation of gene expression are necessary for this process (24). The positive action of GR on gene expression requires interaction of receptor dimers with discrete nucleotide sequences on inducible promoters. The negative action of the receptor is important for the anti-inflammatory and immunosuppressive actions of glucocorticoids.

Modes of Positive Regulation

Positive regulation of genomic transcription was the first described. The most important genes controlled positively gy glucocorticoids are tyrosine aminotransferase and phosphoenol pyruvate carboxykinase genes, which are implicated in the metabolism of the liver (ribonucleases and endonucleases), peptidases, and several receptors including the adrenergic β₂-receptor. When GR

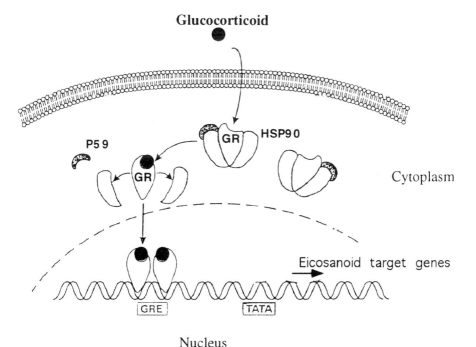

Figure 1 A model illustrating the mechanism of action of glucocorticoid on the expression of eicosanoid target genes. (See text for explanation.)

binds its hormone, it dissociates from the hsp 90–p59 complex and exposes the DNA-binding domain (two zinc fingers) (25). A homodimer of two GR can be coupled to specific DNA sequences GRE (26). The proper contact between the DNA-binding domain of the GR complex and the GRE is not sufficient for inducing transcription. There are two transactivating regions of the receptor, TAF1 and TAF2, which need to be activated by phosphorylation (27). Then a full transcription complex can be formed and RNA polymerase can start transcription (28). Positive regulation can contribute to the anti-inflammatory process. The receptor induces the expression of the inhibitor of NF-κB, IκBα, which binds and reduces activity of NF-κB (29,30). In this case GR uses its transactivation properties to stimulate expression at the IκB promoter. IκBα is responsible for sequestering p65 and p50, the two subunits of NF-κB, in an inactive state in the cytoplasm. Furthermore, positive action is also required for the expression of lipocortin-1, also called anexin-1, a 37-kDa protein (31), which is a potential anti-inflammatory factor by its potentiality to inhibit phospholipase A_2. Its role is confirmed by findings that recombinant lipocortin-1 has acute anti-inflammatory properties and inhibits the release of lipid mediators from the lung (31,32).

Modes of Negative Regulation

Negative transcription of cytokines, growth factors, and proinflammatory enzymes represents the central role of anti-inflammatory and immunosuppressive actions of glucocorticoids. Several mechanisms of overlapping binding sites and protein-protein interactions have been described.

Overlapping Binding Sites

The GR may compete with positive-acting transcription factors for binding to a common site on the promoter region of regulatable genes.

For human osteocalcin gene promoter, for example, studies showed that GR binds to a region overlapping the TATA box, suggesting that the mechanism of transcriptional inhibition in this case is interference with the transcription initiation machinery (33). The TATA box binding factor, TFIID, competes for binding to the same site. Characterization of the glycoprotein, a subunit gene, has shown that transcriptional repression is dependent on the presence of a functional cAMP response element overlapping the GRE (34).

The GR can bind to another type of GRE designated negative GRE (nGRE), which can directly repress the promoter region. Apparently the factor that regulates the activity of the nGRE in the absence of hormone is ubiquitous, since its activity can be found in several cell types. Several lines of evidence suggest that DNA binding to the GR is required for repression of transcription through the nGRE (35). On the promoter region of the interleukin-6 (IL-6) gene there are at least two such GREs (36).

Protein-Protein Interaction

The complex glucocorticoids/GR can bind to the transcription factor–activating protein-1 (AP-1), a heterodimer of two proto-oncogenes c-*jun* and c-*fos*, and block its transcription. AP-1 is a common transcription factor up-regulated during inflammation and proliferation (23). The GR alone, upon binding to DNA, does not regulate transcription in the absence of AP-1. In vitro translation and immunoprecipitation studies showed that the GR physically associates in solution with AP-1 (37). This is the case for human collagenase I (23).

The GR associates in vitro with the p65 and p50 subunits of NF-κB and destroys the DNA-binding activity of these proteins (38). This type of repression occurred for IL-8 gene expression (39).

C. Action on Eicosanoid Target Gene

The effectiveness of glucocorticoids in asthma is probably the result of a combination of inhibitory effects on the inflammatory process through increasing or decreasing gene transcription. Most of these actions result in a reduction in level or activity of proinflammatory mediators. A few anti-inflammatory proteins are thought to be up-regulated by corticoids, for example, lipocortin-1. Lipocortin-1, which is a calcium- and phospholipid-binding protein, is abundant in the lung in epithelial cells, tracheal gland cells, alveolar macrophages, and neutrophils (40). Studies in humans have shown that levels of lipocortin-1 increase in the respiratory tract secretions of healthy volunteers (41) and lung lavage cells of patients after oral administration of therapeutic doses of gluco corticoid (42). The first experiments to demonstrate the existence of the protein showed that an anti-inflammatory protein appeared to mediate the suppression of phospholipase A_2 activity by glucocorticoids, and subsequently eicosanoid synthesis (43,44). But the anti-inflammatory activity of the recombinant and native proteins, both in vivo and in vitro, was not found. Then the discovery that the recombinant protein required refolding into the correct three-dimensional conformation in order to be biologically active stimulated the development of powerful new tools with which to examine the actions of lipocortin-1 (45). It has been shown that lipocortin-1 occupies a specific cell surface binding site on the plasma membrane of the target cells (46), thus indicating that extracellular release is essential for the activity of this protein. How this interaction between lipocortin-1 and its binding site triggers a reduction in inflammation is not entirely clear. It is known that in the A549 cell line, lipocortin-1 reduces eicosanoid production, not by altering expression of cyclooxygenase-2 (COX-2), but by reducing phospholipase A_2 activity, perhaps as a result of modulation of signal transduction processes (47). The mechanism of action of lipocortin-1 in the human lungs remains to be fully elucidated. Lipocortin-1 gene contains a consensus GRE in the promoter, in addition to an AP1 site and other regulatory sequences (48). New evidence suggests that lipocortin-1 may mediate some of the effects of glucocorticoids through putative lipocortin-1 receptors that are located on the surface of phagocytic cells (49).

Corticosteroids have been also described to inhibit the interaction of the genes coding for inducible COX-2 in mononuclear and epithelial cells (50,51). But other studies report that prednisone increases the expression of COX-2 mRNA in blood monocytes from atopic subjects and decreases it in normal subjects (52).

III. Effects of Glucocorticoids on Arachidonic Acid Metabolism In Vitro

The effects of glucocorticoids in vitro on the metabolism of arachidonic acid have been studied in a variety of different cell types and with different steroids. The results described in these studies are controversial and differ depending on the cell type and the way to stimulate, or not to stimulate, the cells (Figure 2).

Studies on rat alveolar macrophages showed that methylprednisolone incubated for 16 hr can inhibit the synthesis of TXB_2, LTB_4, and LTC_4 induced by zymosan. Moreover the same incubation of methylprednisolone for 1 hr significantly inhibits the synthesis of LTB_4 and LTC_4. Some authors have evaluated the ability of glucocorticoids to inhibit arachidonic acid metabolism in rat alveolar macrophages stimulated by hydrogen peroxide as compared to zymosan. After stimulation by hydrogen peroxide, methylprednisolone inhibits TXB_2 only weakly and did not inhibit the release of LTB_4 and LTC_4 (53). In the same way, the synthetic glucocorticoid dexamethasone reduced basal prostacyclin generation only in resident rat macrophages, but not in activated ones. This phenomenon correlates to the presence of a soluble factor that increases prostacyclin generation in resident macrophages but is absent in activated cells (54). Moreover, a recent study on human alveolar macrophages from wheezy infants showed that dexamethasone reduced spontaneous and calcium ionophore A23187 stimulated release of TXB_2 but not A23187 stimulated release of LTB_4 (55). In the same way pretreatment by methylprednisolone of human alveolar macrophages stimulated by A23187 showed an inhibition of immunoreactive cyclooxygenase products to a greater extent than immunoreactive leukotrienes (56). The inhibition of the leukotrienes synthesis suggests the possibility that steroids not only act on the PLA_2 level but also exert a postphospholipase A_2 effect on leukotriene synthesis (57).

A study performed on human blood monocytes showed that budesonide had no significant effect on the release of LTB_4 (58). Blood monocytes are the

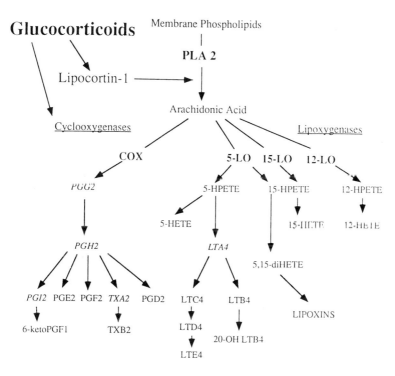

Figure 2 Schematic representation of the arachidonic acid metabolism by cyclooxygenase and lipoxygenases and the potential action of glucocorticoids. (Unstable products are in italics.)

precursors of alveolar macrophages, and in contrast to them, the release of leukotrienes was not affected by the treatment. Moreover, a recent study reports that in peripheral blood monocytes pretreated 24 hr with dexamethasone, dexamethasone caused a concentration-dependent inhibition of PGE_2 production, but had no effect on LTB_4 release (59). These results suggest that the responsiveness of these cells to steroids is dependent on the phase of cell activation-differentiation. Studies of the human promyelocytic U-937 cell line differentiated by 24 hr treatment with phorbol ester myristate show that after treatment for 16 hr with dexamethasone, dexamethasone causes both the release of lipocortin-1 in the cellular supernatant and the inhibition of eicosanoid release (60). The selective release of the lipocortin-1 may explain the inhibition of eicosanoid formation. The in vivo cell responsiveness to glucocorticoids is acquired during cell differentiation from blood monocyte to tissue macrophage.

Vachier et al.

IV. Inhibition of Eicosanoid Biosynthesis In Vivo

It has been postulated that glucocorticoids may inhibit the formation of eicosanoids in vivo, thus explaining their anti-inflammatory actions. Leukotrienes have been investigated in different clinical situations and quantified in biological fluids. Leukotrienes were found by some authors to be increased in asthma at steady state or after a bronchial challenge (61–63). Many studies report that eicosanoids are released in vivo into the alveolar and bronchial space and then recovered in the BAL fluid (64), in the blood (65–67), and in urine (68–72). Nevertheless a few studies report corticoid effects on eicosanoid release in biological fluids. Short-term corticosteroid treatment does not significantly decrease BAL eicosanoids, neither inhaled (73) nor oral (74). In contrast, long-term inhaled corticosteroids decrease LTC_4 levels in BAL (75) and long-term oral corticotherapy is still associated with increased LTE_4 excretion into urine (76). Intravenous prednisolone administered to patients during asthma attacks significantly reduced blood LTB_4 and LTE_4 levels (77).

The formation of eicosanoids was investigated in whole blood and bronchoalveolar lavage cells (BALC) ex vivo in normal subjects. Short-term treatment with prednisone (60 mg/day for 7 days) was not able to induce any reduction of eicosanoid release from stimulated and unstimulated blood (10). This study was able to discriminate between the inhibition in different cell types since there was a profound inhibition of eicosanoid release by BALC. The inhibitory effect was more important on COX-derived products than for LTB_4. Alveolar macrophages are more prone to be affected by glucocorticoids in their release of eicosanoids (57), but there are conflicting results regarding other secretory products of these cells, such as cytokines (78).

The modulation of LTB_4 release by systemic prednisone was investigated using a model of nasal challenge. In the subjects presenting a late response to the allergen challenge, pretreatment with 20 mg of prednisone did not prevent either the occurrence of the late phase or the rise in LTB_4 (79). On the other hand, prednisone has a cell-specific effect on BALC. The effect of oral prednisone was assessed on eicosanoid synthesis by BALC obtained from 14 allergic asthmatic patients. Prednisone treatment was able to inhibit the synthesis of eicosanoids by BALC in vitro. Similarly, Wenzel and colleagues have investigated the clinical and biological effect of a single oral dose of prednisone on the production of LTB_4 by macrophages in asthmatic patients with nocturnal symptoms (80). During the placebo arm of this study, there was no difference in the release of LTB_4 by the alveolar macrophages in vitro between the three different groups of subjects, namely control subjects and asthmatic patients with and without nocturnal symptoms. After administration of prednisone, patients with nocturnal symptoms displayed a clear inhibition by their macrophages to produce LTB_4 in contrast to the patients without nocturnal symptoms and control subjects. The present study suggests that the response of BLAC to glucocorticoids is related to the inflammatory phenotype of the cells. These findings confirm the heterogeneity of macrophages in health and in asthma, the activated cells being more prone to respond to the anti-inflammatory treatment. The effectiveness of glucocorticoids on asthma symptoms might be partly due to their action on macrophages. Blood monocytes are precursors of macrophages and responsible for the maintenance of their pool. They have been shown to be recruited within the airways in asthma (81) and already activated in the blood of symptomatic asthmatic patients (82). In one of our studies, a short-term treatment with high doses of prednisone was not able to alter LTB_4 release from blood monocytes obtained from symptomatic asthmatic patients (83). Using the same cells, we have shown an ex vivo down-regulation of the glucocorticoid receptor gene using the same treatment (84). Thus there is little evidence for a regulating effect of glucocorticoids on eicosanoid synthesis and release at the monocyte level in asthma. These findings can be compared with the absence of intrinsic dysfunction of phospholipase A_2 shown on blood monocytes of asthmatic patients (85).

A characteristic feature of asthma is the infiltration of eosinophils within the airways. These cells are able to synthesize and release the sulfido-leukotrienes LTC_4 (86). Seven-day treatment with 30 mg of prednisolone was shown to decrease the ionophore-induced LTC_4 from a granulocyte preparation obtained from six chronic asthmatic patients (87). Eosinophils purified by percoll density gradient obtained from symptomatic asthmatic patients showed a reduction in their LTC_4 release in vitro after short-term intravenous prednisolone treatment (88).

Neutrophils were found in increased numbers in the airways during the late-phase reaction after an allergen challenge (89), in some patients who died shortly after an exacerbation (90,91), in nocturnal asthma (92), in the sputum of patients with asthma exacerbations (93), and in patients with corticosteroid-dependent asthma (94). But, it seems well established that hyperresponsiveness in human airway tissue can be induced by supernatants of neutrophils stimulated in the presence of varying concentrations of albumin (1).

There are few reports investigating the effects of glucocorticoid treatment on the ability of neutrophils to synthesize eicosanoids. Patients with rheumatoid arthritis used to be treated with a single high dose of glucocorticosteroids. Twenty-four hours after such treatment, it was found that the arachidonic acid metabolism of neutrophils was up-regulated. These cells release higher amounts of the unstable precursor LTA_4 and then LTB_4 and its metabolites (95). The majority of short-term studies with glucocorticoids are consistent with an absence of inhibition of ionophore-induced LTB_4 release by neutrophils in asthma (83,96,97). Nevertheless, some authors report an increase of LTB$_4$ released by neutrophils from asthmatic patients during asthma attack and an inhibition of LTB$_4$ release 48 hr after intravenous prednisolone (98).

V. Conclusions

The mechanism of action of glucocorticoids in asthma is poorly understood. One effect is the inhibition of arachidonic acid metabolism. This elegant hypothesis was sustained by a few studies. Most of them were short-term studies and showed a specific action at the macrophage level without affecting the systemic production of eicosanoids. There is no link between these effects and the clinical severity of the disease. The presence of eicosanoids in sputum and urine of severe asthmatic patients treated by systemic glucocorticoids for a long term raised question about the potency of these drugs to inhibit arachidonic acid metabolism. When inhibitory effects are observed, they are often noted particularly on the generation of TXB and cysteinyl-LT which directly induce deleterious effects on target tissues. These findings might prove to provide a place for other treatments more specifically devoted to inhibiting these mediators, such as leukotrienes antagonists and 5-LO inhibitors.

References

1. Anticevich SZ, Hughes JM, Black JL, Armour CL. Induction of hyperresponsiveness in human airway tissue by neutrophils—mechanism of action. Clin Exp Allergy 1996; 26:549–556.
2. Djukanovic R, Roche WR, Wilson JW, Beasley CR, Twentyman OP, Howarth RH, Holgate ST. Mucosal inflammation in asthma. Am Rev Respir Dis 1990; 142: 434–457.
3. Holgate S. Mediator and cytokine mechanisms in asthma. Thorax 1993; 48: 103–109.
4. Dahlen SE, Hedqvist P, Hammarstrom S, Samuelsson B. Leukotrienes are potent constrictors of human bronchi. Nature 1980; 288:484–486.
5. Samuelsson B. Leukotrienes: mediators of hypersensitivity reactions and inflammation. Science 1983; 220:568–575.
6. Henderson W Jr. The role of leukotrienes in inflammation. Ann Intern Med 1994; 121:684–697.
7. Thien FCK, Walters EH. Eicosanoids and asthma: an update. Prostaglandins Leukot Essent Fatty Acids 1995; 52:271–288.
8. Smith LJ. Leukotrienes in asthma: the potential therapeutic role of antileukotriene agents. Arch Intern Med 1996; 156:2181–2189.
9. Sampson AP. The leukotrienes: mediators of chronic inflammation in asthma. Clin Exp Allergy 1996; 26:995–1004.

10. Sebaldt RJ, Sheller JR, Oates JA, Roberts LJ, Fitzgerald GA. Inhibition of eicosanoid biosynthesis by glucocorticoids in humans. Proc Natl Acad Sci USA 1990; 87:6974–6978.

11. Ballard P, Baxter J, Higgins S. General presence of glucocorticoid receptors in mammalian tissues. Endocrinology 1974; 94:998–1002.

12. Miesfeld R, Godowski P, Maler B, Yamamoto K. Glucocorticoid receptor mutants that define a small region sufficient for enhancer activation. Science 1987; 236: 423–427.

13. Picard D, Yamamoto K. Two signals mediate hormone-dependent nuclear localization of the glucocorticoid receptor. EMBO J 1987; 6:3333–3340.

14. Howard K, Holley S, Yamamoto K, Distelhorst C. Mapping of the hsp 90 binding region of the glucocorticoid receptor. J Biol Chem 1990; 265:11928–11935.

15. Freedman L, Luisi B, Korszun Z. The function and structure of the metal coordination sites within the glucocorticoid receptor DNA binding domain. Nature 1988; 334:543–546.

16. Freedman L, Luisi B. On the mechanism of DNA binding by nuclear hormone receptor: a structural and functional perspective. J Cell Biochem 1993; 51:140–150.

17. Sigler P. Acid blobs and negative noodles. Nature 1988; 333:210–212.

18. Gronemeyer H. Control of transcription activation by steroid hormone receptor. FASEB J 1992; 6:2524–2529.

19. Gustafsson JA, Carlstedt-Duke J, Poellinger L, Okret S, Wikstrom AC, Bronnegard M, Gillner M, Dong Y, Fuxe K, Clintra S, Harfstrand A, Agnat L. Biochemistry, molecular biology, and physiology of the glucorticoid receptor. Endocr Rev 1987; 8:135–234.

20. Rexin M, Bush W, Gehring U. Protein components of the nonactivated glucocorticoid receptor. J Biol Chem 1991; 266:24601–24605.

21. Albers MW, Chang H, Faber LE, Schreiber SL. Association of a 59-kilodalton immunophilin with the glucocorticoid receptor complex. Science 1992; 256:1315–1318.

22. Pratt WP, Sherrer LC, Hutchinson KA, Dalman FC. A model of glucocorticoid receptor unfolding and stabilization by a heat shock protein complex. J Steroid Biochem Mol Biol 1992; 41:223–229.

23. Jonat C, Rahmsdorf HJ, Park KK, Cato ACB, Gebel S, Ponta H, Herrlich P. Antitumour promotion and anti-inflammation: down-regulation of AP-1 (Fos/Jun) activity by glucocorticoid hormone. Cell 1990; 62:1189–1204.

24. Cato ACB, Wade E. Molecular mechanism of anti-inflammatory action of glucocorticoids. BioEssays 1996; 18:371–378.

25. Dahlman-Wright K, Wright A, Carlstedt-Duke J, Gustafsson JA. DNA-binding by the glucocorticoid receptor; a structural and functional analysis. J Steroid Biochem Mol Biol 1992; 41:249–272.

26. Muller M, Renkawitz R. The glucocorticoid receptor. Biochim Biophys Acta 1991; 1088:171–182.

27. Munck A, Mendel DB, Smith LI, Orti E. Glucocorticoid receptors and actions. Am Rev Respir Dis 1990; 141:S2–S10.

28. Beato M, Bruggemeier U, Chalepakis G. Regulation of transcription by glucocorticoids. In: Cohen P, Foulkes IG, ed. The Hormonal Control of Gene Transcription. Amsterdam: Elsevier, 1991:117–128.

29. Scheinman RI, Cogswell PC, Lofquist AK, Baldwin AS. Role of transcriptional activation of IκBα in mediation of immunosuppression by glucocorticoids. Science 1995; 270:283–286.

30. Auphan N, Didonato JA, Rosette C, Helmberg A, Karin M. Immunosuppression by glucocorticoids: inhibition of NF-κB activity through induction of IκB synthesis. Science 1995; 270:286–290.

31. Flower RJ, Rothwell NJ. Lipocortin-1: cellular mechanisms and clinical relevance. Trends Pharmacol Sci 1994; 15:71–76.

32. Cirino G, Flower RJ, Browning JL, Sinclair KL, Pepinsky RB. Recombinant human lipocortin-1 inhibits thromboxane release from guineapig isolated perfused lung. Nature 1987; 328:270–272.

33. Stromstedt PE, Poellinger L, Gustafsson JA, Carlstedt-Duke J. The glucocorticoid receptor binds to a sequence overlapping the TATA box of the human osteocalcin promoter: a potential mechanism for negative regulation. Mol Cell Biol 1991; 11: 3379–3383.

34. Akerblom IE, Slater EP, Beato M. Negative regulation by glucocorticoids through interference with a cAMP responsive enhancer. Science 1988; 241:350–353.

35. Cairns C, Carns W, Okret S. Inhibition of gene expression by steroid hormone receptors via a negative glucocorticoid response element: evidence of the involvement of DNA-binding and agonsitic effects of the antiglucocorticoid/antiprogestin RU486. DNA 1993; 12:695–702.

36. Ray A, Laforge KS, Sehgal PB. On the mechanisms of efficient repression of the interleukin-6 promoter by glucocorticoids: enhancer TATA box and RNA start site occlusion. Mol Cell Biol 1990; 10:5736–5746.

37. Diamond MI, Miner JN, Yoshinaga SK, Yamamoto KR. Transcription factor interactions: selectors of positive or negative regulation from a single DNA element. Science 1990; 249:1266–1272.

38. Ray A, Prefontainr KE. Physical association and functional antagonism between the p65 subunit of transcription factor NF-κB and the glucocorticoid receptor. Proc Natl Acad Sci USA 1994; 91:752–756.

39. Mukaida N. Novel mechanism of glucocorticoid-mediated gene repression. Nuclear factor-κB is target for glucocorticoid-mediated interleukin 8 gene expression. J Biol Chem 1994; 269:13287–13295.

40. Fava RA, McKana J, Cohen SI. Lipocortin 1 is abundant in a restricted number of differentiated cell types in adult organs. J Cell Physiol 1989; 141:284–293.

41. Smith SF, Tetley TD, Datta AK, Smith T, Guz A, Flower RJ. Lipocortin-1 distribution in bronchoalveolar lavage from healthy human lung: effect of prednisolone. J Appl Physiol 1995; 79:121–128.

42. De Caterina R, Sicari R, Giannessi D, Paggiaro PL, Paoletti P, Lazzerini G, Bernini W, Solito E, Parente L. Macrophage-specific eicosanoid synthesis inhibition and lipocortin-1 induction by glucocorticoids. J Appl Physiol 1993; 75:2368–2375.

43. Flower R. Lipocortin and the mechanism of action of the glucocorticoids. Br J Pharmacol 1988; 94:987–1015.

44. Davidson FF, Dennis EA. Biological relevance of lipocortins and related proteins as inhibitors of phospholipase A_2. Biochem Pharmacol 1989; 38:3645–3651.

45. Browning JL, Ward MP, Wallner BP, Pepinski RB. Studies on the structural properties of lipocortin-1 and the regulation of its synthesis by steroids. In: Melli M, Parente L, eds. Cytokines and Lipocortins in Inflammation and Differentiation. New York: Wiley-Liss, 1990:27–45.

46. Goulding NJ, Luying P, Guyre PM. Characteristics of lipocortin 1 binding to the surface of human peripheral blood leukocytes. Biochem Soc Trans 1990; 18:1237–1238.

47. Croxtall JD, Choudhury Q, Tokumoto H, Flower RJ. Lipocortin-1 and the control of arachidonic acid release in cell signalling. Glucocorticoids inhibit G protein–dependent activation of $cPLA_2$ activity. Biochem Pharmacol 1995; 50:465–474.

48. Kovacic RT, Tizard R, Cate RL. Correlation of gene and protein structure of rat and human lipocortin 1. Biochemistry 1991; 30:9015–9021.

49. Goulding NJ, Guyre PM. Glucocorticoids, lipocortin and the immune response. Curr Opin Immunol 1993; 5:108–113.

50. O'Banian MK, Winn VD, Young DA. cDNA cloning and functional activity of a glucocorticoid-regulated inflammatory cyclooxygenase. Proc Natl Acad Sci USA 1992; 89:4888–4892.

51. Mitchell JA, Belvisi MG, Akarasereenont P, Robbins RA, Kwon OJ, Croxtall J, Barnes PJ, Vane JR. Induction of cyclo-oxygenase 2 by cytokines in human pulmonary epithelial cells: regulation by dexamethasone. Br J Pharmacol 1994; 113:1008–1014.

52. Dworski RT, Funk CB, Oates JA, Sheller JR. Prednisone increases PGH-synthase 2 in atopic humans in vivo. Am J Respir Crit Care Med 1997; 155:351–357.

53. Sporn PH, Murphy TM, Peters-Golden M. Glucocorticoids fail to inhibit arachidonic acid metabolism stimulated by hydrogen peroxide in the alveolar macrophages. J Leukoc Biol 1990; 48:81–88.

54. Lum WH, Stawart AG. Regulation of eicosanoid generation in activated macrophages. Int Arch Allergy Appl Immunol 1991; 95:77–85.

55. Azevedo I, deBlic J, Scheinmann P, Vergaftig BB, Bachelet M. Enhanced arachidonic acid metabolism in alveolar macrophages from wheezy infants. Modulation by dexamethasone. Am J Respir Crit Care Med 1995; 152:1208–1214.

56. Balter MS, Eschenbacher WL, Peters-Golden M. Arachidonic acid metabolism in cultured alveolar macrophages from normal, atopic, and asthmatic subjects. Am Rev Respir Dis 1988; 138:1134–1142.

57. Peters-Golden M, Thebert P. Inhibition by methylprednisolone of zymosan-induced leukotriene synthesis in alveolar macrophages. Am Rev Respir Dis 1987; 135:1020–1026.

58. Linden M. The effects of $beta_2$-adrenoceptor agonists and a corticosteroid, budesonide, on the secretion of inflammatory mediators from monocytes. Br J Pharmacol 1992; 107:156–160.

59. Madrestma GS, van Dijk APM, Tak CJAM, Wilson JHP, Zijlsta FJ. Inhibition of the production of mediators of inflammation by corticosteroids is a glucocorticoid receptor-mediated process. Mediat Inflamm 1996; 5:100–103.

60. Solito E, De Caterina R, Giannessi D, Paggiaro PL, Sicari R, Parente L. Studies on the induction of lipocortin-1 by glucocorticoids. Ann Ist Super Sanita 1993; 29:391–394.

61. Nowak D, Grimminger F. Jorres R, Oldigs M, Rabe KF, Seeger W, Magnussen H. Increased LTB4 metabolites and PGD2 in BAL fluid after methacholine challenge in asthmatic subjects. Eur Respir J 1993; 6:405–412.

62. Liu MC, Bleecker ER, Lichtenstein LM, Kagey-Sobotka A, Niv Y, McLemore TL, Permutt S, Proud D, Hubbard WC. Evidence for elevated levels of histamine, prostaglandin D2, and other bronchoconstricting prostaglandins in the airways of subjects with mild asthma. Am Rev Respir Dis 1990; 142:126–132.

63. Mewes T, Riechelmann H, Klimek L. Increased in vitro cysteinyl leukotriene release from blood leukocytes in patients with asthma, nasal polyps, and aspirin intolerance. Allergy 1996; 51:506–510.

64. Chavis C, Arnoux B, Bousquet J. Lipid mediators detection in bronchoalveolar lavage fluid. Paf-acether, cyclooxygenase and lipoxygenase products. European Report on Current Status of Techniques for Assay of Non-Cellular Components in BAL, 1997 (in press).

65. Bernard GR, Korley V, Chee P, Swindell B, Ford-Hutchinson AW, Tagari P. Persistent generation of peptido leukotrienes in patients with the adult respiratory distress syndrome. Am Rev Respir Dis 1991; 144:263–267.

66. Sampson AP, Green CP, Spencer DA, Piper PJ, Price JF. Leukotrienes in the blood and urine of children with acute asthma. Ann NY Acad Sci 1991; 629:437–439.

67. Shindo K, Miyakawa K, Fukumura M. Plasma levels of leukotriene B$_4$ in asthmatic patients. Int J Tissue React 1993; 15:181–184.

68. Asano K, Lilly CM, Odonnell WJ, Israel E, Fischer A, Ransil BJ, Drazen JM. Diurnal variation of urinary leukotriene E(4) and histamine excretion rates in normal subjects and patients with mild-to-moderate asthma. J Allergy Clin Immunol 1995; 96:643–651.

69. Kumlin M, Dahlen B, Bjorck T, Zetterstrom O, Granstrom E, Dahlen SE. Urinary excretion of leukotriuene E4 and 11-dehydro-thromboxane B$_2$ in response to bronchial provocations with allergen, aspirin, leukotriene D$_4$, and histamine in asthmatics. Am Rev Respir Dis 1992; 146:96–103.

70. Bellia V, Bonanno A, Cibella F, Cuttitta G, Mirabella A, Profita M, Vignola AM, Bonsignore G. Urinary leukotriene E(4) in the assessment of nocturnal asthma. J Allergy Clin Immunol 1996; 97:735–741.

71. Fauler J, Frolich JC. Cigarette smoking stimulates cysteinyl leukotriene production in man. Eur J Clin Invest 1997; 27:43–47.

72. Osullivan S, Dahlen B, Dahlen SE, Kumlin M. Increased urinary excretion of the prostaglandin D-2 metabolite 9 alpha,11 beta-prostaglandin F-2 after aspirin challenge supports mast cell activation in aspirin-induced airway obstruction. J Allergy Clin Immunol 1996; 98:421–432.

73. Overbeek SE, Bogard JM, Garrelds IM, Ziljlstra FJ, Mulder PGH, Hoogereden HC. Effects of fluticasone on arachidonic acid metabolites in BAL-fluid and metacholine dose-response curves in non-smoking atopic asthmatics. Mediat Inflamm 1996; 5:224–229.

74. Dworski R, Fitzgerald GA, Oates JA, Sheller JR. Effect of oral prednisone on airway inflammatory mediators in atopic asthma. Am J Respir Crit Care Med 1994; 149:953–959.

75. Oosterhoff Y, Overbeek SE, Douma R, Noordhoek JA, Postma DS, Hoogsteden HC, Zijlstra FJ. Lower leukotriene C-4 levels in bronchoalveolar lavage fluid of asthmatic subjects after 2.5 years of inhaled corticosteroid therapy. Mediat Inflamm 1995; 4:426–430.

76. Vachier I, Kumlin M, Deviller P, Dahlen SE, Bousquet J, Godard P, Chanez P. Urinary LTE_4 and EDN in untreated and steroid-dependent asthmatic patients. Eur Respir J 1996; 9:418S.

77. Shindo K, Fukumura M, Miyakawa K. Plasma levels of leukotriene E_4 during clinical course of bornchial asthma and the effect of oral prednisolone. Chest 1994; 105:1038–1041.

78. Lacronique J, Renon D, Georges D, Henry-Amar M, Marsac J. High-dose beclomethasone: oral steroid sparing effect in severe asthmatic patients. Eur Respir J 1991; 4:807–812.

79. Freeland HS, Pipkorn U, Schleimer RP, Bascom R, Lichtenstein LM, Naclerio RM, Peters SP. Leukotriene B_4 as a mediator of early and late reactions to antigen in humans: the effect of systemic glucocorticoid treatment in vivo. J Allergy Clin Immunol 1989; 83:634–642.

80. Wenzel SE, Trudeau JB, Westcott JY, Beam WR, Martin RJ. Single oral dose of prednisone decreases leukotriene B_4 production by alveolar macrophages from patients with nocturnal asthma but not control subjects: relationship to changes in cellular influx and FEV_1. J Allergy Clin Immunol 1994; 94:870–881.

81. Poston RN, Chanez P, Lacoste JY, Litchfield T, Lee TH, Bousquet J. Immunohistochemical characterization of the cellular infiltration in asthmatic bronchi. Am Rev Respir Dis 1992; 145:918–921.

82. Vachier I, Damon M, Le-Doucen C, de-Paulet AC, Chanez P, Michel FB, Godard P. Increased oxygen species generation in blood monocytes of asthmatic patients. Am Rev Respir Dis 1992; 146:1161–1166.

83. Vachier I, Chavis C, Godard P, Bousquet J, Chanez P. The effects of long term treatment with glucocorticoids on PMN and monocyte LTB_4 production in asthmatic patients. Am J Respir Crit Care Med 1995; 151:A215.

84. Vachier I, Roux S, Chanez P, Loubatière J, Térouanne B, Nicolas J, Godard P. Glucocorticoids induced down-regulation of glucocorticoid receptor mRNA GR expression in asthma. Clin Exp Immunol 1996; 103:311–315.

85. Dooper MW, Timmermans A, Aalbers R, Weersink EJ, de-Monchy JG, Kauffman HF. Production of diacylglycerol and arachidonic acid in peripheral blood mononuclear cells from patients with asthma and healthy controls. Ann Allergy Asthma Immunol 1995; 74:248–254.

86. Roberge CJ, Laviolette M, Boulet LP, Poubelle PE. In vitro leukotriene (LT) C_4 synthesis by blood eosinophils from atopic asthmatics: predominance of eosinophil subpopulations with high potency for LTC_4 generation. Prostaglandins Leukot Essent Fatty Acids 1990; 41:243–249.

87. Gin W, Shaw RJ, Kay AB. Airways reversibility after prednisolone therapy in chronic asthma is associated with alterations in leukocyte function. Am Rev Respir Dis 1985; 132:1199–1203.

88. Shindo K, Hirai I, Koide K, Sumitomo M, Fukumura M. In vivo effect of prednisolone on release of leukotriene C_4 in eosinophils obtained from asthmatic patients. Biochem Biophys Res Commun 1995; 214:869–874.
89. Boschetto P, Zocca E, Bruchi O, Cappellazzo G, Milani GF, Pivirotto F, Mapp CE, Fabbri LM. Importance of airway inflammation for late asthmatic reactions induced by toluene diisocyanate in sensitized subjects. Adv Prostaglandin Thromboxane Leukotriene Res 1987; 17B:1080–1084.
90. Sur S, Hunt LW, Crotty TB, Gleich GJ. Sudden-onset fatal asthma. Mayo Clin Proc 1994; 69:495–496 (editorial).
91. Carroll N, Elliott J, Morton A, James A. The structure of large and small airways in nonfatal and fatal asthma. Am Rev Respir Dis 1993; 147:405–410.
92. Martin RJ, Cicutto LC, Smith HR, Ballard RD, Szefler SJ. Airways inflammation in nocturnal asthma. Am Rev Respir Dis 1991; 143:351–357.
93. Fahy JV, Kim KW, Liu J, Boushey HA. Prominent neutrophilic inflammation in sputum from subjects with asthma exacerbation. J Allergy Clin Immunol 1995; 95:843–852.
94. Chanez P, Paradis L, Vignola A, Vachier I, Vic P, Godard P, Bousquet J. Changes in bronchial inflammation of steroid (GCs) dependent asthmatics. Am J Respir Crit Care Med 1996; 153:A212.
95. Thomas E, Leroux JL, Blotman F, Descomps B, Chavis C. Enhancement of leukotriene A4 biosynthesis in neutrophils from patients with rheumatoid arthritis after a single glucocorticoid dose. Biochem Pharmacol 1995; 49:243nnn248.
96. Paggiaro PL, Bancalari L, Giannessi D, Bernini W, Lazzerini G, Sicari R, Bacci E, Dente FL, Vagaggini B, Decaterina R. Effects of systemic glucocorticosteroids on peripheral neutrophil functions in asthmatic subjects: an ex vivo study. Mediat Inflamm 1995; 4:251nnn256.
97. Schleimer RP, Freeland HS, Peters SP, Brown KE, Derse CP. An assessment of the effects of glucocorticoids on degranulation, chemotaxis, binding to vascular endothelium and formation of leukotriene B_4 by purified human neutrophils. J Pharmacol Exp Ther 1989; 250:598nnn605.
98. Shindo K, Koide K, Fukumura M, Hirai Y. In vivo effect of prednisolone on release of leukotriene B_4 from neutrophils from asthmatic patients. Biochem Biophys Res Commun 1996; 222:759nnn763.

30

Desensitization in Aspirin-Induced Asthma

DONALD D. STEVENSON

Scripps Clinic
La Jolla, California

I. Introduction

We typically think of desensitization as an alteration in the immune response, engineered by repeated exposure to antigens, thus reducing IgE-mediated reactions. Since IgE-mediated mechanisms have not been established as being responsible for aspirin (ASA)-induced respiratory reactions and are considered by most investigators to be unlikely perpetrators of this disease (1), desensitization is used here in its broadest sense and refers to reducing the reactions to ASA by repeated and increasing exposure to ASA until all reactions cease (2).

In 1922, Widal et al. published the first report of successful ASA desensitization (3). By administering small and then increasing daily doses of ASA, they were able to induce tolerance to full therapeutic doses of ASA in one individual, who had previously been shown to react to ASA with a documented respiratory reaction. In 1976, Zeiss and Lockey (4) reported a 72-hr refractory period to ASA after an indomethacin-induced respiratory reaction in a known ASA-sensitive asthmatic patient. In 1977, Bianco et al. (5) reported tolerance to ASA in a known ASA-sensitive asthmatic patient, after repeated bronchial inhalation challenges with ASA-lysine. In 1980, Stevenson et al. (6) reported two ASA-sensitive asthmatic patients who became refractory to ASA after oral ASA challenges had induced typical bronchospastic reactions. Both patients, after achieving the ASA-desensitized state, were then treated with daily ASA over the ensuing months and experienced improvement in their respiratory disease.

II. ASA Desensitization Procedures

All ASA-sensitive asthmatics can be successfully desensitized to ASA (2,7). An example of an oral ASA challenge is presented in Table 1. After oral challenges with increasing doses of ASA, the sensitive patient eventually has a respiratory reaction. As shown in Table 2, respiratory reactions vary, focusing on the upper or lower respiratory tract or various combinations in between. Desensitization is accomplished by reintroducing the dose of ASA that initiated the ASA reaction on the previous day. As soon as a reaction no longer occurs, after repeat exposure to the same dose of ASA, the next highest dose of ASA is given and repeated until further reactions cease. Once a reaction occurs, ASA-desensitizing doses are suspended for that day. The process of escalating ASA doses continues on successive days until the patient can tolerate 650 mg without any reactions. At this point, the patient can take any dose of ASA or nonsteroidal anti-inflammatory drug (NSAID) without any adverse respiratory reaction (6) and at the same time experiences an opening of nasal passages. After ASA desensitization, in the absence of further exposure to ASA, the desensitized state persists for 2–5 days with full sensitivity returning after 7 days (2). Table 3 displays relevant data on a patient undergoing oral ASA challenge, followed by ASA desensitization.

A. Other Procedures to Conduct ASA Desensitization

Inhalation challenges with ASA-lysine are used extensively throughout the world to induce bronchospasm and prove that ASA sensitivity exists in the patient under investigation (5,8–10). Following repeated inhalation challenges,

Table 1 Single-Blind Three-Day Oral ASA Challenge[a]

Time	Day 1	Day 2	Day 3
8:00 A.M.	Placebo	ASA, 30 mg[a]	ASA, 150 mg
11:00 A.M.	Placebo	ASA, 60 mg	ASA, 325 mg
2:00 A.M.	Placebo	ASA, 100 mg	ASA, 650 mg

[a]Individualized: Starting ASA dose may be reduced and timing may be altered.

Table 2 Respiratory Reactions During Oral ASA and NSAID Challenges

Types of reactions	Features of reactions
No reaction	No symptoms and changes in FEV_1 < 15%
Classic	Greater than 20% decrease in FEV_1 associated with naso-ocular reactions
Pure asthma	Greater than 20% decrease in FEV_1 values
Pure rhinitis	Naso-ocular reaction alone
Partial asthma naso-ocular	Decline of 15–20% in FEV_1 values combined with naso-ocular reaction
Laryngospasm	Stridor Flow/volume curve: inspiratory loop flat and notched

patients have been shown to become refractory to further inhalation of ASA-lysine (5). At that point, ASA in oral doses can be introduced without inducing reactions, usually in doses between 150 and 325 mg. Continued daily treatment with ASA can then be started.

In known ASA-sensitive asthmatics, pretreatment with sodium salicylate, which does not induce respiratory reactions in these patients, significantly attenuates the respiratory reactions during oral ASA challenges and in many cases has allowed "silent desensitization" to occur (11). Szmidt et al. (12)

Table 3 An Example of Oral ASA Desensitization

Day	Hour	Substance (dose)	Respiratory responses Nasal	% decline FEV_1
1	8:00 A.M.	Placebo	+	0
	11:00 A.M.	Placebo	+	0
	2:00 P.M.	Placebo	+	4
2	8:00 A.M.	ASA (30 mg)	+ +	12
	11:00 A.M.	ASA (60 mg)	+ + + +	32 (90 min)
3	8:30 A.M.	ASA (60 mg)	+ +	11
	11:30 A.M.	ASA (100 mg)	+ + +	27 (60 min)
4	8:00 A.M.	ASA (100 mg)	0	0
	11:00 A.M.	ASA 9150 mg)	0	12
	2:00 P.M.	ASA (325 mg)	0	0
5	7:00 A.M.	ASA (650 mg)	0	0

induced tolerance (desensitized) in 10 known ASA-sensitive asthmatics by introducing subthreshold doses of ASA orally without inducing respiratory reactions. Patients were instructed to start with ingestion of ASA 20 mg and each day increase the dose by 20 mg, until reaching 300 mg of ASA. None of the patients reacted to the increasing doses of ASA. Therefore, assuming one knows that the patient is ASA sensitive on the basis of a prior oral or inhalation ASA challenge, it is not necessary to induce a respiratory reaction to achieve ASA desensitization. However, failure to establish the diagnosis of ASA-sensitive respiratory sensitivity could result in silent "nondesensitization" in a patient who never was ASA sensitive. From a practical standpoint, an ASA-sensitive asthmatic with concomitant arthritis or need for antiplatelet therapy can be desensitized to ASA and then take daily ASA (at least ASA 81 mg qd) indefinitely or switch to any cross-sensitizing NSAID as long as ASA or NSAID is continued daily.

III. ASA Cross-Sensitivity and Desensitization

A. Strong Inhibitors of COX

All NSAIDs, which inhibit cyclooxygenase (COX) in vitro, cross-react with ASA, producing respiratory reactions (13–16). Furthermore, in ASA-sensitive asthmatics, cross-reactions occur upon first exposure to the new NSAID (15). In 1971, Vane (13) reported that ASA and NSAIDs inhibit formation of prostaglandins. In 1977, Szczeklik et al. (16) reported in vitro experiments demonstrating that ASA and NSAIDs inhibit COX in vitro at different concentrations for each drug. Further, they showed that those NSAIDs which inhibited COX in vitro with the least concentration of drug were the most potent NSAIDs in cross-reacting with ASA. In addition, these potent cross-reacting NSAIDs produced large reactions with very small challenge doses of the NSAID. The reverse was also true. A current list of NSAIDs that cross-react and cross-desensitize with ASA is presented in Table 4. Cross-desensitization occurs between all drugs that inhibit COX (2). Thus, NSAIDs and ASA not only share the pharmacological effect of cross-reactivity but also share the phenomenon of cross-desensitization (7).

B. Weak Inhibitors of COX

Cross-reactivity between ASA and drugs that are weak inhibitors of COX, or do not inhibit COX at all in vitro, is a subject of some controversy. Analgesics, such as acetaminophen, salsalate, choline magnesium trisalicylate, and dextropropoxyphene, have been reported to cause reactions in ASA-sensitive asthmatics by some authors (7). Based on the experimental findings of Vane (14), one would assume that weak inhibitors of COX would either not cross-

Table 4 Nonsteroidal Anti-Inflammatory Drugs that Cross-React and Cross-Desensitize with Aspirin (ASA)

Generic	Brand names
Piroxicam	Feldene
Indomethacin	Indocin
Sulindac	Clinoril
Tolmetin	Tolectin
Ibuprofen	Motrin, Rufen, Advil
Naproxen	Naprosyn
Naproxen sodium	Anaprox, Aleve
Fenoprofen	Nalfon
Meclofenamate	Meclomen
Mefenamic acid	Ponstel
Flurbiprofen	Ansaid
Diflunisal	Dolobid
Ketoprofen	Orudis, Oruval
Diclofenac	Voltaren
Ketoralac	Toradol
Etodolac	Lodine
Nabumetone	Relafen
Oxaprozin	Daypro

react with ASA or would cross-react poorly and only after challenges with large doses of the suspected analgesic. Based on this same reasoning, one would predict that cross-desensitization with weak COX inhibitors, after establishing an ASA-desensitized state with ASA, would also occur. The prediction is that weak inhibitors of COX are not likely to be able to induce the desensitized state in dose ranges consistent with recommended therapeutic doses. The reason for this is that if COX inhibition and induction of respiratory reactions requires large doses of the weak COX inhibitor, even larger doses would be required to induce desensitization. Such doses would be expected to be above standard recommended doses of the drug.

Settipane and Stevenson (17) studied three ASA-sensitive asthmatics, who also gave an associated history of respiratory reactions occurring 2 hr after ingestion of 500–1000 mg acetaminophen (parcetamol). Double-blind, placebo-controlled oral challenges were undertaken. All three patients reacted to provoking doses of 60 mg of ASA. None of the three reacted to acetaminophen 500 mg, but all three experienced bronchospastic reactions after ingesting acetaminophen 1000 mg. Two patients were temporarily desensitized to

1000 and 1500 mg of acetaminophen, but desensitization to 2000 mg could not be sustained and higher doses were not administered because of concern about liver toxicity. Two patients were then desensitized to ASA (650 mg) and were then able to immediately ingest 1000 mg of acetaminophen without adverse effect, demonstrating cross-desensitization.

Salsalate is an anti-inflammatory agent that is used in the treatment of arthritis but is a weak COX inhibitor. Stevenson et al. (18) studied 10 ASA-sensitive asthmatics to evaluate cross-sensitivity to salsalate. We found that two of 10 experienced bronchospastic reactions after ingesting 2 g of salsalate, but not after exposure to lower doses. Repeated challenges with 2 g of salsalate reproduced the same bronchospastic reactions, demonstrating that a weak inhibitor of COX could not desensitize at threshold-provoking doses and suggested that much larger, even toxic doses of the drug would be needed to achieve desensitization. Both patients then underwent ASA challenge and desensitization. Once desensitized to ASA (650 mg), both patients were able to immediately ingest 2 g of salsalate without adverse reactions, demonstrating cross-desensitization. When compared to acetaminophen, the same principles seemed to apply. Salsalate, a weak inhibitor of COX, induced reactions only when large doses of salsalate were used in oral challenges. Even then, reactions appeared in only a small percentage (20%) of ASA-sensitive asthmatics and in these salsalate was a poor inducer of the desensitized state. Nevertheless, both acetaminophen and salsalate have sufficient inhibitory effects on COX to induce mild reactions, particularly when supertherapeutic doses of the drugs are used in challenges. The fact that cross-desensitization occurs between ASA and acetaminophen and salsalate proves that the mechanisms of reaction and desensitization are the same as found with many NSAIDs, which are generally strong inhibitors of COX.

C. Noninhibitors of COX

Azo and nonazo dyes, dextropropoxyphene, hydrocortisone, and sulfites do not cross-react with ASA/NSAID. Stevenson et al. challenged 194 known ASA-sensitive asthmatics with tartrazine and no reactions occurred (19,20). Documentation of a lack of cross-sensitivity between ASA and other dyes and chemicals, nonacetylated salicylates, sulfites, and dextropropoxyphene has been extensively reviewed (21–23). Reports of severe asthma attacks within minutes after receiving hydrocortisone, but not dexamethasone, intravenously (IV) have also appeared in the literature (24–26). Feigenbaum et al. (27) recently reported that 44/45 known ASA-sensitive asthmatics did not react to IV hydrocortisone. One ASA-sensitive asthmatic patient experienced respiratory reactions to both hydrocortisone succinate and methylprednisolone sodium succinate, suggesting an IgE-mediated reaction to the succinate. After ASA desensitization, cross-desensitization to hydrocortisone succinate did not occur, suggesting that ASA-sensitive asthmatics do not experience cross-reactions (or cross-desensitization) between ASA and succinate. Since cross-reactions do not occur between ASA/NSIADs and the above-listed drugs and chemicals, it should not be surprising that cross-desensitization does not occur either.

IV. Treatment with ASA Desensitization

In 1980, Stevenson et al. (6) reported two ASA-sensitive asthmatic subjects who were successfully desensitized to ASA and then treated with daily ASA continuously. Both patients rapidly experienced improvement in nasal patency and one regained her sense of smell. Furthermore, when daily ASA treatment continued over a number of months, nasal airway patency was maintained, regrowth of nasal polyps ceased, and asthma activity diminished. These observations raised some interesting questions. Is it possible to treat the underlying respiratory tract inflammation of ASA disease using the same drug that induces respiratory reactions prior to ASA desensitization? If this were true, what biomolecular events could possibly explain the mechanisms by which this occurred?

Taking into consideration variations in study design, doses of ASA employed, length of treatment with ASA, and criteria for successful clinical outcomes, efficacy has been reported in most studies where treatment with daily ASA was instituted after ASA desensitization had been achieved (6,28–32). One study by Naeije et al. (33) did not show efficacy of ASA treatment in ASA-sensitive asthmatic subjects. However, the usefulness of this study was hampered by small sample size and reliance upon improvement in lung function as the only criteria for improvement. This study was further flawed by low doses of ASA, used for daily treatment and short duration of treatment. Furthermore, the protocol did not allow adjustment of corticosteroid doses downward during treatment with ASA to determine whether lung function could be maintained while systemic steroids were reduced or removed. Lumry et al. (29) demonstrated that ASA treatment of patients with ASA-sensitive rhinosinusitis without asthma, after ASA desensitization, was associated with clearing of hypertrophic rhinitis in 77% of the patients studied.

Stevenson et al. (34) conducted the only double-blind, crossover study of treatment with ASA, after ASA desensitization, in 25 ASA-sensitive asthmatics. During the 3-month treatment arm with daily ASA therapy, patients experienced significant improvement in nasal symptom scores and a reduced use of nasal beclomethasone. However, only half the patients experienced improvement in asthma symptom scores and systemic corticosteroid doses were not significantly reduced during the ASA treatment period. This short-term study employed variable doses of ASA, and recruitment of study subjects was less than projected. Thus the multiple-dose patient samples were of insufficient size to compare subgroups based on treatment doses and outcomes. Retrospectively, it would have been ideal if all 25 patients had been treated with 1300 mg of ASA each day, rather than dividing the 25 patients into treatment subgroups, particularly ASA only 325 mg/day. Furthermore, the time frame of 3 months was insufficient to assess rate of polyp regrowth or need for additional sinus or nasal polyp surgery.

Between 1986 and 1988, we attempted to conduct a long-term, double-blind, placebo-controlled study of ASA desensitization treatment. After 2 years of recruitment, only two patients volunteered to participate. Both underwent ASA oral challenges, followed by successful ASA desensitization. As usually occurs, they immediately noted improvement in their nasal patency at the completion of ASA desensitization. Both started daily treatment with the study drug but disenrolled from the study several weeks later, when nasal congestion returned. In both patients placebo treatment had been randomly assigned. Thus, patients could distinguish between placebo and ASA therapy because of a return of nasal congestion while taking placebo. Furthermore, ASA as a "study drug" is available over-the-counter and not controlled by the investigators, allowing patients the option of not enrolling in a study where placebo treatment would be expected 50% of the time. Finally, the human study committee required full disclosure of therapeutic options, including the opportunity for patients to enroll in an open treatment with ASA in adjusted dosages. Essentially patients elected this last option.

In 1990 Sweet et al. (35) reported the clinical courses of 107 known ASA-sensitive rhinosinusitis asthmatic patients treated with ASA between 1975 and 1988. Forty-two patients avoided aspirin and served as the control group. Thirty-five patients were desensitized to ASA and treated continuously with ASA daily for as long as 8 years. Thirty patients were initially desensitized to ASA and treated with ASA but discontinued ASA after a mean of 2 years. Retrospective analysis of the three groups showed that the patients treated with ASA enjoyed statistically significant reductions in hospitalizations, emergency room visits, outpatient visits, need for additional sinus surgery, need for additional nasal polypectomies, number of upper respiratory infections/sinusitis requiring antibiotics, and improved sense of smell. ASA-desensitized-and-treated patients were also able to significantly reduce systemic corticosteroid maintenance doses, corticosteroid bursts per year, and in the group treated continuously, were able to reduce inhaled corticosteroids when compared to the control group. In the patients who had to discontinue ASA treatment after several years, respiratory disease improved while they were being treated with daily ASA, but reverted back toward pretreatment status after ASA treatment was discontinued. This study showed that ASA desensitization, followed by long-term ASA treatment, improved the clinical course of ASA-sensitive asthma rhinosinusitis and prevented regrowth of nasal polyps while at the same time allowing significant reduction in systemic and inhaled corticosteroids. Side effects from gastritis occurred in 20% of patients treated with ASA. Unfortunately, 30/65 patients who started ASA desensitization therapy discontinued ASA, mostly for misperceived reasons, shrinking the active treatment group to only 35 patients. This made it impossible to subdivide patients into short- and long-term treatment groups to determine whether therapeutic effects were concentrated in the early or late phases of treatment.

In 1996, Stevenson et al. (36) analyzed the clinical courses of an additional 65 ASA-sensitive asthmatics who underwent oral ASA challenges, followed by ASA desensitization between 1988 and 1994. These patients, after ASA oral challenges and standard oral desensitization to ASA, were then treated with daily doses of ASA (650 mg BID) and followed for an average of 3.3 years (range 1–6 years). The following clinical parameters were significantly improved after long-term ASA desensitization treatment: number of sinus infections/year, number of hospitalizations for asthma/year, number of sinus operations/year, improvement in sense of smell, and reduction in use of both nasal topical corticosteroids and systemic corticosteroids. Unchanged after ASA desensitization treatment were number of emergency room visits for asthma/year and use of inhaled corticosteroids. This study showed that the main components of ASA disease, namely aggressive nasal polyp formation and sinusitis, were significantly reduced during long-term ASA desensitization treatment. Concomitantly, nasal and systemic corticosteroids could be successfully reduced or discontinued without the expected increase of inflammatory respiratory disease. Also important, when the 65 patients were subdivided into early and late treatment groups, the results were essentially the same, indicating that therapeutic escape did not occur during long-term treatment with ASA. These data further suggest that early reduction in systemic corticosteroids during the first year of ASA treatment is also not associated with disease escape. For the total group of 65 patients, the need for sinus surgery declined from a pretreatment interval of one operation every 3 years to one every 9 years during treatment with daily ASA.

Future treatment of ASA disease will change significantly, particularly with the addition of 5-LO inhibitors and specific antagonists of LTs (37,38). Although studies that include these new compounds along with ASA desensitization treatment and corticosteroid therapy have not been conducted, there is reason to be optimistic. One study using a Merck LT antagonist, montelukast, in the daily treatment of ASA-sensitive asthmatics measured significant improvement in the clinical course of known ASA-sensitive asthmatics, when compared to placebo treatment (39). Thus combinations of corticosteroids, which inhibit PLA_2 and other effects, ASA desensitization, which inhibits COX-1 and probably PLA_2, combined with specific LT antagonists and inhibitors might significantly improve the clinical outcome of ASA disease. This area of clinical research is likely to uncover new combinations of pharmacological treatment that will further reduce inflammation in the respiratory tract of ASA-sensitive asthmatics.

V. Pathogenesis of ASA Desensitization

In 1967, Vanselow and Smith (40) reported cross-reactions between ASA and an NSAID (indomethacin). Vane (13), in 1971, demonstrated that cross-reactivity between ASA and NSAIds correlates completely with the shared pharmacological effect of COX-1 inhibition. This fact is important in understanding the pathogenesis of ASA- and NSAID-induced reactions and desensitization because simultaneous immune recognition of ASA and the structurally dissimilar NSAIDs is virtually impossible. Furthermore, first-exposure reactions to NSAIds, in known ASA-sensitive asthmatics, occur routinely, a fact that obviates the possibility of prior immune recognition and sensitization. Although anti-ASA or -NSAID IgE antibodies have occasionally been detected, the presence of such antibodies has been inconsistent, controversial, and without correlation in those patients experiencing both ASA and NSAIDs reactions (1).

In the early 1980s, Samuelsson et al. discovered a second metabolic pathway for arachidonate metabolism, the 5-lipoxygenase (5-LO) pathway, where leukotrienes (LTs), LTA_4, LTB_4, LTC_4, LTD_4, and LTE_4 are formed (41). These products are potent mediators of chemotaxis, inflammation, increased vascular permeability, and constriction of bronchial smooth muscles (42). Therefore, in explaining ASA disease and the respiratory reactions to ASA/NSAID, it is logical to hypothesize that arachidonate molecules might be preferentially diverted into the 5-LO pathway, particularly when the COX pathway was blocked by ASA/NSAIds, removing the regulatory effect of PGE_2 on 5-LO (43). This is not to exclude other pathophysiological pathways and mechanisms from playing a role in the reactions and desensitization but merely to focus our thoughts on the central importance of leukotrienes in these reactions. Figure 1 is a graphic presentation of known biochemical events occurring in ASA reactions, acute desensitization (immediately after ingestion of ASA without any reactions), and chronic desensitization treatment (ASA treatment on a daily basis for longer than 2 weeks).

A. Pathogenesis of Acute or Immediate ASA Desensitization

During ASA-induced respiratory reactions, peripheral monocytes from ASA-sensitive asthmatic patients undergoing induced respiratory reactions

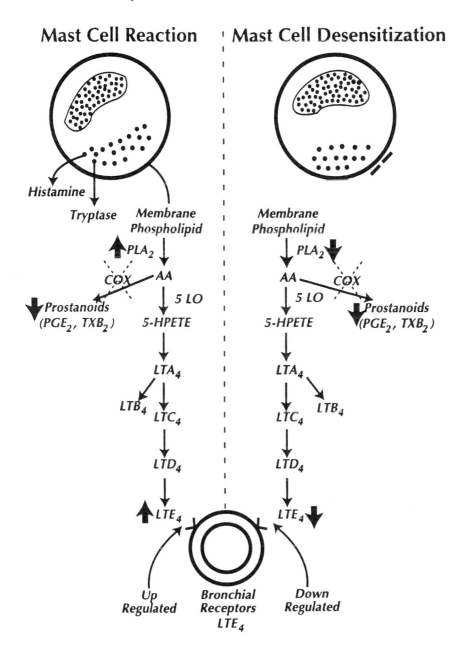

Figure 1 Pathogenesis of ASA reactions and desensitization. The mast cell is a central participant in ASA-induced reactions and ASA desensitization. However, other cells, such as eosinophls, PMNs, and monocytes (macrophages), could participate as they also synthesize prostanoids and LTs.

synthesize increased amounts of leukotrienes. By contrast, after acute ASA desensitization, defined as 3 hr after first ingestion of ASA 650 mg without any adverse effects, peripheral blood monocytes synthesized significantly less thromboxane B_2 but only slightly less LTB_4, the preferential 5-LO product of peripheral monocytes (44). Additionally, nasal LTC_4 and histamine, which had been increased in nasal secretions during ASA-induced respiratory reactions, disappeared at the point of acute desensitization. Similarly, serum histamine and tryptase levels, which were elevated during ASA-induced respiratory reactions, returned to low baseline levels following acute desensitization. During respiratory reactions induced by either oral or inhalation ASA challenges, LTE_4 urine levels were found to be significantly elevated when compared to baseline concentrations (45–47). However, after acute desensitization, urinary LTE_4 concentrations returned to baseline levels (48). Arm et al. (49), on the first day following ASA desensitization, demonstrated a 20-fold decrease in bronchial airway responsiveness to LTE_4, compared to predesensitization responses to inhalation of LTE_4 in ASA-sensitive asthmatics.

B. Chronic or Long-Term ASA Desensitization Treatment

By contrast, after treatment with ASA 650 mg BID for 2 or more weeks, during chronic desensitization, Juergens et al. (44) showed that peripheral monocyte synthesis of LTB_4 declined substantially, to the same level found in normal controls. Nasser et al. (48) reported that during chronic ASA desensitization for 6 months, urine LTE_4 levels declined to lower values, but not to values found in normals. Daffern et al. (unpublished data) showed that treatment with ASA 650 mg BID (twice the daily dose of ASA employed by Nasser et al.) was associated with significant declines in urinary LTE_4 levels in the majority of patients with the mean decrease statistically significant. However, urinary LTE_4 levels from some patients did not change during long-term ASA desensitization treatment. These experiments suggested that ASA desensitization, particularly long-term treatment with higher doses of ASA in some patients, probably inhibits both COX and other enzymes above LTE_4 and probably at the PLA_2 level, leading to diminished synthesis of both prostanoids and LTs. Simultaneously, LTE_4 bronchial receptors remain down-regulated (49), further blunting the effects of any available terminal LTs.

Such an environment would be expected to result in a general decrease in respiratory tract inflammation with a reduction in nasal polyp formation and bronchial hyperirritability.

Acknowledgments

This work was supported by grants from Allergic Disease Center AI-10386 and GCRC Grant M01-RR00833.

References

1. Stevenson DD, Lewis R. Proposed mechanisms of aspirin sensitivity reactions. J Allergy Clin Immunol 1987; 80:788–790 (editorial).
2. Pleskow WW, Stevenson DD, Mathison DA, Simon RA, Schatz M, Zieger RS. Aspirin desensitization in aspirin sensitive asthmatic patients: clinical manifestations and characterization of the refractory period. J Allergy Clin Immunol 1982; 69:11–19.
3. Widal MF, Abrami P, Lermeyez J. Anaphylaxie et idiosyncrasie. Presse Med 1922; 30:189–192.
4. Zeiss CR, Lockey RF. Refractory period to aspirin in a patient with aspirin-induced asthma. J Allergy Clin Immunol 1976; 57:440–448.
5. Bianco SR, M., Petrini G. Aspirin induced tolerance in aspirin-asthma detected by a new challenge test. IRCS J Med Sci 1977; 5:129–136.
6. Stevenson DD, Simon RA, Mathison DA. Aspirin-sensitive asthma: tolerance to aspirin after positive oral aspirin challenges. J Allergy Clin Immunol 1980; 66:82–88.
7. Stevenson DD, Simon RA. Sensitivity to aspirin and nonsteroidal antiinflammatory drugs. In: Middleton EJ, Reed CE, Ellis EF, Adkinson NF Jr, Yunginger JW, Busse WW, eds. Allergy: Principles and Practice. Vol. 2. St. Louis: CV Mosby, 1993:1747–1765.
8. Schmitz-Schumann VM, Juhl E, Costabel U. Analgesic asthma-provocation challenge with acetylsalicyclic acid. Atemw Lungenkrkh Jahrgang 1985; 10:479–485.
9. Phillips GD, Foord R, Holgate ST. Inhaled lysine-aspirin as a bronchoprovocation procedure with aspirin in aspirin-sensitive asthma. J Allergy Clin Immunol 1989; 84:232–241.
10. Park HS. Early and late onset asthmatic responses following lysine-aspirin inhalation in aspirin-sensitive asthmatic patients. Clin Exp Allergy 1995; 25:38–40.
11. Nizankowska E, Dworski R, Soja J, Szczeklik A. Salicylate pre-treatment attenuates intensity of bronchial and nasal symptoms precipitated by aspirin in aspirin-intolerant patients. Clin Exp Allergy 1990; 20:647–652.
12. Szmidt M, Grzelewska-Rzymowska I, Kowalski ML, Rozniecki J. Tolerance to acetylsalicylic acid (ASA) induced in ASA-sensitive asthmatics does not depend on initial adverse reactions. Allergy 1987; 42:182–185.
13. Vane JR. Inhibition of prostaglandin synthesis as a mechanism of action for aspirin-like drugs. Nature New Biol 1971; 231:232–235.
14. Vane JR. The mode of action of aspirin and similar compounds. J Allergy Clin Immunol 1976; 58:691–712.
15. Mathison DA, Stevenson DD. Hypersensitivity to nonsteroidal anti-inflammatory drugs: indications and methods for oral challenge. J Allergy Clin Immunol 1979; 64:669–674.
16. Szczeklik A, Gryglewski RJ, Czerniawska-Mysik G. Clinical patterns of hypersensitivity to nonsteroidal anti-inflammatory drugs and their pathogenesis. J Allergy Clin Immunol 1977; 60(5):276–284.
17. Settipane RA, Stevenson DD. Cross sensitivity with acetaminophen in aspirin sensitive asthmatics. J Allergy Clin Immunol 1989; 84:26–33.

18. Stevenson DD, Hougham A, Schrank P, Goldlust B, Wilson R. Disalcid cross-sensitivity in aspirin sensitive asthmatics. J Allergy Clin Immunol 1990; 86:749–758.
19. Stevenson DD, Simon RA, Lumry WR, Mathison DA. Adverse reactions to tartrazine. J Allergy Clin Immunol 1986; 78:182–191.
20. Stevenson DD, Simon RA, Lumry WR, Mathison DA. Pulmonary reactions to tartrazine. Pediatr Allergy Immunol 1992; 3:222–227.
21. Stevenson DD. Cross-reactivity between aspirin and other drugs/dietary chemicals: a critical review. In: Pichler WJ, Stadler MM, Dahinden CA, Pecoud AR, Frei P, Schneider CH, deWeck AL, eds. Progress in Allergy and Clinical Immunology. Vol. 1. Lewiston, NY: Hogrefe and Huber, 1989:462–473.
22. Manning ME, Stevenson DD. Pseudoallergic drug reactions: aspirin, non-steroidal anti-inflammatory drugs, dyes, additives and preservatives. Immunol Allergy Clin North Am 1991; 11:659–678.
23. Simon RA, Stevenson DD. Adverse reactions to food and drug additives. In: Middleton E Jr, Reed CE, Ellis EF, Adkinson NF Jr, Yunginger JW, Busse WW, eds. Allergy, Principles and Practice. Vol. 2. St. Louis: CV Mosby, 1993:1687–1704.
24. Partridge MR, Gibson GJ. Adverse bronchial reactions to intravenous hydrocortisone in 2 aspirin sensitive patients. Br Med J 1978; 1:1521–1523.
25. Szczeklik A, Nizankowska E, Czerniawska-Mysik G, Sek S. Hydrocortisone and airflow impairment in aspirin-induced asthma. J Allergy Clin Immunol 1985; 76:530–536.
26. Dajani BM, Sliman NA, Shubair KS. Bronchospasm caused by intravenous hydrocortisone sodium succinate (Solu-Cortef) in aspirin sensitive asthmatics. J Allergy Clin Immunol 1981; 68:201–204.
27. Feigenbaum BA, Stevenson DD, Simon RA. Lack of cross-sensitivity to IV hydrocortisone in aspirin-sensitive subjects with asthma. J Allergy Clin Immunol 1995; 96:545–548.
28. Chiu JT. Improvement in aspirin-sensitive asthmatic subjects after rapid aspirin desensitization and aspirin maintenance (ADAM) treatment. J Allergy Clin Immunol 1983; 71(6):560–567.
29. Lumry WR, Curd JG, Zieger RS, Pleskow WW, Stevenson DD. Aspirin-sensitive rhinosinusitis: the clinical syndrome and effects of aspirin administration. J Allergy Clin Immunol 1983; 71:580–587.
30. Nelson RP, Stablein JJ, Lockey RF. Asthma improved by acetylsalicyclic acid and other non-steroidal anti-inflammatory agents. N Engl Reg Allergy Proc 1986; 7(2):117–121.
31. Szczeklik A, Gryglewski RJ, Nizankowska E. Asthma relieved by aspirin and by other cyclooxygenase inhibitors. Thorax 1978; 33(5):664–665.
32. Lockey RF. Aspirin-improved ASA triad. Hosp Pract 1978; 13:129–133.
33. Naeije N, Bracamonte M, Michel O, et al. Effects of chronic aspirin ingestion in aspirin-intolerant asthmatic patients. Ann Allergy 1984; 53(3):262–264.
34. Stevenson DD, Pleskow WW, Simon RA, Mathison DA, Lumry WR, Schatz M, Zieger RS. Aspirin-sensitive rhinosinusitis asthma: a double-blind cross-over study of treatment with aspirin. J Allergy Clin Immunol 1984; 73:500–507.
35. Sweet JA, Stevenson DD, Simon RA, Mathison DA. Long term effects of aspirin desensitization treatment for aspirin sensitive rhinosinusitis asthma. J Allergy Clin Immunol 1990; 86:59–65.

36. Stevenson DD, Hankammer MA, Mathison DA, Christensen SC, Simon RA. Long term ASA desensitization-treatment of aspirin sensitive asthmatic patients: clinical outcome studies. J Allergy Clin Immunol 1996; 98:751–758.

37. Henderson W. New modalities for the pharmacotherapy of asthma: leukotriene inhibitors and antagonists. Immunol Allergy Clin North Am 1996; 16:797–808.

38. Holgate ST, Bradding P, Sampson AP. Leukotriene antagonists and synthesis inhibitors: new directions in asthma therapy. J Allergy Clin Immunol 1996; 98:1–13.

39. Malmstrom KKP, Szczeklik A, Kowalski M, Stevenson DD, Dahlen SE, Haesen R, De Lepeleire I, Ayala C, Shahane A, Zhang J, Reiss TF. Montelukast (MK-0476), a CysLT receptor antagonist, improves asthma control in aspirin-sensitive asthmatic patients. American Thoracic Society, New Orleans, 1997.

40. Vanselow NA, Smith JR. Bronchial asthma induced by indomethacin. Ann Intern Med 1967; 66:568–573.

41. Samuelsson B, Hammarstroem S, Murphy RC, Borgeat P. Leukotrienes and slow reacting substance of anaphylaxis (SRS-A). Allergy 1980; 35:375–381.

42. Volone FH, Boggs JM, Goetzl EJ. Lipid mediators of hypersensitivity and inflammation. In: Middleton E Jr, Reed CE, Ellis EF, Adkinson NF Jr, Yunginger JW, Busse WW, eds. Allergy: Principles and Practice. Vol. 1. St. Louis: CV Mosby, 1993:302–319.

43. Lee TH. Mehcanism of bronchospasm in aspirin-sensitive asthma. Am Rev Respir Dis 1993; 148:1442–1443 (editorial).

44. Juergens UR, Christiansen SC, Stevenson DD, Zuraw BL. Inhibition of monocyte leukotriene B4 production following aspirin desensitization. J Allergy Clin Immunol 1995; 96:148–156.

45. Christie PE, Tagari P, Ford-Hutchinson AW, Charlesson S, Chee P, Arm JP, Lee TH. Urinary leukotriene E4 concentrations increase after aspirin challenge in aspirin-sensitive asthmatic subjects. Am Rev Respir Dis 1991; 143:1025–1029.

46. Christie PE, Tagari P, Ford-Hutchinson AW, Black C, Markendorf A, Schmitz-Schumann M, Lee TH. Urinary leukotriene E_4 after lysine-aspirin inhalation in asthmatic subjects. Am Rev Respir Dis 1992; 146:1531–1534.

47. Sladek K, Szczeklik A. Cysteinyl leukotrienes overproduction and mast cell activation in aspirin-provoked bronchospasm in asthma. Eur Respir J 1993; 6:391–399.

48. Nasser SMS, Patel M, Bell GS, Lee TH. The effect of aspirin desensitization on urinary leukotriene E_4 concentration in aspirin-sensitive asthma. Am J Respir Crit Care Med 1995; 115:1326–1330.

49. Arm JP, O'Hickey SP, Spur BW, Lee TH. Airway responsiveness to histamine and leukotriene E_4 in subjects with aspirin-induced asthma. Am Rev Respir Dis 1989; 140:148–153.

AUTHOR INDEX

Italic numbers give the page on which the complete reference is listed.

A

Aalbers, R., 515, *521*
Aanesen, J.P., 481, *490*
Abbadie, C., 152, *160*
Abe, K., 37, *44*
Abe, M., 289, *297*
Abe, T., 37, *44*
Abelli, L., *237, 249*
Abraham, N.G., 27, 34, *39, 43*, 60, *74*
Abrahamsohn, P.A., 149, *159*
Abrami, P., 317, 318, *332*, 352, 361, *364, 368*, 523, *535*
Abramin, P., 440, *449*, 452, *470*
Abramovitz, M., 23, 98, *108*, 146, 147, *157*
Abramowitz, M., 374, *387*
Abramson, M.J., 204, *211*, 222, *228*
Acker, M., 115, *125*
Ackerman, R.C., 149, *159*
Ackerman, S.J., 188, *198*, 395, *413*
Ackerman, V., 382, *389*
Ackermann, E., 95, *106*
Adachi, M., 454, 457, 467, *470*
Adamek, L., 302, 303, 304, 307, 308, *312*, 372–79, 381, 382, 383, *385*

Adams, G.K., 358, 359, *366*
Adams, J., 279, *282*
Adamson, S.L., 7, *19*
Adcock, I.M., 114–19, 121, 122, *124*, *125*, *126*, 302, *311*
Adcock, J.J., 241, *251*
Adelroth, E., 259, 263, 265, *268, 270*, *271*, 397, *413*
Adkinson, F., Jr., 319, *332*, 499, *504*
Adkinson, N.F., Jr., 285, 286, *296*, 372, 380, *386*, 460, *471*
Adler, K.B., 235, *247*
Adra, C.N., 204, *211*
Advenier, C., 115, *125*, 427, *435*
Agnat, L., 508, *517*
Agrawal, D.K., 393, 394, 404, 408, *411*, *412, 418*
Agrawal, K.P., 284, *293*
Aguilar-Santelises, M., 191, *200*
Ahern, D., 65, *74*
Ahlstedt, S., 216, 219, *225*
Ahnen, D.J., 149, 150, 154, *159, 160*
Aikawa, T., 397, *414*
Aizawa, H., 114, *124*, 265, *270*
Aizawa, T., 397, *414*
Akai, Y., 5, *18*, 146, *156*

Akaike, T., 240, *251*
Akarasereenont, P., 6, 9, *19*, *21*, 114, 115, 119, *124*, *126*, 130, *141*, 146, *157*, 232, *246*, 285, *295*, 302, *311*, 354, 355, *365*, 512, *519*
Akerblom, I.E., 510, *518*
Akermans, R., 283, *293*
Akolkar, P., 208, *213*
Akutsu, I., 402, *416*
Alander, C., 132, *142*
Alander, D.B., 146, *156*
Albano, M., 13, 16, *22*
Albers, M.W., 508, *517*
Albert, R.K., 197, *200*
Alberts, D.S., 149, 150, 154, *159*, *160*
Albrecht, J.H., 49, *69*
Ale-Martinez, J.E., 149, *159*
Alessandrini, P., 79, *88*
Alexander, A.G., 441, *450*
Alexander, M., 138, *143*
Alexander, R., 95, *106*
Ali, A., 405, *417*
Aljabi, D., 284, *293*
Allan, D., 344, *350*
Allegra, L., 347, *350*, 420, 424, 425, 429, 431, *432*, *434*, 468, *471*, 498, *504*
Allen, M., 97, *107*
Alonso, F., 94, *105*
Alper, C., 206, *212*
Alton, E.W.F.W., 429, *436*
Altounyan, R.E.C., 397, *413*
Amaral-Marques, R., 456, 459, *470*
Ameisen, J.C., 301, *311*, 440, *449*, *450*
Amelung, P.J., 205, *212*, 222, *228*
Amin, A.R., 232, *245*
Aminlari, M., 239, *251*
An, S.-J., 34, *43*
Anderson, G.P., 188, 193, *199*
Anderson, M., 479, *489*
Anderson, P., 352, 353, 354, 355, 358, *364*, 381, *388*
Anderson, R., 301, *310*
Anderson, R.D., 136, 137, *142*
Anderson, S.D., 216, 222, *224*, 259, *264*, *269*, *270*, 427, 431, *435*, *437*

Anderson, W.H., 235, *247*
Andersson, B., 479, *489*
Andersson, M., 477, 479, *489*
Andersson, R., 352, 353, 354, 355, 358, *364*, 381, *388*
Anderton, R.C., *269*
Andrade, W.P., 441, *450*
Andreasson, K.I., 7, *20*, 133, *142*, 146, *156*
Andreatta-Van Leyen, S., 33, *42*
Andri, G., 13, 16, *22*
Andri, L., 13, 16, *22*
Angeli, P., 62, *74*
Anggärd, E., 29, *40*, 79, *88*
Ansari, A.A., 206, 209, *212*, *213*
Anticevich, S.Z., 507, 515, *516*
Antonipillai, I., 27, 34, *39*
Anwar, A.R., 401, *416*
Aoyama, T., 53, *71*
Appleby, S.B., 118, *126*
Appleton, I., 6, *19*, 135, *142*, 233, *246*
Arai, I., 7, *20*, 122, *127*, 131, *141*
Arai, S., *23*
Arakawa, T., 118, *126*, 137, *142*
Aranda, J.V., 7, *19*
Archakov, A.I., 68, *75*
Arcoleo, E., 232, 234, *245*
Arfors, K.E., 321, *333*
Arita, H., 95, *106*, 284, *294*
Arm, J.P., 56, *72*, 197, *200*, 285, *294*, 296, 303, 304, 308, *312*, *313*, *314*, 321, 322, 324, 327, *333*, *334*, *335*, 337, *348*, 357, 361, *365*, 371, 383, *384*, *389*, 393, 394, 408, *410*, *411*, 424, 429, *434*, 440, *449*, 496, 497, *504*, 534, *537*
Arm, M.P., 355, 358, 361, *365*
Armandola, M.C., 12, *22*
Armetti, L., 91, 96, *104*, 306, *314*, 321, *333*, 347, *350*, 360, 361, *367*, 371, *385*, 422, 424, 425, 429, *433*, *434*
Armour, C.L., 116, *125*, 507, 515, *516*
Arnberg, H., 237, *249*
Arnelle, D., 237, *249*
Arner, B., 361, *368*
Arnetti, L., 427, *435*

Arnold, J.L., 53, *71*
Arnoux, B., 514, *520*
Arrasmith, M., 93, *105*
Arroyave, C.M., 358, *366*
Arruda, L.K., 222, *227*
Arsura, M., 153, *160*
Asai, K., 148, *159*
Asano, K., 6, *19*, 235, *247*, 287, *297*, 303, *312*, 514, *520*
Asfaha, S., 292, *298*
Askenase, P.W., 35, *43*
Asmis, R., 394, *412*
Assoufi, B., 217, 219, 220, 221, 223, 226, 289, *298*, 373, 382, *386*, *388*
Atkins, M.B., 28, *40*
Atkinson, D.L., 222, *228*
Attali, P., 148, *158*
Atuur, M., 232, *245*
Aubier, M., 237, *250*
Augusti-Vidal, A., 300, *310*, 457, 467, *471*
Auphan, N., *127*, 510, *518*
Auriault, C., 301, *311*
Aursudkij, B., 400, *414*
Austen, K.F., 28, *40*, 56, *72*, 99, *108*, 188, 197, *199*, *200*, 253, *257*, 285, 286, *294*, *296*, 302, 303, 304, 307, 308, *312*, *313*, 321, *333*, 338, *349*, 358–61, *366*, 372–79, 381, 382, 383, *385*, *386*, *387*, *388*, *389*, 392, 393, 394, 397, 400, 401, *409*, *410*, *411*, *412*, *413*, *414*, *415*, *418*
Austgen, M., 442, *450*
Autuori, F., 148, *159*
Averill, F.J., 284, *294*
Avontuur, J.A., 274, *281*
Awad, J.A., 78, 79, *87*, *88*, 111, *123*
Awdeh, Z., 206, *212*
Awni, W.M., 188, *199*
Ayala, C., 531, *537*
Azevedo, I., 512, *519*
Azzawi, M., 373, 382, *386*, *388*

B

Baas, A., 95, *106*
Babcock, G.T., 171, *185*

Bacci, E., 515, *522*
Bach, C., 146, *157*
Bach, M.K., 321, *333*, 400, *414*
Bachelet, M., 512, *519*
Bachert, C., 482, 483, *490*
Backer, V., 217, 224, *226*, *229*
Badr, K.F., 30, *41*, 77, 78, 79, *87*, *88*, 287, *297*
Baenkler, H., 91, 96, *104*
Bahkle, Y.S., 232, *246*
Baier, L.D., 232, 233, *245*
Bailey, T.J., 256, *258*
Bailie, M., 98, 102, *108*
Baker, A.J., 285, 288, *295*, 362, *368*
Baker, J., 99, *108*
Baker, J.R., 286, *296*
Baker, P.N., 232, 233, 234, *246*
Bakhle, Y.S., 5, *19*, 119, *126*
Balazy, M., 27, 28, 30, 31, 32, *39*, *40*, *41*, *42*, 50, 51, 58, 59, 60, 62, 63, 65, 66, *70*, *72*, *73*, *74*, *75*
Baldasaro, M., 304, *313*, 383, *389*, 393, *410*
Baldwin, A.S., 119, *127*, 510, *518*
Ball, J.G., 236, *248*
Ballard, P., 508, *517*
Ballard, R.D., 515, *522*
Ballif, B.A., 149, *159*
Ballioni, P., 300, *310*
Balsinde, J., 95, *106*
Balter, M.S., 285, 286, *295*, 512, *519*
Balvisi, M.G., 111, *123*
Bambauer, R., 442, *450*
Bancalari, L., 515, *522*
Bandouvakis, J., 259, 264, *268*
Banerjee, M., 78, *87*
Banres, P.J., 117, *125*
Bao, Y., 32, *42*
Baptist, J.E., 456, 458, 460, *470*
Baranowski, S.L., 397, *414*
Barbado, A., 456, 459, *470*
Barbee, R.A., 218, 221, 223, *226*
Bardin, P.G., 231, *245*
Barkans, J., 217, 219–23, *225*, *226*, *227*, 382, *389*

Barker, J., 302, 308, *311*, 329, *335*, 338, 342, 344, *349*, 372–76, *385*, 495, 498, *503*, *504*

Barnèon, G., 216, 219, *225*

Barner, A., 11, *22*

Barnes, C.A., 7, *20*, 133, *142*, 146, *156*

Barnes, N.C., 117, *125*, 362, *368*, 397, *413*, 441, *450*

Barnes, P.J., 6, 16, *19*, *23*, 111, 113–19, 121, 122, *123*, *124*, *125*, *126*, *127*, 217, *225*, 235, 237, 239, 240, *247*, *249*, *251*, 265, *270*, 285, *295*, 302, *311*, 400, 403, 405, *414*, *416*, *417*, 426, 427, 430, 431, *435*, *437*, 512, *519*

Barnet, H.N., 317, 318, *332*

Barnett, J., 2, *17*, 146, *157*, 163, 164, 169, 170, 178, 179, 181, *184*

Barratt, J.T., 149, *159*

Barrow, S.E., 287, *297*

Bartosik, A., 441, *450*

Bascom, R., 235, *247*, 287, *297*, 360, *367*, 514, *521*

Basomba, A., 429, *436*, 468, *471*

Bass, D., 95, *106*

Battistini, B., 115, *125*

Baxter, J., 508, *517*

Bayburt, T., 94, *105*

Bayol, A., 360, *367*

Bazan, N., 7, *20*, 302, *311*

Beall, D., 481, 482, *490*

Beam, W.R., 288, *297*, 514, *521*

Bean, D.K., 308, *315*, 495, *503*

Beasley, C.R., 238, *250*, 507, *516*

Beasley, R.W., 188, *198*, 222, *228*, 373, *386*

Beato, M., 510, *517*, *518*

Beaty, T.H., 205, *212*, 222, *228*

Beck, L., 481, 482, *490*

Beckman, J.S., 234, *246*

Bedard, P., 479, *490*

Bednar, M.M., 62, *74*

Beers, R.F., 223, *229*, 299, 300, 302, 304, *309*, 309, 318, *332*, 361, *368*, 451, 463, *470*

Begishvili, T., 188, *198*, 222, *228*

Beharry, K., 7, *19*

Beiche, F., 7, *20*

Beier, D.R., 188, *198*

Bel, E.H., *271*

Bell, G.S., 308, *314*, 324, 327, 328, *334*, *335*, 357, 361, *365*, 371, 379, *384*, *388*, 424, 429, *434*, 534, *537*

Bell, J.I., 206, 208, 209, *213*

Belley, M., 362, *368*

Bellia, V., 514, *520*

Bellini, A., 382, *389*

Belloni, P., 273, *281*

Belosludtsev, Y., 62, *74*

Belvisi, M.G., 6, *19*, 114, 115, 116, 117, 119, *124*, *125*, 237, 239, 240, *249*, 285, *295*, 302, *311*, 512, *519*

Bennett, A., *23*, 421, *433*

Bennett, A.R., 373, *387*

Bennett, C.F., 284, *294*

Bennett, D., 274, *281*

Bennett, J., 115, *125*

Bennett, P., 7, 8, *20*

Benoit, R.R., 8, *21*

Benson, M.K., *269*

Bentley, A.M., 219, 221, *226*, 289, *298*, 382, *389*

Benveniste, J., 235, *247*, 360, *367*

Ben-Yaakov, M., 401, *415*

Berger, M., 27, 34, *39*, 457, *470*

Bernard, G.R., 514, *520*

Berni, F., 431, *437*

Bernini, W., 511, 515, *518*, *522*

Bernstein, J.M., 473, 477, 486, *488*, *489*

Bernstrom, K., 65, *75*

Berti, F., 426, 427, *434*, *435*

Bessler, W., 273, *281*

Bestynska, A., 421, *433*

Betail, M., 218, *226*

Betteridge, D.J., 79, *88*

Bewtra, A.K., 222, *228*

Bezian, J.H., 301, *311*

Bhat, K.N., 358, *366*

Bhatt, R.K., 56, 65, *72*, *74*

Bhattacharyya, D.K., 173, 179, *185*, *186*

Bhattacharyya, S., 210, *214*

Bianco, I., 95, *106*

Bianco, S., 91, 96, *104*, 300, 301, 302,
304, 306, *310*, *311*, *312*, *313*, *314*,
321, *333*, 347, *350*, 351, 352, 357,
358, 360, 361, *364*, *366*, *367*, 371,
380, *385*, *388*, 420, 421, 422,
424–31, *432*, *433*, *434*, *435*, *436*,
438, 468, *471*, 498, *504*
Bianco, S.R., 523, 524, 525, *535*
Bias, W.B., 206, *212*
Biberfeld, P., 191, *200*
Bigby, B.G., 265, *270*
Bigby, T., 99, *108*, 286, 287, *296*, *297*
Bigerna, B., 374, *387*
Bilaniuk, L.T., 468, *472*
Billiar, T.R., 274, *281*
Bina, J.C., 401, *415*
Bingham, C.O. III, 285, *296*
Binks, S.M., 263, *270*
Birch, P.J., 9, *21*
Bischoff, S.C., 342, *349*, 382, *389*, 401,
416
Bishai, I., 7, *19*
Bishai, P.M., 421, *433*
Bishop-Bailey, D., 117, *125*, 135, *142*,
233, *246*
Bito, L.Z., 33, *42*
Bittolo Bon, G., 79, *88*
Björck, T., 113, *123*, 303, *312*, 323, *334*,
337, *348*, 355, 358, 361, 362, *365*,
368, 371, 372, *384*, 496, 497, *504*,
514, *520*
Bjork, J., 321, *333*
Bjornsdottir, U., 408, *418*
Black, C., 322, 323, *333*, *334*, 337, *348*,
358, *366*, 534, *537*
Black, J.L., 116, *125*, 507, 515, *516*
Black, P., 266, *271*, 287, *296*, *297*
Blair, I.A., 30, *41*, 60, 62, 63, 65, *73*, 75,
77, 78, *87*, 253, *257*, 306, *314*, 360,
367
Blanco, C., 299, *310*
Blaser, K., 217, 218, 221, *225*
Bleecker, E.R., 112, *123*, 205, *212*, 222,
228, 286, *296*, 514, *520*
Blobel, G., 167, *184*
Block, F.J., 113, *123*, 287, *297*

Blömer, K., 209, *214*
Blomjous, F.J., 238, *250*
Blomqvist, H., 304, *313*, 324, 326, *334*,
353, 355, 356, 358, 362, *364*, *369*,
372, *385*, 424, 429, *434*, 502, *505*
Blotman, F., 288, *297*, 515, *522*
Blouin, R.A., 50, *70*
Blumenstein, B.A., 441, *450*
Blumenthal, M.N., 206, *212*, 454, 457,
464, *470*
Bochenek, G., 207, *213*, 223, *229*, 300,
304, 308, *310*, *313*, *315*, 326, *334*, 362,
369, 441, *450*, 464, *471*, 502, *505*
Bode, F., 217, 218, 221, 225
Boeglin, W.E., 53, 60, 62, *71*, 73
Boelens, H., 395, *413*
Boer, L., 217, 218, 221, *225*
Bogardus, A.M., 256, *258*
Bögel, R., 11, *22*
Boggs, M.J., 532, *537*
Bohman, S.O., 29, *40*
Bolcskei, P., 91, 96, *104*
Bonanno, A., 514, *520*
Bonne, C., 301, *311*
Bonney, R., 101, *108*
Bonsignore, G., 514, *520*
Bonta, I.L., 397, *414*
Bonventre, J.V., 29, *40*, *41*
Boreus, L.O., 301, *310*
Boréus, L.O., 352, 353, 354, 355, 358,
364, 381, *388*
Borgeat, P., 27, *39*, 372, 380, *386*, 393,
394, 402, *410*, *411*, *412*, *416*, 479,
490, 532, *537*
Bories, C., 148, *158*
Bork, P., 169, *185*
Boschetto, P., 216, *225*, 515, *522*
Boss, H.J., 78, *87*
Bosse, M., 395, 401, *413*
Bosserman, M.K., 236, *248*
Bosso, J.V., 329, *335*, 343, *350*, 358, *367*
Böttcher, I., 12, *22*
Botting, J., 302, *311*
Botting, R.M., 8, *21*, 119, *126*, 138,
143, 232, 233, *245*, 419, 421, 424,
431, *432*

Bouali, F., 152, *160*
Boucher, R.C., 188, *198*, 426, *434*
Boughton Smith, N.K., 274, *281*
Bouhuys, A., 235, *247*, 248
Boulet, L.P., 395, 401, 408, *413*, *417*, 515, *521*
Boullet, C., 360, *367*
Bouman, K., 204, *211*
Bourne, H.R., 253, *257*
Boushey, H.A., 265, *270*, 426, *434*, 515, 522
Bousquet, J., 216, 219, *225*, 235, 239, *247*, *251*, 287, 288, *297*, 302, 304, *311*, *313*, 381, *388*, 447, *450*, 514, 515, *520*, *521*, 522
Bouta, I.L., 380, *388*
Boutwell, R.K., 148, *159*
Boyce, J., 383, *389*, 392, 393, *409*, *410*
Boyce, S., 13, 14, *22*, 122, *127*
Boyer, W.C., 171, *185*
Braam, B., 33, *42*
Bracamonte, M., 529, *536*
Bradbury, M.J., 284, *294*
Bradding, P., 382, *389*, 531, *537*
Bradford, T.R., 343, *350*
Bradley, B., 219, 221, *226*
Bradley, B.L., 373, 382, *386*, *388*
Bradley, J., 94, *105*
Bradshaw, W.S., 149, 150, 152, 153, *160*
Brain, E.A., 222, *228*
Braman, S.S., 218, *226*
Branch, D.W., 146, *156*
Brandtzaeg, P., 373, *387*, 481, 482, *490*
Brannon, T.S., 25, 34, *39*, 237, *249*
Braquet, P., 192, *200*, 393, 394, *410*, *411*
Brasch, F., 6, *19*
Brash, A.R., 53, 60, 62, 63, *71*, *73*, 286, *296*, 394, *412*
Brattsand, R., 408, *417*
Braun, J.J., 475, *488*
Braunstein, G., 235, *247*
Bray, W.M., 400, *414*
Brayton, P., 303, 305, *312*
Breazeale, D.R., 205, *212*, 222, *228*

Breder, C.D., 7, *20*
Bredt, D.S., 237, *249*, *250*
Breiteneder, H., 206, *212*
Brendel, K., 149, 150, 154, *159*, *160*
Bresnahan, B.A., 37, *44*
Breuer, D.K., 9, *21*, 26, *39*, 146, *157*, 172, 173, 174, *185*, *186*
Brewster, C.E.P., 494, *503*
Breyer, M.D., 5, *18*, 256, *258*
Breyer, R.M., 256, *258*
Brideau, C., 13, 14, *22*, 122, *127*
Brigham, K.L., 140, *144*
Brink, C., 235, *247*, 360, *367*
Britten, K.M., 361, 373, 382, *387*, *389*
Britton, J.R., 426, *435*
Brock, T., 94, 98, 102, 103, *105*, *108*, 286, *296*
Brocklehurst, W., 265, *271*
Brodkey, F.D., 222, *228*
Broekman, M.J., 56, *72*
Bromberg, P.A., 6, *19*
Bronnegard, M., 508, *517*
Brown, C.R., 118, 119, 121, *126*
Brown, D.M., 149, *159*
Brown, G.P., 80, *88*
Brown, K., 95, *106*
Brown, K.E., 515, *522*
Brown, M.J., 265, *270*
Brown, R., 118, *126*
Browner, M.F., 2, *17*, 163, 164, 169, 170, 178, 179, 181, *184*
Browning, J.L., 510, 511, *518*, *519*
Bruchi, O., 515, *522*
Bruggemeier, U., 510, *517*
Brugger, R., 52, *70*
Bruijnzeel, P.L., 393, 394, 395, 408, *411*, *412*, *417*
Bruining, H.A., 274, *281*
Brun, J., 218, *226*
Brun, R., 103, *109*
Brun, R.P., 36, *43*, 147, *158*
Brune, K., 7, *20*
Brunelleschi, S., 235, *247*
Brunner, T., 342, *349*
Bruynzeel, P., 372, *386*, 393, 394, *411*, *412*

Bucciarelli, A., 79, *88*
Buchanan, S.K., 182, *186*
Buchstein, H.F., 320, *332*
Buckle, V., 208, *213*
Buckler, A.J., 153, *160*
Buitkus, K.L., 113, *123*, 287, *297*
Buja, L.M., 140, *144*
Bulbena, O., 303, 305, *312*, 323, *334*,
    337, 347, *348*, 358, 360, *366*, 380,
    381, 388, 496, 497, *504*
Bunting, S., 3, *17*, 52, *71*
Buntix, A., *271*, 362, *368*
Burch, R.A., 284, *293*, 402, *416*
Burck, W.H., 275, *282*
Burdick, M., 98, *108*
Burdick, M.D., 285, 292, *295*
Buret, A., 292, *298*
Burk, R.F., 77, 78, *87*
Burke, K.M., 222, *228*
Burke, L.A., 393, 394, 408, *411*
Burns, G.B., 358, 359, *366*
Burrows, B., 218, 221, 223, *226, 227*
Burt, R.W., 149, 150, 154, *159, 160*
Buschi, A., 427, *435*
Bush, R.K., 362, *368*
Bush, W., 508, *517*
Busse, R., 273, *281*
Busse, W.W., 188, 193, *198, 199*, 231,
    245, 287, *297*, 303, *312*, 362, *368*,
    408, *418*
Butcher, S., 6, *19*
Buters, J.T.M., 68, *75*
Butler, G.B., 235, *247*
Butt, J.C., 219, *227*
Buttery, L., *237, 239, 250, 251*
Buytenhek, M., 161, *183*
Bynoe, T.C., 237, *249*

C

Cabanieu, G., 301, *311*
Caen, J., 301, *311*
Cairns, C., 510, *518*
Cairns, J., 192, *200*
CaJacob, C.A., 49, 53, *69*

Calenda, A., 192, *200*
Calhoun, W.J., 238, *250*, 268, *271*
Callan, O.H., 176, 178, *186*
Calle, E.E., 148, *158*
Callery, C.P., 358, 360, *366*
Callery, J.C., 91, *104*, 304, 305, *313*,
    324, 329, *334, 335*, 337, 343, *348*,
    357, *365*, 371, *384*, 428, *435*, 496,
    497, 498, 502, *504*
Cambert, C., 393, *410*
Cameron, M.J., 344, *350*
Camp, R.D.R., 400, *414*
Campbell, A.M., 235, *247*, 477, *489*
Campbell, I.D., 169, *185*
Campbell, M.D., 77, *87*
Campos, A., 429, *436*, 468, *471*
Canet, E., 50, *70*
Cannon, P.J., 28, *40*
Cao, C., 7, *20*
Capdevila, J., 25, 27, 30, 34, *38, 41*, 46,
    58, 59, 60, 62, 63, 65, *69, 73, 75*
Caplin, I., 475, *488*
Cappellazzo, G., 515, *522*
Capriotti, A., 93, *105*
Capron, A., 286, *296*, 301, *311*, 429,
    436, 440, 442, 444, 447, 448, *449*,
    450
Capron, M., 442, *450*
Car, B.D., 8–9, *20*, 139, *143*, 146, *157*,
    285, 292, *295*
Caramori, G., 222, *228*
Cardarelli, N., 374, *387*
Cardillo, R., 402, *416*
Carew, T.E., 129, *143*
Carey, D., 116, *125*
Carillo, T., 299, *310*
Carlstedt-Duke, J., 508, 510, *517, 518*
Carlton, D.P., 130, *141*
Carns, W., 510, *518*
Carrión, T., 495, 496, *503*
Carroll, M.A., 28, 30, 31, 33, 34, *40*,
    41, 42, 43, 60, 62, 63, 66, *73, 74, 75*
Carroll, N., 515, *522*
Carson, J.L., 8, 9, *21*
Carter, J.D., 6, *19*
Carter, M.C., 222, *227*

Cartier, A., 56, *72*, *269*
Cartwright, M., 4, *18*
Casadevall, J., 500, *505*
Casale, T.B., 342, *349*
Casals Stenzel, J., 279, *282*
Case, J.P., 26, 34, *39*
Cashman, J.R., 393, *410*
Castillo, J.A., 300, *310*, 457, 467, *471*, 500, *504*
Castillo, R., 299, *310*
Castle, L., 51, *70*
Castonguay, A., 148, *159*
Cate, R.L., 512, *519*
Catella, D.T., 62, *74*
Catella, F., 59, *73*
Cato, A.C.B., 509, 511, *517*
Caughey, G.H., 393, *410*
Cauna, N., 477, 478, *489*
Cavaliere, A., 374, *387*
Cech, A., 274, *281*
Cederbaum, A.I., 51, *70*
Celestin, J., 342, *349*
Cerrina, J., 360, *367*
Ceuppens, J., 253, *257*
Chacos, N., 59, *73*
Chafee, F.H., 223, *229*, 319, 320, *332*, 452, 457, 458, 460, 464, 469, *470*
Chalepakis, G., 510, *517*
Champagne, K., 395, 401, *413*
Champion, E., 362, *368*
Chan, C.C., 13, 14, *22*, 122, *127*, 400, *414*
Chan, H., 221, 223, *227*
Chan, S., 307, *314*
Chanarin, N., 397, 400, *413*
Chand, N., 408, *418*
Chanez, P., 216, 219, *225*, 235, 237, 239, *247*, *249*, *251*, 447, *450*, 514, 515, *521*
Chang, H., 508, *517*
Chang, M.S., 53, *71*
Chanmugam, P., 146, *156*
Channon, J., 94, *105*
Chan-Yeung, M., 221, 222, 223, *227*, *269*
Chanz, P., 515, *522*

Chao, P.W.H., 56, *72*
Chapman, M.D., 222, *227*
Chapman, R.W., 219, *227*
Chaprin, D., 222, *228*
Charette, L., 362, *368*
Charleson, P., 28, *40*
Charleson, S., 4, *18*, 56, *72*, 92, 97, *104*, 374, *387*
Charlesson, S., 303, *312*, 322, *333*, 337, *348*, 355, 358, 361, *365*, 371, *384*, 440, *449*, 496, 497, *504*, 534, *537*
Charpin, J., 222, *228*
Chaud, M., 233, *246*
Chaudry, N.B., 113, *124*
Chauhan, K., 63, *74*
Chavis, C., 288, *297*, 372, *386*, 514, 515, *520*, *521*, *522*
Chee, C., 237, *249*
Chee, J., 496, 497, *504*
Chee, P., 303, *312*, 322, *333*, 337, *348*, 355, 358, 361, *365*, 371, *384*, 440, *449*, 514, *520*, 534, *537*
Chekraborty, I., 8, *21*
Chemtob, S., 7, *19*
Chen, J., 36, *43*, 103, *109*, 147, *158*
Chen, X., 188, 193, *199*
Chen, X.-S., 98, *108*
Cheng, W., 274, *282*
Chensue, S.W., 253, *257*
Cherwitz, D.L., 49, *69*
Cheung, P.S., 9–10, *21*
Chi, E., 94, *105*
Chi, E.Y., 197, *200*
Chiang, G.K.S., 197, *200*
Chiang, M.-Y., 284, *294*
Chida, M., 6, *19*
Childres, C.E., 236, *248*
Chilton, F., 95, *106*
Chilton, F.H., 132, *141*, 284, 286, *293*, *294*, *296*, 360, *367*
Chinery, R., 96, 103, *107*
Chinn, R.A., 400, *414*
Chiou, M., 146, *157*
Chipman, J.G., 3, *17*, 25, 34, *39*, 130, *141*, 145, 146, 147, 148, 152, *155*, *156*, *159*, 162, *183*, 285, *294*

Chiu, J.T., 529, *536*
Chopin, C., 300, *310*
Choudhury, Q., 114, *124*, 511, *519*
Choudry, N.B., *269*
Chow, A.W., 400, *414*
Chow, J., 2, *17*, 146, *157*, 163, 164, 169, 170, 178, 179, 181, *184*
Chrisensen, S.C., 531, *537*
Christiansen, S.C., 300, 308, *310*, *314*, 534, *537*
Christie, P.E., 302, 303, 304, 308, *311*, *312*, *313*, *315*, 322, 323, 324, 327, 329, *333*, *334*, *335*, 337, 338, 342, 344, *348*, *349*, 355, 357–61, *365*, *366*, *367*, 371–76, 378, 380, 381, *384*, *385*, 424, 425, 429, *434*, 440, *449*, 495–98, *503*, *504*, 534, *537*
Christman, B.W., 140, *144*, 253, *257*, 306, *314*
Christman, J.W., 253, *257*, 306, *314*
Christophers, E., 204, *211*
Chua, K.-Y., 222, *227*
Chulada, P.C., 4, 7, *18*, *20*, 138, 139, *143*, 146, *157*, 285, *294*
Chumley, P., 273, 274, 280, *281*
Chung, D., 198, *200*, 393, 394, *411*
Chung, K.F., 111, 113, 118, *123*, *124*, *126*, 400, *414*, 427, 431, *435*, *437*
Church, M.K., 306, *314*, 358, 359, 361, *366*, 373, 380, 381, *387*, *388*, 403, *417*
Churcher, Y., 344, *350*
Churchill, L., 9, 10, 11, *21*, 235, *247*, 360, *367*
Ciabattoni, G., 78, 79, 80, 82, *87*, *88*
Ciaccia, A., 221, *227*
Cibella, F., 514, *520*
Cicutto, L.C., 515, *522*
Cidlowski, J.A., 119, *127*
Cillari, E., 232, 234, *245*
Cipollone, F., 9, *21*, 80, 82, 84, *88*
Cirino, G., 510, *518*
Ciyotani, A., 239, *250*
Claesson, H.E., 191, 192, *200*, 358, *365*
Clair, I.A., 63, *74*
Claria, J., 147, *158*

Clark, D.A., 28, *40*
Clark, J.D., 29, 30, *40*, *41*, 94, *105*, 374, *387*
Clark, J.E., 50, *70*
Clark, T.J., 393, 394, *411*
Clement, P., 305, *313*
Cline, M.G., 218, 221, 223, *226*
Clintra, S., 508, *517*
Clubb, F.J., 140, *144*
Cmiel, A., 306, *314*, 321, *333*, 347, *350*, 360, *367*, 421, 424, *433*, *434*
Coburn, A.S., 302, 303, 304, 307, 308, *312*
Cocco, G., 420, *433*
Coceani, F., 7, *19*
Cockcroft, D.W., 193, *200*, 216, 222, *224*, *225*, 259, *268*, *269*, *271*, 284, *293*
Coffey, M.J., 94, 98, 103, *105*, *108*, 286, *296*
Coffey, R.J., 96, 103, *107*, 148, *158*
Coffman, R.L., 188, 193, *199*
Cogan, M.G., 33, *42*
Coggon, D., 224, *229*
Cogswell, P.C., *127*, 510, *518*
Cohan, V.L., 285, 286, *296*
Cohen, S.I., 511, *518*
Cohn, H., 91, *104*
Cohn, J., 188, *199*, 286, *296*, 304, 305, *313*, 329, *335*, 337, 340, 342, 343, *348*, *349*, 357, 358, 360, 362, *365*, *366*, *368*, 371, *384*, 428, *435*, 496, 497, 498, 502, *504*
Cole, M., 397, *413*
Cole, P.J., 285, 286, *295*, 360, *367*
Coleman, R.A., 36, *37*, *43*, 253, 256, *257*
Coles, S.T., 400, *414*
Colin-Jones, D.G., 8, *21*
Collée, J.M., 204, *211*
Colley, D.G., 394, *412*
Collins, J.V., 373, 382, *386*, *388*
Collins, L.J., 37, *44*
Collins, R.J., 8–9, *20*, 146, *157*, 285, 292, *295*
Collmer, D., 7, *20*

Comtois, J.F., 395, 401, *413*
Conanan, N.D., 113, *124*, 307, *314*
Conary, J.T., 140, *144*
Conde-Frieboes, K., 95, *106*
Conrad, D.J., 287, *297*, 393, *410*
Conraux, C., 475, *488*
Contel, N.R., 8–9, *20*, 139, *143*, 146, *157*, 285, 292, *295*
Conway, M., 475, *488*
Cooins, R.J., 139, *143*
Cookson, W.O.C.M., 203–10, *211, 212, 213, 214*, 222, *228*, 269, 308, *315*
Coon, M.J., 47, 48, 68, *69*
Cooper, C., 34, 35, *43*
Copeland, N., 98, *108*
Copeland, R.A., 173, *185*
Corey, E.J., 28, *40*, 86, *89*, 338, *349*, 372, *386*, 393, 397, 400, 409, *410, 413, 414*
Corne, J.M., 218, *226*
Cornélis, F., 208, 209, *213*
Coroneos, E., 6, *19*
Correia, M.A., 50, *70*
Corrigan, C.J., 217, 219, 220, 221, 223, *226, 227*
Corriu, C., 50, *70*
Corry, D.B., 188, 195, 197, *199*
Costabel, U., 524, *535*
Costantini, F., 79, *88*
Costello, J.F., 395, 397, *413*
Coulet, M., 218, *226*
Couret, I., 235, *247*
Coutts, A.A., 400, *414*
Covington, M.B., 8–9, *20*, 139, *143*, 146, *157*, 285, 292, *295*
Cowburn, A.S., 372–79, 381, 382, 383, *385*
Cox, M., 98, *108*
Cox, M.E., 374, *387*
Coyle, A.J., 188, 193, *198, 199*
Craddock, C.F., *269*
Craik, C.S., 393, *410*
Cramer, W., 182, *186*
Crastes-de-Paulet, A., 372, *386*
Crea, A.E., 393, 394, 401, 408, *411, 415*

Creely, D.P., *23*, 122, *127*, 146, *157*, 163, *184*
Créminon, C., 9, *21*, 78, 79, 80, 82, 84, 87, *88*, 302, *311*, 381, *388*
Crews, B.C., 51, *70*, 234, *246*
Crittenden, N.J., 393, 394, *410*
Crofford, L.J., 26, 34, *39*, 285, 292, *295*
Cromlish, W., *23*
Cromwell, O., 393, 394, 401, 402, *410, 411, 416*
Cross, A.H., 233, *246*
Crotty, T.B., 515, *522*
Croxtall, J., 6, *19*, 114, 115, 119, *124, 126*, 135, *142*, 233, *246*, 285, *295*, 302, *311*, 511, 512, *519*
Crzelewska-Rzymowska, I., 329, *335*
Cuccurullo, F., 82, *88*
Cuff, M.T., *269*
Cullen, K., 224, *229*
Culp, S., *23*
Cunningham, D.D., 234, *246*
Cunningham, J.N., 274, *282*
Cunningham, L., 495, *503*
Curd, J., 358, *366*
Curd, J.G., 460, *471*, 529, *536*
Curley, F.J., 441, *450*
Currie, M.G., 34, *43*, 119, *126*, 232, 233, 235, *245, 246*
Cuss, F.M., 219, *227*, 235, *247*
Cuttitta, G., 514, *520*
Cybulsky, M., 138, *143*, 198, *200*
Czerniak, P.M., 8–9, *20*, 139, *143*, 146, *157*, 285, 292, *295*
Czerniawska-Mysik, G., 299, 301, 302, 304, *309, 311*, 320, *332, 333*, 351, 357, 361, 363, *364*, 371, *385*, 421, 423, *433*, 440, *449*, 457, 459, 468, *471, 472*, 526, 528, *535, 536*
Czuk, C.I., 393, 394, *410*
Czuk, E.I., 393, 394, *410*

D

Daffonchio, L., 427, 430, *435*
D'Agostino, P., 232, 234, *245*

Dahinden, C.A., 342, *349*, 382, *389*, 394, 401, *412*, *416*
Dahl, R., 429, *436*, 468, *472*
Dahlén, B., 113, *123*, 301, 303, 304, *310*, *312*, *313*, 323, 324, 326, *334*, 337, 343, *348*, *350*, 352–56, 358, 359, 361, 362, *364*, *365*, *367*, *368*, *369*, 371, 372, 380, 381, *384*, *385*, *388*, 420, 424, 425, 428, 429, *433*, *434*, *436*, 496, 497, 500, 502, *504*, *505*, 514, *520*
Dahlen, S.-E., 56, *72*, 113, *123*, 303, 304, *312*, *313*, 321, 323, 324, 326, *333*, *334*, *337*, 343, *348*, *350*, 353, 355, 356, 358–62, *364*, *365*, *366*, *367*, *368*, *369*, 371, 372, 380, *384*, *385*, *388*, 397, *413*, 424, 425, 428, 429, *434*, *436*, 496, 497, 502, *504*, *505*, 507, 514, *516*, *520*, *521*, 531, *537*
Dahlman-Wright, K., 510, *517*
Dailey, L.A., 6, *19*
Dajani, B.M., 500, *505*, 528, *536*
Dakhama, A., 408, *417*
Dallman, M.F., 284, *294*
Dalman, F.C., 508, *517*
Dal Vecchio, L., 216, *225*
Daly, J.M., 274, *281*
Dama, A.R., 13, 16, *22*
Damiani, P., 274, *282*
Damodaran, C., 206, *212*
Damon, M., 372, *386*
Damonte, C., 300, *310*, 358, *366*
Damonte, M.C., 420, *433*
Damoon, M., 515, *521*
Damstrup, L., 96, 103, *107*
Daniel, V., 96, 103, *107*
Daniel, V.C., 77, *87*
Daniels, S.E., 204, 210, *211*, *214*
Daphna-Iken, D., 232, 233, *245*
Darbyshe, J.F., 50, *70*
Das, S.K., 8, *21*
Datta, A.K., 511, *518*
Davì, G., 79, *88*
David, J.R., 401, *415*
Davidge, S.T., 232, 233, 234, *246*

Davidson, A.E., 397, *413*
Davidson, D.A., 285, 286, *296*
Davidson, F.F., 511, *518*
Davidson, R., 401, *415*
Davidson, T.M., 494, *503*
Davies, B.H., 113, *124*, 264, *270*
Davies, R.J., 121, *127*, 218, *226*, 477, *489*
Davis, R.J., 30, *41*
Davson, H., 33, *42*
Dawson, T.M., 237, *250*
Deal, E.C., *269*
Deam, S., 344, *350*
deBlic, J., 512, *519*
De Boer, M., 393, *411*
de Brum-Fernandes, A.J., 392, *409*
De Carli, M., 217, 223, *226*
De Caterina, R., 511, 513, 515, *518*, *519*, *522*
De Cesare, D., 79, *88*
De Clerck, F., 236, 238, 239, *248*
Dehaven, R.N., 362, *368*
Deibert, K., 233, 235, *246*
De Jongste, J.C., 397, *414*
De Kimpe, S.J., 239, *251*
Dekker, J.W., 204, 206, 207, *211*, *213*, 308, *315*
De Klerk, N.H., 205, *212*
Delage, C., 218, *226*
Delamere, F., 115, *125*
Delaney, J.C., 223, *229*, 320, *333*, 429, *436*, 460, *471*
Delanty, N., 79, *88*
Delany, J.C., 468, *472*
DeLepeleire, I., 362, *368*, 531, *537*
Delgado, J., 299, *310*
D'Elios, M.M., 217, 223, *226*
Delneste, Y., 223, *228*, 309, *315*, 442, 447, 448, *450*
Del Prete, G.F., 217, 223, *226*
Demarcq, J.M., 300, *310*
De Marzo, N., 216, 219, 221, *225*, *227*
Demedts, N.J., 430, *437*
Demetris, A.J., 274, *281*
Demetz, M.G., 427, *435*
Demoly, P., 287, 288, *297*, 302, *311*, 381, *388*

de Monchy, J.G., *269*, 393, 394, 395, *411*, *413*, 515, *521*
Dempsey, P., 96, 103, *107*
DeMuzio, J., 402, *416*
Denburg, J., 308, *315*, 479, 482, 486, *489*, *490*, 494, 495, 496, *503*
Deneffe, G., 427, *435*
Denison, M.S., 49, *69*
Denison, T.R., 456, 458, 460, *470*
Dennis, E., 95, *106*
Dennis, E.A., 284, *293*, 511, *518*
Dent, G., 403, 405, 407, *416*, *417*
Dente, F.L., 515, *522*
DeNucci, G., 232, 233, 234, *245*
Denyer, L.H., 253, *257*
de-Paulet, A.C., 515, *521*
De Raeve, H.R., 237, *250*
Derse, C.P., 515, *522*
De Sanctis, G.T., 188, *198*
Descharmes, A., 301, *311*
Descomps, B., 288, *297*, 515, *522*
Dessanger, J.-F., 284, *293*
Dessein, A.J., 401, *415*
Deutschl, H., 501, *505*
Devalia, J.L., 121, *127*, 477, *489*
Devchand, P., 27, 28, *40*, 103, *109*
Deviller, P., 514, *521*
Devillier, P., 115, *125*
Devlin, R.B., 6, *19*, 235, *247*
de Vries, H.G., 204, *211*
De Vries, K., 395, *413*
De Weck, A.L., 382, *389*, 401, *416*
De Wildt, D.J., 236, *248*
DeWitt, D., 7, *20*, 96, 97, *106*, *107*, 146, 147, 152, *155*, *158*
DeWitt, D.L., 3, 9, *17*, *21*, *23*, 26, 30, 35, *39*, *41*, *43*, 79, 80, *88*, 117, *125*, 129, 130, 136, *140*, *141*, *142*, 146, 147, *156*, *157*, *158*, 161, 164, 170, 174, 179, *183*, *184*, *185*, *186*, 285, 289, *294*, 295, *298*
Dey, S.K., 8, *21*
Diamant, Z., *271*
Diamond, M.I., 511, *518*
Diamond, P., 358, 359, *366*
Didonato, J.A., *127*, 510, *518*

Diehl, R.E., 97, *108*
Dieli, M., 232, 234, *245*
Dietz, R., 170, 171, *185*
di Giamberardino, M., 82, *88*
di Giovine, F.S., 209, *214*
Dik, I.E.M., 236, 237, *248*, *249*
Dinchuk, J.E., 4, 8–9, *18*, *20*, 139, *143*, 146, *157*, 285, 292, *295*
Di Pierso, J.F., 401, *415*
DiRienzo, V., 500, *504*
Dirksen, A., 217, 224, *226*, *229*
Di Rosa, M., 233, *246*
Dishman, E., 30, *41*, 60, 63, 65, *73*, 75
DiSilvestre, D.A., 188, *198*
Di Stefano, A., 217, 219, 221, 223, *226*, 227
Dixon, C.M.S., 113, *123*
Dixon, M., 397, *413*
Dixon, R.A.F., 28, *40*, 97, *108*
Djukanovic, R., 188, *198*, 217, 219, 225, *227*, 238, *250*, 361, 373, 382, *387*, *389*, 494, *503*, 507, *516*
Docherty, J.C., 380, *388*
Dohi, Y., 304, *313*, 357, 361, *365*, 371, *384*
Doig, M.V., 400, *414*
Doizoe, T., 357, 361, *365*
Dollery, C.T., 113, *123*, *271*, 285, 286, 287, *295*, *296*, *297*, 322, *333*, 360, 362, *367*, *368*
Dolovich, J., *269*, 308, *315*, 475, 479, 482, 486, *488*, *489*, *490*, 494, 495, 496, *503*
Domagala, B., 441, *450*
Dompeling, E., 283, *293*
Donello, J.E., 256, *258*
Dong, Y., 508, *517*
Dooper, M.W., 515, *521*
Doppierio, S., 427, 430, *435*
Dougherty, H.W., 253, *257*, 380, *388*
Dougherty, W.H., 306, *314*
Douglas, I., 400, *414*
Douglas, J.G., 33, 34, *42*
Douglas, J.S., 235, *247*, 248
Douglas, R.G., 239, *251*
Doull, I., 188, *198*, 222, 228

Douma, R., 514, *520*
Dow, L., 224, *229*
Dracon, M., 442, 444, *450*
Drake-Lee, A., 475, 479, *488*, *489*, *490*
Drazen, J., 91, *104*, 237, *249*, 361, 375, *388*
Drazen, J.D., 358, 360, *366*
Drazen, J.M., 6, *19*, 28, *40*, 188, 197, *198*, *199*, *200*, 235, 237, *247*, *249*, 287, *297*, 303, *304*, *305*, *312*, *313*, 321, 324, 329, *333*, *334*, *335*, 337, 343, *348*, 357, 362, *365*, *368*, 371, *384*, 392, 395, 397, *409*, *413*, 428, *435*, 496, *497*, *498*, 502, *504*, 514, *520*
Dredge, D.R., 188, *198*
Drettner, B., 501, *505*
Drouhin, F., 148, *158*
D'Souza, M.F., 218, *226*
Du, T., 191, *199*
Duarte, C., 456, 459, *470*
Dubay, G.R., 34, *42*
Dube, L., 304, *313*, 326, *334*, 362, *369*, 502, *505*
DuBois, R., 96, 103, *107*
DuBois, R.N., 5, *18*, 59, *73*, 135, *142*, 146, 148, 149, *156*, *158*, *159*, *160*
Dubowitz, M., 204, *211*
Dudley, D.J., 7, *20*, 146, *156*
Duff, G.W., 209, *214*
Dugas, B., 192, *200*
Duhamel, O., 148, *158*
Duiverman, E., 283, *293*
DuMaine, J., 232, 233, *245*
Dunn, C.E., 34, *43*
Dunn, J., 179, *186*
Dunn, M.J., 33, 34, *42*
Dunnett, C., 259, *268*
Duplaga, M., 223, *228*, 309, *315*, 419, 424, *432*, 441, 442, 449, *450*, 469, *472*
Dupuy, P.M., 237, *249*
Durham, S., 289, *298*
Durham, S.K., 273, 280, *281*
Durham, S.R., 217, 219, 220–23, *225*, *226*, *227*, *269*, 289, *298*, 373, 382, *386*, *388*, *389*, 496, *503*

Durkop, H., 374, *387*
Durmuller, U., 96, *107*
Durocher, A., 300, *310*
Duroux, P., 283, *292*
Duyao, M., 153, *160*
Duysinx, B., 219, *227*
Dvorak, A., 92, 96, *104*, *107*
Dvorak, H., 92, *104*
Dwivedi, R., 6, *19*
Dworski, J., 496, 497, 498, *503*
Dworski, R., 91, *104*, 113, *123*, 253, 257, 286, 287, 288, 289, *296*, *297*, 298, 303, 305, 306, 307, 309, *312*, *313*, *314*, 321, *323*, *328*, *333*, 337, 339, 342, 343, 347, *348*, 359, 360, 361, *367*, 371, 378, 380, 381, 382, *384*, 408, *417*, 419, 421, 428, *432*, *433*, 496, 497, 498, *504*, 512, 514, *519*, *520*, 525, *535*
Dyczek, A., 207, *213*, 223, *228*, 308, 309, *315*, 419, 424, *432*, 441, 442, 449, *450*

E

Eakins, K.E., 3, *17*
Eberhardt, C., 222, *228*
Eberhart, C.E., 148, *158*
Ebner, C., 206, *212*
Edenius, C., 358, *365*
Edmunds, A.T., *269*
Edwin, S.S., 7, *20*, 146, *156*
Egan, R.W., 130, *140*, 219, *227*
Eguchi, N., 96, *107*
Ehrlich-Kautzky, E., *206*, *212*, 222, *228*
Eidelman, D.H., 191, *199*
Einarsson, O., 122, *127*
Eisenbrey, A.B., 476, *489*
Eitelbach, F., 374, *387*
Ekabo, O.K., 176, 178, *186*
Elder, D.J.E., 149, 150, *160*
Elias, J.A., 122, *127*
Eling, T., 95, *106*, 132, *141*
Elliott, E.V., 397, *413*
Elliott, G.R., 380, *388*

Elliott, J., 515, *522*
Ellis, J.L., 113, *124*, 191, *199*, 307, *314*,
   397, *413*
Elsas, M.I., 401, *415*
Elsas, P., 401, *415*
Elsas, R., 401, *415*
Elwood, W., 113, *124*, 427, *435*
Elzas, M., 56, *72*
Emami Nouri, E., 12, *22*
Emanueli, C., 238, *250*
Enander, I., 216, 219, *225*
Endo, K., 56, *72*
Endo, T., 136, *142*
Eng, V.M., 8–9, *20*, 139, *143*, 146, *157*
Engelberts, D., 7, *19*
Engelhardt, G., 11, *22*
Engels, F., 235, 236, *248*
Engl, V.M., 285, 292, *295*
Engul, A., 122, *127*
Enomoto, T., 454, 457, 467, *470*
Enrietto, P.J., 152, *160*
Entingh, A.J., 148, *159*
Epstein, J.D., *269*
Erger, R.A., 342, *349*
Erickson, R.R., 49, *69*
Erij, D., 63, *74*
Eriksen, P., 197, *200*
Erikson, R.I., 146, 147, *156*
Erikson, R.L., 3, *17*, 25, 34, *39*, 130,
   141, 147, *158*, 162, *183*, 285, *294*
Erjefält, J.S., 477, 479, *489*
Erle, D.J., 188, 195, 197, *199*
Erlich-Kautzky, E., 205, *212*
Erlij, D., 31, 34, *41*, *42*
Ermler, U., 182, *186*
Erzurum, S.C., 237, *250*
Escalante, B., 31, 34, *41*, *42*, *43*, 63,
   74
Esch, B. van, 236, 239, *248*
Eschenbacher, W.L., 285, 286, *295*,
   426, *434*, 512, *519*
Eshenaur, S.C., 50, *70*
Estabrook, R.W., 47, 48, 53, 59, *69*, *71*,
   73
Ethier, D., 56, *72*, 92, 97, *104*
Euchenhofer, C., 118, *126*

Evans, J., 4, *18*, 92, 97, 102, *104*, *108*,
   109, 361, 375, *388*
Evans, J.F., 4, *18*, *23*, 28, *40*, 148, *159*
Evans, J.N., 235, *247*
Evans, P.M., 403, *416*
Evans, R., 103, *109*
Evans, R.M., 36, *43*, 147, *158*
Evans, S., 308, *315*, 475, *488*
Evans, T.W., 16, *23*, 114, 119, *124*, 400,
   414
Evett, G.E., 145, 148, 152, *155*, *159*
Ewart, S.L., 188, *198*
Ewert, D.L., 149, *160*

F

Fabbri, L.M., 216, 217, 219, 221, 222,
   223, *224*, *225*, *226*, *227*, *228*, 264,
   265, *270*, 515, *522*
Faber, L.E., 508, *517*
Fabian, I., 401, *415*
Fabra, J.M., 495, 496, *503*
Fackler, J.C., 237, *249*
Fae, I., 206, *212*
Fagan, D., 129, *140*
Fagan, J.M., 130, *141*
Fahlstadius, P., 53, *71*
Fahy, J.V., 515, *522*
Fai, V., 431, *437*
Fairbairn, C.E., 256, *258*
Fairbairn, D.W., 149, *160*
Fais, G., 500, *504*
Falck, J.R., 25, 27, 28, 30, 31, 34, *38*,
   40, *41*, *42*, 46, 51, 56, 58, 59, 60, 62,
   63, 65, 66, *69*, *70*, *72*, *73*, *74*, *75*
Falgueyret, J.P., *23*, 146, 147, *157*
Falini, B., 374, *387*
Falliers, C.J., 320, *332*, 454, 456, 457,
   460, 464, *470*
Fantone, J.C., 253, *257*
Farina, P.R., 9, 10, 11, *21*
Farmer, S.G., 115, *125*
Farr, R.S., 223, *229*, 320, *332*, 457, 460,
   468, *470*, *471*
Fasano, M.B., 132, *141*, 286, *296*

Fasoli, A., 401, *415*
Fauci, A.S., 394, *412*
Fauler, J., 514, *520*
Faulks, R.D., 140, *144*
Faureau, I., 53, *71*
Faux, J.A., 203, 204, 208, 210, *211*, *213*, *214*
Fava, R.A., 511, *518*
Favalli, C., 148, *159*
Featherstone, R.L., 6, *19*
Feelisch, M., 234, *246*
Fehr, P., 96, *107*
Feigenbaum, B.A., 500, *505*, 528, *536*
Feinberg, S.M., 452, 460, 463, 467, 469, *470*
Feinmark, S.J., 28, *40*
Feinstein, A.R., 320, *332*
Feletou, M., 50, *70*
Felkner, R.H., 284, *294*
Feltenmark, S., 191, *200*
Feng, Y., 149, *159*
Fenna, R.E., 164, *184*
Fennessy, M.R., 191, *199*
Ferhanoglu, B., 3, *18*
Ferland, C., 395, 401, 408, *413*, *417*
Fernandes, L.B., 115, *125*
Fernandez, J.C., 495, 496, *503*
Fernandez, M.D., 495, 496, *503*
Fernandez-Caldas, E., 222, *227*
Ferreira, F., 206, *212*
Ferreira, S.H., 5, *19*
Ferrenbach, S., 148, *158*
Ferreri, N.R., 33, 34, 35, *42*, *43*, 303, 305, *312*, 322, 323, 327, 329, *334*, 337, 343, *348*, 358, 360, *366*, 496, *504*
Ferretti, B., 431, *437*
Feyereisen, R., 47, 48, *69*
Ficado, C., 323, *334*
Fiers, W., 401, *415*
Figini, M., 238, *250*
Filep, J., 115, *125*
Finger, E., 198, *200*
Finkelman, F.D., 188, 191, 193, *199*, *200*
Finnerty, J.P., 263, 264, 265, *270*

Finotto, S., 482, *490*, 494, 495, 496, *503*
Fischer, A., 91, *104*, 237, *249*, 287, *297*, 303, *312*, 514, *520*
Fischer, A.R., 188, *199*, 304, 305, *313*, 324, 329, *334*, *335*, 337, 343, *348*, 357, *365*, 371, *384*, 428, *435*, 496, 497, 498, 502, *504*
Fischer, C., 54, *75*
Fischer, D., 148, *158*
Fischer, G.F., 206, *212*
Fischer, J.E., 274, *282*
Fish, J., 362, *368*
Fish, J.E., 285, 286, 289, *295*, 296
Fisher, A.R., 358, 360, *366*
Fisher, C., 86, *89*
Fitgerald, G.A., 514, *520*
Fitzgerald, D.J., 59, *73*
FitzGerald, G.A., 3, *17*, 36, *43*, 56, 59, 72, 73, 78, 79, 80, 82, 86, *87*, 88, *89*, 113, *123*, 129, *140*, 286, 287, 288, *296*, *297*, 323, *334*, 355, 358, 361, 362, *365*, *368*, 408, *417*, 507, 514, *517*
Fitzharris, P., 393, *411*
Fitzpatrick, F.A., 25, 27, 34, *38*, 46, 52, 63, 65, *69*, *71*, *74*, *75*, 103, *109*
Fitzsimmons, B., 56, *72*
Flanders, W.D., 148, *158*
Flannery, E.M., 221, 223, *227*
Flarup, M., 458, *471*
Fleming, I., 273, 276, *280*
Flenghi, L., 374, *387*
Flensborg, E.W., 475, 478, *489*
Fletcher, B.S., 3, *17*, 136, 137, *142*, 146, 147, *156*, 162, *183*, 285, *294*
Flower, R.J., 9, *21*, 114, 119, *124*, *126*, 130, *141*, 146, *157*, 161, 172, 173, *183*, 354, 355, *365*, 510, 511, *518*, *519*
Flynn, J.T., 285, 286, 289, *295*
Focht, R.J., 8–9, *20*, 139, *143*, 146, *157*, 285, 292, *295*
Foegh, M.L., 393, *410*
Fogstrup, J., 486, *490*
Folco, G.C., 56, *72*, 91, 96, *104*, 303, 306, *312*, *314*, 321, *333*, 347, *350*,

[Folco, G.C.]
360, 361, *367*, 371, *385*, 419, 424,
425, 427, 429, *432*, *434*, *435*
Folgering, H., 283, *293*
Folkerts, G., 231, 234–40, *245*, *246*,
247, *248*, *249*, *250*, *251*
Folkerts, H.F., 236, 238, 239, *248*
Folkesson, H.G., 188, 195, 197, *199*
Fölster-Holst, R., 204, *211*
Fontana, A., 303, *312*, 419, *432*
Fonteh, A., 95, *105*, *106*, 132, *141*, 284,
286, *294*, *296*
Fontino, M., 206, *212*
Foord, R., 304, *313*, 353, *364*, 524, *535*
Forbes, A.B., 204, *211*, 222, *228*
Ford, D., 95, *106*
Ford-Hutchinson, A.W., 6, 13, 14, *19*,
22, *23*, 26, 28, 34, *39*, *40*, 97, *108*,
122, *127*, 303, *312*, 322, 323, *333*,
334, 337, *348*, 355, 358, 361, 362,
365, *366*, *368*, 371, *384*, 392, 400,
401, 405, *409*, *414*, *415*, *417*, 440,
449, 496, 497, *504*, 514, *520*, 534,
537
Forman, B., 103, *109*
Forman, B.M., 36, *43*, 147, *158*
Förstermann, U., 118, *126*
Fortin, R., 28, *40*
Foster, A., 400, *414*
Foster, D.W., 338, *349*, 372, *386*, 393,
409, *410*
Foster, P.S., 188, 195, 197, *199*
Foster, S., 324, *334*, 357, *365*, 371, *384*,
424, 429, *434*
Fotuhi, M., 237, *250*
Fournier, E., 440, *449*
Fournier, M., 237, *250*, 372, 380, *386*
Fowler, A.A., 372, *386*
Fox, C.C., 285, 286, *296*
Fox, J., 33, *42*
Franchi, A.M., 233, *246*
Francis, A., 317, 318, *332*
Frank, J., 4, *18*
Franke, 318, *332*
Frantz, R., 188, *199*
Franzuso, G., 118, *126*

Freche, C., 432, *438*
Freedman, L., 508, *517*
Freeland, H.S., 287, *297*, 514, 515, *521*,
522
Freeman, B.A., 273, 274, 280, *281*
Freeman, G.J., 374, *387*, 393, *409*
Freeman, T.M., 206, *212*
Fregonese, L., 13, 16, *22*
Frei, B., 78, 79, 82, *87*
Freiburghaus, J., 394, *412*
Freidhoff, L.R., 205, 206, *212*, 222,
228
Freire, J., 146, *157*
French, C.L., 441, *450*
Frenette, R., 362, *368*
Frew, A.J., 221, 223, *227*
Frey, B.M., 284, *294*
Frey, F.J., 284, *294*
Frey, M., 442, *450*
Friedhoff, L.R., 206, *212*
Friedlaender, S., 452, 460, 463, 467,
469, *470*
Friedman, B.S., *271*
Friedman, F.K., 68, *75*
Friend, D., 99, *108*
Friend, D.S., 361, 376, *388*, 392, *409*
Friend, J.L., 284, *293*
Fries, J.T., 8, 9, *21*
Frith, P.A., 259, *268*, *269*
Fritsch, W., 204, *211*
Fritzsch, G., 182, *186*
Frobert, Y., 80, *88*
Frölich, J.C., 54, *75*, 514, *520*
Fronek, Z., 209, *214*
Frossard, N., 115, *125*
Frostell, C.G., 237, *249*
Fruteau de Laclos, B., 393, *410*
Fryer, A.D., 307, *314*
Fu, J.Y., 3, *17*, 192, *200*, 285, *295*
Fu, L., 287, *297*
Fuchimoto, S., 50, *69*
Fujii-Kuriyama, Y., 47, 48, 56, *69*, *72*
Fujimoto, N., 96, *107*
Fujimura, M., *335*
Fujita, S., 102, *108*
Fukuda, T., 382, *389*, 402, *416*

Fukumura, M., 402, 408, *416*, *417*, 514, 515, 516, *520*, *521*, 522
Fukunaga, M., 78, *87*
Fukuo, K., 232, 233, *246*
Fuller, R.W., 113, 114, *123*, *124*, 263, 269, 271, 284–88, *293*, *295*, *296*, 297, 322, *333*, 362, *368*, *369*, 408, *417*
Fulton, D., 38, *44*, 50, 60, *70*, *73*
Funae, Y., 53, *71*
Funare, Y., 47, *69*
Funk, C., 98, 99, *108*
Funk, C.B, 512, *519*
Funk, C.D., 3, 9, *17*, *21*, 26, *39*, 129, *140*, 146, *157*, 174, *186*, 192, *200*, 287, 288, 289, *297*
Funk, D.C., 36, *43*
Funk, L.B., 3, *17*, 129, *140*
Furchgott, R.F., 38, *44*
Furci, L., 36, *43*
Furth, E., 93, *105*
Furuyama, J., 204, *211*
Fusco, O., 9, *21*, 80, 84, *88*
Fusetti, G., 12, *22*
Futaki, N., 7, *20*, *23*, 122, *127*, 131, *141*
Fuxe, K., 508, *517*

G

Gaa, S.T., 34, 35, *43*
Gaddy, J.N., 362, *368*
Gagne, G.D., 237, *249*
Galavage, M., 101, *108*
Galens, S., 401, *416*
Gallagher, H., 274, *281*
Galli, S.J., 192, *200*
Gallin, E., 427, *435*
Gambacorta, M., 374, *387*
Gambaro, G., 91, 96, *104*, 301, 304, 306, *311*, *313*, *314*, 321, *333*, 347, *350*, 360, 361, *367*, 371, *385*, 421, 422, 424–27, 429, 431, *433*, *434*, *435*, *436*, *437*
Gammelgaard, N., 486, *490*
Ganci, A., 9, *21*, 80, 84, *88*

Gangal, S.V., 284, *293*
Gappett-Struebe, M., 146, 152, *155*
Garaci, E., 148, *159*
Garavito, M., 173, *185*
Garavito, R.M., 2, *17*, 45, *68*, 79, 80, *88*, 130, *140*, 145, 146, 147, 152, *155*, *157*, 162, 163, 164, 166, 167, 174, 176, 178, 179, *184*, *186*
Garcia Rodriguez, L.A., 8, *21*
Garcia-Zepeda, E.A., 342, *349*
Gardner, C.R., 273, 280, *281*
Garland, L.G., 241, *251*
Garrison, H.A., 476, *489*
Gartmann, J., 442, *450*
Gasson, J.C., 401, *415*
Gaston, B., 237, *249*
Gatta, A., 62, *74*
Gauldie, J., 495, 496, *503*
Gaur, S.N., 284, *293*
Gauthier, J.Y., 28, *40*, 362, *368*
Gavett, S.H., 188, 193, *199*
Gaya, A., 495, 496, *503*
Gazel, P., 301, *311*
Gaziano, J.M., 78, 79, 82, *87*
Gearing, A.J., 401, *415*
Gebel, S., 509, 511, *517*
Geddes, D., 429, *436*
Gehring, U., 508, *517*
Geiger, K.M., 408, *418*
Geiman, J.M., 239, *251*
Geisslinger, G., 7, *20*
Gelb, A.F., *269*
Gelb, M., 94, *105*
Gelboir, H.V., 53, *71*
Gelder, C.M., 119, *126*
Gelfand, E.W., 188, 192, 193, *199*
Geller-Bernstein, C., 401, *415*
Gelpi, E., 303, 305, *312*, 323, *334*, 337, 347, *348*, 358, 360, *366*, 380, 381, *388*, 432, *437*, 496, 497, *504*
Gene, R.-M., 284, *293*
Georges, D., 514, *521*
Gerar, N.P., 192, *200*
Gerard, C., 237, *249*
Gerard, N.P., 395, *413*

Gergel, D., 51, *70*
Gerritsen, J., 204, *211*, 283, *293*
Geuens, G.M.A., 236, 238, 239, *248*
Ghanayem, B.I., 4, 7, *18*, *20*, 138, 139, *143*, 146, *157*, 285, *294*
Ghavanian, N., 216, 219, *225*
Ghezzo, H., 191, *199*
Ghio, A.J., 6, *19*
Ghosh, B., 205, *212*
Ghosh, D., 97, *107*
Ghosh, S., 152, *160*
Giannaras, J., 173, *185*
Giannessi, D., 511, 513, 515, *518*, *519*, *522*
Giardello, G.M., 148, *158*
Giardiello, F.M., 148, *158*
Gibb, W., 7, 8, *20*
Gibson, G.J., 423, *433*, 528, *536*
Gibson, P.G., 259, *268*
Giembycz, M.A., 113, *124*, 403, 405, *416*, *417*
Gierse, J.K., 2, *17*, *23*, 122, *127*, 146, *157*, 163, 164, 174, 178, 180, 181, *184*, *186*
Gil, D.W., 256, *258*
Gilbert, I.A., 188, *198*
Gildehaus, D., 146, *157*
Giles, R.E., 362, *368*
Gillam, I., 264, *270*
Gillard, J.W., 28, *40*, 97, *108*
Gillies, B., 284, 288, *293*, 362, *369*, 408, *417*
Gillner, M., 508, *517*
Gilman, A., 236, *248*
Gilrov, D.W., 6, *19*
Gimbrone, M.A., Jr., 138, *143*
Gimeno, M., 233, *246*
Gin, W., 515, *521*
Giraldo, B., 454, 457, 464, *470*
Girard, Y., 56, *72*
Glasgow, W., 95, *106*
Glass, M., 188, *199*
Glassberg, M.K., 122, *127*
Glatt, M., 12, *22*
Gleich, G.J., 476, *489*, 515, *522*
Glennie, M.J., 373, *387*
Glezen, W.P., 239, *251*

Glover, S., 94, *105*
Godard, P., 216, 219, *225*, 283, 287, 288, *292*, *297*, 302, *311*, 372, 381, *386*, *388*, 401, *415*, 514, 515, *521*, *522*
Godfrey, S., *269*
Godowski, P., 508, *517*
Godstein, R.A., 188, *198*
Goetz, D.W., 206, *212*
Goetzl, E.J., 400, *414*, 532, *537*
Goldberg, A.L., 130, *141*
Goldberg, H., 30, *41*
Golde, D.W., 401, *415*
Goldenberg, M., 101, *108*
Goldie, R.G., 115, *125*
Goldlust, B., 528, *536*
Goldstein, B.M., 218, *226*
Goldthwait, D.A., 33, 34, *42*
Goller, N.L., 273, 280, *281*
Golub, M., 27, 34, *39*
Gomes, M.J., 456, 459, *470*
Gomperts, B.D., 344, *350*
Gong, H., Jr., *269*
Gonzales, F.J., 53, *71*
Gonzalez, F., 103, *109*
Gonzalez, F.J., 27, 28, *40*, 47, 48, 49, *69*
Gonzalo, J.-A., 198, *200*
Goodman, L.S., 236, *248*
Goodwin, J.S., 253, *257*
Gopaul, N.K., 79, *88*
Goppelt-Struebe, M., 7, *20*
Gordon, J., 192, *200*
Gordon, J.A., 30, *41*, 66, *75*
Gordon, R., 13, 14, *22*, 122, *127*
Gorman, R.R., 56, *72*
Gorry, S.A., 8–9, *20*, 139, *143*, 285, 292, *295*
Gosset, P., 223, *228*, 286, *296*, 309, *315*, 442, 447, 448, *450*
Gottlieb, D.J., 224, *229*
Goulding, E.H., 4, 7, *18*, *20*, 138, 139, *143*, 146, *157*, 285, *294*
Goulding, N.J., 511, 512, *519*
Grace, A., 475, *488*
Graf, M., 51, *70*
Graf, P.D., 264, *270*

Graham, A.G., 9, 10, 11, *21*
Graham-Lorence, S., 59, *73*
Granger, D.N., 138, *143*
Granstrom, E., 56, *72*, 113, *123*, 303, *312*, 323, *334*, 337, *348*, 355, 358, 361, *365*, 371, 372, *384*, 496, 497, *504*, 514, *520*
Grant, J.A., 217, 219–23, *225*
Gras-Masse, H., 223, *228*, 309, *315*, 442, *450*
Grass, D.S., 284, *294*
Grassi, J., 80, *88*, 344, *350*
Gravel, S., 198, *200*, 393, 394, *411*
Graves-Deal, R., 96, 103, *107*
Gray, E.J., 222, *227*
Gray, G.A., 273, 276, *280*
Gray, P.W., 222, *228*
Greaves, M.W., 400, *414*
Greco, A., 9, *21*, 80, 82, 84, *88*
Green, C.P., 514, *520*
Green, F.H.Y., 219, *227*
Green, S.A., 209, *214*, 222, *228*
Gregersen, P.K., 208, *213*
Gregg, I., 216, 222, *225*, *228*
Greiff, L., 477, 479, *489*
Grcim, H., 46, 49, 68, *69*
Grelbein, M.V., 49, *69*
Grelli, S., 148, *159*
Griendling, K., 94, *105*
Griffin, J.E. III, 29, *40*
Griffin, M., 8, 9, *21*, 397, *413*
Griffith, O.W., 279, *282*
Griglewsky, R.J., 421, *433*
Grilli, M., 150, 152, *160*
Grimminger, F., 514, *520*
Grob, P., 9, 10, 11, *21*, 442, *450*
Grobholz, J.K., 188, *198*
Groden, J., 4, *18*, 148, *159*
Grodzinska, L., 235, *247*, 284, *294*
Gronemeyer, H., 508, *517*
Gronich, J.H., 29, *40*, *41*
Gross, C.E., 62, *74*
Gross, P.H., 149, 150, 154, *159*, *160*
Gross, R., 95, *106*
Gross, S., 232, 233, *246*
Gross, S.S., 34, *43*, 50, 51, *70*, 279, *282*

Grossman, C.J., 9, *21*
Grossman, J., 362, *368*
Grouix, B., 116, *125*
Gruart, V., 442, *450*
Gruenert, D.C., 429, *436*
Gruetter, G.A., 236, *248*
Grugni, A.A., 347, *350*, 420, 424, 429, 431, *432*, 468, *471*, 498, *504*
Grunberger, D., 393, *410*
Grunewald, J., 208, *213*
Grunstein, M.M., 116, *125*
Gryglewski, R.J., 3, *17*, 52, *71*, 232, 233, 235, *245*, *247*, 284, *294*, 299, 301, 302, *304*, *309*, *311*, 320, *332*, *333*, 351, 354, 357, 361, 363, *364*, *365*, 371, *385*, 440, *449*, 457, 459, *471*, 526, 529, *535*
Grzegorczyk, J., 305, *313*, 329, *335*, 498, *504*
Grzelewska-Rzymowska, I., 307, *314*, 358, *366*, 456, 460, 464, 469, *470*, 525, *535*
Gualberto, A., 119, *127*
Gualde, N., 301, *311*
Guan, H., 32, *42*
Guay, D., 13, 14, *22*, 122, *127*
Gudat, F., 96, *107*
Guengerich, F.P., 47, 48, 53, 59, 60, 63, *69*, *71*, *73*
Guenounou, M., 239, *251*
Guerin, J.-C., 283, *292*
Guez, S., 301, *311*
Guidot, D.M., 280, *282*
Gulwani-Akolar, B., 208, *213*
Gunsalus, I.C., 47, 48, *69*
Guo, F.H., 237, *250*
Gupta, S., 284, *293*
Gustafson-Svard, C., 4, *18*, 148, *159*
Gustafsson, J.A., 68, *75*, 508, 510, *517*, *518*
Gutierrez, H.H., 273, 274, 280, *281*
Gutierrez-Ramos, J.-C., 198, *200*
Gutthann, S.P., 8, 9, *21*
Guyre, P.M., 511, 512, *519*
Guz, A., 511, *518*
Gwaltney, J., 122, *127*

H

Haahtela, T., 231, 238, *245*, 268, *271*, 283, *292–93*, 321, *333*, 342, *349*, 361, 373, 383, *386*, *387*, *389*
Haas, F., 475, *488*
Habib, A., 80, *88*
Haby, M.M., 222, *227*
Haddad, E., 115, 116, 119, *125*
Haeggström, J., 98, 99, *108*, 358, *365*
Haeggstrom, J.Z., 27, *40*
Haesen, R., 531, *537*
Hague, A., 149, 150, *160*
Hajibeigi, A., 131, 132, 133, *141*
Hajjar, D.P., 235, *247*
Hakeda, Y., 132, *142*, 146, *156*
Hale, S.E., 47, *69*
Haley, K., 361, 375, *388*
Hall, C., 95, *106*
Hall, C.B., 239, *251*
Hallböök, O., 4, *18*, 148, *159*
Halonen, M., 218, 221, 223, *226*
Halstensen, T.S., 373, *387*
Halushka, P.V., 79, *87*
Ham, E.A., 253, *257*, 306, *314*, 380, *388*
Hamann, K.J., 396, 397, *413*, *414*
Hamasaka, Y., 7, *20*, 131, *141*
Hamashima, Y., 478, *489*
Hamberg, M., 27, *39*, 53, 56, *71*, *72*, 170, *185*
Hamberger, C., 284, *293*
Hamboodiri, M.M., 4, *18*
Hamelink, M.L., 372, *386*, 393, 394, 408, *411*, *412*, *417*
Hamid, Q., 237, 239, *249*, *251*, 289, *298*, 308, *315*, 382, *389*, 495, 496, *503*
Hamielec, C.M., 264, *270*
Hamilos, D., 305, 308, *314*, *315*, 495, 496, *503*
Hamilton, A.L., *271*
Hammarstrom, S., 27, *39*, 321, *333*, 397, *413*, 507, *516*, 520, 532, *537*
Hampe, C.L., 203, *211*
Hamzeh, Y.S., 500, *505*
Hancock, B., 4, *18*

Handa, M., 357, 361, *365*
Hanif, R., 149, *159*
Hanifin, J.M., 307, *314*
Hankammer, M.A., 308, *314*, 531, *537*
Hannun, Y.A., 29, *40*
Hansel, T.T., 217, 218, 221, *225*
Hansen, J.A., 209, *214*, 319, *332*
Hanss, J.G., 46, 53, *69*
Hansson, G., 56, *72*
Hara, N., 114, *124*
Hara, S., 52, *70*, 137, *142*, 289, *297*
Harada, T., 456, 464, 468, 469, *470*
Harada, Y., 6, *19*
Haraldsen, G., 481, 482, *490*
Harbrecht, B.G., 274, *281*
Harding, C., 209, *213*
Hardman, R., 132, *141*
Hardwick, J.P., 53, *71*
Hardy, C.C., 113, 114, *123*, *124*, 259, 264, *269*
Hardy, P., 7, *19*
Harfstrand, A., 508, *517*
Hargreave, F.E., 193, *200*, 216, *225*, 259, 264, *268*, *269*, 283, *292*, 397, *413*
Harlan, J.E., 170, *185*
Harley, J.B., 394, *412*
Harmon, A.T., 239, *251*
Harmon, M.W., 239, *251*
Harnett, J.C., 457, *470*
Harrap, S.B., 204, *211*, 222, *228*
Harris, R.C., 5, *18*, 146, *156*
Hart, F.D., 2, *16*
Hart, L., 118, *126*
Hartwig, S., 501, *505*
Harvey, C., 393, *411*
Harvey, V., 92, *104*
Hashimoto, L., 208, *213*
Hashimoto, T., 204, *211*
Hashiramoto, A., 148, *159*
Hasselgren, P.O., 274, *282*
Hatanaka, K., 6, *19*
Hatzelmann, A., 62, *74*, 306, *314*, 361, 380, 381, *388*, 403, *417*
Haurand, M., 52, *71*
Hauschildt, S., 273, *281*

Hauser, S.D., 2, 13, *17*, 22, *23*, 122, 127, 135, *142*, 146, *156*, *157*, 163, 180, *184*, *186*, 285, *295*
Hauser, U., 482, *490*
Havu, V.K., 462, *471*
Hawkey, C., 8, 9, *21*, 96, 103, *107*
Hawksworth, R.J., 303, *312*, 322, *333*, 357, 361, *365*, 372, *385*
Hay, D.W.P., 115, *125*, 188, *199*, 371, *381*
Hayaishi, O., 7, *19*, 96, *107*, 129, *140*, 161, *183*
Hayashi, Y., 36, 37, *43*
Haye, R., 481, 482, *490*
Haye-Legrand, I., 360, *367*
Hayes, E.C., 372, 380, *386*
Haynes, T.J., 475, *488*
Hazen, S., 95, *106*
Hearn, L., 92, 97, *104*
Heath, C.W., 4, *18*, 148, *158*
Hebert, J., 372, 380, *386*, 393, *410*, 479, *490*
Hecker, G., 253, *257*
Hecker, M., 52, *70*, *71*, 86, *89*
Hedenstierna, G., 237, *249*
Hedenstrom, H., 237, *249*
Hedqvist, P., 56, *72*, 235, *247*, 321, *333*, 360, *367*, 397, *413*, 507, *516*, 520
Heibein, J., 92, 97, *104*
Heidvall, K., 358, *365*
Heino, M., 231, 238, *245*, 373, *386*
Heinzel, F.P., 209, *213*
Helmberg, A., *127*, 510, *518*
Helvig, C., 59, *73*
Hemler, M., 1, *16*, 129, *140*, 161, *172*, 173, *183*
Hempel, S., 117, *125*
Henderson, J.L., 274, *282*
Henderson, W., Jr., 507, *516*, 531, *537*
Henderson, W.R., 197, *200*, 307, *314*, 338, 342, *349*, 394, 408, 409, *412*, *418*
Hendrick, D.J., 218, *226*
Henney, C.S., 253, *257*
Henricks, P.A.J., 234, 236, 237, 240, *246*, *248*, *249*, *251*

Henriksen, J.M., 265, *270*
Henry, D., 8, 9, *21*
Henry-Amar, M., 283, *292*, 514, *521*
Henson, J.E., 188, 192, *199*
Henson, P., 94, *105*
Henson, P.M., 393, *410*
Herbert, F.A., 218, *226*
Herbison, G.P., 221, 223, *227*
Herpin-Richard, N., 284, *293*
Herrlich, P., 509, 511, *517*
Herrnreiter, A., 400, 401, *414*, *416*
Herschman, H., 95, *106*
Herschman, H.R., 3, *17*, 81, *88*, 130, 136, *141*, *142*, 146, 147, *156*, *158*, 162, *183*, 285, *294*, *295*
Herschman, W.R., 136, 137, *142*
Herwerden, L., 204, *211*
Heusser, C.H., 382, *389*
Hewitt, C.J., 221, 223, *227*
Heymann, P.W., 222, *227*
Hicks, D.J., 149, 150, *160*
Higgins, D.A., *271*
Higgins, S., 508, *517*
Higgs, E.A., 138, *143*
Higgs, G.A., 2, 3, *16*, *17*
Highland, E., 287, *297*
Higuchi, S., 7, *20*, *23*, 122, *127*, 131, *141*
Hill, D.B., 50, *70*
Hill, E., 62, 63, *74*, 132, *141*, 393, *410*
Hill, K.E., 77, 78, *87*
Hill, M.R., 204, 208, 210, *211*, *212*, *213*, *214*
Hill, R., 122, *127*
Hill, R.G., 13, 14, *22*
Hill, S., 8, 9, *21*
Hill, W.A., 237, *249*
Hinderer, K.H., 477, 478, *489*
Hirai, I., 515, *521*
Hirai, Y., 402, 408, *416*, *417*, 516, *522*
Hirata, K., 394, *412*
Hirata, M., 36, 37, *43*, *44*
Hirata, T., 37, *44*
Hirose, T., 114, *124*
Hirshman, C.A., 237, *249*
Hirst, J.J., 8, *21*
Hirst, S.J., 115, 116, 119, 122, *125*, *127*

Hitch, D., 479, *489*
Hla, T., 9, *21*, 26, 34, *39*, 118, 121, *126*, *127*, 130, *141*, 146, 148, *157*, *159*, 174, *186*
Ho, J.C., 147, *158*
Hodges, M.K., 395, *413*
Hodulik, C.R., 286, *296*
Hoff, T., 146, 152, *155*
Hoffman, M., 300, *310*
Hoffman, N.E., 343, *349*
Hofmann, H., 234, *246*
Hogan, S.P., 188, 195, 197, *199*
Hoganson, C.W., 171, *185*
Hogg, J.C., 188, *198*
Högman, M., 237, *249*
Hoigne, R.A., 299, 302, *310*
Holdaway, M.D., 221, 223, *227*
Holgate, S.T., 5, *19*, 113, 114, *123*, *124*, 216–19, 224, *225*, *226*, *227*, *229*, 259, 263, 264, 265, *269*, *270*, 302, 303, 304, 307, 308, *312*, *313*, 353, 358, 359, 361, *364*, *366*, 372–79, 381, 382, 383, *385*, *386*, *387*, *389*, 494, *503*, 507, *516*, 524, 531, *535*, *537*
Holgate, T., 188, *198*, 222, *228*
Holland, E., 115, *125*
Holley, K.E., 476, *489*
Holley, S., 508, *517*
Holmberg, K., 501, 502, *505*
Holopainen, E., 469, *472*
Holroyd, K.J., 222, *228*
Holroyde, M.C., 397, *413*
Holt, P.G., 209, *213*
Holtzman, J.L., 49, *69*
Holtzman, M.J., 147, *157*, 264, 265, *270*
Homma, D., 11, *22*
Honda, A., 256, *258*
Hong, S.-C.L., 284, *294*
Honold, G., 209, *214*
Hoogsteden, H.C., 514, *520*
Hoover, G.E., 217, *225*
Hope, B.T., 237, *250*
Hopfer, U., 33, 34, *42*
Hopkin, J.M., 203, 204, 206, 208, *211*, *212*, *213*

Hori, T., 35, *43*, 96, *107*, 136, *142*, 147, *158*, 285, *294*
Horiguchi, T., 357, 361, *365*
Horiguchi, Y., 96, 99, *107*, *108*
Horikoshi, S., 454, 457, 467, *470*
Horn, B.R., 447, *450*
Horn, M.E.C., 222, *228*
Horton, R., 27, 34, *39*
Hougham, A., 528, *536*
Howard, K., 508, *517*
Howarth, P.H., 115, *125*, 237, 238, 239, *249*, *250*, *251*, 361, 373, 382, *387*, *389*, 494, *503*
Howarth, R.H., 507, *516*
Howell, C.J., 393, 394, 401, *411*, *415*
Howie, K., 479, *489*
Howland, W.C., 303, 305, *312*, 322, 323, 327, 329, *334*, 337, 343, *348*, 358, 360, *366*, 496, *504*
Hoyle, K., 284, *293*
Hsi, L.C., 170, 171, *185*
Huang, D., 182, *186*
Huang, D.D., 28, 30, 31, *40*, 62, 66, *74*, 75
Huang, S.K., 188, *199*
Hubbard, R.C., 13, *22*
Hubbard, W.C., 112, *123*, 235, *247*, 284, 286, *294*, *296*, 360, *367*, 514, *520*
Hudson, I., 218, *226*
Huggins, E.M., 117, *125*
Hughes, J.M., 507, 515, *516*
Hughes, M.D., 283, *293*
Hui, K.P., 362, *368*
Huisman, E., 274, *281*
Humbert, M., 217, 219–23, *225*, *226*, 227
Humes, J., 101, *108*
Hunninghake, G.W., 80, *88*, 117, *125*
Hunt, J.A., 233, *246*
Hunt, L.W., 515, *522*
Hupp, K., 204, *211*
Hutcheson, I.R., 274, *281*
Hutchinson, K.A., 508, *517*
Hwang, D., 146, *156*
Hwang, P.M., 237, *250*

Hybertson, B.M., 280, *282*
Hylander, R.D., 206, *212*
Hyslop, P., 94, *105*
Hyzy, R., 102, *109*

I

Iacobelli, S., 9, *21*, 80, 84, *88*
Ialenti, A., 233, *246*
Ianaro, A., 233, *246*
Ichihashi, K., 454, 457, 467, *470*
Ichikawa, A., 37, *43*, 256, *258*
Ieroni, M.G., 304, *313*
Igarashi, Y., 303, 304, 305, *312*, *313*,
    337, 343, *348*, 358, 360, *366*, 428,
    435, 496, 497, 498, 502, *504*
Ihara, H., 52, *71*
Ihrig-Biedert, I., 118, *126*
Iizuka, H., 7, *20*, 131, *141*
Ijiri, S., 240, *251*
Ikai, K., 96, 99, *107*, *108*
Iles, J., 65, *74*
Imai, T., 454, 457, 467, *470*
Imaizumi, T., 222, *228*
Imaoka, S., 47, 53, *69*, *71*
Imig, J.D., 34, *43*
In, K.H., 287, *297*
Inase, N., 146, *155*
Ince, C., 274, *281*
Ingram, C.G., *269*
Ingram, R.H., Jr., *269*
Inman, M., 113, *123*, 263, 265, *270*,
    271
Inoue, H., 52, *70*, 137, *142*
Inoue, K., 95, *106*
Inoue, T., 232, 233, *246*
Inoue, Y., 263, *269*
Irani, A.A., 308, *315*
Irani, A.M., 343, *350*, 373, 382, *386*,
    388
Irifune, M., 456, 464, 468, 469, *470*
Irish, J.M., 33, *42*
Irvin, C.G., 188, 192, *198*, *199*
Irvine, R.F., 29, *40*
Irwin, R.S., 441, *450*

Isakson, P.C., 13, *22*, *23*, 122, *127*, 135,
    142, 146, *156*, *157*, 285, *295*
Iseki, S., 133, *142*
Ishizaki, J., 95, *106*
Islam, N., 56, *72*
Isobe, R., 56, *72*
Israel, B.C., 50, *70*
Israel, E., 91, *104*, 188, *199*, 287, *297*,
    303, 304, 305, *312*, *313*, 324, 329,
    334, *335*, 337, 343, *348*, 357, 358,
    360, *362*, *365*, *366*, *368*, 371, *384*,
    428, *435*, 496, 497, 498, 502, *504*,
    514, *520*
Itabachi, S., 397, *414*
Ito, K., 394, 401, *411*, *412*
Ives, D., 146, *157*, 163, 178, 181, *184*
Izumi, T., 27, 31, *40*, 393, *410*

J

Jack, R., 99, *108*
Jack, R.M., 361, 376, *388*, 392, *409*
Jackowski, S., 94, *105*
Jacob, C.O., 209, *214*
Jacobsen, M., 373, 382, *386*, *388*
Jacobson, H.R., 5, *18*, *30*, *41*, 59, *73*,
    146, *156*
Jacobson, M.R., 496, *503*
Jacoby, D.B., 307, *314*
Jaegar, J.J., *269*
Jaffee, B.D., 8–9, *20*, 139, *143*, 146,
    157, 285, 292, *295*
Jaffuel, D., 287, 288, *297*, 302, *311*,
    381, *388*
Jager, L., *217*, 218, 223, *225*
Jahnsen, F.L., 373, *387*, 481, 482, *490*
Jakobsson, P.J., 191, 192, *200*
Jakubowski, J., 94, *105*
Jalbert, G., 148, *159*
James, A., 210, *214*, 515, *522*
James, A.L., 204, 205, 208, *211*, *212*,
    213
Janson, C.H., 208, *213*
Janssen, M., 236, 239, 240, *248*, *251*
Jansson, I., 53, *71*

Jantti Alanko, S., 469, *472*
Järvinen, M., 283, *292–93*
Jasper, D.R., 13, *22*
Javdan, P., 238, *250*
Jayadev, S., 29, *40*
Jeffery, P.K., 219, 221, *226*, 373, 382, *386*, *388*, 429, *436*
Jenkins, N., 98, *108*
Jennette, J.C., 5, *18*, 139, *143*, 146, 157, 285, 292, *294*
Jetton, T., 96, 103, *107*
Jewell, C.M., 119, *127*
Ji, C., 146, *157*, 179, *186*
Jick, H., 8, *21*
Jines, G.L., 265, *270*
Johansson, S.G.O., 462, *471*
Johns, R.A., 237, 239, *250*, *251*
Johnson, E.F., 47, 48, *69*
Johnson, H.G., 393, 394, 400, *410*, *414*
Johnson, P.R., 116, *125*
Johnston, J.J., 8–9, *20*, 139, *143*, 146, 157, 285, 292, *295*
Johnston, K., 372, *386*
Johnston, S.L., 231, *245*, 397, 400, *413*
Jonas, M., 94, *105*, 197, *200*
Jonat, C., 509, 511, *517*
Jondal, M., 191, *200*
Jones, C.R., 50, *70*
Jones, D.A., 4, *18*, 130, *141*, 148, *159*
Jones, F., 197, *200*
Jones, G.L., 264, *270*
Jones, P.P., 253, *257*
Jones, S.A., 7, *19*
Jones, S.L., 138, *143*
Jones, T.R., 362, *368*
Jones, V., 479, *490*
Jongejan, R.C., 397, *414*
Joos, G.F., 362, *368*
Jordana, G., 308, *315*, 475, *488*
Jordana, M., 482, 486, *490*, 494, 495, 496, *503*
Jörg, A., 394, *412*
Jornvall, H., 27, *39*, 374, *387*
Jorres, R., 514, *520*
Joseph, M., 301, *311*, 429, *436*, 440, 442, 444, 447, 448, *449*, *450*

Josephs, L.K., 216, *225*
Jothy, S., 148, *159*
Jubran, A., 279, *282*
Juergens, U.R., 308, *314*, 534, *537*
Juhl, E., 300, *310*, 524, *535*
Julier, C., 208, 209, *213*
Jullian, E., 284, *293*
Julou Schaeffer, G., 273, 276, *280*
Jung, M.C., 209, *214*
Juniper, E.F., 216, 222, *224*, 259, *268*, 283, *292*
Jurivich, D., 95, *106*
Jutzler, G.A., 442, *450*

K

Kabrun, N., 152, *160*
Kaever, V., 146, 152, *155*
Kageyama, R., 36, 37, *43*
Kagey-Sobotka, A., 112, *123*, 286, *296*, 514, *520*
Kaghad, M., 204, *211*
Kahn, R.M., 307, *314*
Kaiser, H.B., 362, *368*
Kajita, T., 395, *412*, *413*
Kakizuka, A., 37, *44*
Kaldunski, M., 34, *43*
Kaliner, M.A., 235, *247*, 253, *257*, 303, 304, 305, *312*, *313*, 321, *333*, 337, 343, *348*, 358, 360, *366*, 398, 400, *414*, 428, *435*, 496, 497, 498, 502, *504*
Kalliel, J.N., 218, *226*
Kallos, P., 223, *229*
Kalt, C., 301, *311*
Kaminsky, D.A., 340, 342, *349*
Kanai, N., 32, *42*, 486, *490*
Kane, G.C., 286, *296*
Kaneko, T., 96, *107*
Kang, K.H., 78, *87*
Karahalios, P., 362, *368*
Karara, A., 30, *41*, 46, 58, 59, 60, 65, *69*, *73*, *75*
Kargman, S., 4, *18*, *23*, 97, *107*, 146, 147, 148, *157*, *159*

Karin, M., 118, 122, *126, 127*, 510, *518*
Karlsson, W., 501, 502, *505*
Karthein, R., 170, 171, *185*
Karuzina, I.I., 68, *75*
Kashiwarbara, Y., 118, *126*
Kasper, M., 96, *107*
Kastalerz, L., 304, *313*
Kato, H., 148, *159*
Katori, M., 6, *19*
Katsuyama, M., 256, *258*
Kauffman, H.F., 112, *123*, 269, 393, 394, 395, *411, 413*, 515, *521*
Kaufman, W.E., 7, *20*, 133, *142*, 146, *156*
Kaulbach, H., 303, 305, *312*
Kava, T., 231, 238, *245*, 283, *292–93*, 373, *386*
Kawabori, S., 308, *315*
Kawaguchi, H., 132, *142*, 146, *156*
Kawahito, Y., 148, *159*
Kawai, M., 204, *212*
Kawamura, M., 6, *19*
Kawikova, I., 111, *123*
Kay, A.B., 188, 193, *199*, 217, 219–23, *225, 226, 227, 229*, 289, *298*, 373, *382, 386, 388, 389*, 393, 394, 400, 401, 402, *410, 411, 414, 416*, 441, *450*, 496, *503*, 515, *521*
Kayembe, J.M., 219, *227*
Kayganich, K., 65, *75*
Kedzie, K.M., 256, *258*
Keen, M., 233, *246*
Keith, P.K., 475, *488*
Keith, R.A., 362, *368*
Keller, H., 27, 28, *40*, 103, *109*
Keller, S.L., 255, *257*
Kelloff, G., 148, *159*
Kelly, R.W., 344, *350*
Kelly, W., 218, *226*
Kelner, M.J., 232, 233, *245*
Kelsey, C.R., 285, 286, *295*, 360, *367*
Kemendy, D.M., 308, *315*
Kemeny, D.M., 206, *213*
Kemp, J., 287, *297*
Kemp, J.P., 362, *368*
Kempner, E., 95, *106*

Kennedy, B., 116, *125*
Kennedy, B.P., *23*, 146, 147, *157*
Kennedy, M.E., 3, *17*, 129, *140*
Kent, K.C., 37, *44*
Kern, E.B., 476, *489*
Kerrebijn, K.F., 283, *293*, 397, *414*
Kester, M., 6, *19*
Kharitonov, S.A., 239, *251*
Khatsenko, O.G., 34, *43*, 50, 51, *70*
Khosla, M.C., 33, *42*
Kijne, A.M., 372, *386*, 393, 394, *411, 412*
Kijne, G.M., 394, *412*
Kikawa, Y., *263, 269*
Kikuta, Y., 56, *72*
Kilbourn, R.G., 273, 279, *281, 282*
Killian, D.N., 193, *200*, 259, *268*
Kim, C.-J., 286, *296*
Kim, H.S., 4, 7, *18, 20*, 138, 139, *143*, 285, *294*
Kim, K.W., 515, *522*
Kimmitt, P., 217, 219, 220, 221, 223, *226*
Kimura, S., 148, *159*
Kindt, T.J., 208, *213*
Kinet, J.P., 204, *211*
King, G.A., 140, *144*
King, M., 188, *198*
Kingsleigh-Smith, D.J., 429, *436*
Kinnes, D.A., 253, *257*
Kinoshita, 56, *72*
Kips, J.C., 362, *368*
Kirkland, S., 96, 103, *107*
Kirkwood, T.B.L., 208, *213*
Kishino, J., 95, *106*
Kishore, V., 30, *11*, 65, *75*
Kistelhorst, C., 508, *517*
Kitajima, S., 289, *297*
Kitzler, J., 132, *141*
Kiuchi, H., 304, *313*, 357, 361, *365*, 371, *384*
Kiviranta, K., 283, *292–93*
Klebanoff, S.J., 409, *418*
Klein, D.E., 319, 320, *332*, 452, 457, *470*
Klein, T., 5, 6, *18, 19, 23*

Kleinert, H., 118, *126*
Kletter, Y., 401, *415*
Kliewer, S., 103, *109*
Klimek, L., 514, *520*
Kline, P.A., 283, *292*
Kliphuis, J.W., 204, *211*
Kluckman, K.D., 4, 5, 7, *18*, *20*, 138, 139, *143*, 146, *157*, 285, 292, *294*
Knapp, H.R., 287, *297*, 323, *334*, 355, 358, 361, *365*
Knapp, K.R., 255, *257*
Knigge, K.M., 237, *250*
Knight, D.A., 113, *124*
Knight, R.K., 360, *367*
Knol, E.F., 403, *416*
Knol, K., 283, *293*
Knoll, E., 27, 34, *39*
Knopf, J.L., 29, 30, *41*, 94, *105*, 374, *387*
Knowles, M.R., 188, *198*
Knowles, R.G., 273, *281*
Knox, A., 115, 122, *125*, *127*, 426, *435*
Kobayashi, H., 204, *211*
Koboldt, C., 2, *17*, *23*, 122, *127*, 146, *157*, 180, *186*
Kobzik, L., 237, *249*
Koch, C., 217, *226*
Kodansky, D., 499, *504*
Koedam, J.A., 393, *411*
Koenderman, L., 394, *412*
Koeter, G.H., 395, *413*
Koh, E., 232, 233, *246*
Kohler, J., 273, *281*
Koide, K., 402, 408, *416*, *417*, 515, 516, *521*, *522*
Kok, P.T., 372, *386*, 393, 394, 408, *411*, *412*, *417*
Kolb, J.P., 192, *200*
Koley, A.P., 68, *75*
Kolls, J., 273, *281*
Kondo, M., 148, *159*, 239, *250*
Kondo, T., 56, *72*
Konishi, A., 96, *107*
Konishi, Y., 357, 361, *365*
Konno, K., 239, *250*
Koo, M., 209, *214*

Koop, D.R., 51, 58, 63, *70*, *72*
Kopp, E., 152, *160*
Koppenol, W.H., 234, *246*
Korbut, R., 284, *294*
Koregel, C., 405, *417*
Korley, V., 514, *520*
Korszun, Z., 508, *517*
Kortholm, B., 486, *490*
Koskinen, S., 283, *292-93*
Kosturkov, G., 457, 459, *470*
Koudstaal, P.J., 80, *88*
Koutsos, M.I., 149, *159*
Kovacic, R.T., 512, *519*
Kowalski, M.L., 303, 304, 305, 307, *312*, *313*, *314*, 329, *335*, 358, *366*, 456, 460, 464, 469, *470*, 498, *504*, 525, 531, *535*, *537*
Kowon, O.J., 114, 115, 119, *124*
Kraemer, S.A., 136, *142*
Kraft, D., 206, *212*
Kraig, R.P., 7, *20*
Kramer, R., 94, *105*
Krauss, A.H., 342, *349*, 383, *389*
Krell, R.D., 362, *368*
Kremer, L., 198, *200*
Kreukniet, J., 393, 408, *411*, *417*
Krieger, M., 342, *349*
Krishnan, V.J., 118, *126*
Krishnaswamy, G., 205, *212*, 222, *228*
Kriz, R.W., 29, *41*, 94, *105*, 374, *387*
Kroegel, C., 113, *124*, 217, 218, 223, *225*, *228*, 380, *388*, 396, 405, *413*, *417*
Kromer, B.M., 78, *87*
Krueger, M.A., 49, *69*
Krutzch, M., 149, 150, 154, *159*, *160*
Krzanowski, J.J., 235, *247*
Kubes, P., 138, *143*
Kudo, I., 95, *106*
Kuehl, F.A., Jr., 28, *40*, 101, *108*, 130, *140*, 253, *257*, 306, *314*, 380, *388*
Kuga, S., 289, *297*
Kuhn, H., 27, *39*, 287, *297*
Kuhn, J.P., 468, *472*
Kuitert, L.M., 114, 115, 117, 118, 119, *124*, *125*, 302, *311*

Kujubu, D.A., 3, *17*, 130, 136, *141*,
   142, 146, 147, *156*, 162, *183*, 285,
   294, *295*
Kuklinski, P., 468, *472*
Kulchak, A.L., 149, *160*
Kulling, G., 222, *228*
Kulmacz, R.J., 96, *107*, 130, *140*, 153,
   160, 170, 171, 173, 174, 179, *185*,
   186, 234, 235, *247*
Kulp, G.V.P., 284, *293*, 402, *416*
Kumabashiri, I., *335*
Kumagami, H., 329, *335*
Kumazawa, T., *329*, *335*
Kume, K., 27, 31, *40*
Kume, N., 138, *143*
Kumegawa, M., 136, *142*
Kumlin, B., 371, 372, *384*
Kumlin, M., 113, *123*, 303, 304, *312*,
   313, 323, 324, 326, *334*, 337, 343,
   348, *350*, 353, 355, 356, 358, 359,
   361, 362, *364*, *365*, *366*, *367*, *368*,
   369, 372, 380, *385*, *388*, 424, 428,
   429, *434*, *436*, 496, 497, 502, *504*,
   505, 514, *520*, *521*
Kummer, W., 237, *249*
Kuna, P., 304, *313*
Kunkel, S.L., 253, *257*, 285, 292, *295*
Kuo, L., 239, *251*
Kupfer, D., 53, *71*
Kuramitsu, K., 304, *313*, 357, 361, *365*,
   371, *384*
Kurlak, L., 393, *411*
Kurre, U., 98, *108*
Kurumball, R.G., 146, *157*, 163, 164,
   174, 178, 180, 181, *184*
Kusnierz, J.P., 442, *450*
Kusunose, E., 47, 56, *69*, *72*
Kusunose, M., 47, 56, *69*, *72*
Kutchera, W., 4, *18*, 148, *159*
Kutin, J.J., 204, *211*, 222, *228*
Kvon, M., 460, *471*
Kwan, M.Y., *23*, 146, 147, *157*
Kwoh, D.K., 320, *332*
Kwon, O.J., 6, *19*, 118, 121, *126*, 237,
   250, 285, *295*, 302, *311*, 512, *519*
Kwong, E., 4, *18*

L

Labarre, C., 239, *251*
Labat, C., 235, *247*, 360, *367*
Labayle, D., 148, *158*
Lacoste, J.Y., 216, 219, *225*, 447, *450*,
   515, *521*
Lacronique, J., 514, *521*
Ladenius, A.R.C., 238, *250*
Laethem, C.L., 51, 58, 63, *70*
Laethem, R.M., 51, 58, 63, *70*, *72*
Laforge, K.S., 510, *518*
Lagrue, G., 442, *450*
Lal, C.K., *373*, *387*
Laitinen, A., 231, 238, *245*, 268, *271*,
   321, *333*, 342, *349*, 361, 373, 383,
   386, *387*, *389*
Laitinen, L.A., 231, 238, *245*, 268, *271*,
   283, *292–93*, 321, *333*, 342, *349*,
   361, 373, 383, *386*, *387*, *389*
Lakkis, F.G., 287, *297*
Lam, B.K., 28, *40*, 99, *108*, 302, 303,
   304, 307, 308, *312*, *313*, 361, 372–79,
   381, 382, 383, *385*, *387*, *388*, *389*,
   392, 393, 394, *409*, *410*, *412*
Lam, S., *221*, *223*, *227*
Lamb, G., 274, *281*
Lamm, W.J.E., 197, *200*
Lampe, F., 188, *198*, 222, 224, *228*, *229*
Lan, S., 269
Landau, L.T., 218, *226*
Lander, E.S., 188, *198*
Lander, H.M., 235, *247*
Landino, L.M., 51, *70*, 234, *246*
Landon, D.N., 360, *367*
Landry, M.L., 122, *127*
Lands, W.E., 1, *16*, 129, *140*, 161, 172,
   173, *183*, *185*
Lane, C.G., 264, 265, *270*
Lane, S.J., 116, *125*, 372, 380, 381, *385*
Laneuville, O., 9, *21*, 26, *39*, 146, *157*,
   172, 173, 174, 179, *185*, *186*
Lang, L., 204, *211*
Lange, P., 224, *229*
Langenbach, R., 4, 5, 7, *18*, *20*, 138,
   139, *143*, 146, *157*, 285, 292, *294*

Langman, M.J.S., 8, *21*
Laniado Schwartzman, M., 34, *43*
Lanigan, A., 204, *211*, 222, *228*
Lanni, C., 362, *368*
Lanteaume, A., 222, *228*
Lantz, M.E., 8, *21*
Laporte, J., 392, *409*
Laposata, M., 93, *105*
Lapp, P., 479, *489*
Larchè, M., 219, 221, *227*
Larkin, S., 111, *123*, 233, 234, *246*
Larkin, V.A., 280, *282*
Larrick, J., 253, *257*
Larsen, G.L., 188, 192, *198*, 286, *296*, 372, *386*
Larsen, P.L., 474, 476, 477, 478, *488*, *489*
Larsson, C., 29, *40*, 324, *334*, 353, 355, 356, 358, *364*, 372, *385*, 424, 429, *434*
Larsson, L., 304, *313*, 326, *334*, 361, *368*, 502, *505*
Larsson, P., 191, *200*
Lasalle, P., 309, *315*
Laskin, J.D., 273, 280, *281*
Lassalle, P., 223, *228*, 429, *436*, 442, 444, 447, 448, *450*
Lassegue, B., 94, *105*
Lathrop, G.M., 204, 210, *211*, *214*
Lau, L.C., 263, *270*
Lau, S., 237, *249*
Laurent, C., 501, *505*
Lauwen, A.P.M., 380, *388*
Lavins, B.J., 268, *271*
Laviolette, M., 393, 394, 395, 401, 402, 408, *410*, *411*, *413*, *416*, *417*, 515, *521*
Lawrence, S., 188, *198*, 222, *228*
Lawson, D.H., 8, *21*
Lawson, J.A., 59, 60, 62, 63, *73*, 78, 79, 80, 82, *87*, *88*, 394, *412*
Lawson, W., 470, *472*
Lazarus, S.C., 146, *155*
Lazzerini, G., 511, 515, *518*, *522*
Lea, R., 495, 496, *503*
Leahy, K., 13, *22*, 135, *142*, 146, *156*, 162, *183*, 285, *295*

Leaves, N.I., 210, *214*
Leblanc, R., 273, *281*
Le Breton, G.C., 37, *44*
Leckie, A.J.B., 317, *332*
Lecomte, M., 146, *157*, 173, 179, *185*, *186*
Leder, P., 342, *349*
Ledford, A., 5, *18*, 139, *143*, 146, *157*, 285, 292, *294*
Ledford, D., 287, *297*, 362, *368*
Le-Doucen, C., 515, *521*
Lee, C.A., 4, 5, 7, *18*, *20*, 138, 139, *143*, 146, *157*, 285, 292, *294*
Lee, C.W., 338, *349*, 372, *386*, 393, 409, *410*
Lee, H., 153, *160*
Lee, J., 56, *72*
Lee, J.B., 32, *42*
Lee, L., 13, *22*, 135, *142*, 146, *156*
Lee, R.H., 303, *312*
Lee, S.H., 146, *156*
Lee, T.H., 56, *72*, 116, *125*, 206, *213*, 268, *271*, 302, 303, 304, 308, *311*, *312*, *313*, *314*, *315*, 321–24, 327, 328, 329, *333*, *334*, *335*, 337, 338, 342, 344, *348*, *349*, 355, 357–61, *365*, *366*, *367*, 371–76, 378–81, 383, *384*, *385*, *388*, *389*, 393, 394, 397, 400, 401, 408, *411*, *413*, *414*, *415*, 419, 424, 425, 429, *432*, *434*, 440, *449*, 495–98, *503*, *504*, 515, *521*, 532, 534, *537*
Lee, T.L., 342, *349*
Lees, J., 7, *19*
Leff, A.R., 284, *293*, 397, 400, 401, 402, 403, 405, 407, *414*, *416*, *417*
Leger, S., 362, *368*
Legrand, A., 301, *311*
Lehman, J., 95, *106*
Lehman, P.A., 408, *418*
Lehmann, J., 103, *109*
Lehtonen, K., 283, *292–93*
Lei, M., 191, *199*
Lei, Z.M., 7, *20*
Leikauf, G.D., 265, *270*
Leitao, M.C., 456, 459, *470*

Leitch, A.G., 397, *413*
Lelias, J.-M., 204, *211*
Lemke, S.M., 236, *248*
Lenhard, J., 103, *109*
Lenzi, H.L., 401, *415*
Leonard, C.A., 476, *489*
Leone, A., 274, *281*
Lepley, R.A., 103, *109*
Lequeux, N., 302, *311*, 381, *388*
Lermoyez, J., 317, 318, *332*, 352, 361, *364*, *368*, 440, *449*, 452, *470*, 523, *535*
Leroux, J.L., *288*, *297*, 515, *522*
Leroy, O., 300, *310*
Leslie, C., 94, 98, *105*, *108*
Leslie, C.A., 235, *247*
le Souef, P., 204, 208, 210, *211*, *213*, *214*
Lessof, M.H., 393, 394, *411*
Leszczynska-Piziak, J., 232, *245*
Leukotriene, A., 27, *39*, 192, *200*
Leung, D.Y.M., 308, *315*, 495, 496, *503*
Levasseur-Acker, G.M., 432, *438*
Leveille, C., 28, *40*
Leveridge, J., 208, *213*
Levi, R., 279, *282*
Levin, B., 148, *158*
Levine, B.B., 206, *212*
Levine, L., 284, *294*
Levine, S.J., 121, *127*
Levine, T.M., 146, *155*
Levitt, R.C., 188, *198*, 205, *212*, 222, *228*
Levy, D.B., 147, *158*
Levy, L.O., 146, *156*
Lewis, A.J., 235, *247*
Lewis, D.B., 197, *200*
Lewis, G.D., 209, *214*
Lewis, I., 479, *490*
Lewis, R., 523, 532, *535*
Lewis, R.A., 28, *40*, 114, *124*, 188, *199*, 286, *296*, 302, *311*, 338, *349*, 358, 359, 360, *366*, 372, *386*, 393, 394, 400, 401, 409, *410*, *411*, *414*, *415*, *418*
Li, A., 204, *211*

Li, C., 98, *108*
Li, C.S., 13, 14, *22*, 122, *127*
Li, D.Y., 7, *19*
Li, J., 146, *156*
Li, P., 96, *107*
Li, X., 7, *20*, 188, *199*
Li, Z., 30, *41*
Lianos, E.A., 37, *44*
Liao, J.C., 239, *251*
Lichtenstein, L., 92, *104*
Lichtenstein, L.M., 112, *123*, 253, *257*, 285, 286, 287, *296*, *297*, 358, 359, *366*, 372, 380, *385*, *386*, 514, *520*, *521*
Lidholdt, T., 473, 486, *488*, *490*
Lidholt, T., 501, *505*
Liftin, C.D., 285, 292, *294*
Liggett, S.B., 209, *214*, 222, *228*
Lilja, I., 4, *18*, 148, *159*
Lilly, C., 91, *104*
Lilly, C.M., 6, *19*, 235, *247*, 303, 304, 305, *312*, *313*, 324, 329, *334*, *335*, 337, 343, *348*, 357, 358, 360, *365*, *366*, 371, *384*, 428, *435*, 496, 497, 498, 502, *504*, 514, *520*
Lim, B., 204, *211*
Lim, L.L.-Y., 8, 9, *21*
Lim, R.W., 3, *17*, 146, 147, *156*, 162, *183*, 285, *294*
Lin, A., 94, *105*
Lin, A.Y., 29, 30, *41*, 374, *387*
Lin, K.-L., 222, *227*
Lin, K.T., 65, *74*
Lin, L., 32, *42*, 94, *105*
Lin, L.-L., 29, 30, *40*, *41*, 374, *387*
Linardic, M., 29, *40*
Lindbom, L., 360, *367*
Linden, M., 501, *505*, 512, *519*
Lindenthal, U., 91, 96, *104*
Lindgren, J.A., 56, *72*, 321, *333*, 358, *365*
Lindholdt, T., 486, *490*
Lindqvist, N., 501, *505*
Lindsay, A.R.G., 429, *436*
Lindsay, D.A., 264, *270*
Lindsay, J., 317, *332*

Lindsay, M.A., 405, *417*
Liou, S., 146, *156*
Liston, T.E., 359, *367*
Litchfield, T., 515, *521*
Liu, F.Y., 33, *42*
Liu, J., 515, *522*
Liu, M.C., 112, *123*, 284, 286, *294*, *296*, 514, *520*
Liu, S.F., 16, *23*, 114, 119, *124*
Lloyd, C.M., 198, *200*
Lobbecke, E.A., 223, *229*
Lockart, A., 432, *438*
Lockey, R., 460, *471*
Lockey, R.F., 319, 326, *332*, *334*, 352, *364*, 501, *505*, 523, 529, *535*, *536*
Locksley, R.M., 188, 195, 197, *199*, 209, *213*
Loeter, G.H., 112, *123*
Lofquist, A.K., *127*, 510, *518*
Loftin, C.D., 4, 5, 7, *18*, *20*, 138, 139, *143*, 146, *157*, 285, *294*
Logan, R., 8, 9, *21*
Lokuta, A.J., 34, 35, *43*
Loll, P.J., 2, *17*, 45, *68*, 130, *140*, 145, 152, *155*, 162, 163, 164, 166, 174, 176, 178, 179, *184*, *186*
Longmire, A.W., 78, 79, 82, *87*
Lonigro, A.J., 32, *42*
Loose-Mitchell, D.S., 3, *18*, 131, 132, 133, 140, *141*, *144*, 153, *160*
Loper, J.C., 47, 48, *69*
Lopez, E., 495, 496, *503*
Loscalzo, J., 237, *249*
Lottspeich, F., 52, *70*
Lotvall, J.O., 113, *124*, 427, *435*
Loubatière, J., 515, *521*
Louis, R., 219, *227*
Loveridge, J., 208, 209, *213*
Lovijärvi, A., 283, *293*
Lowe, D., 475, *488*
Lowenstein, C.J., 237, *249*
Lu, J.-L., 239, *251*
Lu, M., 62, *74*
Lu, R., 32, *42*
Lu, X., 149, 150, 152, 153, *160*
Lucas, F.S., 9, *21*

Luckhoff, A., 273, *281*
Luisi, B., 508, *517*
Luk, G.D., 4, *18*
Lum, W.H., 512, *519*
Lumin, S., 60, 63, *73*
Lumry, W., 304, *313*
Lumry, W.R., 460, *471*, 501, *505*, 528, 529, *536*
Lund, J., 68, *75*
Lund, V., 473, 486, *488*, *490*, *491*
Lundberg, J.M., 274, 280, *282*
Luong, C., 2, *17*, 163, 164, 169, 170, 178, 179, 181, *184*
Lupulescu, A., 148, *158*
Lurd, J.G., 501, *505*
Luster, A.D., 342, *349*
Luttmann, W., 396, *413*
Luying, P., 511, *519*
Lympany, P., 206, *213*, 308, *315*
Lynch, J., 203, 204, *211*
Lynch, S.M., 78, 79, 82, *87*

M

Ma, Y.M., 50, *70*
Maas, R.L., 394, *412*
Maccache, P.H., 402, *416*
MacCarthy, A., 208, *213*
MacDermot, J., 285, 286, *295*, 360, *367*
MacDonald, A.J., 393, 402, *411*
MacGlashan, D.W., 358, 359, *366*, 372, 380, *385*, *386*
Maciag, T., 26, 34, *39*
Macica, C., 62, *74*
Mackay, G.A., 430, *436*
Mackay, I.S., 486, *491*, 496, *503*
Mackenzie, R., 146, *157*
Maclauf, J., 344, *350*
Maclouf, J., 9, *21*, 56, *71*, 80, 82, 84, *88*, 322, *333*, 358, *365*, 440, *449*
MacMillan, A., 424, 429, *434*
MacMillan, D.K., 393, *410*
MacMillan, R., 324, *334*, 357, *365*, 371, *384*
McAllister, K., 401, 402, 403, *416*

McBride, H.M., 373, *387*
McCall, C.E., 117, *125*
McCall, T., 239, *250*
McCann, S.M., 233, *246*
McCauley, E., 253, *257*, 380, *388*
McClain, C.J., 50, *70*
McDevitt, H.O., 209, *214*
McDonald, J.J., 2, *17*, 146, *157*, 180, *186*
McDonald, J.R., 223, *229*, 457, *470*
McDowell, T.L., 209, *214*
McFadden, C.A., 188, *199*
McFadden, E.R., *269*, 358, *366*, 397, *413*, 441, *450*
McFarlane, C.S., 362, *368*
McGeady, S.J., 216, *225*
McGiff, J.C., 25, 27–4, *38*, *39*, 40, *41*, *42*, *43*, *44*, 46, 50, 53, 58, 60, 62, 63, 65, 66, *69*, *70*, *71*, *73*, *74*, *75*
McGill, K.A., *199*
McGrail, S.H., 37, *44*
McIntyre, T.M., 4, *18*, 130, *141*, 148, *159*, 222, *228*
McKana, J., 511, *518*
McKanna, J.A., 5, *18*, 146, *156*
McKay, D., 33, 34, *42*
McKinnon, K., 235, *247*
McLaren, W.J., 8, *21*
McLaughlin, M.K., 232, 233, 234, *246*
McLauhlan, P., 479, *490*
McLemore, T.L., 112, *123*, 286, *296*, 514, *520*
McMenamin, C., 209, *213*
McNatt, J., 140, *144*
McNeill, R.S., *269*
McNish, R., 94, 97, 98, 102, *105*, *108*, *109*
McParland, C.P., 284, *293*
Madden, M., 6, *19*, 95, *105*, 235, *247*
Maddox, Y.T., 393, *410*
Madhun, Z.T., 33, 34, *42*
Madrestma, G.S., 513, *519*
Maeda, N., 329, *335*
Maekawa, M., 47, *69*
Maestrelli, P., 217, 219, 221, 222, 223, *226*, *227*, *228*

Maggi, E., 209, *213*
Maghni, K., 394, *412*
Magni, E., 12, *22*
Magnussen, H., 397, 401, 405, 407, *414*, *416*, *417*, 514, *520*
Mahauthaman, R., 393, 394, *411*
Mahboubi, K., 38, *44*, 50, *70*
Mahler, J.F., 4, 5, 7, *18*, *20*, 138, 139, *143*, 146, *157*, 285, 292, *294*
Mahmic, A., 222, *227*
Maier, J.A.M., 26, 34, *39*
Majima, M., 6, *19*
Makino, S., 382, *389*, 402, *416*
Makita, K., 46, *58*, 60, *69*
Makita, N., 78, *87*
Makker, H.K., 263, *270*
Maler, B., 508, *517*
Malik, K.U., 32, *42*, 53, *71*
Malinski, T., 273, *281*
Mallet, A.I., 79, *88*
Malmberg, H., 469, *472*
Malmstrom, K., 304, *313*, 531, *537*
Malo, J.L., 56, *72*, 216, 222, 224, *227*, 266, *271*
Maltby, N.H., 287, *296*, 322, *333*
Manabe, H., 408, *418*
Mancini, J., 4, 13, 14, *18*, *22*, *23*, 28, *40*, 102, *109*, 122, *127*, 146, 147, 148, *157*, *159*, 374, *387*
Mandel, Jl.J., 34, *42*
Manetta, J., 94, *105*
Manna, S., 59, *73*
Manning, M.E., 528, *536*
Manning, P., 284, *293*
Manning, P.J., 56, *72*, 113, *124*, 259, 263, 264, 265, 266, *268*, *269*, *270*, *271*, 347, *350*, 360, *367*
Manning, P.M., 265, *270*
Manning, P.T., 285, *295*
Manso, G., 285, 288, *295*, 362, *368*
Mansuy, D., 46, *68*
Manzetti, G.W., 477, 478, *489*
Mao, X.Q., 204, *212*
Mapp, C.E., 216, 217, 219, 221, 223, *225*, *226*, *227*, 515, *522*
Marcheselli, V.L., 7, *20*

Marcinkiewicz, E., 301, *311*
Marcus, A., 148, *158*
Marcus, A.J., 56, *72*
Marfat, A., 28, *40*
Margiotta, P., 31, *41*, 60, 66, *73*, *75*
Margolskee, D.J., 263, 265, *269*, *270*,
    304, *313*, 324, *334*, 353, 355, 356,
    358, 361, 362, *364*, *368*, 372, *385*,
    424, 425, 429, *434*
Marini, G., 79, *88*
Marini, M., 382, *389*
Markendorf, A., 322, 323, *333*, *334*,
    337, *348*, 358, *366*, 534, *537*
Markowitz, A., 68, *75*
Marnett, L.J., 51, *70*, 129, *140*, 146,
    148, *156*, *158*, 170, *185*, 234, *246*
Marney, S.R., Jr., 113, *123*, 287, *297*
Marom, Z., 321, *333*, 400, *414*
Marques, D., 456, 459, *470*
Marquette, C.H., 300, *310*, 429, *436*
Marsac, J., 235, *247*, 514, *521*
Marsh, D.G., 203, 204, 205, 206, *211*,
    212, 222, *228*, 319, *332*, 460, *471*
Marshall, J., 495, 496, *503*
Marshall, L., 95, *106*
Marshall, P.J., 171, *185*
Marshall, T., 94, *105*
Martelli, M., 374, *387*
Martelli, N.A., 339, *349*, 429, *436*, 468,
    471
Martin, A.J., 218, *226*
Martin, J.G., 191, *199*
Martin, M.V., 60, 63, *73*
Martin, R.J., 209, *214*, 222, *228*, 288,
    297, 340, 342, *349*, 514, 515, *521*,
    522
Martin, T.R., 188, 192, *198*, *200*
Martinez, A.C., 198, *200*
Martinez, F.D., 218, 221, 223, *226*
Martinez, S., 182, *186*
Martinson, M.E., 383, *389*
Maruyama, N., 397, *414*
Masferrer, J., 3, 13, *17*, *22*, 27, 34, *39*,
    43, 60, *74*, 119, *126*, 135, *142*, 146,
    156, 232, 233, 235, *245*, *246*, 285,
    295

Masi, C., 420, *433*
Mason, H.S., 49, *69*
Masson, P., 362, *368*
Mastalerz, L., 300, 306, *310*, *314*, 321,
    326, *333*, *334*, 347, *350*, 360, 362,
    367, *369*, 424, *434*, 469, *472*, 502,
    505
Masters, B.S., 47, 49, 50, 53, *69*, *70*
Mastino, A., 148, *159*
Mastyugin, V., 58, 62, *73*
Mathe, A.A., 235, *247*
Mathison, D.A., 223, *229*, 300, 308,
    310, *314*, 320, 327, *332*, *334*, 352,
    364, 457, *470*, 501, *505*, 523, 524,
    526, 528, 529, 530, 531, *535*, *536*,
    537
Matijevic-Aleksic, N., 130, 140, *141*
Matsuda, T., 335
Matsumoto, K., 96, *107*
Matsumoto, R., 285, *294*, *296*
Matsumoto, T., 374, *387*
Matsumura, K., 7, *20*
Matsunaga, T., 456, 464, 468, 469, *470*
Matsunami, N., 4, *18*, 148, *159*
Matsuura, T., 454, 457, 467, *470*
Matsuzaki, G., 394, *411*
Matthaei, K.I., 188, 195, 197, *199*
Matthay, M.A., 188, 195, 197, *199*
Matthiesen, F., 206, *213*
Matthys, H., 217, 218, *225*, 380, *388*,
    405, *417*
Mattila, L., 462, *471*
Mattoli, S., 382, *389*, 401, *415*
Mattoso, V.L., 401, *415*
Maunsbach, A.B., 29, *40*
Maurand, M., 52, *71*
Maxwell, P., 30, *41*
May, M.A., 253, *257*
Mayer, 317, *332*
Mayer, B., 237, *249*
Mayer, D., 400, 401, 403, *414*, *416*
Meade, E.A., *23*, 117, *125*, 130, 136,
    141, *142*, 147, *157*, 285, *294*
Medina, J., 99, *108*
Medina, J.F., 192, *200*
Meese, C.O., 86, *89*

Mehlisch, D.R., 13, *22*
Mehta, D., 284, *293*
Meidell, R.S., 140, *144*
Melillo, E., 113, *124*, 265, *271*, 347, *350*, 360, *367*, 420, *433*
Melillo, G., 420, *433*
Mellon, J.J., 193, *200*, 259, *268*
Memo, M., 150, 152, *160*
Menard, L., 402, *416*
Mencia-Huerta, J.M., 192, *200*
Menconi, M.J., 280, *282*
Mendel, D.B., 510, *517*
Meng, Q., 115, *125*, 217, 219, 221, *226*, *289*, *298*, *382*, *389*
Mentzer, S., 361, 375, *388*
Menz, G., 217, 219–23, *225*, *226*, *227*, 300, *310*
Merchant, M., 188, *198*
Merlie, J.P., 129, *140*
Merrett, M., 273, *281*
Messer, G., 209, *214*
Metcalfe, D.D., 188, *198*
Mewes, T., 514, *520*
Meyer, G., 427, 430, *435*
Meyers, D.A., 188, *198*, 206, *212*, 222, *228*
Meyrick, B.O., 140, *144*
Mezzetti, A., 79, *88*
Miadonna, A., 303, *312*, 419, *432*
Michalska, Z., 301, *311*
Micheal, G.J., 237, *250*
Michel, F.B., 216, 219, *225*, 235, *247*, 287, 288, *297*, 302, *311*, 372, 381, *386*, *388*, 515, *521*
Michel, H., 162, 182, *184*, *186*
Michel, O., *529*, *536*
Micka, K., 442, *450*
Miesfeld, R., 508, *517*
Mifune, J., *335*
Milani, G.F., 219, 221, *227*, 515, *522*
Milano, S., 232, 234, *245*
Mileva, Z., 457, 459, *470*
Milewski, M., 300, 309, *310*, *315*, 441, *450*, 469, *472*
Millar, J.S., *269*

Miller, A., *2*, *17*, *163*, 164, 169, 170, 178, 179, 181, *184*
Miller, D., 97, *108*
Miller, D.K., 28, *40*
Miller, F.F., 319, *332*
Miller, K.B., 32, *42*
Miller, M.F., 237, *249*
Milona, M.N., 374, *387*
Milona, N., 29, *41*, 94, *105*
Milovic, J.E., 8, *21*
Milton, A.S., 7, *20*
Minakama, S., 56, *72*
Minamikawa, T., 102, *108*
Mincek, N.V., 149, *159*
Miner, J.N., 511, *518*
Minnard, E.A., 274, *281*
Minotti, G., 79, *88*
Minton, T.A., 77, 78, 79, *87*
Mioskowski, C., 62, *74*
Mirabella, A., 514, *520*
Mirone, C., 303, *312*, 419, *432*
Mishima, T., 395, *412*
Misik, V., 51, *70*
Misko, T.P., 34, *43*, 119, *126*, 232, 233, 235, *245*, *246*
Mita, H., 395, *412*, *413*
Mita, S., 454, 457, 467, *470*
Mitchell, J.A., 6, 9, *19*, *21*, 111, 114, 115, 116, 117, 119, *123*, *124*, *125*, *126*, 130, 135, *141*, *142*, 146, *157*, 232, 233, 234, *245*, *246*, 285, *295*, 302, *311*, 354, 355, *365*, 512, *519*
Mitchell, K.D., 33, *42*
Mitchell, M.D., 7, *20*, 146, *156*
Mitzner, W., 188, *198*
Miura, Y., 454, 457, 467, *470*
Miyagawa, H., 408, *418*
Miyakawa, K., 514, *520*, *521*
Miyamoto, T., 129, *140*, 161, *183*
Miyanomae, T., 263, *269*
Miyashiro, J.M., 146, *157*
Miyata, A., 52, *70*, *71*
Mizukami, Y., 56, *72*
Mizuno, N., 96, *107*
Moavero, N.E., 347, *350*, 420, 424, 429, 431, *432*, 468, *471*, 498, *504*

Mock, B.A., 204, *211*
Mode, A., 68, *75*
Modi, M., 263, 265, *270*, *271*
Moest, D.R., 238, *250*
Moffatt, M.F., 204, 208, 209, *211*, *213*, *214*
Mogensen, C., 478, *489*
Mohamed, S., 431, *437*
Mohapatra, S., 209, *213*
Mohr, S., 146, *155*
Moises, H.-W., 204, *211*
Molema, J., 283, *293*
Molimard, M., 427, 432, *435*, *438*
Molina, C., 218, *226*
Moncada, S., 3, *17*, 52, *71*, 138, *143*, 273, 274, 280, *281*
Moneret-Vautrin, D.A., 301, *311*
Monick, M.M., 117, *125*
Monik, M.M., 80, *88*
Montalbetti, N., 303, *312*, 419, *432*
Montealegre, F., 222, *227*
Montefort, S., 382, *389*
Montserrat, J.M., 300, 303, 305, *310*, *312*, 323, *334*, 337, 347, *348*, 358, 360, *366*, 380, 381, *388*, 457, 467, *471*, 496, 497, *504*
Moore, A.R., 6, *19*
Moore, K., 322, *333*
Moore, K.P., 79, *88*
Moore, S.A., 66, *75*
Moqbel, R., 393, 402, *411*
Mor, S., 401, *415*
Moran, N., 36, *43*
Morgan, D.W., 235, *247*
Morgan, E., 92, 96, *104*, *107*
Morgans, D.J., 179, *186*
Morham, S.G., 4, 5, 7, *18*, *20*, 138, 139, *143*, 146, *157*, 285, 292, *294*
Moride, Y., 8, 9, *21*
Morimoto, K., 204, *211*, *212*, 256, *258*
Morimoto, R., 95, *106*
Morimoto, S., 232, 233, *246*
Morita, I., 35, *43*, 96, *107*, 136, *142*, 147, *158*, 169, *184*, 285, *294*
Morris, D., 103, *109*
Morris, M.M., 259, *268*, 397, *413*

Morrison, A., 232, 233, *245*
Morrison, P., 204, *211*
Morrow, J., 96, 103, *107*
Morrow, J.D., 51, *70*, 77, 78, 79, 82, *87*, *88*, 111, *123*, 146, *156*, 234, *246*, 287, *297*
Morton, A., 515, *522*
Morton, B.E., 397, *414*
Morton, D.R., 321, *333*, 400, *414*
Morton, H.E., 97, *108*
Morton, N.E., 188, *198*, 222, *228*
Moss, P., 209, *213*
Moss, P.A.H., 208, *213*
Motojima, S., 382, *389*, 402, *416*
Mudd, J., 129, *140*
Mueller, R., 382, *389*
Muerhoff, S.A., 49, 53, *69*
Muijsers, R.B.R., 234, *246*
Mukai, S., 148, *159*
Mukaida, N., 511, *518*
Mukherjee, E., 97, *107*
Mukhopadhyay, A., 95, *106*
Mukundan, C.R., 77, *87*
Mul, F.P., 403, *416*
Mulder, M.F., 274, *281*
Mulkins, M., 287, *297*
Mullane, K.M., 25, 27, 34, *38*
Mullarkey, M.F., 319, *332*, 441, *450*
Mullee, M.A., 216, *225*
Muller, E., 392, *409*
Müller, K.-M., 6, *19*
Muller, M., 510, *517*
Mullin, M., 237, *249*
Mullins, M.D., 255, *257*
Mullol, J., 432, *438*, 495, 496, 500, *503*, *505*
Mulsch, A., 273, *281*
Munafo, D., 99, *108*, 287, *297*
Munck, A., 510, *517*
Mundel, P., 237, *249*
Munkonge, F., 429, *436*
Muñoz, N.M., 397, 400, 401, 402, 403, 405, 407, *414*, *416*, *417*
Murad, F., 237, *249*
Murakami, M., 95, *106*, 285, *294*, *296*
Murdoch, W.J., 149, *159*

Murdock, K.Y., 284, *293*
Murota, S., 96, *107*
Murphy, M., 8, *21*
Murphy, R., 532, *537*
Murphy, R.C., 27, 34, *39*, *43*, 46, 56,
  59, 60, 62, 63, 65, *69*, *71*, *72*, *73*, *74*,
  75, 322, *333*, 358, *365*, 393, *410*
Murphy, T.M., 512, *519*
Murray, J.J., 255, *257*, 286, 287, *296*,
  297, *362*, *368*
Musial, J., 223, *228*, 309, *315*, 419, 424,
  432, 441, 442, 449, *450*
Musk, A.W., 204, 205, 208, 210, *211*,
  212, *213*, *214*
Mutha, S.S., 209, *213*
Muto, M., 206, *213*
Myers, D.A., 203, 204, 205, *211*, *212*
Myers, P.R., 232, 233, *246*
Mygind, N., 473, 474, 475, 478, 486,
  488, *489*, *490*, 501, *505*

N

Naama, H., 274, *281*
Nabe, M., 408, *418*
Naclerio, R.M., 284, 287, *293*, *297*,
  372, 380, *385*, *386*, 486, *491*, 514,
  521
Nadel, J., 188, *198*
Nadel, J.A., 264, 265, *270*, 393, 400,
  410, *414*
Nadler, J.L., 27, 34, *39*
Naeije, N., 529, *536*
Nagano, T., 456, 464, *468*, 469, *470*
Nagata, M., 304, *313*, 357, 361, *365*,
  371, *384*
Nagy, L., 400, *414*
Nair, N.M., 222, *228*
Nairn, J.R., *269*
Nakamura, Y., 204, *211*
Nakane, M., 237, *249*
Nakanishi, S., 36, 37, *43*
Nakano, T., 284, *294*
Nakashima, H., 289, *297*
Nakashima, T., 478, *489*

Nalefski, E.A., 29, 30, *40*
Naline, E., 432, *438*
Namba, T., 256, *258*
Namboodri, M.M., 148, *158*
Nanmour, T.M., 77, 78, *87*
Napier, F.E., 430, *436*
Narko, K., 26, 34, *39*, 118, 121, *126*, *127*
Narumiya, S., 36, 37, *43*, *44*, 97, *107*,
  256, *257*, *258*
Nasjletti, A., 32, *42*, 62, *74*
Naspitz, C.K., 222, *227*
Nassar, G.M., 287, *297*
Nasser, S.M.S., 302, 308, *311*, *314*, 324,
  327, *328*, 329, *334*, *335*, 338, *342*,
  344, *349*, 357, 359, 360, *365*, *367*,
  372, 380, 381, *385*, 424, 429, *434*,
  495, 498, *503*, *504*, 534, *537*
Nastainczyk, W., 170, 171, *185*
Natarajan, R., 27, 34, *39*
Nathan, C., 118, *126*
Natoli, C., 9, *21*, 80, 84, *88*
Naumann, T., 98, *108*
Nava, E., 273, *281*
Navar, L.G., 33, *42*
Nayyar, S., 479, *490*
Nebert, D.W., 47, 48, *69*
Needleman, P., 3, *17*, 34, *43*, 119, *126*,
  129, *140*, 232, 233, 235, *245*, *246*,
  285, *295*
Neeley, S.P., 284, *293*, 401, 402, *416*
Neely, J.D., 205, *212*, 222, *228*
Negishi, M., 37, *43*, 256, *258*
Neill, K.H., 400, *414*
Neill, M.A., 409, *418*
Neilson, K., 118, *126*
Nelson, D.R., 47, 48, *69*
Nelson, H.S., 300, *310*
Nelson, R.P., 529, *536*
Nelson, S., 273, *281*
Nemenoff, R.A., 29, *40*, *41*
Nemoto, Y., 289, *297*
Nevalainen, T.J., 284, *294*
Newball, H., 259, 264, *268*, 358, 359,
  366
Newman, J.H., 78, *87*
Newman, S.P., 114, 119, *124*, *126*

Newton, R., 16, *23*, 114–19, *124*, *125*, *126*, 302, *311*
Ney, P., 253, *257*
Ng, K.K.F., 32, *42*
Nguyen, B., 146, *157*
Nials, A.T., 253, *257*
Niankowska, E., 284, *293*
Nichizuka, Y., 29, *40*
Nichol, G., 113, *123*
Nicholson, D.W., 392, 401, 405, *409*, *415*, *417*
Nicolas, J., 515, *521*
Nicolson, G.L., 169, *184*
Nicosia, S., 56, *72*
Nielson, K., 130, *141*
Nieves, A.L., 342, *349*, 383, *389*
Nieves, B., 273, 274, 280, *281*
Niho, Y., 289, *297*
Nii, Y., 400, *414*
Niiro, H., 289, *297*
Nijkamp, F.P., 231, 234–40, *245*, *246*, *247*, *248*, *249*, *250*, *251*
Nikander, K., 283, *292–93*
Ninis, R.W., 50, *70*
Nish, W.A., 206, *212*
Nishigaki, N., 256, *258*
Nishimura, Y., 206, *213*
Nishioka, S., *335*
Nisperos, B., 319, *332*
Niv, Y., 112, *123*, 286, *296*, 514, *520*
Nix, A., 113, *123*
Nizankowska, E., 91, *104*, 207, *213*, 223, *228*, 300–309, *310*, *311*, *312*, *313*, *314*, *315*, 321, 323, 326, 328, *333*, *334*, 337, 339, 342, 343, 347, *348*, *350*, 359–62, *367*, *369*, 371–83, *384*, *385*, 419, 421, 423, 424, 428, *432*, *433*, *434*, 441, 442, 449, *450*, 464, 469, *471*, *472*, 496–99, 502, *503*, *504*, *505*, 525, 528, 529, *535*, *536*
Nizankowska, G., 223, *229*
Noah, T.L., 235, *247*
Nogami, H., 114, *124*
Noguchi, Y., 240, *251*
Nomot, T.E., 204, *212*

Noordhoek, J.A., 514, *520*
Norman, P.S., 319, *332*, 460, *471*, 499, *504*
Norris, A.A., 429, *436*
Norrs, A., 429, *436*
North, A.J., 25, 34, *39*, 237, *249*
Nourooz-Zadeh, J., 79, *88*
Noveral, J.P., 116, *125*
Nowak, D., 514, *520*
Nozawa, K., 27, 34, *39*
Nucera, E., 500, *504*
Nucero, E., 300, *310*
Nugent, K.P., 4, *18*
Nugent, M.J., 13, *22*
Nugteren, D.H., 161, *183*
Numao, T., 402, *416*
Numokawa, Y., 138, *143*
Nüsing, R., 5, 6, *18*, *19*, *23*, 96, *107*, 146, *155*

O

Oae, S., 237, *249*
Oates, J., 91, *104*, 305, 307, 309, *313*, 337, 339, 342, 343, 347, *348*, 361, 371, 378, 380, 381, 382, *384*, 496, 497, 498, *504*
Oates, J.A., 60, 62, 63, *73*, 78, 79, 82, 87, 286, 287, 288, *296*, *297*, 303, *312*, 321, 323, 328, *333*, 337, 339, 343, *348*, 358–62, *366*, *367*, *368*, 371, 381, *384*, 394, 408, *412*, *417*, 419, 428, *432*, 496, 497, 498, *503*, 507, 512, 514, *517*, *519*, *520*
O'Banion, M.K., 3, *17*, 146, 147, *156*, 285, *295*, 512, *519*
O'Brien, W.F., 8, *21*
O'Byrne, P.M., 56, *72*, 113, 114, *123*, *124*, 216, 222, *224*, 242, *251*, 259, 263, 264, 265, *268*, *269*, *270*, *271*, 283, 284, *292*, *293*, 347, *350*, 360, *367*, 397, *413*
Ocetkiewicz, A., 284, *294*
O'Connor, B.J., 431, *437*
O'Connor, G.T., 224, *229*

Odlander, B., 191, 192, *200*
O'Donnell, W.J., 303, *312*, 514, *520*
Oesterhelt, D., 162, *184*
Offerhaus, G.J.A., 148, *158*
Ogihara, T., 232, 233, *246*
Ogino, K., 6, *19*
Ogino, M., 6, *19*
Ogino, N., 129, *140*, 161, *183*
Ogino, S., 456, 464, 468, 469, *470*
Ogle, C., 274, *282*
Oglesby, T.D., 56, *72*
Ogorochi, T., 97, *107*
Ohara, O., 284, *294*
Ohashi, K., 140, *143*
Ohashi, Y., 382, *389*
O'Hearn, D.J., 188, *199*
O'Hickey, S.P., 308, *314*, 327, *335*, 357, 361, *365*, 534, *537*
Ohmori, K., 408, *418*
Ohno, I., 482, *490*, 494, 495, 496, *503*
Ohno, T., 6, *19*
Oho, J.C., 136, *142*
Ohta, N., 206, *213*
Ojo, T.C., 94, *105*
Okada, T., 454, 457, 467, *470*
Okanlami, D.A., 307, *314*
Okano, H., 99, *108*
Okawachi, I., 456, 464, 468, 469, *470*
Okita, R.T., 47, 56, *69*, *72*
Okret, S., 508, 510, *517*, *518*
Okudaira, H., 394, *411*
Okuma, M., 37, *44*
Olazon, I., 441, *450*
Oldigs, M., 514, *520*
Olinsky, A., 218, *226*
Oliverio, S., 148, *159*
Oliw, E.H., 46, 53, 59, 60, 62, 63, *69*, *71*, *73*
Ollerenshaw, S.L., 373, *386*
Olson, D.M., 8, *21*
Olsson, I., 373, *387*
Omata, K., 34, *43*
Omura, T., 45, *68*
O'Neill, G.P., 4, 6, *18*, *19*, *23*, 26, 34, *39*, 146, 147, 148, *157*, *159*
O'Neill, K.L., 149, *160*

Oosterhoff, Y., 112, *123*, 514, *520*
Oosterhout, A.J.M., 238, *250*
Opas, E., 97, *108*
Opdenakker, G., 217, 219, 221, *226*
Orehek, J., 235, *247*, *248*
Orita, K., 50, *69*
Orloff, J., 4, *18*
Orti, E., 510, *517*
Ortiz de Montellano, P.R., 34, *43*, 45, 46, 49, 50, 53, *68*, *69*, *70*
Ortolani, C., 303, *312*, 419, *432*
Os, M., 478, *489*
Osawa, Y., 50, *70*
Osen, E., 146, *157*
O'Shaughnessy, K.M., *271*, 284, 287, 288, *293*, *297*, 362, *368*, *369*, 408, *417*
Oshima, H., 4, *18*
Oshima, M., 4, *18*
O'Sullivan, 359, 361, *367*
O'Sullivan, B.P., 280, *282*
O'Sullivan, M., 117, *125*
O'Sullivan, S., 343, *350*, 380, *388*, 428, *436*, 514, *520*
Otes, J.A., 287, 288, 289, *297*
Otomo, S., 7, *20*, *23*, 122, *127*, 131, *141*
Otsuka, T., 289, *297*
Otto, J., 25, 26, 30, 33, 34, 35, *38*, *43*, 96, *107*, 147, *158*, 164, 169, *184*, 285, *294*, 317, *332*
Ouellet, M., *23*, 146, 147, *157*
Overbeek, S., 514, *520*
Owen, W.F. Jr., 392, 394, 401, 409, *411*, *412*, *415*
Ownbey, R.T., 342, *349*
Oyekan, A., 50, 62, 66, *70*

P

Pace, D., 263, 265, *270*, *271*
Pacini, R., 374, *387*
Paddupakkam, R.K., 460, 465, *471*
Padovano, A., 420, *433*
Padovano, R., 82, *88*
Pagano, P.J., 32, *42*

Page, C.P., 111, *123*
Paggiaro, P.L., 511, 513, 515, *518*, *519*, *522*
Pain, M., 218, *226*
Paine, R., 98, *108*
Pais, J.M., 12, *22*
Pajak, A., 441, *450*
Pak, J., 209, *214*, 222, *228*
Pak, J.P., 146, *157*
Palmer, G., 170, 171, 174, *185*
Palmer, J., 148, *158*
Palmer, J.B., 235, *247*
Palmer, R.M.J., 138, *143*
Pamukcu, R., 149, 150, 154, *159*, *160*
Panah, S., 9–10, *21*
Panara, M.R., 9, *21*, 80, 82, 84, *88*
Pancré, V., 440, *449*
Panczenko, B., 235, *247*, 284, *294*
Panhuysen, C.I.M., 205, *212*, 222, *228*
Paoletti, P., 511, *518*
Pape, G.R., 209, *214*
Paradis, L., 515, *522*
Paradiso, A.M., 235, *247*
Paranka, N.S., 149, 150, 154, *159*, *160*
Paraskeva, C., 149, 150, *160*
Parè, P., 222, *227*
Parente, L., 511, 513, *518*, *519*
Pariente, A., 148, *158*
Pariente, R., 237, *250*
Park, H.S., 422, *433*, 524, *535*
Park, K.K., 509, 511, *517*
Park, S.S., 49, *69*
Parker, R.E., 140, *144*
Parker, W.A. Jr., 206, *212*
Parnham, M.J., 14, 15, *22*
Parratt, J.R., 273, 276, 279, *280*
Parronchi, P., 209, *213*
Parsons, S., 392, 409
Parsons, W.G. III, 393, *410*
Parthasarathy, S., 129, 138, *143*
Partridge, M.R., 423, *433*, 528, *536*
Pasargiklian, M., 347, *350*, 358, *366*, 420, 421, 424, 426, 429, 431, *432*, *433*, *434*, *435*, 468, *471*, 498, *504*
Passalacqua, G., 13, 16, *22*

Pastor, C., 274, *282*
Patel, I., 103, *109*
Patel, I.R., 232, *245*
Patel, M., 308, *314*, 327, 328, *335*, 361, 379, *388*, 534, *537*
Patel, S., 115, *125*
Patriarca, G., 300, *310*, 500, *504*
Patrignani, P., 9, *21*, 80, 82, 84, *88*
Patrono, C., 9, *21*, 78, 79, 80, 82, 84, *87*, *88*
Patry, C., 392, *409*
Pattemore, P.K., 231, *245*
Paul, J.E., 219, *227*
Paul, W.E., 188, 191, *198*, *200*
Pauletti, D., 9, 10, 11, *21*
Paul-Eugene, N., 192, *200*
Paulmichl, M., 429, *436*
Pauwels, R., 304, *313*, 362, *368*
Pavlovic, D., 237, *250*
Pavord, I.D., 96, *107*, 113, 115, 122, *124*, *125*, 255, *257*, 306, 307, *314*, 347, *350*, 360, 361, *367*, 371, 380, *385*, 431, *437*
Payen, D., 274, *282*
Pazdur, R., 148, *158*
Pearce, F.L., 430, *436*
Pearce, S.F.A., 235, *247*
Pearlman, H., 362, *368*
Pearson, D.J., 301, *311*
Peat, J.K., 222, 224, *227*, *229*
Pecht, I., 429, *436*
Pedersen, C.B., 501, *505*
Pedersen, M., 217, *226*
Pedrosa Ribeiro, C.M., 34, *42*
Pelaez, A., 429, *436*
Pelaez, Z., 468, *471*
Pellegrino, S., 500, *504*
Pelletier, G., 372, 380, *386*, 479, *490*
Peltonen, L., 462, *471*
Pengelly, D., 475, *488*
Penneton, M., 13, 14, *22*, 122, *127*
Penning, T.D., 146, *157*
Penrose, J.F., 28, *40*, 99, *108*, 302, 303, 304, 307, 308, *312*, *313*, 361, 372–79, 381, 382, 383, *385*, *387*, *388*, 389, 392, 393, *409*, *410*

Pepinsky, R.B., 510, 511, *518*, *519*
Pepperl, D.J., 256, *258*
Pepys, J., 218, *226*
Peri, K.G., 7, *19*
Perin, P.V., 216, *225*
Perin, S., 239, *251*
Perkins, R.S., 403, 405, *416*, *417*
Perkins, W., 13, *22*, 135, *142*, 146, *156*
Permutt, S., 112, *123*, 286, *296*, 514, *520*
Perrier, H., 374, *387*
Perrin, D.M., 136, *142*
Persson, C.G.A., 477, 479, *489*
Persson, T., 283, *292–93*
Peters, J., 103, *109*
Peters, J.M., 27, 28, *40*
Peters, M.J., 119, *126*
Peters, S.P., 285, 286, 289, *295*, *296*, 358, 359, *366*, 372, 380, *385*, *386*, 514, 515, *521*, *522*
Petersen, J., 401, *415*
Petersen, M., 474, *488*
Peters-Golden, M., 94, 97, 98, 102, 103, *105*, *108*, *109*, 146, *156*, 285, 286, 289, 292, *295*, *296*, 298, 512, 514, *519*
Peterson, C., 373, *387*
Peterson, J.A., 59, *73*
Petres, S.P., 287, *297*
Petrigine, G., 498, *504*
Petrigni, G., 300, 302, *310*, *312*, 347, *350*, 380, *388*, 420–24, 429, 431, *432*, *433*, *434*, 468, *471*
Petrini, G., 351, 352, 357, *364*, 523, 524, 525, *535*
Petros, A., 274, *281*
Pfeilschifter, J., 5, *18*, *23*
Pfister, R., 217, 219–23, *225*, *226*, *227*, 302, 308, *311*, 329, *335*, 338, 342, 344, *349*, 359, 360, 361, *367*, 372–76, 378, 380, 381, *385*, 495, 498, *503*, *504*
Phare, S.M., 94, *105*
Phelan, P., 218, *226*
Phillipin, B., 237, *249*
Phillips, G.D., 304, *313*, 353, *364*, 524, *535*

Phillips, R.K.S., 4, *18*
Philpot, R., 132, *141*
Phipps, R.P., 149, *159*, 253, *257*
Piacentini, G.L., 398, *414*
Piacentini, M., 148, *159*
Piazza, G.A., 149, 150, 154, *159*, *160*
Picado, C., 300, 303, 304, 305, *310*, *312*, *313*, 337, 347, *348*, 358, 360, *366*, 380, 381, *388*, 432, *438*, 457, 467, *471*, 495, 496, 497, 500, *503*, *504*, *505*
Picard, D., 508, *517*
Picard, S., 393, 394, *410*, *411*
Pickering, S.A.W., 233, *246*
Pickett, W.C., 400, *414*
Pickl, W.F., 206, *212*
Picot, D., 2, *17*, 45, *68*, 130, *140*, 145, 152, *155*, 162, 163, 164, 166, 167, 174, 176, 178, 179, *184*, *186*
Piechuta, H., 362, *368*
Piera, C., 432, *438*
Pierce, K.L., 256, *258*
PierFranco, S., 150, 152, *160*
Pieroni, M., 91, 96, *104*, 301, 304, 306, *311*, *313*, *314*, 321, *333*, 347, *350*, 360, 361, *367*, 371, *385*, *421*, *422*, 424–31, *433*, *434*, *435*, *436*, *437*, *438*
Pierson, W., 362, *368*
Pietroni, M.G., 302, *312*
Pike, K.D., 206, *213*
Pilar Garcia, M., 31, *42*
Pilbeam, C.C., 132, *142*, 146, *156*
Pile, K., 207, 209, *213*, 308, *315*
Pileri, S., 374, *387*
Pilote, S., 402, *416*
Pina, J., 456, 459, *470*
Pinis, G., 304, *313*, 326, *334*, 362, *369*, 441, *450*, 502, *505*
Piper, P.J., 395, 397, *413*, 514, *520*
Pipkorn, U., 287, *297*, 372, 380, *385*, *386*, 514, *521*
Pirson, F., 222, *228*
Pittas, A., 149, *159*
Pivirotto, F., 219, 221, *227*, 515, *522*
Pizzi, M., 150, 152, *160*

Platts-Mills, T.A.E., 217, 222, *225*, *227*
Plaza, V., 303, 305, *312*, 323, *334*, 337, 347, *348*, 358, 360, *366*, 380, 381, *388*, 496, 497, *504*
Pleskow, W.W., 352, 358, *364*, *366*, 460, *471*, 501, *505*, 523, 524, 526, 529, *535*, *536*
Pober, J., 94, *105*
Poellinger, L., 508, 510, *517*, *518*
Poggi, S., 374, *387*
Polak, J.M., 115, *125*
Pollice, M., 286, *296*
Pollock, J.S., 237, *249*
Polosa, R., 264, *270*
Polson, J.B., 235, *247*
Pomerantz, K.B., 235, *247*
Pong, A.S., 3, *17*, 129, *140*
Poniatowska, M., 305, *313*, 329, *335*, 498, *504*
Ponomarev, M., 182, *186*
Ponta, H., 509, 511, *517*
Porter, T.D., 48, 68, *69*
Portman, O.W., 138, *143*
Posnett, D.N., 208, *213*
Post, T.J., 402, *416*
Postma, D.S., 112, *123*, 205, *212*, 222, *228*, 514, *520*
Poston, R.N., 515, *521*
Poubelle, F.P., 515, *521*
Poubelle, P.E., 395, *413*
Powell, W.S., 198, *200*, 393, 394, *411*
Pradelles, P., 80, *88*, 238, *250*, 344, *350*
Prakash, C., 60, 63, *73*, *74*, 253, *257*, 306, *314*
Prakash, O., 206, *212*
Pramanik, B., 30, *41*
Prasit, P., 13, 14, *22*, 374, *387*
Prat, J., 303, 305, *312*, 323, *334*, 337, 347, *348*, 358, 360, *366*, 380, 381, *388*, 432, *437*, 496, 497, *504*
Praticò, D., 79, 80, 86, *88*, *89*
Pratt, W.P., 508, *517*
Praxton, J., 130, *140*
Prefontaine, K.E., 119, *126*, 511, *518*
Preissler, U., 237, *249*

Prescott, S.M., 4, *18*, 130, *141*, 148, *159*, 222, 228
Price, J., 479, *489*, *490*
Price, J.F., 514, *520*
Prickman, L.E., 320, *332*
Pride, N.B., 113, *124*
Prin, L., 442, *450*
Proctor, K.G., 25, 27, 34, *38*
Profita, M., 514, *520*
Proud, D., 112, *123*, 235, *247*, 286, *296*, 360, *367*, 514, *520*
Prough, R.A., 59, *73*
Prytz, S., 501, *505*
Pucci, M.L., 32, *42*
Puett, D., 122, *127*
Pujol, J.L., 401, *415*
Pype, J.L., 427, 430, *435*, *437*

Q

Qiao, L., 149, *159*
Qiu, Z., 94, *105*
Quanjer, P.H., 216, 222, *224*
Quero, A.M., 239, *251*
Quilley, J., 29, 38, *40*, *44*, 50, 60, *70*, *73*
Quinn, M.T., 129, 138, *143*
Quinones, S., 273, 280, *281*
Quiralte, J., 299, *310*
Quirce, S., 222, *227*
Qvortrup, K., 477, *489*

R

Ra, C., 204, *211*
Raatgeep, R.C., 397, *414*
Rabasseda, X., 13, *22*
Rabbri, L., 217, 223, *226*
Rabe, K.F., 397, 401, 403, 405, 407, *414*, *416*, *417*, 514, *520*
Rabinovitch, H., 393, *410*
Rackemann, F.M., 217, *225*
Radermecker, M., 219, *227*
Radhika, A., 148, *158*, *159*

Radmark, O., 27, *39*, 99, *108*, 191, 192, 200, 374, *387*, 393, *410*
Radomski, M., 301, *311*
Rafferty, J., 274, *282*
Raffestin, B., 360, *367*
Rahm, A.L.K., 149, 150, 154, *159*
Rahm, K., 149, *160*
Rahmsdorf, H.J., 509, 511, *517*
Raible, D.G., 393, 402, *411*, *416*
Raij, L., 274, *281*
Raine, D.A., 300, *310*
Rainey, D.K., 429, *436*
Rainsford, K.D., 233, 234, *246*
Raiss, L.G., 132, *142*, 146, *156*
Ramanadham, S., 95, *106*
Ramden, P., 237, *249*
Ramesha, C., 2, *17*, 29, *41*, 94, *105*, 163, 164, 169, 170, 178, 179, 181, *184*, 374, *387*
Ramis, I., 303, 305, *312*, 323, *334*, 337, 347, *348*, 358, 360, *366*, 380, 381, *388*, 432, *438*, 496, 497, *504*
Ramon, P., 442, 444, *450*
Ramsdale, E.H., 259, *268*, 283, *292*
Ramwell, P.W., 393, *410*
Rand, T.H., 394, *412*
Randle, D.L., 320, *332*, 464, *471*
Rands, E., 97, *108*
Rangwala, S.H., 2, *17*, *23*, 122, *127*, 180, *186*
Ransay, A.J., 188, 195, 197, *199*
Ransil, B.J., 303, *312*, 514, *520*
Rao, B.S., 206, *212*
Rao, C.V., 7, *20*, 148, *159*
Rao, G., 94, 95, *105*, *106*
Rao, P.V., 206, *212*
Rasberg, B., 304, *313*, 326, *334*, 362, *369*, 502, *505*
Rasmussen, N., 477, *489*
Rasori, R., 13, 14, *22*
Rasp, G., 343, *350*
Raud, J., 360, *367*
Ravalese, J. III, 401, *415*
Raven, J., 204, *211*, 222, *228*
Ravenscraft, M.D., 79, *88*
Rawlins, M.D., 8, *21*

Ray, A., 119, 122, *126*, *127*, 510, 511, 518
Ray, B.S., 188, 192, *199*
Raychowdhury, M.K., 37, *44*
Raz, A., 3, *17*, 285, *295*
Razen, J.M., 192, *200*
Reddy, B.S., 148, *159*
Reddy, K.M., 62, *74*
Reddy, N., 132, *141*
Reddy, S., 95, *106*
Reddy, S.T., 81, *88*, 147, *158*, 285, *294*
Redington, A., 237, *249*
Redington, A.F., 115, *125*
Reece, E.R., 188, *198*
Reed, D., 150, 152, 153, *160*
Reed, H.E., 238, *250*
Reed, W., 6, *19*
Refini, M., 422, 426, *433*, *434*
Refini, R.M., 91, 96, *104*, 301, 302, 304, 306, *311*, *312*, *313*, *314*, 321, *333*, 347, *350*, 360, 361, *367*, 371, 380, *385*, *388*, 421, 424–31, *433*, *434*, *435*, *436*, *438*
Regan, J.W., 256, *258*
Regier, M., 94, 96, *105*, *106*, *107*
Regier, M.K., 30, 35, *41*, *43*, 136, *142*, 147, *158*, 169, *184*, 285, *294*
Regnard, J., 432, *438*
Regoli, D., 115, *125*
Reich, N.O., 49, 53, *69*
Reid, L.M., 400, *414*
Reid, M.J., 206, *212*
Reijnart, I., 236, 238, 239, *248*
Reilly, J., 237, *249*, 361, 375, *388*
Reilly, M., 79, *88*
Reinikainen, K., 283, *292–93*
Reinsprecht, M., 429, *436*
Reiss, T.F., 304, *313*, 531, *537*
Reisz, P., 51, *70*
Remick, D., 253, *257*
Ren, Y., 153, *160*
Renaud, J.P., 46, *68*
Rengasamy, A., 237, 239, *250*, *251*
Renkawitz, R., 510, *517*
Renon, D., 283, *292*, 514, *521*
Renz, H., 188, 192, *199*

Repine, J.E., 280, *282*
Repine, M.J., 280, *282*
Resau, J.H., 235, *247*, 360, *367*
Resch, K., 146, 152, *155*
Resnick, M.B., 342, *349*
Rettori, V., 233, *246*
Reuter, B.K., 292, *298*
Rex, J., 7, *19*
Rexin, M., 508, *517*
Rhangwala, S.H., 146, *157*
Rhoden, K.J., 115, *125*
Riano, H.F., 4, *18*
Ricci, M., 217, 219, 223, *226*, *227*
Ricciardolo, F.L.M., 238, *250*
Rice, G.E., 8, *21*
Rice, H.M., 148, *159*
Rice, T.W., 237, *250*
Richard, J., 479, *490*
Richards, J.S., 3, *17*, 135, *142*, 146, *156*
Richardson, C., 98, *108*
Richmond, R., 360, *367*
Riddick, C.A., 286, 287, *296*, *297*
Riechelmann, H., 514, *520*
Rieke, C.J., 173, *185*
Riendeau, D., 4, 13, 14, *18*, *22*
Riethmüller, G., 209, *214*
Rifkind, A.B., 34, *43*, 50, 51, *70*
Rigas, B., 149, *159*
Rihs, S., 395, *412*
Rinaldi, M., 303, *312*, 419, *432*
Ring, W.L., 286, 287, *296*, *297*
Ristimaki, A., 26, 34, *39*, 118, 121, *126*, *127*
Ritter, J.M., 322, *333*
Rivenson, A., 148, *159*
Rivera, A., 273, 274, 280, *281*
Riveros-Moreno, V., 237, *249*
Rizzo, M.C., 222, *227*
Robbins, R.A., 6, *19*, 114, 115, 119, *124*, 237, *250*, 285, *295*, 302, *311*, 512, *519*
Roberge, C.J., 395, *413*, 515, *521*
Roberts, E., 94, *105*
Roberts, J.A., 373, 382, *386*, *389*
Roberts, J.M., 232, 233, 234, *246*
Roberts, L.J., 111, *123*, 146, *156*, 507, 514, *517*

Roberts, L.J.I., 358, 359, *366*, *367*
Roberts, L.J. II, 77, 78, 79, 82, *87*, *88*, 111, *123*, 255, *257*, 286, 287, 288, *296*, *297*, 358, 359, 360, 362, *366*, *368*, 393, 394, *410*, *412*
Roberts, L.J. III, 287, *297*
Roberts, R., 259, 264, *268*, *269*
Robertson, D.L., 3, *17*, 25, 34, *39*, 130, *141*, 146, 147, 148, *156*, *158*, *159*, 162, *183*, 285, *294*
Robin, E.C., 27, 34, *39*
Robin, E.D., 447, *450*
Robinson, C., 113, 114, *123*, *124*, 259, 264, *269*, 358, 359, *366*
Robinson, D.S., 217, 219, 220, 221, 223, *226*, *227*, 289, *298*, 382, *389*
Robinson, M.A., 208, *213*
Robinson, R.C., 68, *75*
Robuschi, M., 91, 96, *104*, 300, 301, 302, 304, 306, *310*, *311*, *312*, *313*, *314*, 321, *333*, 347, *350*, 351, 352, 357, 358, 360, 361, *364*, *366*, *367*, 371, 380, *385*, *388*, 420–27, 429, 430, 431, *432*, *433*, *434*, *435*, *436*, *438*, 468, *471*, 498, *504*
Roca-Ferrer, J., 495, 496, *503*
Roche, W.R., 238, *250*, 361, 373, *386*, *387*, 494, *503*, 507, *516*
Rocheleau, H., 408, *417*
Rock, C., 94, *105*
Rodger, I.W., 13, 14, *22*
Rodkey, J., 28, *40*
Rodriguez, L.A.G., 8, 9, *21*
Rodwell, L.T., 431, *437*
Roebber, M., 206, *212*
Roehlig, F., 309, *315*
Rogers, D.F., 400, *414*
Rogers, T.B., 34, 35, *43*
Rokach, J., 56, *72*, 266, *271*, 362, *368*
Rola-Pleszczynski, M., 192, *200*, 392, *409*
Rollins, T., 92, 96, *104*
Romagnani, S., 209, *213*, 217, 223, *226*
Roman, R.J., 34, *43*, 50, 58, 62, *70*, *73*
Romar, A., 429, *436*, 468, *471*
Rome, L.H., 173, *185*

Romero, M., 33, *42*
Roos, D., 403, *416*
Roper, R.L., 253, *257*
Rosello, J., 303, 305, *312*, 323, *334*,
  337, 347, *348*, 358, 360, *366*, 380,
  381, *388*, 496, 497, *504*
Rosen, A., 192, *200*
Rosen, R., 28, *40*
Rosenberg, A.M., 337, *348*
Rosenberg, L., 148, *158*
Rosenberg, M., 91, *104*
Rosenberg, M.A., 304, 305, *313*, 324,
  329, *334, 335*, 337, 343, *348*, 357,
  358, 360, *365, 366*, 371, *384*, 428,
  435, 496, 497, 498, 502, *504*
Rosenberg, W.M.C., 206, 208, *213*
Rosenbusch, J.P., 162, *184*
Rosenkranz, B., 54, *75*
Rosenthal, R., 362, *368*
Rosenthal, R.R., 499, *504*
Rosenwasser, L.J., 188, 193, *199*
Rosette, C., *127*, 510, *518*
Roshak, A., 284, *293*
Rossellò-Cafatau, J., 432, *438*
Rossi, A.G., 393, 394, *411*
Rossoni, G., 426, 427, *434, 435*
Rosteiro, F.M., 12, *22*
Rostgaard, J., 477, *489*
Rot, A., 342, *349*
Roth, H.J., 394, *412*
Rothenberg, M.E., 342, *349*, 401, *415*
Rothwell, N.J., 510, *518*
Rotondo, M.T., 82, *88*
Rottoli, L., 426, 428, 429, *435*
Roubin, R., 401, *415*
Rouse, C., 343, *350*
Roux, S., 515, *521*
Rouzer, C., 28, *40*
Rouzer, C.A., 97, *107, 108*, 374, *387*
Rowley, J.D., 204, *211*
Roy, P., 13, 14, *22*
Rozman, M., 495, 496, *503*
Rozniecki, I., 358, *366*
Rozniecki, J., 303, 305, 307, *312, 314*,
  329, *335*, 456, 460, 464, 469, *470*,
  525, *535*

Ruan, K., 96, *107*
Ruan, K.-H., 140, *143*, 153, *160*
Ruangyuttikarn, W., 49, *69*
Rubin, P., 91, *104*, 304, 305, *313*, 324,
  329, *334, 335*, 337, 343, *348*, 357,
  358, 360, 362, *365, 366, 368*, 371,
  384, 428, *435*, 496, 497, 498, 502,
  504
Rucknagel, D.L., 319, *332*, 460, *471*
Rudack, C., 482, *490*
Ruddle, N.H., 35, *43*
Rudehill, A., 274, 280, *282*
Rudent, A., 239, *251*
Ruf, H.H., 170, *171, 185*
Ruffin, R.E., *269*
Rühlmann, E., 405, 407, *417*
Ruhno, J., 479, *489*
Rundcratz, H., 501, *505*
Runge, M., 95, *106*
Rupniak, N.M.J., 14, *22*
Rutgers, B., 112, *123*
Rutherford, B.C., 284, *293*
Ryan, G., 204, 208, *211, 213*, 259, *268*
Ryan, G.E., 210, *214*
Ryan, G.R., 205, *212*
Rybalova, S., 28, 30, 31, *40*, 62, *74*
Rychlicka, J., 358, *366*
Ryeom, S., 92, *104*

S

Sabattini, E., 374, *387*
Sacerdoti, D., 62, *74*
Sadeghi-Hashjin, G., 234, 236, 237,
  240, *246, 248, 249, 251*
Sadick, M.D., 209, *213*
Sadowski, H.B., 3, *17*, 146, 147, *156*
Sadowski, S., 28, *40*, 101, *108*
Saetta, M., 217, 219, 221, 223, *226, 227*
Safier, L.B., 56, *72*
Saga, T., 357, 361, *365*
Saito, H., 395, *412, 413*
Saito, M., 6, *19*
Sakakibara, H., 357, 361, *365*
Sakamoto, T., 113, *124*

Sakamoto, Y., 99, *108*, 304, *313*, 357, 361, *365*, 371, *384*

Sala, A., 34, *43*, 56, *71*, 72, 91, 96, *104*, 303, 306, *312*, *314*, 321, 322, *333*, 347, *350*, 361, 371, *385*, 393, *410*, 419, 422, 424, 425, 427, 429, *432*, *433*, *434*, *435*

Sala, P., 360, *367*

Salari, H., 372, 380, *386*, 393, *410*, 479, *490*

Salén, E.B., 361, *368*

Salkine, M.L., 218, *226*

Salmeron, S., 283, *292*

Salome, C.M., 259, *268*

Salter, M., 273, *281*

Salvador, E.V., 33, *42*

Salvemini, D., 34, *43*, 119, *126*, 232, 233, 235, *245*, *246*

Samet, J., 6, *19*, 95, *105*, *106*, 132, *141*, 286, *296*

Sampson, A.P., 302, 303, 304, 307, 308, *312*, 371–79, 381, 382, 383, *384*, *385*, 395, *413*, 507, 514, *516*, *520*, 531, *537*

Samter, M., 223, *229*, 299, 300, 302, 304, *309*, 309, 318, *332*, 361, *368*, 451, 463, *470*, *471*

Samuelsson, B., 27, *39*, *40*, 56, *72*, 170, *185*, 188, 191, 192, *199*, *200*, 266, *271*, 321, *333*, 374, *387*, 393, 397, *410*, *413*, 507, *516*, 520, 532, *537*

Sandford, A., 222, *227*

Sandford, A.J., 204, *211*

Sanduja, R., 3, *18*

Sanduja, S.K., 130, 140, *141*, *143*

Sano, H., 26, 34, *39*, 148, *159*

Sansonetti, M., 222, *228*

Santini, G., 82, *88*

Saper, C.B., 7, *20*

Sapsford, R.J., 477, *489*

Sarge, K., 95, *106*

Saroea, H.G., 113, *123*

Sasaki, H., 397, *414*

Sasaki, S., 204, *212*

Sasazuki, T., 206, *213*

Satchawatcharaphong, C., 9–10, *21*

Sato, R., 45, 47, 48, *68*, *69*

Satoh, K., 222, *228*

Saulnier, F., 300, *310*

Saunders, M.A., 115, 116, 117, 119, *125*

Sautebin, L., 233, *246*

Sauter, G., 96, *107*

Savage, R., 8, 9, *21*

Savelkoul, H.F.J., 238, *250*

Scanlon, P.D., 397, *413*

Schafer, D., 91, 96, *104*

Schall, T.J., 342, *349*

Schapowal, A.G., 469, *472*

Scharschmidt, L.A., 33, 34, *42*

Schatz, M., 352, *364*, 529, *536*

Schaub, E., 420, *433*

Scheffer, H., 204, *211*

Scheiner, O., 206, *212*

Scheinman, R.I., 119, *127*, 510, *518*

Scheinmann, P., 512, *519*

Schellenberg, R.R., 393, *410*

Schenkman, J.B., 46, 49, 53, 68, *69*, *71*

Scherrer, M., 457, *470*

Scheuerer, S., 7, *20*

Schiavino, D., 500, *504*

Schieber, E.B., 30, *41*, 62, 65, *74*

Schievella, A., 94, *105*

Schinder, H., 429, *436*

Schindler, M., 30, 35, *41*, *43*, 96, *106*, *107*, 136, *142*, 147, *158*, 169, *184*, 285, *294*

Schindler, U., 234, *246*

Schlegel, K., 11, *22*

Schleimer, R.P., 92, *104*, 285, 286, 287, *296*, *297*, 358, 359, *366*, 372, 380, *385*, *386*, 514, 515, *521*, *522*

Schlimmer, P., 442, *450*

Schlumberger, H.D., 223, *229*, 301, *310*

Schmidt, H.H.H.W., 234, 237, *246*, *249*

Schmiege, L.M., 239, *251*

Schmitz-Schumann, M., 207, *213*, 300, 302, 308, 309, *310*, *311*, *315*, 327, 329, *335*, 337, 338, 342, 344, *348*, *349*, 359, 360, 361, *367*, 372–76, 378, 380, 381, *385*, 420, *433*, 440, *449*, 469, *472*, 495, 498, *503*, *504*, 534, *537*

Schmitz-Schumann, V.M., 524, *535*
Schnedier, W.P., 53, *71*
Schnitzer, Chr., 11, *22*
Schnitzler, C., 11, *22*
Schoeffel, R.E., 264, *270*
Schotman, E., 289, *298*, 308, *315*, 495, 496, *503*
Schou, C., 205, 206, 208, *212*, *213*, 222, *228*
Schrank, P., 300, *310*, 528, *536*
Schreiber, J., 218, *226*
Schreiber, S.L., 508, *517*
Schreuers, A.J.M., 238, *250*
Schrör, K., 253, *257*
Schudt, C., 306, *314*, 361, 380, 381, *388*, 403, *417*
Schueler, V.J., 30, *41*
Schulman, E.S., 358, 359, *366*, 402, *416*
Schulz, R., 273, *281*
Schuster, A., 393, *410*
Schuster, V.L., 32, *42*
Schwartz, J.I., 263, 265, *269*
Schwartz, L.B., 308, *315*, 329, *335*, 339, 343, 344, *349*, *350*, 358, *367*, 372, 373, 382, *386*, *388*
Schwartzman, M.L., 27, 31, 33, *39*, *41*, *42*, 46, 58, 60, 62, 63, *69*, *73*, *74*
Schweizer, A., 12, *22*
Schwenke, D.C., 129, *143*
Sciulli, M.G., 82, *88*
Scoggan, K.A., 392, 401, *409*, *415*
Scott, D.W., 149, *159*
Scott, S., 92, 97, *104*
Scuri, M., 302, *312*, 380, *388*, 431, *437*
Seale, J.P., 431, *437*
Seamark, R.F., 344, *350*
Sears, M.R., 205, *212*, 221, 223, *227*
Sebaldt, R.J., 288, *297*, 362, *368*, 507, 514, *517*
Sedgwick, J.B., 408, *418*
Seeds, M., 95, *106*
Seeger, W., 514, *520*
Segal, A., 287, *297*
Segal, A.T., 362, *368*
Sehgal, P.B., 510, *518*
Sehmi, R., 393, 394, *411*

Seibert, K., 2, 3, 13, *17*, *22*, *23*, 34, *43*, 119, 122, *126*, *127*, 135, *142*, 146, *156*, *157*, 162, 180, *183*, *186*, 232, 233, 235, *245*, 285, *295*
Sek, S., 423, *433*, 528, *536*
Sekizawa, K., 397, *414*
Selroos, O., 283, *292–93*, 408, *417*
Selvakumar, B., 206, *212*
Senna, G.E., 13, 16, *22*
Serafin, A., 223, *228*, 309, *315*, 419, 424, *432*, 441, 442, 449, *450*
Serafin, W.E., 255, *257*
Sergant, M., 447, 448, *450*
Serhan, C., 98, *108*
Serhan, C.N., 147, *158*
Serwonska, M., 300, 304, *310*, 313, 468, *472*
Sestini, P., 91, 96, *104*, 301, 302, 304, 306, *311*, *312*, *313*, *314*, 321, *333*, 347, *350*, 360, 361, *367*, 371, 380, *385*, *388*, 421, 422, 424–31, *433*, *434*, *435*, *436*, *438*
Seth, A., 30, *41*
Setoguchi, K., 240, *251*
Settipane, G.A., 218, 223, *226*, *229*, 319, 320, *332*, 452, *457*, 458, 460, 464, 465, 469, *470*, *471*, 473, 474, 475, 479, 486, *488*
Settipane, R.A., 300, *310*, 527, *535*
Shahane, A., 304, *313*, 531, *537*
Shapiro, J., 91, *104*, 324, *334*, 337, *348*, 357, *365*, 371, *384*
Shapiro, S., 148, *158*
Sharkey, K.A., 292, *298*
Sharp, P.A., 203, 204, *211*
Shaskin, P., 191, *200*
Shatz, M., 523, 524, 526, *535*
Shaul, P., 237, *249*
Shaul, P.W., 25, 34, *39*
Shaw, A.E., 204, *211*
Shaw, R.J., 393, *410*, *411*, 515, *521*
Shearer, M.A., 430, *436*
Shedlofsky, S.I., 50, *70*
Sheffer, A.L., 215, 216, 217, 222, *224*, 358, *366*, 394, 409, *411*
Shelhamer, J.H., 321, *333*, 400, *414*

Sheller, E., 496, 497, 498, *503*
Sheller, J.R., 91, *104*, 113, *123*, 286,
    287, 288, 289, *296*, *297*, *298*, 303,
    305, 307, 309, *312*, *313*, 321, 323,
    328, *333*, 337, 339, 342, 343, 347,
    348, 359, 360, 361, 362, *367*, *368*,
    371, 378, 380, 381, 382, *384*, 408,
    417, 419, 428, *432*, 496, 497, 498,
    504, 507, 512, 514, *517*, *519*, 520
Shelly, C., 102, *109*
Shen, S.Y., 65, *74*
Shepherd, G.C., 253, *257*
Sheppard, D., 426, *434*
Sherrer, L.C., 508, *517*
Shida, T., 395, *412*, *413*
Shievella, A.R., 29, 30, *40*
Shiff, S.I., 149, *159*
Shigyo, M., 114, *124*
Shih, C., 86, *89*
Shih, N.-Y., 86, *89*
Shi-Hua Li, 307, *314*
Shiiki, S., 50, *69*
Shimizu, T., 27, 31, *39*, *40*, 374, *387*
Shimoji, K., 86, *89*
Shimokawa, T., 130, *140*, 170, 179,
    185, *186*
Shindo, K., 99, *108*, 402, 408, *416*, *417*,
    514, 515, 516, *520*, *521*, *522*
Shinhama, K., 237, *249*
Shipley, M.E., 400, *414*
Shipp, E., 59, *73*
Shirakawa, T.S., 204, *211*, *212*
Shirasaki, H., 119, *126*
Shirley, M.A., 56, *72*
Shish, C.-K., 9, 10, 11, *21*
Shore, S.A., 237, *249*
Shornick, L.P., 147, *157*
Shou, J., 274, *281*
Shuaib Nasser, S.M., 361, 371–76, 378,
    379, 381, *384*, *385*, *388*
Shubair, K.S., 500, *505*, 528, *536*
Shultz, P.J., 274, *281*
Shuman, T., 393, *410*
Shute, J.K., 306, *314*, 361, 380, 381,
    388, 403, *417*
Shutenko, Z.S., 234, *246*

Shyr, Y., 78, 79, 82, *87*
Sibbald, B., 222, *228*
Sicari, R., 511, 513, 515, *518*, *519*, *522*
Siconolfi, A., 274, *282*
Siddhanta, A.K., 30, *41*
Siebenlist, U., 118, *126*
Siegel, S.C., 362, *368*
Siegelman, M.H., 198, *200*
Sierra-Honigmann, M., 94, *105*
Sigal, E., 287, *297*, 393, *410*
Sigal, I.S., 28, *40*
Sigler, P., 508, *517*
Silberstein, D.S., 401, *415*
Silver, J., 208, *213*
Silver, R.M., 146, *156*
Simi, B., 148, *159*
Simmon, D.L., 135, *142*
Simmons, D.L., 3, 7, *17*, *20*, 25, 34, *39*,
    130, *141*, 145–50, 152, 153, *155*,
    156, *158*, *159*, *160*, 162, *183*, 285,
    294
Simmons, R.L., 274, *281*
Simon, H.U., 469, *472*
Simon, R.A., 300, 308, *310*, *314*, 327,
    334, 352, 358, *364*, *366*, 468, *472*,
    500, 501, *505*, 523, 524, 526, 528,
    529, 530, 531, *535*, *536*, *537*
Simons, R.L., 239, *251*
Simonson, S.G., 268, *271*
Simony-Lafontaine, J., 216, 219, *225*
Simoone, P., 358, *366*, 421, *433*
Sinclair, K.L., 510, *518*
Singel, D.J., 237, *249*
Singer, I., 92, 97, 98, 103, *104*, *108*
Singer, I.I., 286, *296*
Singer, S.J., 169, *184*
Sinicrope, F.A., 148, *158*
Sirois, J., 3, *17*, 135, *142*, 146, *156*
Sirois, P., 115, *125*, 392, 394, *409*, *412*
Sirous, J., 146, *156*
Sistonen, L., 95, *106*
Siwarski, D., 204, *211*
Sjödahl, R., 4, *18*, 148, *159*
Skorecki, K., 30, *41*
Sladek, K., 91, *104*, 113, *123*, 287, *297*,
    302–5, 307, 308, 309, *312*, *313*, 321,

[Sladek, K.]
   323, 328, 329, *333*, *334*, 337, 339,
   342, 343, 347, *348*, *349*, 355, 358–61,
   365, *367*, 371–83, *384*, *385*, 419,
   425, 428, *432*, *434*, 441, *450*, 496,
   497, 498, *503*, *504*, 534, *537*
Slater, D.M., 7, 8, *20*, 114, 115, 119,
   124, 302, *311*
Slater, E.P., 510, *518*
Sliman, N A , 500, *505*, 528, *536*
Sliwinska-Kowalska, M., 303, 305, *312*
Sloan, S.I., 339, 343, 344, *349*
Sloan, S.J., 305, *314*
Smardova, J., 152, *160*
Smith, A.P., 223, *229*
Smith, C.H., 357, 361, *365*
Smith, C.J., 146, *156*
Smith, C.M., 303, 304, *312*, *313*, 322,
   324, *333*, *334*, 355, 361, *365*, 371,
   372, *384*, *385*, 424, 429, *434*
Smith, H.R., 188, 192, *199*, 286, *296*,
   372, *386*, 515, *522*
Smith, J., 182, *186*
Smith, J.R., 320, *333*, 532, *537*
Smith, L.I., 510, *517*
Smith, L.J., 188, *199*, 507, *516*
Smith, M.J.H., 400, *414*
Smith, S., 218, *226*
Smith, S.F., 511, *518*
Smith, S.N., 429, *436*
Smith, T., 511, *518*
Smith, W., 92, 94, 96, 97, *104*, *105*,
   106, *107*, 147, *158*, 285, *294*
Smith, W.G., 285, *295*
Smith, W.L., 1, 9, *16*, *21*, *23*, 25, 26, 30,
   33–37, *38*, *39*, *41*, *43*, 63, *74*, 79, 80,
   88, 129, 130, 136, *140*, *141*, *142*,
   146, 147, *157*, *158*, 161, 164, 169,
   170, 171, 173, 174, 179, *183*, *184*,
   185, *186*, 256, *257*, 285, *294*, *295*
Smithies, O., 4, 5, 7, *18*, *20*, 138, 139,
   143, 285, 292, *294*
Smitz, J., 305, *313*
Smyth, E., 79, *88*
Snapper, C.M., 191, *200*
Snyder, D.W., 362, *368*

Snyder, S.H., 237, *250*
So, O.Y., 176, 178, *186*
Soberman, R.J., 56, *72*, 188, *199*, 286,
   296, 374, *387*, 394, 401, 409, *411*,
   412, *415*
Sockson, W.O.C.M., 204, *211*
Soderman, D.D., 253, *257*, 380, *388*
Sofia, M., 280, *282*
Sofia, R.D., 408, *418*
Sogawa, K., 56, *72*
Soja, J., 91, *104*, 303, 305, 307, 309,
   312, *313*, 321, 323, 328, *333*, 337,
   339, 342, 343, 347, *348*, 359, 360,
   361, *367*, 371–383, *384*, *385*, 419,
   428, *432*, 441, *450*, 496, 497, 498,
   503, *504*, 525, *535*
Solito, E., 511, 513, *518*, *519*
Soloperto, M., 401, *415*
Solway, J., 397, *413*
Sonenshein, G.E., 153, *160*
Song, K., 94, *105*
Song, Y.L., 308, *315*
Songu-Mize, E., 33, *42*
Sørensen, H., 475, 478, *489*, 501, *505*
Soter, N.A., 358, 359, *366*, 400, *414*
Sousa, A.R., 302, 308, *311*, 329, *335*,
   338, 342, 344, *349*, 359, 360, 361,
   367, 372–76, 378, 380, 381, *385*,
   495, 498, *503*, *504*
Sovijärvi, A., 283, *292–93*
Soyoola, E., 146, *156*
Spada, C.S., 342, *349*, 383, *389*
Spady, D., 65, *75*
Spaethe, S.M., 284, *293*, 402, *416*
Spagnotto, S., 304, *313*, 421, 422, 426,
   427, 431, *433*, *434*, *435*, *437*
Spahn, J., 475, *488*
Span, P., 236, 238, 239, *248*
Spannhake, E.W., 285, 286, 289,
   295
Sparrow, D., 224, *229*, 253, *257*
Spaziani, E.P., 8, *21*
Spearman, M.E., 59, *73*
Spector, A.A., 30, *41*, 66, *75*
Spector, J., 99, *108*, 304, *313*, 361, 376,
   383, *388*, *389*, 392, 393, *409*, *410*

Spector, S.L., 188, *199*, 223, *229*, 320, *332*, 457, 460, 468, *470*, *471*
Speer, F., 320, *332*, 456, 458, 460, *470*
Spencer, D.A., 514, *520*
Spengler, M., 253, *257*
Spengler, R., 253, *257*
Spengler, U., 209, *214*
Sperl, G., 149, 150, 154, *159*, *160*
Spiegelberg, H.L., 303, 305, *312*, 322, 323, 327, 329, *334*, 337, 343, *348*, 358, 360, *366*, 496, *504*
Spiegelman, B., 36, *43*, 103, *109*, 147, *158*
Spigelman, A.D., 4, *18*
Spink, W.W., 454, 457, 464, *470*
Sporik, R.B., 222, *227*
Sporn, P.H., 512, *519*
Spring, J., 431, *437*
Springall, D.R., 115, *125*, 237, 239, *249*, *250*, *251*
Spruce, K.E., 324, *334*, 357, *365*, 371, *384*, 424, 429, *434*
Spry, C.J.F., 373, *387*, 393, 394, *411*, *412*
Spur, B., 56, *72*, 308, *314*, 374, *387*
Spur, B.W., 268, *271*, 321, 327, *333*, 335, 342, *349*, 357, 361, *365*, 383, *389*, 393, 394, 408, *411*, 534, *537*
Sriramarao, P., 206, *212*
Stablein, J.J., 529, *536*
Stadel, J.M., 284, *293*
Stadler, J., 274, *281*
Stafforini, D.M., 222, *228*
Stahl, P., 95, *106*
Staiano-Coico, L., 149, *159*
Stallings, W.C., 146, *157*
Stammberger, H., 476, *489*
Staneva-Stoianowva, M., 457, 459, *470*
Stanworth, D., 479, *490*
Starr, T., 35, *43*
Statman, R., 274, *282*
Statt, C., 6, *19*
Stawart, A.G., 512, *519*
Stec, D.E., 58, 62, *73*
Stechschulte, D.J., 253, *257*

Steel, L., 235, *247*
Steele, V., 148, *159*
Stefanski, E., 116, *125*
Steffenrud, S., 479, *490*
Stegeman, R.A., 146, *157*
Stehelin, D., 152, *160*
Stein, H., 374, *387*
Stein, S.H., 253, *257*
Steinberg, D., 129, 138, *143*
Steinhilber, D., 191, 192, *200*, 394, *412*
Stellato, C., 481, 482, *490*
Stember, R.H., 206, *212*
Stenius-Aarniala, B., 283, *292–93*
Stensvad, F., 304, *313*, 326, *334*, 361, 362, *368*, *369*, 502, *505*
Sterk, P.J., 187, 188, *198*, 216, 222, *224*, 231, *245*
Stern, N., 27, 34, *39*
Stevens, A.M., 146, *157*, 163, 164, 174, 178, 180, 181, *184*
Stevens, C.A., 238, *250*
Stevens, R.L., 401, *415*
Stevens, W.H., 264, *270*, *271*
Stevenson, D.D., 223, *229*, 299, 300, 302–5, 307, 308, *310*, *311*, *312*, *313*, *314*, 320, 322, 323, 326, 327, 329, *332*, *334*, *335*, 337, 339, 343, *348*, *349*, *350*, 352, 358, 360, *364*, *366*, *367*, 457, 460, 468, *470*, *471*, *472*, 496, 500, 501, *504*, *505*, 523, 524, 526–32, 534, *535*, *536*, *537*
Stewart, A.G., 191, *199*
Stewart, G.A., 113, *124*
Stewart, G.R., 239, *251*
Stoclet, J.C., 273, 276, *280*
Stokes, J.B., 4, *18*
Stolley, P.D., 148, *158*
Stone, R.A., 113, *123*
Storz, Chr., 219, 221, *226*
Stout, B.K., 393, 394, *410*
Strader, C.D., 28, *40*
Strand, J.C., 32, *42*
Strandberg, K., 235, *247*
Strauss, R.H., *269*
Strauss, W.E., 78, 79, 82, *87*
Strban, M., 264, *270*

Strek, M.E., 284, *293*, 397, 402, *414*, *416*
Stretton, C.D., 115, *125*
Striano, J.A., 32, *42*
Strieter, R., 98, *108*
Strieter, R.M., 285, 292, *295*
Stromstedt, P.E., 510, *518*
Stuart-Smith, K., 237, *249*
Stuehr, D.J., 237, *250*
Stuppy, R., 95, *106*
Suarez, B.K., 203, *211*
Suarez-Mendez, V.J., 301, *311*
Subers, E., 101, *108*
Suburo, A., 233, *246*
Sudderick, R.M., 496, *503*
Suetsugu, S., 357, 361, *365*
Suga, M., 240, *251*
Sugarbaker, D., 237, *249*
Sugerbaker, D., 361, 375, *388*
Sugimoto, Y., 37, *43*, 256, *258*
Sugiyama, H., 394, 408, *411*, *418*
Sui, Z., 34, *43*, 50, *70*
Suko, M., 394, *411*
Sultzman, L., 94, *105*
Sultzman, L.A., 29, *41*
Sultzman, L.S., 374, *387*
Sumimoto, H., 56, *72*
Sumitomo, M., 402, 408, *416*, *417*, 515, *521*
Summer, W., 273, *281*
Summers, E., 263, 265, *270*, *271*
Sun, F.F., 32, *42*, 53, *71*, 393, 394, *410*
Sun, M., 7, 8, *20*
Sun, W., 146, *156*
Sunday, M., 361, 375, *388*
Sur, S., 515, *522*
Suzuki, M., 138, *143*, 357, 361, *365*
Svahn, T., 283, *292–93*
Svensson, C., 477, 479, *489*
Swann, B.P., 233, 234, *246*
Swanson, E.W., 477, 478, *489*
Swanson, L.J., 304, *313*, 326, *334*, 362, *369*, 502, *505*
Swanson, M.E., 284, *294*
Swanston, A., 475, *488*

Sweet, J.A., 530, *536*
Sweet, J.M., 327, *334*, 501, *505*
Sweetman, B.J., 358, 359, 360, *366*
Sweifel, B., 285, *295*
Swierkosz, T.A., 119, *126*, 232, 233, *245*, *246*
Swift, L., 65, *75*
Swindell, B., 514, *520*
Swinney, D.C., 176, 178, *186*
Swystun, V.A., 284, *293*
Sydbom, A., 358, 360, *366*, *367*
Symons, J.A., 209, *214*
Szabó, C., 273, 274, 276, *280*
Szarek, J.L., 235, *247*
Szczeklik, A., 56, 72, 91, *104*, 207, *213*, 223, *228*, *229*, 284, *293*, 299, 300–309, *309*, *310*, *311*, *312*, *313*, *314*, *315*, 320, 321, 323, 326, 329, 332, *333*, *334*, 337, 339, 342, 343, 347, *348*, *349*, *350*, 351, 357–63, *364*, *367*, *369*, 371–83, *384*, *385*, 419, 421, 423, 424, 425, 428, *432*, *433*, *434*, 440, 441, 442, *449*, 449, *450*, 457, 459, 464, 468, 469, *471*, *472*, 496–99, 502, *503*, *504*, *505*, 525, 526, 528, 529, *531*, *534*, *535*, *536*, *537*
Szefler, S.F., 515, *522*
Szentivanyi, A., 235, *247*
Szmidt, M., 307, *314*, 329, *335*, 358, *366*, 456, 460, 464, 469, *470*, 525, *535*

T

Tabe, K., 304, *313*, 357, 361, *365*, 371, *384*
Taborda-Barata, L., 217, 219, 220–23, *225*
Tadjkarimi, S., 111, *123*, 237, *249*
Tadokoro, K., 394, 401, *412*
Tagari, P., 13, 14, *22*, 303, *312*, 322, 323, *333*, *334*, 337, *348*, 355, 358, 361, *365*, *366*, 371, *384*, 440, *449*, 496, 497, *504*, 514, *520*, 534, *537*

Tai, P.C., 373, *387*
Tak, C.J.A.M., 513, *519*
Takafuji, S., 382, *389*, 394, 401, *412*, *416*
Takahashi, A., 102, *108*
Takahashi, K., 30, *41*, 78, *87*, 111, *123*
Takahashi, N., 37, *44*
Takahashi, S., *23*, 122, *127*, 131, *141*
Takahashi, T., 27, 31, *40*, 111, *123*
Takahashi, Y., 136, *142*
Takai, S., 204, *211*
Takai, T., 129, *140*
Takamatsu, S., 222, *228*
Takamura, H., 329, *335*
Takasaki, K., 329, *335*
Takemura, H., 239, *250*
Taketani, Y., 6, *19*, 136, *142*
Taketo, M.M., 4, *18*
Takeuchi, K., 37, *44*
Takishima, T., 397, *414*
Takizawa, H., 62, *74*
Tamagata, K., 146, *156*
Tamaoki, J., 239, *250*
Tammivaara, R., 283, *292–93*
Tamura, G., 397, *414*
Tamura, N., 393, 394, 404, *411*, *412*
Tan, E.M., 320, *332*, 358, *366*
Tanabe, T., 52, *70*, *71*, 129, 131, 137, *140*, *141*, *142*, 166, *184*, 289, *297*
Tanaka, S., 47, *69*, 138, *143*
Tanaka, Y., 289, *297*
Tang, J.-L., 132, 133, 138, *141*, *143*
Tang, W., 122, *127*
Taniguchi, N., 395, *412*, *413*
Taniyama, Y., 37, *44*
Tanner, M.A., 232, 233, *246*
Tashkin, D.P., *269*
Tattersfield, A.E., 96, *107*, 113, 114, 122, *123*, *124*, 255, *257*, 259, 264, *269*, 306, 307, *314*, 347, *350*, 360, 361, *367*, 371, 380, *385*, 426, 431, *435*, *437*
Tauber, A., 253, *257*
Tavares, I.A., *23*, 421, *433*
Tay, A., 30, *41*

Taylor, A.A., 239, *251*
Taylor, B.M., 53, *71*, 393, 394, *410*
Taylor, G.W., 46, 53, *69*, 263, 266, *269*, *271*, 287, *296*, *297*, 322, *333*
Taylor, I., 287, *296*
Taylor, I.K., 263, *269*, *271*, 285, 287, 288, *295*, *297*, 362, *368*
Taytard, A., 283, *292*
Tazawa, R., 136, *142*
Tedeschi, A., 303, *312*, 419, *432*
Teisseire, B., 274, *282*
Temple, D.M., 427, 430, *435*, *436*
ten Kate, L.P., 204, *211*
Tenor, H., 306, *314*, 361, 380, 381, *388*, 403, *417*
Tentori, L., 148, *159*
Terao, S., 52, *71*
Teraoka, H., 284, *294*
Térouanne, B., 515, *521*
Terpstra, G.K., 393, *411*
Terragno, N.A., 32, *42*
Terries, M.H., 494, *503*
Tetley, T.D., 511, *518*
Tetsuka, T., 232, 233, *245*
Thebert, P., 512, 514, *519*
Theodore, J., 447, *450*
Theoharides, A.D., 53, *71*
Thiele, B.-J., 27, *39*
Thiele, J., 374, *387*
Thiemermann, C., 9, *21*, 119, *126*, 130, *141*, 146, *157*, 232, 233, *246*, 273, 274, 279, *280*, *281*, 354, 355, *365*
Thien, F.C., 303, *312*, 322, *333*, 357, 361, *365*, 372, *385*, 507, *516*
Thijs, L.G., 274, *281*
Thomas, E., 288, *297*, 515, *522*
Thomas, M., 253, *257*
Thomas, P.S., 319, *332*
Thomas, R.U., 395, *413*
Thompson, D.C., 191, *199*
Thompson, P.J., 113, *124*
Thomson, H., 263, 265, *270*
Thomson, H.W., 263, *270*
Thomson, N.C., 259, 264, *268*, *269*
Thorel, T., 429, *436*

Thornton-Manning, J.R., 49, *69*
Thun, M., 148, *158*
Thun, M.J., 4, *18*, 148, *158*
Thunissen, F.B.J.M., 237, *250*
Thurman, M.J., 49, *69*
Tiano, H.F., 5, 7, *18*, *20*, 138, 139, *143*, 146, *157*, 285, 292, *294*
Tiao, G., 274, *282*
Tielemans, W., 239, *251*
Tien, Y., 197, *200*
Timmermans, A., 515, *521*
Timmers, M.C., *271*
Timmons, M.D., 51, *70*, 234, *246*
Tinkleman, D., 287, *297*, *362*, *368*
Tippins, J.R., 78, *87*
Tizard, R., 512, *519*
Tjoelker, L.W., 222, *228*
Toda, M., 402, *416*
Toelle, B.G., 222, *227*
Toews, G.B., 102, *109*
Toh, H., 166, *184*
Tohkin, M., 95, *106*
Tokumoto, H., 511, *519*
Tokuyama, K., 113, *124*
Tollino, M., 286, *296*
Tomioka, H., 408, *418*
Tomlinson, A., 6, *19*, 135, *142*, 233, *246*
Tomoda, K., 329, *335*
Tone, Y., 137, *142*
Tong, X., 32, *42*
Tonnel, A.B., 223, *228*, 286, *296*, 300, 301, 309, *310*, *311*, *315*, 429, *436*, 440, 442, 444, 447, 448, *449*, *450*
Tontonoz, P., 36, *43*, 103, *109*, 147, *158*
Toogood, J.H., 321, *333*
Tool, A.T., 403, *416*
Tooley, M., *269*
Torphy, T.J., 188, *199*, 371, *384*
Tos, M., 473, 474, 476, 478, 484, 486, *488*, *489*, *490*
Toth, P., 7, *20*
Tough, S.C., 219, *227*
Touqui, L., 284, *293*
Tovey, E., 222, *227*
Townley, R.G., 222, *228*, 393, 394, 404, 408, *411*, *412*, *418*

Tracey, M., 224, *229*
Trautman, M.S., 7, *20*, 146, *156*
Trendelenburg, F., 442, *450*
Trepanier, L., 408, *417*
Trevethick, M.A., 9, *21*
Triggiani, M., 284, *294*
Trotter, J.L., 233, *246*
Trousset, M., 148, *158*
Truan, G., 59, *73*
Trudeau, J.B., 288, *297*, 340, 342, 343, *349*, *514*, *521*
Trzaskos, J.M., 4, 8–9, *18*, *20*, 139, *143*, 285, 292, *295*
Tsai, A., 170, 171, *185*, *234*, 235, *247*
Tsai, A.-L., 3, *18*, 130, 140, *141*, 171, 174, *185*
Tsang, B.K., 146, *156*
Tsicopulos, A., 429, *436*
Tsing, S., 146, *157*
Tsuda, M., 357, 361, *365*
Tsuji, H., 329, *335*
Tsujii, M., 135, *142*, 149, *160*
Tsurumoto, H., 329, *335*
Tsutsumi, E., 37, *44*
Tu, Y.-P., 188, 192, *198*
Tuck, M.L., 27, 34, *39*
Turk, J., 95, *106*, 147, *157*, 394, *412*
Turki, J., 209, *214*, 222, *228*
Turner, N., 266, *271*, 287, *296*
Turner-Warwick, M., 222, *228*
Twentyman, O.P., 238, *250*, 507, *516*
Twort, C.H., 122, *127*
Tygstrup, I., 475, 478, *489*
Tzizik, D., 96, *107*

U

Uchida, D., 188, *198*
Udholm, S., 458, *471*
Ueda, N., 118, *126*, 137, *142*
Ueki, I.F., 265, *270*, 393, *410*
Uglik, S.F., 232, 233, *245*
Uhlig, S., 6, *19*, 280, *282*
Ujihara, M., 96, 97, *107*
Ullman, H.L., 56, *72*

Ullrich, V., 5, 6, *18*, *19*, *23*, 51, 52, 62,
    70, *71*, *74*, 86, *89*, 96, *107*, 146, *155*
Ulrik, C.S., 217, 224, *226*, *229*
Ulsøe, C., 486, *490*
Umeda, H., 357, 361, *365*
Umland, S.P., 219, *227*
Undem, B.J., 188, 191, *199*, 285, 286,
    296, 371, *384*, 397, *413*
Uozumi, N., 27, 31, *40*
Upmacis, R.K., 235, *247*
Urade, Y., 96, *107*
Usandivaras, G., 429, *436*, 468, *471*
Ushikubi, F., 36, 37, *43*, *44*
Utzmann, R., 11, *22*

V

Vacheron, F., 239, *251*
Vachier, I., 514, 515, *521*, *522*
Vadas, P., 116, *125*
Vagaggini, B., 515, *522*
Vaghi, A., 91, 96, *104*, 301, 302, 304,
    306, *311*, *312*, *313*, *314*, 347, *350*,
    358, 360, 361, *366*, *367*, 371, 380,
    385, *388*, 421–27, 429, 430, 431,
    433, *434*, *435*, *436*, *438*
Vagliasindi, M., 421, 431, *433*, *437*
Vailes, L.D., 222, *227*
Valente, D., 303, *312*, 419, *432*
Valentovic, M.A., 236, *248*
Vallance, P., 239, *250*, 273, 274, 280,
    281
Vallee, B.L., 27, *40*
Vallin, P., 427, 430, *435*
Van Ark, I., 238, 240, *250*, *251*
Van Damme, J., 217, 219, 221, *226*
Van de Loo, P.G.F., 235, 236, 237,
    248, *249*
van den Bos, G.C., 274, *281*
van den Bosch, H., 116, *125*
Vandenbunder, B., 152, *160*
van der Baan, B., 474, 479, *488*
van der Belt, B., 395, *413*
Van der Linde, H.J., 235, 237–40, *247*,
    248, *249*, *250*, *251*

Van der Linden, P.-W.G., 343, *350*
VanderMeer, T.J., 280, *282*
Van der Ouderaa, F.J., 161, *183*
Van Der Straeten, M.E., 362, *368*
van der Veen, H., *271*
Van der Veer, J.J., 317, 318, *332*
Van der Zwan, J.K., 343, *350*
van Dijk, A.P.M., 513, *519*
Van Dorp, D.A., 161, *183*
Vane, J.R., 2, 3, 4, 6, 8, 9, *16*, *17*, *18*,
    19, *21*, 34, *43*, 50, 51, 52, *70*, *71*,
    114, 115, 119, *124*, *126*, 130, 135,
    138, *141*, *142*, *143*, 146, *157*, 161,
    172, 173, *183*, 232, 233, *245*, *246*,
    273, 274, 279, *280*, 280, 285, *295*,
    302, *311*, 354, 355, 361, *365*, 374,
    388, 419, 421, 424, 431, *432*, 512,
    519, 526, 532, *535*
Van Eerdewegh, P., 203, *211*
van Essen-Zandvliet, E.E., 283, *293*
van Grunsven, P.M., 283, *293*
van Herderweden, L., 222, *228*
van Herwaarden, C.L.A., 283, *293*
Van Heuven-Nolsen, D., 236, 239,
    248, *251*
Vanhoutte, P.M., 50, *70*, 235, *247*
van Kesel, A., 447, *450*
van Kooten, F., 80, *88*
van Lambalgen, A.A., 274, *281*
Van Leeuwen, B.H., 383, *389*
Van Leeuwen, W.S., 457, 463, 467, *470*
van Metre, T.E., 460, *471*
van Schayck, C.P., 283, *293*
Vanselow, N.A., 319, 320, *332*, *333*,
    460, *471*, 532, *537*
van Weel, C., 283, *293*
Vanzieleghem, M., 283, *292*, 479, *489*
Vardey, C.J., 253, *257*
Vargaftig, B.B., 179, *186*, 284, *293*
Vargö, A.K., 501, *505*
Varma, D.R., 7, *19*
Varney, V.A., 496, *503*
Varnum, B.C., 3, *17*, 146, 147, *156*,
    162, *183*, 285, *294*
Vaseghi, T., 239, *251*
Vassali, G., 382, *389*

Vaughan, J.H., 320, *332*
Vazquez, M., 27, 28, *40*, 103, *109*
Veldink, G.A., 393, 394, *411*, *412*
Venge, P., 216, 219, *225*, *269*, 373, *387*
Vergaftig, B.B., 512, *519*
Verhagen, J., 372, *386*, 393, 394, 395, *411*, *412*
Verheyen, A.K.C.P., 235, 236, 238, 239, 240, *247*, *248*, *250*, *251*
Verhoeven, A.J., 403, *416*
Verkade, P.E., 56, *72*
Verleden, G.M., 427, 430, *435*, *437*
Verma, A.K., 148, *159*
Vervloet, D., 222, *228*
Vessey, M.P., 8, *21*
Vic, P., 515, *522*
Vicaut, E., 274, *282*
Vickers, P., 13, 14, *22*, 92, 97, 98, *104*, *108*, 361, 375, *388*
Vickers, P.J., *23*, 28, *40*, 148, *159*, 374, *387*
Vielh, P., 148, *158*
Vignola, A.M., 235, *247*, 514, 515, *520*, *522*
Vikka, V., 268, *271*
Vikoukal, E., 206, *212*
Vilkka, V., 321, *333*, 342, *349*, 383, *389*
Villa, L.M., 427, *435*
Villamanzo, I.G., 429, *436*, 468, *471*
Villar, A., 224, *229*
Vincent, S.R., 237, *250*
Violi, F., 79, *88*
Virchow, C., 300, 309, *310*, *315*, 420, *433*, 440, *449*
Virchow, J.C. Jr., 217, 218, 221, 223, *225*, *228*, 395, 396, *412*, *413*
Vishwanath, B.S., 284, *294*
Visser, J.J., 274, *281*
Vita, A.J., 397, 402, 403, *414*, *416*
Vittori, E., 382, *389*
Vliegenthart, J.F., 393, *411*
Voelkel, N.F., 6, *19*, 52, 56, *71*, 322, *333*, 372, *386*
Volone, F.H., 532, *537*
Volovitz, B., 401, *415*
von Bethmann, A., 6, *19*

Von Maur, K., 319, *332*
Von Metre, T.E. Jr., 319, *332*
Vorng, H., 429, *436*, 440, *449*
Vouloumanos, N., 5, *18*, 139, *143*, 146, *157*, 285, 292, *294*
Voznesensky, O., 132, *142*, 146, *156*
Vyas, P., 232, *245*

W

Waalkens, H.J., 283, *293*
Waddel, K.A., 360, *367*
Wade, E., 509, *517*
Wade, M.L., 52, *71*
Wagenman, M., 482, *490*
Wagner, M., 91, 96, *104*
Wahli, W., 27, 28, *40*, 103, *109*
Wainwright, P., 8, *21*
Walenga, R.W., 6, *19*
Walfort, M.J., 400, *414*
Walker, C., 153, *160*, 217, 218, 221, 223, *225*, *228*, 395, 396, *412*, *413*
Wallace, J.L., 292, *298*
Wallace, R.E., 284, *294*
Wallaert, B., 223, *228*, 300, 309, *310*, *315*, 440, 442, 447, 448, *449*, *450*
Wallner, B.P., 511, *519*
Walls, A., 329, *335*, 338, 344, *349*, 359, 360, 361, *367*, 372, 373, 378, *385*, *387*
Walsh, G.M., 393, 401, *411*, *416*
Walters, E.H., 113, *124*, 204, *211*, 222, *228*, 264, 265, *270*, 507, *516*
Walton, C.H.A., 320, *332*, 464, *471*
Wandzilak, M., 301, *311*
Wang, H., 280, *282*
Wang, H.E., 34, 35, *43*
Wang, J., 8, *21*
Wang, L.-H., 131, 132, 136, 140, *141*, *142*, *143*, 173, *185*
Wang, M.H., 58, 62, *73*
Wang, N.S., 191, *199*
Wang, W.H., 62, *74*
Wang, Z., 78, 79, 80, 82, *87*
Wang, Z.Y., 374, *387*

Wangaard, C.H., 223, *229*, 320, *332*, 460, 468, *471*
Wanner, A., 122, *127*
Ward, J.K., 237, *249*
Ward, M.P., 511, *519*
Ward, P.S., 287, *297*
Wardlaw, A.J., 401, *416*
Ware, J.A., 37, *44*
Warner, G.L., 149, *159*
Warner, J.A., 396, *413*
Warner, M., 68, *75*
Warner, T.D., 119, *126*, 232, 233, *245*, *246*
Warnock, M.L., 188, 195, 197, *199*
Warren, J.B., 237, *250*
Warren, M.S., 305, *314*, 339, 340, 343, 344, *349*
Warringa, R.A., 408, *417*
Warshauer, M.E., 148, *158*
Wartmann, M., 30, *41*
Wasserman, S.I., 358, *366*
Wassink, G.A., 393, *411*
Watanabe, Y., 7, *20*
Waterman, M.R., 47, 48, *69*
Watson, M., 188, *198*, 222, *228*
Watson, N., 397, *414*
Watson, R.M., 113, *124*, 263, 264, 265, *269*, *270*, *271*, 347, *350*, 360, *367*
Watt, G.D., 222, *228*
Waxman, D.J., 47, 48, 60, 63, *69*, *73*
Wayoff, M., 301, *311*
Webb, C., 383, *389*
Webb, D.R., 319, *332*
Webb, J.K., 14, *22*
Weber, P., 51, *70*
Weber, R.W., 300, *310*
Weber, Th., 219, *227*
Weersink, E.J., 515, *521*
Wei, C., 234, 235, *247*
Wei, S., 59, 65, *73*, *75*
Weil, J., 8, *21*
Weimer, K.E., 54, *75*
Weimer, N., 218, *226*
Weir, T., 222, *227*
Weiss, E.H., 209, *214*
Weiss, J.W., 397, *413*

Weiss, M., 403, *416*
Weiss, R.M., 53, *71*
Weiss, S.T., 224, *229*
Weissenbach, J., 204, *211*
Weissenbach, R., 12, *22*
Weissmann, G., 232, *245*
Weitzberg, E., 274, 280, *282*
Weksler, B., 287, 288, *297*, 302, *311*, 381, *388*
Weldon, D., 216, *225*
Weller, P., 92, 96, *104*, *107*
Weller, P.F., 338, 342, *349*, 372, *386*, 393, 395, 409, *410*, *413*
Wellings, R., 263, *269*, 284, 288, *293*, 362, *369*, 408, *417*
Wells, A., 479, *490*
Wells, L.B., 25, 34, *39*, 237, *249*
Welsh, K.I., 206, *213*, 308, *315*
Welsh, M., 426, *434*
Wendel, A., 6, *19*, 280, *282*
Wenzel, A., 265, *270*
Wenzel, S.E., 286, 288, *296*, *297*, 305, *314*, 339, 340, 342, 343, 344, *349*, 362, *368*, 372, *386*, 514, *521*
Werner, H., 12, *22*
Westcott, J.Y., 286, 288, *296*, *297*, 305, *314*, 339, 340, 342, 343, 344, *349*, 372, *386*, 514, *521*
Westlund, P., 56, *72*
Westwick, J., 405, *417*
Wetterholm, A., 27, *40*, 192, *200*
Wetzel, C.E., 441, *450*
Wey, H., 427, *435*
Wheatley, L.M., 217, 222, *225*
Wheelan, P., 56, *72*
Wheeldon, A., 253, *257*
Whisman, B.A., 206, *212*
White, M.A., 358, 360, *366*
White, M.V., 303, 304, 305, *312*, *313*, 337, 343, *348*, 428, *435*, 496, 497, 498, 502, *504*
White, R.L., 4, *18*, 148, *159*
White, S.R., 284, *293*, 397, 402, *414*, *416*
Whitlock, J.P. Jr., 49, *69*
Whittle, B.J., 274, *281*

Whittle, B.J.R., 3, 4, *17, 18*
Widal, F., 317, 318, *332*, 352, 361, *364, 368*, 452, *470*
Widal, M.F., 440, *449*, 523, *535*
Widdicombe, J.H., 265, *270*
Wiener-Kronish, J.P., 188, 195, 197, *199*
Wigle, D.T., 219, *227*
Wigzell, H., 208, *213*
Wikstrom, A.C., 508, *517*
Wilborn, J., 98, *108*, 146, *156*, 285, 289, 292, *295, 298*
Wilder, R.L., 26, 34, *39*, 148, *159*
Wilkinson, J.R., 393, 394, 408, *411*
Willerson, J.T., 140, *144*
Williams, A.J., 324, *334*, 357, *365*, 371, *384*, 424, 429, *434, 436*
Williams, D.E., 47, 49, 53, *69*
Williams, F.S., 397, *414*
Williams, H., 362, *368*
Williams, J., 96, *107*, 113, *124*, 255, *257*, 347, *350*, 360, *367*
Williams, J.M., 173, *185*
Williams, K.L., 268, *271*
Williams, R., 79, *88*
Williams, T.J., 111, *123*, 233, 234, *246*
Williams, V.C., 263, 265, *269*, 324, *334*, 353, 355, 356, 358, 362, *364, 368*, 372, *385*, 424, 429, *434*
Willis, D., 6, *19*
Willoughby, D.A., 6, *19*, 135, *142*
Wills-Karp, M., 188, 193, *199*
Willson, T., 103, *109*
Wilson, A.G., 209, *214*
Wilson, A.J., 237, *250*
Wilson, J., 494, *503*
Wilson, J.H.P., 513, *519*
Wilson, J.W., 238, *250*, 361, 373, *387*, 507, *516*
Wilson, M.J., 149, *159*
Wilson, R., 528, *536*
Wilson, S.J., 361, 373, *387*
Wilson, T.W., 380, *388*
Wink, D.A., 50, *70*

Winn, V., 3, *17*, 146, 147, *156*
Winn, V.D., 285, *295*, 512, *519*
Wiseman, J., 9, *21*
Wisniewski, A., 431, *437*
Wizemann, T.M., 273, 280, *281*
Wladislavosky-Wasserman, P., 476, *489*
Wloch, M., 116, *125*
Wojciechowska, B., 303, 305, *312, 313*, 329, *335*, 498, *504*
Wojtulewski, J.A., 2, *16*
Wolff, M.H., 56, *72*
Wolff, S.P., 79, *88*
Wolkoff, A.W., 32, *42*
Wollin, L., 280, *282*
Wong, C., 96, *107*
Wong, C.S., 113, *124*, 255, *257*, 347, *350*, 360, *367*
Wong, D., 308, *315*
Wong, D.-Y., 305, *313*
Wong, E., 13, 14, *22*, 98, *108*, 374, *387*
Wong, G.G., 495, *503*
Wong, M.H., 8, *21*
Wong, P.H., 53, *71*
Wong, P.Y., 32, *42*, 56, 65, *72, 74*, 79, *87*
Wong, S., 475, *488*
Wong, Z.Y.H., 204, *211*, 222, *228*
Wood, R., 308, *315*, 495, 496, *503*
Wood-Baker, R., 263, 265, *270*
Woods, J., 92, 97, 98, 103, *104, 108*, 401, *415*
Woods, J.W., 286, *296*
Woodward, D.F., 256, *258*, 383, *389*
Woolcock, A.J., 217, 222, 224, *225, 227, 229*, 259, *268*, 373, *386*
Woolley, K.L., 113, *124*, 265, *271*, 347, *350*, 360, *367*
Wordsworth, B.P., 206, *213*
Workman, R., 286, *296*
Worley, P.F., 7, *20*, 133, *142*, 146, *156*
Wright, A., 510, *517*
Wu, K., 96, *107*
Wu, K.K., 3, *18*, 130–33, 135, 136, 138, 140, *141, 142, 143, 144*
Wu, L.C., 237, *249*

Wu, M., 153, *160*
Wu, Y., 122, *127*
Wuthric, B., 429, *436*
Wyche, A., 3, *17*
Wyile, G., *271*

X

Xaubet, A., 432, *438*, 495, 496, *503*
Xiao, G., 171, *185*
Xie, J., 273, *281*
Xie, Q., 118, *126*
Xie, W., 3, *17*, 25, 34, *39*, 130, 136,
    137, *141*, *142*, 145, 146, 147, 148,
    150, 152, 153, *155*, *156*, *158*, *159*,
    160, 285, *294*
Xie, W.L., 162, *183*
Xu, J., 205, *212*, 222, *228*
Xu, K., 28, *40*, 99, *108*, 304, *313*, 361,
    376, 383, *388*, *389*, 392, 393, *409*,
    410
Xu, L.J., 191, *199*
Xu, N., 172, 173, *185*
Xu, X., 94, *105*
Xu, X.-M., 131, 132, 133, 136, 140,
    141, *142*, *143*, *144*
Xu, X.P., 232, 233, *246*
Xue, C., 237, *250*

Y

Yacoub, M.H., 111, 115, 116, 119,
    123, *125*, 237, *249*
Yadagiri, P., 31, *41*, 63, *74*
Yamagata, K., 7, *20*, 133, *142*
Yamamoto, H., 304, *313*, 357, 361,
    365, 371, *384*
Yamamoto, K., 6, *19*, 118, *126*, 137,
    142, 304, *313*, 357, 361, *365*, 371,
    384, 508, 511, *517*, *518*
Yamamoto, M., 204, *211*
Yamamoto, S., 6, *19*, 27, *39*, 56, 72,
    118, *126*, 129, 136, 137, *140*, *142*,
    161, 166, *183*, *184*

Yamaoka, K.A., 192, *200*
Yamashita, K., 60, *73*
Yamashita, T., 329, *335*
Yan, J., 59, *73*
Yan, K., 259, *268*
Yan, Y.T., 65, *74*, 79, *87*
Yanagawa, N., 27, 34, *39*
Yang, C.S., 58, 62, *73*
Yang, M., 209, *213*
Yankaskas, J.R., 477, *489*
Yannoni, Y., 147, *158*
Yasruel, Z., 495, *503*
Yates, D., 239, *251*
Yayashi, H., 96, *107*
Yee, Y.K., 362, *368*
Yeola, S., 60, 62, *73*
Yergey, J., *23*, 146, 147, *157*
Yin, K., 79, *87*
Ying, S., 217, 219, 220–23, *225*, *226*,
    227, 289, *298*, 496, *503*
Yochida, K., 394, *411*
Yokomizo, T., 27, 31, *40*
Yokota, Y., 36, 37, *43*
Yokoyama, C., 52, *70*, *71*, 129, 131,
    137, *140*, *141*, *142*, 166, *184*
Yokoyama, M., *23*, 122, *127*, 131, 141
Yoshida, H., 222, *228*
Yoshida, S., 408, *418*
Yoshikawa, K., 7, *20*, 131, *141*
Yoshimi, R., 329, *335*
Yoshimoto, T., 27, *39*, 166, *184*, 374,
    387, 394, 409, *411*
Yoshinaga, S.K., 511, *518*
Yoss, E.B., 285, 286, 289, *295*
Yost, G.S., 49, *69*
Youlten, L.J., 393, 394, *411*
Young, A., 210, *214*
Young, D.A., 3, *17*, 146, 147, *156*, 285,
    295, 512, *519*
Young, I.G., 188, 195, 197, *199*, 383,
    389
Young, I.R., 8, *21*
Young, J.M., 9–10, *21*
Young, R.N., 362, *368*
Young, R.P., 203, 204, 206, 208, *211*,
    213

Yu, S., 13, *22*
Yui, Y., 395, *412*, *413*
Yukawa, M., 37, *44*
Yunis, E., 206, *212*

Z

Zackert, W.E., 77, *87*
Zakar, T., 8, *21*
Zamboni, R., 362, *368*
Zamel, N., *269*
Zanber, A.G., 148, *158*
Zandecki, M., 447, 448, *450*
Zanetti, M.E., 253, *257*, 380, *388*
Zang, E., 148, *159*
Zaphiropoulos, P.G., 68, *75*
Zapol, W.M., 237, *249*
Zawadzki, J.V., 38, *44*
Zeiger, R.S., 352, *364*, 460, *471*, 501, *505*
Zeiss, C.R., 326, *334*, 352, *364*, 501, *505*, 523, *535*
Zeldin, D., 46, 58, 60, *69*
Zeller, C., 457, *470*
Zembowicz, A., 138, *143*
Zeng, J., 164, *184*
Zetterström, O., 113, *123*, 301, 303, 304, *310*, *312*, *313*, 323, 324, 326, *334*, 337, *348*, 352–56, 358, 361, 362, *364*, *365*, *368*, *369*, 371, 372, 381, *384*, *385*, *388*, 420, 424, 425,

[Zetterström, O.]
429, *433*, *434*, 462, *471*, 496, 497, 500, 502, *504*, *505*, 514, *520*
Zhang, C.D., 62, *74*
Zhang, J., 531, *537*
Zhang, J.Y., 60, 63, *73*, *74*
Zhang, Y., 13, *22*, 135, *142*, 146, *156*, 162, *183*, 197, *200*
Zhao, Y., 34, *43*
Zheng, Y.M., 240, *251*
Zhong, H., 146, *156*
Zhu, X., 400, 401, 405, 407, *414*, *416*, *417*
Zhu, Y., 30, 31, *41*, 62, 65, *74*, *75*
Zhu, Z., 122, *127*
Zieger, R.S., 523, 524, 526, 529, *535*, *536*
Zijlstra, F.J., 112, *123*, 513, 514, *519*, *520*
Zimmer, T., 253, *257*
Zimmerman, G.A., 4, *18*, 130, *141*, 148, *159*, 222, *228*
Zimmerman, R.A., 468, *472*
Zintzaras, E., 208, *213*
Zocca, E., 515, *522*
Zoldhelyi, P., 140, *144*
Zorn, T.M., 149, *159*
Zou, A.-P., 34, *43*, 50, *70*
Zou, M.H., 52, *71*
Zuccari, G., 427, *435*
Zuraw, B.L., 308, *314*, 534, *537*
Zusman, R., 4, *18*
Zweifel, B.S., 3, *17*, 285, *295*

SUBJECT INDEX

A

Accolate, 265
Acetaminophen, 527
Acetylcholine, 264
Acetylsalicylate, 423
Acute Respiratory Distress Syndrome, 273
Acylhydrolase, 29
Adenylate cyclase, 33
Adhesion molecules, 481
Adipocyte, 37
β-Agonists, 363
AIA (*see* Aspirin-induced asthma)
AIANE (European Network on Aspirin-induced Asthma)
  database, 452
  patients, 452
  structure, 452
Airway
  absorption of aspirin, 352, 355
  hyperresponsiveness, 187, 231, 236
    stimuli, 259, 426
  inflammation, 187, 308, 355, 363
  obstruction, 187, 362
    inhibitors, 424
    measurement, 192

Allergens challenge, 261, 286
  environmental, 261
Aminopeptidase, 27
Angiotensin II
  and 12(S)-HETE, 27
Antigen-presenting cells, 191
Anti-inflammatory drugs (*see* Nonsteroidal anti-inflammatory drugs)
Antinuclear antibodies, 441
Antioxidants, 84
Aortic coarctation model of hypertension, 32
Apoptosis, 135, 145
Arachidonic acid (AA), 25, 45, 79, 84, 91
  arachidonyl peroxyl radical isomers, 77
  functional pools, 101
  metabolites, 362
  oxidative pathways in platelets, 301
  peroxidation, 77
  reacylation mechanism, 29
  regulation of metabolism, 284
  second messenger, 29
Aspirin, 2, 146, 173, 299
  adverse reactions, 299
  and apoptosis, 150

[Aspirin]
concentrations, 339
desensitization, 302, 320, 326, 358, 526
and inflammation, 317
mechanism of action, 129
pharmacokinetics, 355
treatment with, 317
Aspirin challenge, 303, 351, 378, 500
and aspirin-induced asthma, 222
aspirin provocation tests, 300
cumulative dose, 356
inhalation, 337, 420
nasal, 300, 304
nasal secretions, 305
oral, 300, 337, 339, 420
provocative dose (PD_{20}), 322, 353, 361
segmental bronchial challenge, 305, 360
Aspirin-induced asthma (AIA), 16, 111, 122, 202, 299, 351, 440
and allergy, 301
and atopy, 300, 320
and autoimmunity, 441
and BAL fluid, 320, 328
and bronchial biopsy, 302, 338, 371, 373
bronchospastic reaction, 299, 317, 355, 421
clinical symptoms, 300, 319
and cysteinyl leukotrienes, 321, 340
desensitization, 307, 501, 523, 531
pathogenesis, 532, 533
procedures, 524
respiratory reactions, 525
diagnosis, 222, 300, 463
and dyes, 528
and eosinophils, 300, 329, 342
epidemiology, 318, 439
family history, 300
genetics of, 192, 207, 299, 308
and hydrocortisone, 528
immunosupression, 441
indomethacin, 431
and inhibitors of COX, 526

[Aspirin-induced asthma (AIA)]
and lymphocytes, 338
and macrophages, 338
and mast cells, 343
mediators, 304, 338, 347
histamine, 343
PGD_2, 338
and neutrophils, 338
pathogenesis, 299, 308, 318, 320, 331, 357, 419
chronic viral infection, 440
cyclooxygenase theory, 301
over expression of LTC_4 synthase, 304
platelets, 301, 440
prostaglandins, 320, 344
protective activity, 3,
cromones, 429
furosemide, 429
prostanoids, 344
treatment, 300, 318
Aspirin intolerance (see NSAIDs)
incidence, 457
provocation tests, 500
and pulmonary function tests, 463
symptoms, 364, 454
anaphylactic shock, 253, 458
angioedema, 458
bronchial asthma, 456
dyspnea, 458
loss of smell, 468
nasal blockage, 458, 468
nasal polyps, 454, 460
rash, 458
redness of head and neck, 458
rhinorrhea, 456, 458, 468, 481, 499
rhinosinusitis, 454, 458, 468, 494, 499
sneezing, 468
urticaria, 458
treatment, 485, 500, 529
antihistamines, 468
corticosteroids, 464
cromoglycates, 468
methyloxanthines, 468
and viral infection, 309, 460

Aspirin-intolerant asthmatics (*see* Aspirin-induced asthma)
Aspirin provocation test (*see* Aspirin challenge)
Aspirin-sensitive asthma (*see* Aspirin-induced asthma)
Asthma, 5, 111, 187
  aspirin intolerant (*see* Aspirin-induced asthma)
  aspirin tolerant, 307
    bronchial biopsy, 373
  atopic, 188, 201
  definition, 215
  diagnosis, 216
  extrinsic, 217
  and genetics, 201, 204, 209
  intrinsic
    clinical features, 223
    epidemiology, 217
    etiology, 222
  occupational, 221
  pathophysiology, 114, 191
  and prostanoids, 377
  role of afferent nervous system, 191
  symptoms, 259
  and viral infection, 231
Atopic asthma (*see* Asthma)
Atopy
  and aspirin-induced asthma, 300, 320
  and aspirin intolerance, 461
  and cytokines, 289
  and lymphocytes, 289
  markers, 222

B

Bradykinin, 4, 33, 238
Bronchial asthma (*see* Asthma)
Bronchial hyperresponsiveness (*see* Airway hyperresponsiveness)
Bronchial mucosa, 338
Bronchoalveolar lavage (BAL), 112, 193, 286, 342, 337, 305
  and asthma, 221, 320, 328
  and aspirin-induced asthma, 320, 328

[Bronchoalveolar lavage (BAL)]
  eosinophils, 340
  leukotrienes, 340
Bronchodilation, 352, 361

C

Carbon monoxide, 51
Carrageenin, 14
Celecoxib, 11, 13
Ceramide, 29
Chloroperoxidase, 46
Chromones
  mode of action, 429
Chromosomes, 204
Cinalukast, 263
Colon cancer, 4, 148
Corticosteroids (*see* Glucocortico-steroids)
Cyclic AMP, 253
  response element, 136
Cyclooxygenase (COX) 1, 25, 79, 91, 284, 351, 496, 511
  active site, 1, 166
  activity, 302
  and aspirin-induced asthma, 301
  and bronchoconstriction, 302
  cellular expression, 287
  constitutive isoform, 302
  dimer formation, 169
  drugs, 145, 147, 301, 308, 318, 320, 339, 532
  genes, 129, 138, 309
  glycosylation sites, 164
  inhibition, 164, 285, 302, 320, 331, 337, 354, 363
  isoforms, 25, 285, 302
    activity ratio, 8
  localization, 95
  mechanism of action, 170
  products, 284, 306
  structure
    biochemical, 164
    three-dimensional, 2, 161, 309

Cyclooxygenase-1(COX-1), 25, 45,
    129, 232, 285, 302, 374, 383
  arachidonic acid, 2
  regulation of expression, 26, 360
  structure, 2, 130
  suicidal autoinactivation, 130
Cyclooxygenase-2 (COX-2), 25, 45, 79,
    111, 130, 232, 285, 302, 374,
    383
  and asthmatic, 114
  baculovirus transfer vector for, 163
  functions, 4, 138, 146
  induction, 3, 135
  localization, 114, 136
  regulation of expression, 117, 126,
    133, 360
    inhibitions, 3, 122
  structure, 2
Cysteinyl leukotrienes (Cys LTs), 28,
    91, 188, 240, 302, 340, 358,
    497
  antagonists, 324, 355, 400, 531
  bronchoconstrictors, 321
  cellular source, 395
  excretion, 288, 303, 306, 321, 355
  function, 321, 395
  infusion, 321
  inhalation, 321, 357
  and mast cells, 323, 328
  products, 321, 392, 534
Cysteinyl LT_1 receptor antagonist,
    265, 268
Cytochrome P450 (CYP450), 25, 45,
    49
  mixed function oxidase system, 50
  dependent monooxygenase, 25
Cytokines, 114, 481
  and nasal polyps, 481

D

Dexamethasone, 3, 84, 148, 285
Dibromododecenoic acid, 50
Diclofenac, 11, 146
DUP-697, 173

E

Early asthmatic response, 261
Eicosanoids, 25, 77, 91, 497
  gene expression regulation, 288
  mediators, 337
  metabolism, 513
  synthesis pathways, 91, 102, 374, 514
Electron paramagnetic resonance
    spectroscopy (EPR), 170
Endothelial cell, 28,
  antibodies against, 442
  injury, 280
Endothelin, 122
Endothelium-derived relaxing factor
    (EDRF) (*see* Nitric oxide)
Endotoxin (*see* Lipopolysaccharide)
Enzymes
  calcium activation, 29, 102
  localization for eicosanoid formation,
    91, 99
  membrane association, 92
Eosinophils,113, 188, 219, 221 304,
    391, 338
  and antileukotriene drugs, 402
  and antioxidants, 409
  and asthma, 329
  and CD25, 447
  chemoattractants, 342, 515
  and glucocorticosteroids, 408
  GM-CSF, 401
  heterogeneity, 394
  and leukotrienes, 329
  mediators
    cytokines, 396
    ECP, 339, 396, 498
    EDN, 396
    EPO, 396
    MBP, 396
    PAF, 394, 403
    VIP, 396
  and nasal polyps, 496
  priming, 401
  protein kinase C/protein tyrosine
    kinase inhibitors, 404
Eotaxin, 198, 342

15R-Epilipoxins, 147
Epoxides, 30
Epoxyalcohols, 53
Epoxyeicosatrienoic acid (EET), 46, 58
Epoxygenase, 58
Exercise-induced bronchoconstriction, 260
    and cysteinyl leukotrienes, 262

F

Flurbiprofen, 2, 173, 265
Furosemide, 32
    protective activity in bronchocon-
        striction, 426

G

Genetics of asthma, 201
Glucocorticoid response element (GRE), 137
Glucocorticosteroids, 3, 28, 119, 122, 264, 362
    anti-inflammatory action, 508
    and aspirin-induced asthma, 464
    cyclooxygenase inhibition, 285
    effectiveness, 283
    lipoxygenase inhibition, 286
    mode of action, 511
    receptor, 508
    regulation, 509
Glutathione, 28
G-protein-coupled receptors, 29
Granulocyte macrophage colony-
        stimulating factor (GM-CSF), 219, 401

H

Histamine, 4, 241, 264, 338, 534
Human leukocyte antigen (HLA), 205
    and leukotrienes, 192
    and nasal polyps, 308

Hydrogen peroxide, 52
Hydroperoxy-eicosatrienoic acid (HPETE), 27, 45, 53
Hydroxyeicosatetraenoic acid (HETE), 27, 45, 53, 286
    12(R)-HETE, 27
    12(S)-HETE, 27
    15-HETE, 130, 147, 179, 296, 497
    molecules, 47, 53
    second messengers, 27
Hydroxyl radical, 52
Hypochlorite, 52

I

Ibuprofen, 2, 173
IgE, 188
    receptors, 204, 222
    specific, 222
    total, 222
Immediate early genes, 136
Indomethacin, 2, 32
Inflammation, 27, 139, 187
    cells, 342
Interferon, 191, 221, 284
Interleukins (IL)
    IL-1, 29, 232
    IL-1α, 132
    IL-1β, 6, 111
    IL-2, 221
        receptor, 448
    IL-3, 219, 342, 401, 495
    IL-4, 188, 191, 219, 289
    IL-5, 188, 219, 342, 382, 401, 447, 495
        receptor, 188
    IL-8, 81, 342, 495
    IL-12, 188
Iodosuprofen, 176
Ion
    channels, 33, 426
    exchangers
        Cl^-/HCO_3^-, 426
        Na^+/H^+, 426
    pump, 426
    transporter, 426, 429

Isocyanates, 221
Isoprostane, 77
  biosynthesis, 84, 86
  cigarette smoking, 86
  free radical-catalyzed mechanism, 77

L

Late asthmatic response, 261
Leukocyte margination, 280
Leukotriene A_4 (LTA_4), 91, 358
  hydrolase, 27, 99, 102, 304, 374, 375, 383
  localization, 99
Leukotriene B_4 (LTB_4), 192, 308, 340, 497
Leukotriene C_4 synthase
  and aspirin-induced asthma, 304, 373
Leukotriene C_4, D_4, E_4 (*see* Cysteinyl leukotrienes)
Leukotrienes (LTs) (*see also* Cysteinyl leukotrienes), 53, 91, 187, 280, 351
  antileukotriene drugs, 356, 357, 361, 363
  and asthma (*see* Aspirin-induced asthma)
  biosynthesis, 363
  catabolism
    oxidation, 27
  cells expressing, 286, 304
  and glucocorticosteroids, 286
  mediators, 302, 357
  production, 303, 342
    bronchial lavage, 322
    nasal lavage, 322
    urine, 322
  transcellular metabolism, 27
Lipase
  arachidonyl selective, 29
Lipocortin, 511
Lipopolysaccharide, 3, 80,114, 137, 273
  histological changes in lungs, 277
Lipoxins, 56

Lipoxygenase (LOX), 25, 91
  genetics, 303
  isoforms
    5-lipoxygenase (*see* 5-lipoxy-genase)
    12-lipoxygenase, 26
    15-lipoxygenase, 26, 303
  products, 286, 301
5-Lipoxygenase (5-LO), 16, 91, 187, 374, 375, 383
  deficient mice, 193
  expression in cells, 28
  gene polymorphism, 287
  inhibitor, 240, 337, 357, 363, 531
    ZD2138, 324
    Zileuton, 397
  pathway enzymes, 376
  products, 286
  translocation, 28, 342
Lipoxygenase-5 activating protein (FLAP), 28, 91, 374, 375, 383
  localization, 97
Loop diuretics
  protective activity against broncho-constriction, 429
Lymphocytes, 84
  B-lymphocytes, 191
  T-lymphocytes, 219, 307, 338, 448
    receptor (TCR), 205
    and nasal polyps, 496
Lysine–aspirin, 351, 420
Lysophosphatidylcholine (lysoPC), 33, 138

M

Macrophages, 3, 113, 195
  MIP, 1, 198
Mast cell, 113, 188, 219
  activation, 358
  aspirin intolerance, 498
  enzymes
    protease, 7, 188
    tryptase, 498
Meiosis, 202

Meloxicam, 10, 122
Metacholinc, 264
  hyperresponsiveness, 193, 259
Microsomes, 48
Misoprostol, 255
Mitogen-activated protein kinase, 30
Mitosis, 147
MK-0679, 324
MK-476 (*see* Montelukast)
MK-571, 263, 265
MK-966, 11, 14
Monocytes, 3, 80, 84
  chemotactic protein 3 (MCP-3),
    219
Montelukast (MK-476), 188, 531
Mouse strains, 187
  129 Sv, 195
  C57BL/6, 195
Multiple organ failure syndrome,
    273

N

Nasal polyposis (nasal polyps), 352,
    474
  and allergy, 474
  anatomy, 476, 494
  and aspirin, 494
  and aspirin-induced asthma, 460,
    485
  and bacterial infection,475
  blood eosinophil count, 300
  cells, 474, 479, 482
  diagnosis, 485
  mediators,482, 495
  symptoms, 337, 481, 499
  treatment, 485, 501
Neutrophils, 52, 84, 279
Nicotinamide adenosinediphosphate
    reduced form (NADPH),
    52
Nimesulide, 10, 122, 402, 421
Nitric oxide (NO), 6, 32, 50, 119, 138,
    231, 273

[Nitric oxide (NO)]
  and bronchial hyperresponsiveness,
    234
  cytoprotection, 280
  function, 232
  gas, 274
  and guanyl cyclase, 237
  and PGE$_2$, 231, 234, 243
Nitric oxide synthase (NO synthase,
    NOS) ,46
  constitutive, 232
  inducible, 232, 273
  inhibitors, 119, 273
    side effects, 274
Nitrogen dioxide, 59
Nonsteroidal anti-inflammatory drugs
    (NSAIDs), 1, 32, 130, 145,
    383
  and aspirin-induced asthma, 300,
    421
  obstructive responses, 424
  pyrazolones, 421, 459
  side effects, 11
Norepinephrine, 29
NS-398, 173
Nuclear factor-κB, 30, 116, 152, 231,
    243
Nucleobindin, 149

O

Oncogenes, 148
  Bcl$_2$, 152
  c-*myc*, 153
  p53, 153
Oxidants, 121

P

Peroxidase, 25, 45
Peroxisomal oxidation, 27
Peroxisome-proliferator-activated
    receptors, 27, 147

Peroxynitrite, 52, 273
Prostacyclin (PGI$_2$), 1, 32, 113
  synthase, 51, 97, 136
  metabolism, 285
Prostaglandin endoperoxide synthase
  (PGHS) (*see* Cyclooxy-
  genase)
Prostaglandins
  prostaglandin D$_2$ (PGD$_2$), 4, 113,
    393, 497
    metabolism, 359
    synthase localization, 96
  prostaglandin E$_1$ (PGE$_1$), 264
  prostaglandin E$_2$ (PGE$_2$), 2, 113,
    380
    function, 253, 425
    receptors, 253
    synthase localization, 97
  prostaglandin F$_2$, (PGF$_2$), 4, 113
  prostaglandin G$_2$, (PGG$_2$), 25
  prostaglandin H$_2$, (PGH$_2$), 25, 45,
    91, 301
Phosphatidylcholine (PC), 31, 65
Phosphatidylethanolamine (PE), 31,
  65
Phosphatidylinositol, 33, 65
Phospholipase A$_2$ (PLA$_2$), 29, 78, 91,
  232, 284
  calcium-independent, 94
  cytosolic, 94, 374
  lysophospholipases, 284
  secretory, 94, 284
  translocation, 30
Phospholipids, 28, 84
Phosphorylation
  serine, 30
  tyrosine, 30
Phorbol 12-myristate 13-acetate
  (PMA), 132
Piroxicam, 8, 300
Platelet-activating factor (PAF),
  280
Platelet-derived growth factor
  (PDGF), 122
Platelets, 28, 78, 280
Polyunsaturated fatty acids, 29, 50

Pranlukast, 188
Prostaglandin H synthase (*see*
  Cyclooxygenase)
Protein kinase C, 30
  inhibitors, 133
Pyrazolones, 459
  patterns of reaction, 421
  symptoms, 459

R

RANTES, 198, 219, 342, 459
Rhinoviruses, 121
RS-104897, 178
RS-57067, 180

S

Salicylate, 150, 179, 525, 544
Salsalate, 528
SC-558, 146, 180
Septic shock, 273
Shear stress response element,
  132
Signal translocation, 30
SK&F-104,353, 324
Slow-reacting substance of anaphy-
  laxis (SRS-A) (*see* Cysteinyl
  leukotrienes)
Sphingomyelin hydrolysis, 29
Sulindac, 4
Superoxide, 52, 273

T

TATA box, 131
Thromboxane TXA$_2$, 1, 111, 280,
  393
  metabolism, 497
  receptors, 78
  synthase, 51, 96
Transforming growth factor (TGF),
  148

Tumor necrosis factor alpha (TNFα),
    6, 29, 111, 148, 209, 233

V

Vasopressin, 4
Viral infection, 307
    and aspirin-induced asthma,
        440
    and asthma, 231

X

X-ray crystallography, 162

Z

Zafirlukast, 188, 263
Zaprinast, 237
Zileuton, 188, 397
Zomepirac, 178